Manipal Manual of
Orthopaedics

Manipal Manual of Orthopaedics

Second Edition

As per the Competency Based Medical Education Curriculum (NMC)

Vivek Pandey MBBS MS (Orthopaedics)
Professor, Unit Head
Trauma, Joint Replacement, Sports Medicine, and
Arthroscopy Division
Department of Orthopaedic Surgery
Kasturba Medical College
Manipal Academy of Higher Education
Manipal, Karnataka, India

Foreword
P Sripathi Rao

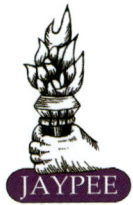

JAYPEE BROTHERS MEDICAL PUBLISHERS
The Health Sciences Publisher
New Delhi | London

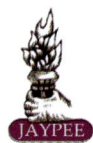 **Jaypee Brothers Medical Publishers (P) Ltd**

Headquarters
Jaypee Brothers Medical Publishers (P) Ltd
EMCA House, 23/23-B
Ansari Road, Daryaganj
New Delhi 110 002, India
Landline: +91-11-23272143, +91-11-23272703
+91-11-23282021, +91-11-23245672
Email: jaypee@jaypeebrothers.com

Corporate Office
Jaypee Brothers Medical Publishers (P) Ltd
4838/24, Ansari Road, Daryaganj
New Delhi 110 002, India
Phone: +91-11-43574357
Fax: +91-11-43574314
Email: jaypee@jaypeebrothers.com

Overseas Office
J.P. Medical Ltd
83 Victoria Street, London
SW1H 0HW (UK)
Phone: +44 20 3170 8910
Fax: +44 (0)20 3008 6180
Email: info@jpmedpub.com

Website: www.jaypeebrothers.com
Website: www.jaypeedigital.com

© 2023, Jaypee Brothers Medical Publishers

The views and opinions expressed in this book are solely those of the original contributor(s)/author(s) and do not necessarily represent those of editor(s) and publisher of the book.

All rights reserved. No part of this publication may be reproduced, stored or transmitted in any form or by any means, electronic, mechanical, photocopying, recording or otherwise, without the prior permission in writing of the publishers.

All brand names and product names used in this book are trade names, service marks, trademarks or registered trademarks of their respective owners. the publisher is not associated with any product or vendor mentioned in this book.

Medical knowledge and practice change constantly. This book is designed to provide accurate, authoritative information about the subject matter in question. However, readers are advised to check the most current information available on procedures included and check information from the manufacturer of each product to be administered, to verify the recommended dose, formula, method and duration of administration, adverse effects and contraindications. It is the responsibility of the practitioner to take all appropriate safety precautions. Neither the publisher nor the author(s)/editor(s) assume any liability for any injury and/or damage to persons or property arising from or related to use of material in this book.

This book is sold on the understanding that the publisher is not engaged in providing professional medical services. If such advice or services are required, the services of a competent medical professional should be sought.

Every effort has been made where necessary to contact holders of copyright to obtain permission to reproduce copyright material. If any have been inadvertently overlooked, the publisher will be pleased to make the necessary arrangements at the first opportunity.

Inquiries for bulk sales may be solicited at: jaypee@jaypeebrothers.com

Manipal Manual of Orthopaedics

First Edition: 2019

Second Edition: **2023**

ISBN: 978-93-5696-178-4

Printed at Nutech Print Services - India

Dedicated to

My Parents
Kuldip Narain Pandey and Manju Pandey

My wife
Deeksha

and son
Krish

My brother and his family
Abhishek, Susanne, Demira and Maya

My Teachers and Students!

Foreword

A textbook for use by an undergraduate medical student should be both comprehensive and comprehensible. The demands of the Competency Based Medical Education dictate that the book should be comprehensive and yet precise. Too much detail at the expense of understanding and recall would also be counterproductive.

The latest edition of the Manipal Manual of Orthopaedics is a compilation of the three essential principles of undergraduate teaching—how to teach, what to teach and very importantly what not to teach. This book enhances comprehension and recall through highlights, boxes, illustrations and flowcharts. It not only meets the demands of CBME but goes beyond it. In short, it is just what the doctor ordered!

P Sripathi Rao MBBS MS (Orth) FRCS
Former Dean KMC, Manipal
Former Consultant and Director
Medcare Orthopaedics and Spine Hospital, Dubai, UAE

Preface to the Second Edition

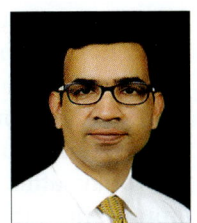

The second edition of *Manipal Manual of Orthopaedics* is presented with great delight. This book's 1st edition received great praise from readers, including students, residents and teachers.

In the past few years, orthopaedics has advanced quickly with the emergence of new surgical methods, tools, and technologies. This second version of the manual has undergone a complete revision and update to consider these improvements in the orthopaedics sector. National Medical Council, India has recently revamped medical education as competency-based medical education (CBME). The CBME guidelines were taken into consideration when structuring this version.

The book covers a wide range of orthopaedic conditions essential for undergraduate orthopaedic training, including everything from fundamental anatomy and physiology to the current surgical methods. It is intended to provide a thorough reference for medical students, residents and practicing orthopaedic surgeons. Each topic is covered briefly and clearly in the book, and to aid comprehension, there are also clinical photos, figures, radiographs and flowcharts. Adding crucial ideas in 'note' and 'important' boxes would enable students to enhance the knowledge required for postgraduate exams.

I want to thank all contributors who made this edition possible sincerely. The development of this second edition would not have been possible without their commitment and knowledge. I also want to express our gratitude to the readers for their insightful comments and ideas, which have enabled us to enhance the content and appearance of this manual.

I anticipate that the second edition of the *Manipal Manual of Orthopaedics* will be equally well-regarded as the first and useful tool for students and orthopaedic surgeons in training.

In order to improvise the further editions, I would humbly request you all to provide a feedback and suggestions on vivekortho@yahoo.co.in.

Vivek Pandey

Preface to the First Edition

One pertinent question always came to my mind as an undergraduate student of 90s that how much I am supposed to read and understand in orthopaedics as it was a minor subject and part of general surgery in final MBBS exams. There were few books around, which gave ample information about the conditions. However, I felt difficult to retain all the information stuffed and more difficult to recollect and write in exams.

Today, after 15 years, orthopaedics is a superspecialty in itself and information in and around this subject has become voluminous, but it has still remained a part of surgery with similar objectives for MBBS students. As a teacher and practitioner of the same subject, I always remain guarded on one aspect while teaching that 'how much to teach and how much to leave'. Over the years of teaching has made me realize that succinct precise information for undergraduates is more than enough. Too much stuffing of material in the book spoils the readability. Every single condition in orthopaedics is not important to be taught to undergraduates. Moreover, excess information cannot be revised and recollected during examinations.

Hence, I decided to pen down the entire orthopaedics in a precise and focused way for undergraduates. I wrote the trauma section of this book two years back for my students and uploaded on my website which was very well appreciated by the students. After that, I decided to complete it even for cold orthopaedics. the idea was to come out with a comprehensive manual of orthopaedics, which would include entire important text material while filtering out matters which are not-so-important for an undergraduate. the students can always refer reference textbooks for any further clarifications.

After all the chapters were written, each major section was reviewed by the specialist surgeons in the field to make it perfect for reading and understanding. However, despite multiple revisions of each chapter, paragraphs, word and reviews by another specialist, there is a possibility of some inadvertent error and unwanted omissions. I would welcome all suggestions and constructive criticism in its future reprints and revised editions.

If this simplified, structured, filled in with tips and pearls and pictorial academic material could help a student in understanding the nuances of entire orthopaedics in precise manner, I would feel blessed and consider my humble endeavor successful.

Vivek Pandey

Acknowledgments

It gives me immense pleasure to acknowledge the efforts of every individual who motivated and helped me in accomplishing my academic work on the second edition of *Manipal Manual of Orthopaedics*. I am deeply indebted to my alma mater, Kasturba Medical College (KMC), Manipal, Karnataka, India, and its organizational support, creating an excellent academic and clinical environment for teaching.

At the outset, I would acknowledge the blessings and guidance of my parents in all endeavors. My father, Dr KN Pandey, a Georgian (KGMC, Lucknow) has never let my guard down, whether in life or profession! He continues to inspire me with simplified and structured teaching. On the other hand, my mother has been a pillar of strength. As almost all academic work happens at home, taking away our personal time and space, I appreciate the support of my wife, Deeksha Pandey (Prof OBG, KMC, Manipal) and my son Krish Pandey. Krish has been instrumental in giving me countless ideas to improve the design and presentation of the book.

It is a fact that none of my books has ever been designed without the guidance of my senior Prof Kiran Acharya (KMC, Manipal), who always gives me invaluable inputs at each stage of the book regarding cover, layouts, color, font, and presentation with his unmatchable taste!

I am blessed to have great teachers like Prof(s) Sripathi Rao, Benjamin Joseph, SP Mohanti, and Sharath Rao, who inspire me with their impeccable knowledge and teaching style. Special thanks to Prof Vineet Sharma from KGMC, Lucknow, who always encouraged me to teach younger colleagues and spread knowledge. I would also like to thank my Prof(s) Anil Bhat, Shyamasunder Bhat and Monappa Naik, all luminaries in their fields who contributed significantly to numerous chapters.

I owe several respectable colleagues who offered to evaluate chapters to make sure that each portion is up to the mark. I want to start by expressing my gratitude to Dr Navaneeth Kamath (Consultant Musculoskeletal Oncologist, Mangalore, India) for his detailed, insightful comments on the part on bone tumors. He diligently fixed any mistakes and ensured that every word in that section was accurate. Dr Amrath, one of my other colleagues, also improved the tumor section. I appreciate the assistance in structuring the spine section from Prof Shyamasunder Bhat, Dr Raghuraj K and Dr Madhav Pai. I appreciate my colleague Dr Ashwath's review of the chapter on nerve injury (Professor, Hand Surgery, KMC Manipal).

One of the most skilled paediatric orthopaedic surgeons and an avid researcher, Prof Hitesh Shah (Paediatric orthopaedic surgery, KMC, Manipal) has reviewed the paediatric section. I also thank Dr Siddharth Kamath (Paediatric orthopaedic surgery, KMC, Manipal) for reviewing paediatric orthopaedic section and providing several critical inputs.

I also acknowledge the valuable contributions made in the trauma division by Dr Sandeep Vijayan and Dr Saktthi S (KMC, Manipal). I am also thankful for the contribution of Dr Suvajit Podder (Assistant Professor, Department of Anesthesia, KMC, Manipal) and Dr Akshay Dhanda (Registrar, Aster RV Hospital, Bengaluru) in the section on procedural skills. I also thank my Twitter colleague, Dr Anantika Sharma, who provided various suggestions, which have been incorporated into the book.

Acknowledgments

Although it is the hard work of the author and multiple reviewers, this edition would not have existed if M/s Jaypee Brothers Medical Publishers, New Delhi, India, and their staff had not assisted. I appreciate the hard work put forward by Shri Jitendar P Vij (Group Chairman), Mr Ankit Vij (Managing Director), Mr MS Mani (Group President), Dr Madhu Choudhary (Director-Educational Publishing), Ms Pooja Bhandari (Director-Production) and Dr Aditya Tayal (Team Lead–UG Publishing) in delivering the revised version.

How to get the improved content in the second edition? Ask users of 1st edition! I want to thank all of the innumerable students, interns, and residents who provided essential feedback for this edition's potential improvements. I also want to thank all the students who have supported first edition of this book and helped it become one of the most significant and trustworthy books in orthopaedics! Most importantly, I owe my gratitude to the patients I have treated over the past 20 years, whose reflections may be found on every page of this book.

Contents

Chapter No.	Chapter Name	Competency No.	Page No.
	Section 1: Skeletal Trauma and Polytrauma		
1.	**Principles of Triage** • A Note on Geriatric Triaging *10*	OR1.1	3
2.	**Shock and its Management**	OR1.2	13
3.	**Soft Tissue Injuries–Part 1**	OR1.3	19
4.	**Soft Tissue Injuries–Part 2**	OR1.4	24
5.	**Dislocation of Major Joints** • Introduction to Dislocations *28* • Dislocations around the Shoulder *33* • Acute Anterior Dislocation of the Shoulder Joint *34* • Recurrent Anterior Dislocation of Shoulder *37* • Posterior Dislocation of the Shoulder Joint *39* • Acromioclavicular Joint Dislocation *41* • Elbow Dislocations *44* • Common Dislocations around the Wrist *46* • Hip Dislocation *47* • Posterior Dislocation of the Hip Joint *48* • Anterior Dislocation of Hip Joint *51* • Central Fracture Dislocation of the Hip *52* • Dislocation around the Knee *53* • Knee Dislocation *53* • Patella Dislocation *55*	OR1.5	28
	Section 2: Fractures and Ligament Injuries		
6.	**Basics of Orthopaedics**	OR2.01	61
7.	**Introduction to Fractures**	OR2.02	69
8.	**Fracture in Children and Physeal Injuries** • Peculiarities of Bone and Fractures in Children *83* • Physeal Injuries *83*	OR2.03	83
9.	**Fracture Clavicle** • Fracture Clavicle Mid-Shaft *88* • Lateral Third Clavicle Fracture *90* • Medial Third Clavicle Fracture *91*	OR2.1	87
10.	**Fractures around the Shoulder** • Fracture Proximal Humerus *92* • Fracture Greater Tuberosity of the Humerus *96* • Fracture Scapula *97*	OR2.2	92
11.	**Relief of Joint Pain** • Pathogenesis of Joint Pain *99*	OR2.3	99

Chapter No.	Chapter Name	Competency No.	Page No.
12.	**Fracture Shaft Humerus, Supracondylar Humerus and Other Fractures around Elbow** • Fracture Shaft Humerus *103* • Fracture Supracondylar Humerus *106* • Intercondylar Fracture of Humerus *115* • Lateral Condyle Fracture *117* • Fracture Olecranon *119* • Radial Head Fracture *121* • Pulled Elbow (Nursemaid Elbow) *122*	OR2.4	103
13.	**Fracture of Forearm Bone, Galeazzi and Monteggia Fracture** • Fracture of Radius Ulna Shaft *124* • Monteggia Fracture Dislocation *126* • Galeazzi Fracture Dislocation (Piedmont's Fracture) *128*	OR2.5	124
14.	**Fractures around the Wrist and Hand** • Colles' Fracture *131* • Smith's Fracture (Reverse Colles') *135* • Barton Fracture *136* • Chauffeur's Fracture/Hutchinson Fracture/Backfire Fracture *137* • Scaphoid Fracture *138* • Metacarpal and Phalangeal Fractures *140*	OR2.6	131
15.	**Fracture Pelvis**	OR2.7	143
16.	**Injuries of the Spine and Spinal Cord** • Acute Spinal Cord Injury *155* • Urinary Bladder Innervation, Function and Dysfunction *159* • Spine/Vertebral Injuries *162* • Specific Fractures of the Spine *169*	OR2.8	150
17.	**Fracture Acetabulum**	OR2.9	173
18.	**Fracture Femur Neck and Intertrochanteric Femur** • Fracture Femur Neck *177* • Fracture Intertrochantric Femur *184*	OR2.10	177
19.	**Fracture around Knee—Patella, Distal Femur and Proximal Tibia** • Fracture Patella *187* • Distal Femur Fracture *191* • Tibial Plateau Fracture *193*	OR2.11	187
20.	**Fracture Shaft Femur and Subtrochanteric Femur** • Fracture Shaft Femur *197* • Fracture Subtrochanteric Femur *200*	OR2.12	197
21.	**Fractures of Both Bone Leg, Tibial Plafond, Calcaneum and Small Bones of Foot** • Fractures of Shaft Tibia Fibula *201* • Fracture Fibula *203* • Fractures of Tibial Plafond/Pilon *204* • Fracture of Calcaneum *206* • Fracture of Talus *210* • Lisfranc's Injury (Tarsometatarsal Dislocation) *212* • Fracture of Metatarsals *214*	OR2.13	201

Chapter No.	Chapter Name	Competency No.	Page No.
22.	**Fracture of the Ankle** • Pott's/Bimalleolar Fracture 217	OR2.14	217
23.	**Complications of Fracture** • Volkmann's Ischemia (Compartment Syndrome) 222 • Fat Embolism Syndrome (FES) 225 • Injury to Major Blood Vessels 229 • Deep Vein Thrombosis (DVT) 230 • Pulmonary Thromboembolism (PTE) 231 • Myositis Ossificans (MO) 232 • Nonunion of Fracture 238 • Delayed Union 241 • Malunion 242 • Joint Stiffness 244 • Limb Shortening 245	OR2.15	221
24.	**Open Fracture**	OR2.16	248
25.	**Ligament Injury of Knee, Ankle and Other Sports Injuries** • General Description of Ligament Injury 255 • Ligament and Meniscal Injury of the Knee 257 • Anterior Cruciate Ligament (ACL) Tear 257 • Posterior Cruciate Ligament (PCL) Tear 261 • Meniscal Injuries 263 • Collateral Ligaments of the Knee 266 • Ankle Ligament Injury/Sprain 269 • Miscellaneous Sports Injuries 271	OR2.17	255
	Section 3: Musculoskeletal Infection		
26.	**Osteomyelitis** • Osteomyelitis 279 • Acute Bacterial (Pyogenic) Osteomyelitis 280 • Chronic Osteomyelitis 287 • Brodie's Abscess and Garre's Sclerosing Osteomyelitis 293	OR3.1	279
27.	**Septic Arthritis** • Septic Arthritis 295 • Tom Smith Arthritis 300	OR3.1	295
28.	**HIV Infections and Orthopaedics**	OR3.1	301
29.	**Spirochetal Infections of Bones and Joints**	OR3.1	304
	Section 4: Mycobacterial Musculoskelatal Infections		
30.	**Skeletal Tuberculosis** • Tuberculosis of the Hip Joint 312 • Tuberculosis of the Knee Joint 318 • Tuberculosis of the Spine 320 • Tuberculosis of Shoulder 327 • Tubercular Osteomyelitis 327 • Hansen's Disease 327	OR3.1, OR4.1	309

Chapter No.	Chapter Name	Competency No.	Page No.
Section 5: Arthritis			
31.	**Overview of Arthritis, Osteoarthrosis Knee** • Osteoarthritis/Osteoarthrosis *335* • Primary Degenerative Osteoarthrosis of the Knee *338*	OR5.1	333
32.	**Rheumatoid Arthritis**	OR5.1	343
33.	**Seronegative Arthritis and Other Arthritis** • Psoriatic Arthritis *357* • Reactive Arthritis/Reiter's Syndrome *359* • Enteropathic Arthritis *361* • Crystalline Arthritis: Gout *362* • Crystalline Arthritis: Pseudogout *365* • Neuropathic/Charcot's Arthropathy *367* • Miscellaneous Arthritis *370*	OR5.1	352
Section 6: Degenerative Conditions of the Spine			
34.	**Approach to Neck and Low Back Pain** • Intervertebral Disc Prolapse (IVDP) *377* • Cauda Equina Syndrome (CES) *387* • Conus Medullaris Syndrome (CMS) *388* • Spondylosis *388* • Spondylolysis and Spondylolisthesis *390* • Lumbar Canal Stenosis *393*	OR6.1	377
Section 7: Metabolic Diseases of the Bone			
35.	**Metabolic Diseases of the Bone** • Brief Review of Role of Calcium, Phosphorus, Magnesium, Vitamin D and their Regulations *399* • Rickets *400* • Osteomalacia *408* • Osteoporosis *410* • Osteosclerosis Disorders *416* • Osteopetrosis/Albers-Schönberg Disease/Marble Bone Disease *416* • Paget's Disease/Osteitis Deformans *418* • Fluorosis *421* • Hyperparathyroidism *423* • Scurvy *426*	OR7.1	399
Section 8: Neuromuscular Disorders			
36.	**Neuromuscular Disorders** • Poliomyelitis *431* • Myopathies *433* • Duchenne Muscular Dystrophy *434*	OR8.1	431

Chapter No.	Chapter Name	Competency No.	Page No.
	Section 9: Cerebral Palsy		
37.	**Cerebral Palsy**	OR9.1	439
	Section 10: Bone Tumors		
38.	**Basics of Bone Tumors**	OR10.1	447
39.	**Benign Bone Tumors and Tumor-like Lesions** • Osteochondroma (Solitary Exostosis) *456* • Multiple Exostoses/Diaphyseal Aclasis/Hereditary Multiple Exostosis *458* • Unicameral Bone Cyst/Simple Bone Cyst *459* • Aneurysmal Bone Cyst (ABC) *460* • Fibrous Dysplasia *461* • Osteoid Osteoma *463* • Osteoma *465* • Giant Cell Tumor of Bone (GCTB) *465* • Enchondroma (Chondroma) *468* • Chondroblastoma/Codman's Tumor *469*	OR10.1	456
40.	**Malignant Bone Tumors** • Osteosarcoma *470* • Ewing's Sarcoma *473* • Multiple Myeloma/Kahler's Disease *475* • Chondrosarcoma *477*	OR10.1	470
	Section 11: Peripheral Nerve and Brachial Plexus Injuries		
41.	**Approach to Peripheral Nerve Injuries**	OR11.1	481
42.	**Specific Nerve Injuries** • Common Nerve Injuries *494*	OR11.1	494
43.	**Brachial Plexus Injury**	OR11.1	512
	Section 12: Congenital and Other Pediatric Disorders		
44.	**Congenital and Other Pediatric Disorders** • Congenital Talipes Equinus Varus (CTEV) *521* • Congenital Vertical Talus *530* • Developmental Dysplasia of Hip *531* • Multiple Congenital Contractures *539* • Coxa Vara *540* • Slipped Capital Femoral Epiphysis (SCFE) *541* • Perthes' Disease and Other Osteochondrosis *544* • Perthes' Disease (Legg-Calve-Perthes Disease) *545* • Flat Foot/Pes Planus *551* • Pes Cavus *554* • Spina Bifida *554* • Skeletal Dysplasias *557* • Congenital Pseudoarthrosis of Tibia (CPT) *561* • Congenital Knee Dislocation *562*	OR12.1	521

Chapter No.	Chapter Name	Competency No.	Page No.
	Section 13: Regional Conditions		
45.	**Upper Limb Disorders** • Frozen Shoulder *565* • Rotator Cuff Tendinopathy/Tendinitis *567* • Acute Calcific Rotator Cuff Tendinitis *568* • Rotator Cuff Tear *569* • Painful Arc Syndrome *571* • Tennis Elbow (Lateral Epicondylitis) *572* • Golfer's Elbow (Medial Epicondylitis) *574* • De Quervain's Tenosynovitis *575* • Carpal Tunnel Syndrome *576* • Dupuytren's Contracture *578* • Ganglion *579* • Compound Palmar Ganglion *581* • Trigger Finger *581*	—	565
46.	**Spine and Lower Limb Disorders** • Torticollis *583* • Congenital Torticollis *583* • Kyphosis *585* • Scoliosis *586* • Cervical Rib *592* • Avascular Necrosis of the Femoral Head *593* • Femoroacetabular Impingement (FAI) *596* • Baker's Cyst *597* • Genu Varum and Valgum *598* • Genu Valgum (Knock Knee) *599* • Genu Varum/Bow Legs *601* • Osteochondritis Dessicans (OCD) Knee *602* • Synovial Chondromatosis *604* • Discoid Meniscus *605* • Osgood–Schlatter Disease *606* • Chondromalacia Patella *606* • Plantar Fasciitis *607* • Morton's Neuroma *609* • Retrocalcaneal Bursitis (Hump-Bump/Haglund's Deformity) *609* • Various Toe Deformities *610* • Various Bursitis *610*	—	583

Chapter No.	Chapter Name	Competency No.	Page No.
	Section 14: Miscellaneous Topics		
47.	**Common Procedural Skills** • Casts in Orthopaedics 613 • Splints in Orthopaedics 620 • Lower Limb Splint 620 • Upper Limb Splint 624 • Spine 625 • Strappings 626 • Traction 628 • Intravenous Cannulation 634 • Peripheral Venous IV Cannulation 634 • Central Line Cannulation 636 • Urinary Catheterization 638 • Endotracheal Intubation 640	OR13.1, OR13.2	613
48.	**Overview of Common Orthopaedic Procedures** • Closed Reduction, Open Reduction, Internal Fixation, External Fixation 645 • Methods of Joint Reconstruction 647 • Arthroplasty 647 • Arthrodesis 648 • Osteotomy 649 • Bone Grafting 650 • Tendon Transfer Procedure 651 • Arthroscopy 652 • Amputations 653 • Tourniquets 656 • Synovial Fluid Analysis 657	OR13.1, OR13.2	645
49.	**Overview of Physiotherapy**	—	658
50.	**Basics of Imaging in Orthopaedics**	—	662
Index			667

List of Abbreviations

#	Fracture	LRTI	Lower respiratory tract infection
ACL	Anterior cruciate ligament	MRI	Magnetic resonance imaging
AFO	Ankle foot orthosis	MTB	*Mycobacterium tuberculosis*
AP	Anteroposterior	NCV	Nerve conduction velocity
ATLS	Advanced trauma life support	OA	Osteoarthrosis/Osteoarthritis
ATT	Antitubercular treatment	ORIF	Open reduction and internal fixation
AVN	Avascular necrosis	PBM	Peak bone mass
BMD	Bone mineral density	PCL	Posterior cruciate ligament
C/S	Culture and sensitivity	POP	Plaster of Paris
CR	Closed reduction	RTA	Road traffic accident
CRIF	Closed reduction and internal fixation	RTI	Respiratory tract infection
CT	Computed tomography	SRUJ	Superior radioulnar joint
DEXA	Dual energy X-ray absorptiometry	SSG	Split-thickness skin graft
DRUJ	Distal radioulnar joint	URTI	Upper respiratory tract infection
EMG	Electromyography	UTI	Urinary tract infection
GA	General anesthesia	VIC	Volkmann ischemic contracture
IF	Internal fixation		

How to Make Best Use of Manipal Manual of Orthopaedics

This newer edition of the *Manipal Manual of Orthopaedics* contains all the necessary knowledge required for undergraduate orthopaedic knowledge and the syllabus covered in the examination in a precise yet comprehensive manner. All the essential topics mandated by CBME are covered comprehensively in the book. However, the unnecessary details have been trimmed to keep the content simple and interesting. There is no end to the knowledge and learning process, but the crux of undergraduate teaching is to stick to the principle that "***one must know what not to teach***".

- Though the book covers all topics according to the CBME, students must follow their institutional teaching to note the more frequently asked topics in their university/college.
- This book also covers all other relevant topics for postgraduate entrance examinations. Many of such relevant fact facts are mentioned in notes and important boxes.
- For any desirable ***advanced reading***: If a student feels that he/she needs to learn more about a particular topic, they can always refer to reference book, such as Apley's Textbook of Orthopaedics.
- The ***manual illustrates the investigations in must-know-fashion*** so that one can remember all appropriate investigations with their relevance.
- The ***treatment principles*** are outlined along with a brief description of the procedure and ***appropriate flowchart*** wherever necessary. However, the treatment details have been trimmed as undergraduates do not need to know the detailed procedure of most conditions. Further, the treatment for certain conditions can be debated as the protocols vary in various institutions, and medicine is often a shade of grey, not black and white.
- There are places left at the end of the chapter where one can write notes as a supplement.
- This book does not intend to teach history taking or examination of a system or joint. Hence, the examination methods in the textbook are not addressed in detail, and mostly the name of tests is mentioned. However, we have provided a *free online version* of the textbook "**Musculoskeletal Examination for Undergraduates**" ***by Dr Vivek Pandey, published by Jaypee Brothers Medical Publishers, New Delhi***. The latter book carries a comprehensive coverage of the entire orthopaedic examination in an illustrative and pictorial manner.
  The same book is in print format too. The print format carries important clinical examination videos.
- Students can also visit the Diginerve website/app for the ***online orthopaedic lectures*** by Vivek Pandey.
  https://www.diginerve.com/course/orthopaedics-for-undergrads/
- Another book by the author, "*Manipal Practical Orthopaedics*" is extremely handy for clinical case discussion and viva in orthopaedics. The contents of this book have immensely helped students in practical and theory exams.

  I would humbly request and appreciate it if you could mail your feedback at vivekortho@yahoo.co.in to improve the forthcoming editions.

SECTION 1

Skeletal Trauma and Polytrauma

SECTION OUTLINE

1. Principles of Triage
2. Shock and its Management
3. Soft Tissue Injuries—Part 1
4. Soft Tissue Injuries—Part 2
5. Dislocation of Major Joints

Skeletal Trauma and Polytrauma

1

CHAPTER 1

Principles of Triage

Trauma is the leading cause of death and disability in the first four decades. The implications of trauma can be a significant burden to any nation's progress with its disparity between life expectancy and quality of life.

Trauma is defined as the "study of medical problems associated with physical injury," while an injury is defined as "the adverse effect of a physical force."

The managament of an injured individual starts from the time of trauma at the site up to the time patient reaches the hospital. The injuries could vary from mild to severe and life or limb-threatening. Therefore, the trauma management team must adopt a systematic approach to ensure an optimal outcome for the injured person. **Flowchart 1.1** shows the sequence of patient care from the time of injury to the hospital.

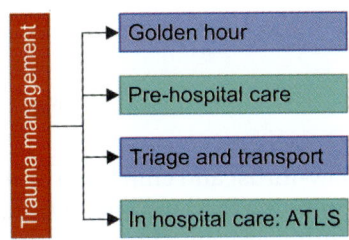

Flowchart 1.1: Sequence of patient care from the site of trauma to the hospital.

(ATLS: Advanced trauma life support)

GOLDEN HOUR

Golden hour refers to the 1st-hour post-injury. A patient's prognosis significantly lies in the attention given and management done during this time, especially in a seriously injured patient. Prompt and sensible first aid measures and efficient subsequent arrangements for further management can help reduce the morbidity and mortality associated with these injuries.

Further, a polytrauma patient involved in any high-velocity injury (road traffic accident, stuck under a collapsed structure) must be tackled in a quick and systemic approach to reduce mortality and morbidity. **Figure 1.1** shows the timeline in a polytrauma patient, including immediate response at the site of trauma, triaging, disentanglement and extrication, transportation, stabilization in the accident and emergency department, and surgical intervention.

PRE-HOSPITAL CARE

Pre-hospital care involves the first aid and emergency care provided either by the bystanders present at the site of the accident or the emergency team who arrived after the call. The local bystanders must immediately call for help while providing the initial first aid to the patient. The management of a patient by a bystander includes:
- Immediate call for help
- In-line immobilization of the cervical spine. Avoid unnecessary patient movement, especially of the spine, to prevent injury (suspected or proven) to the spine and spinal cord

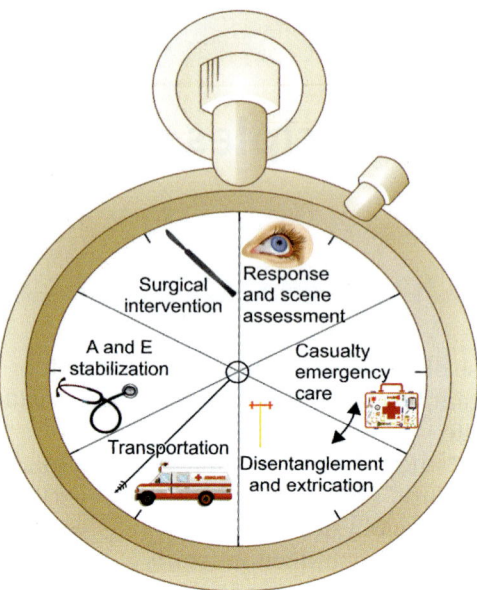

Fig. 1.1: Timeline of a polytrauma patient.

- Jaw-thrust and chin lift to clear the airway, if they are aware of it
- Splinting the limb with a firm, linear object such as an umbrella, folded newspaper, stick, cardboard, etc. **(Fig. 1.2)**.
- Applying compression over an actively bleeding injured site **(Fig. 1.3)**.
- Arranging for safe transport to a trauma center at the earliest.

In case the emergency team of trained personnel has arrived at the site of injury, they provide pre-hospital care to the injured persons as they are well-trained in extraction and resuscitative measures. A trained team enhances the care of the injured person by the following steps:

- Immediately assess the patient with ATLS protocol (airway, breathing, circulation). Standard cardiopulmonary resuscitation can be started if the patient is not responsive with an absent pulse and spontaneous breathing
- Place the patient on a hard board/stretcher and apply cervical collar
- Oxygen delivery through the nasal cannula or bag and mask

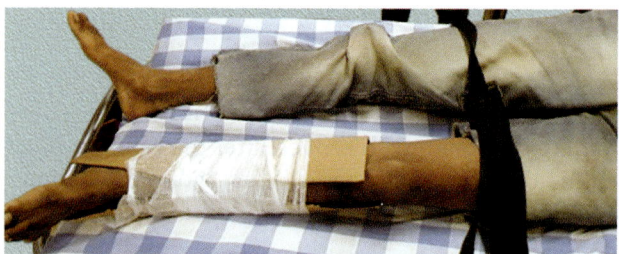

Fig. 1.2: Splintage of left leg with cardboard and cotton bandages.

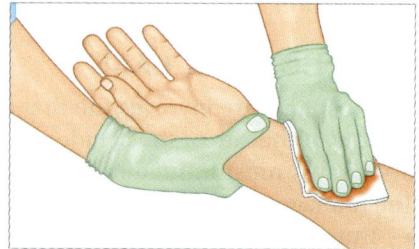

Fig. 1.3: Compression over the bleeding site.

- Secure an intravenous (IV) line and start intravenous fluids (crystalloids)
- Pressure bandage/tourniquet over actively bleeding site.

TRIAGE

Triaging in trauma refers to the process by which emergency medical personnel sort and prioritize accident victims at the scene. Triaging is intended to identify those accident victims most in need of immediate care to make the best use of limited treatment and transport resources. It also refers to the process used in the emergency departments to determine the order in which the presenting patient will be seen. The patient can be triaged in four categories—red, yellow, green, and black.

Accurate triage ensures that limited medical resources are directed towards achieving the maximum positive impact for the largest number of people. In contrast, incorrect triaging may fail to identify patients needing urgent intervention (under-triage)—also risks overwhelming healthcare facilities with patients who do not require time or necessary treatment.

There are two types of triaging—triage sieve and triage sort.

1. **Triage sieve:** It is a quick method of triaging persons based upon several observations, such as whether the person is conscious, can breathe with a regular palpable pulse, capillary refill, and walk independently.
2. **Triage sort:** It is a more systematic way to triage a patient using vital assessments and scores such as respiratory rate, systolic blood pressure, and Glasgow coma score.

Both triaging systems enable emergency personnel to designate patients into four color-coded (RED-YELLOW-GREEN-BLACK) priority strategies **(Table 1.1)**.

Further, to make the triaging process seamless, American College of Surgeons Committee on Trauma (ACS-COT) has recommended an advanced *four-step approach*:
- Step 1-Physiologic criteria
- Step 2-Anatomic criteria

Table 1.1: Triaging.

Color	Triage priority	Type of Injury	Examples
Red	Red-Immediate	Life-threatening	- Tension hemopneumothorax - Fracture pelvis with uncontrolled bleeding and hypotension - Convulsions
Yellow	Yellow-Urgent	- Serious but stable patient and not in any imminent danger - Requires observation	- Fracture femur - Stable liver laceration
Green	Green-Minor	- The patient who will require treatment at some point	- Fracture distal radius
Black	Black-Deceased/Unsurvivable	- Deceased or patients with extensive injuries who will not be able to survive given the care available	- Massive open head injury with GCS 3 - 95% of third-degree burns

(GCS 3: Glasgow Coma Scale 3)

- Step 3-Mechanism of injury
- Step 4-Special consideration.

The decision based upon these criteria to field triage the person and shift them to a trauma center is made by emergency medical personnel.

Step 1-Physiologic criteria: It is intended to allow for rapid identification of critically injured patients by assessing the level of consciousness (Glasgow Coma Scale) and measuring vital signs (systolic blood pressure and respiratory rate). Step 1 criteria are:
- Glasgow Coma Scale ≤13, or
- SBP of <90 mmHg, or
- Respiratory rate of <10 or >29 breaths per minute (<20 in infants aged <1 year), or need for ventilatory support.

Step 2-Anatomic criteria: The criteria pertaining to the chest and extremity injuries are included. Step 2 guidelines recognize that certain patients may have normal physiology, but specific anatomic injuries might require the highest level of care within the defined trauma system. Step 2 criteria are:
- All penetrating injuries to the head, neck, torso, and extremities proximal to the elbow or knee
- Chest wall instability or deformity (e.g., flail chest)
- Two or more proximal long-bone fractures
- Crushed, degloved, mangled, or pulseless extremity
- Amputation proximal to wrist or ankle
- Pelvic fractures
- Open or depressed skull fractures
- Paralysis.

Step 3-Mechanism of injury: It comprises
- Falls
  - Adults: >20 feet (one story = 10 feet)
  - Children: >10 feet or two to three times the height of the child
- High-risk auto crash
  - Intrusion, including roof: >12 inches occupant site; >18 inches any site
  - Ejection (partial or complete) from automobile
  - Death in the same passenger compartment
  - Vehicle telemetry data consistent with a high risk for injury
- Automobile versus pedestrian/bicyclist thrown, run over, or with significant (>20 mph) impact; or
- Motorcycle crash >20 mph.

Step 4-Special consideration: In this step, emergency medical personnel must determine whether persons who have not met steps 1, 2, or 3 have underlying conditions or comorbid factors that place them at higher risk of injury. Injured persons who meet step four criteria might require trauma center care.
- Older adults
  - Risk for injury/death increases after the age of 55 years
  - SBP <110 might represent shock after the age of 65 years
  - Low impact mechanisms (e.g., ground-level falls) might result in severe injury

- Children should be triaged preferentially to pediatric capable trauma centers
- Anticoagulants and bleeding disorders: Patients with head injuries are at high risk for rapid deterioration
- Burns
    - Without other trauma mechanisms: triage to burn facility
    - With trauma mechanism: triage to the trauma center
- Pregnancy >20 weeks
- Emergency medical service provider judgment.

TRANSPORT TO THE HOSPITAL

- Transport to the hospital should be done as early as possible, especially in a seriously injured person with life or limb-threatening injuries. The transport can be done by road or air ambulance. Long-distance transfer to the hospital can be done by air ambulance.
- During the transport, the ambulance should be well-equipped to support the patient's life, such as the facility to continue IV fluids, oxygen, cardiac monitors, infusion pumps, and a defibrillator.
- The ambulance team must alert the nearest trauma center regarding the arrival of the critical patient(s) to ensure that necessary specialists are available to provide immediate care.

IN-HOSPITAL CARE—ATLS PROTOCOL

Once the patient is admitted in the hospital, the patient should be evaluated on a standard Advanced Trauma Life Support (ATLS). **ATLS** was initially introduced in 1978 by the American College of Surgeons, a standardized algorithm for initial stabilization and subsequent management of injured patients. It has evolved drastically over the years based on the varied consensus of the medical experts managing patients in triage. The guideline comprises:

- Initial management is in the form of a rapid primary evaluation and resuscitation of vital functions. Primary survey is performed based on the popular acronym **ABCDE**—*Airway, Breathing, Circulation, Disability,* and *Exposure.*
- After the primary survey, the patient must be subjected to secondary and tertiary surveys.

1. Primary Survey

The five tenets of the primary survey (ABCDE) are briefly discussed here.

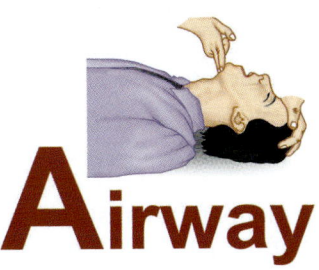
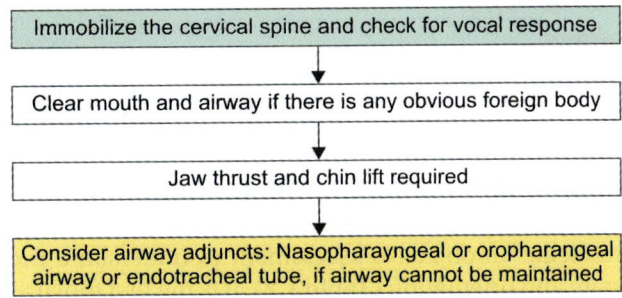

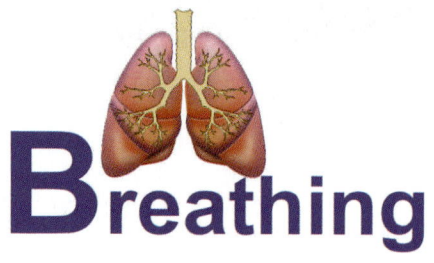
Breathing

- High flow oxygen through the nasal cannula/mask
- Inspect, percuss and auscultate chest
- Check for tension pneumothorax (prominent neck vein, tracheal shift, hyperresonant note on percussion, and absent breath sounds)—immediately decompress if suspected
- Insert chest tube for hemothorax/pneumothorax
- Major vessel bleeding within the chest should be controlled

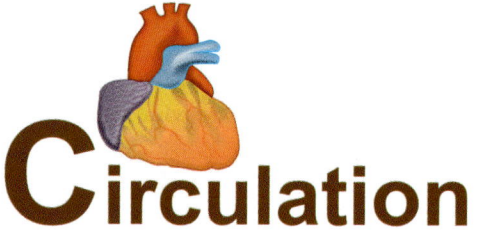
Circulation

- Check pulse and blood pressure. Control external bleeding
- Secure one/two large bore cannulae and start IV fluid (crystalloid)
- Assess blood loss and replenish volume with blood transfusion as early as possible

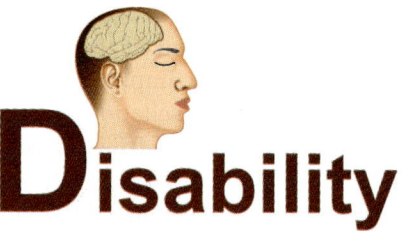
Disability

Disability implies neurological assessment, which should be rapidly assessed using **'AVPU'** command
Alert
Voice response
Pain response
Unresponsive
- Pupils are monitored for size and reactivity
- Assess disability with Glasgow coma scale (GCS). GCS should be repeated at regular intervals to note any deterioration

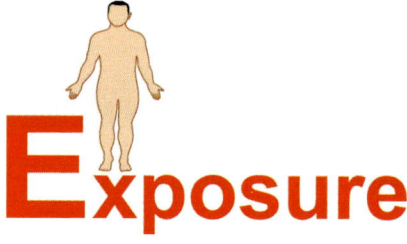
Exposure

The patient must be exposed fully (bearing the dignity of patient in mind) to assess other injuries especially spine, chest, abdomen, and pelvis and examined front and back using a carefully controlled leg roll (50% of body area). Also assess temperature and take measures to prevent hypothermia, if present

Glasgow Coma Scale (GCS) for Disability Assessment:
GCS was published in 1974 by Prof Graham Teasdale and Prof Bryan Jennett (neurosurgeons) to create an objective assessment to understand the impairment of the patient's conscious state and orientation **(Table 1.2)**. It is the first tool used as part of the ATLS guidelines. Normal GCS is 15, while the poorest is 3.

Table 1.2: Glasgow coma score.

Feature	Response	Score
Best eye response	Open spontaneously	4
	Open to verbal command	3
	Open to pain	2
	No eye opening	1
Best verbal response	Oriented	5
	Confused	4
	Inappropriate words	3
	Incomprehensible sound	2
	No verbal response	1
Best motor response	Obeys command	6
	Localizes pain	5
	Withdraws from pain	4
	Flexion from pain	3
	Extension to pain	2
	No motor response	1

Box 1.1: AMPLE assessment.

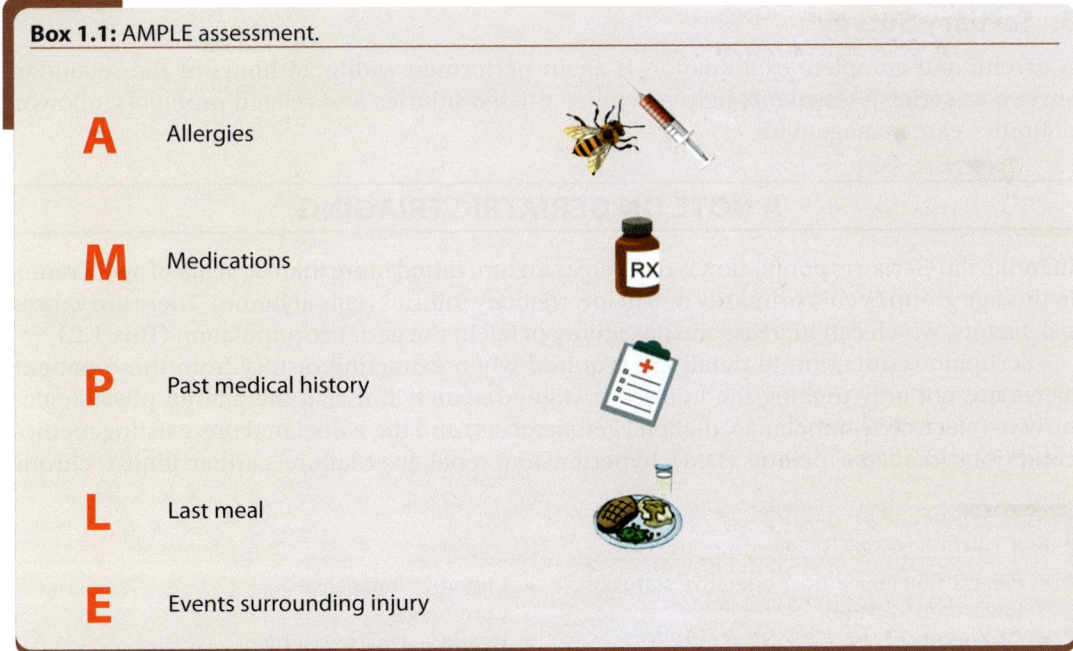

- **A** Allergies
- **M** Medications
- **P** Past medical history
- **L** Last meal
- **E** Events surrounding injury

Adjuncts to the Primary Survey

After a quick primary survey, a brief history is taken along with AMPLE **(Box 1.1)**. Other adjuncts are relevant investigations like X-rays [trauma series (spine, pelvis, chest) and other limb X-ray, if applicable], FAST (Focused Assessment with Sonography in Trauma) which is an abdominal four quadrant scan to look for free fluid/blood, blood tests [hemoglobin, packed cell volume (PCV), renal and liver function tests], pulse oximetry, arterial blood gas analysis, and electrocardiogram (ECG). Some patients may require additional support by inserting a urinary catheter or Ryle's tube.

2. Secondary Survey

Patients are only subjected to a secondary survey if they are conscious, oriented, and hemodynamically stable.

It comprises a thorough head-to-toe examination of the patient with an accurate assessment of the distal neurovascular status. It is usually performed after a successful resuscitation maneuver and stabilization of the vital parameters. The history and physical examination are repeated if the initial attempt is inconclusive.

X-rays/CT/MRI indicated by examination for additional information is obtained. If at any time during the secondary survey, the patient deteriorates, another primary survey is carried out, as a potential life threat may be present.

Important note: The patient should be removed from the rigid spine board (during the primary survey) and placed on a firm mattress as soon as reasonably feasible, as the spine board can rapidly cause skin breakdown and pain while a firm mattress provides equivalent stability for suspected spinal fractures.

3. Tertiary Survey

A careful and complete examination is again performed within 24 hours of the secondary survey, as serial assessments help recognize missed injuries and related problems, allowing definitive care management.

A NOTE ON GERIATRIC TRIAGING

In India, the Geriatric population is defined as an individual more than 60 years of age. Trauma in this age group occurs primarily due to low-velocity injuries (falls at home). There are various risk factors, which can increase the possibility of fall in the geriatric population **(Box 1.2)**.

Scrupulous attention to detail are required when extracting history from these patients as we are not only treating the injuries sustained acutely but also the altered physiological reserve (electrolyte imbalance, diabetic ketoacidosis) and the associated pre-existing medical conditions [diabetes mellitus (DM), hypertension, renal, liver failure, cardiac illness, chronic

---

Box 1.2: Risk Factors for fall.

- Pre-existing injury (post-operative status of lower limb fracture)
- Osteoporosis
- History of syncope/Parkinson's disease
- Postural hypotension
- Medications
- Hypoglycemia
- Cognitive imbalance
- Continence
- Hearing/visual impairment
- Improper footwear
- Non-conducive environment like slippery floor

steroid intake, peripheral vascular disease, chronic venous insufficiency, and osteoporosis], that can hinder with healing and prognosis.

At the Time/Scene of the Injury

The elderly patient should be screened and referred to a multidisciplinary center equipped with adequately trained surgical staff and optimal rehabilitation services.

In Triage

- The local and systemic injuries should be noted.
- A detailed history of the patient's ambulatory status before injury would give an idea of the prognosis and aid in the decision-making of the management.
- Vitals (temperature, heart rate, blood pressure, respiration rate), ABG, ECG, chest X-ray, and cognitive assessment must be performed.
- The focused assessment with sonography in trauma (FAST) scan is reliable for detecting bleeding within the abdominal/pelvic cavity.
- In an unresponsive patient, immobilize the cervical spine with a hard cervical collar before shifting for imaging.
- Monitoring the hydration status and urine output is crucial.
- Adequate analgesics should be given.
- Elderly patients are susceptible to hemorrhage and can suffer from hypovolemic shock with lesser blood loss than young patients.
- Fragility fractures around the dorsal spine are prevalent and primarily missed in this age group. It should be screened again.
- If imaging was not performed for any reason, documentation must be done in their best interests after counseling the attendees.
- Patients are to be catheterized only in cases of head injury associated with intubation, hemodynamic instability, who cannot be relied upon adequate oral feeds, or in those patients where input-output monitoring is essential; to avoid UTIs.
- Deep vein thrombosis prophylaxis should be started if not contraindicated.
- Always confirm that there is no pressure sore at the time of admission, as these patients are very prone to the same.

Fundamental principles in the management of elderly patients:
- Age, comorbid conditions and chronic drug intake can alter the physiological presentation of the patient.
- Meticulous evaluation by an experienced clinician/surgeon is a must. Injuries are often missed or identified only retrospectively, as the trauma mechanism is usually unclear.
- Assessment to identify the presence of pain. For individuals with cognitive impairment—non-verbal pain manifestation should be elicited.
- Analgesia: Refrain from NSAID exploitation as most patients have medical contraindications (GI ulcers, renal failure, cardiac illness, liver failure). Limit to the lowest dose or concise course.
- Timely reversal of anticoagulant therapy to plan for surgery, if otherwise fit.
- The involvement of a geriatrician in patient care is vital to understanding their needs and improving outcomes.
- Risk vs benefit ratio to decide on interventional management.

Limb Injuries

- Initial imaging and appropriate temporary stabilization (splint/POP slab/Ex-fix) guidelines are similar to any patient-age-independent.
- However, decision-making regarding managing limb fractures is slightly different in the geriatric population as their bone stock and pre-existing co-morbidities tend to curtail treatment options for the surgeon. Although the surgical fixation, especially displaced lower limb fractures, enables early mobilization of these patients to avoid complications of recumbency (bedsore, hypostatic pneumonia, urinary tract infection, and deep vein thrombosis), the co-morbidities may not allow surgical intervention. Therefore, with the patient's best interest in mind, these fractures could be managed conservatively.

Notes

CHAPTER 2

Shock and its Management

DEFINITION

Shock is the systemic state of *prolonged inadequacy in tissue perfusion* due to primary circulatory failure.

Adequate oxygenation to the cells is vital for cellular respiration and metabolism. Any etiology that affects circulation and tissue perfusion would lead to cellular death and organ dysfunction.

Several important factors are responsible for blood circulation in the body, such as:
- Adequacy of cardiac pump
- Adequate blood volume
- No obstruction or congestion to the vessels
- Resisted peripheral vasculature and protected capillaries

Table 2.1 helps understand how affection in anyone of these factors manifests as a shock.

Table 2.1: Normal mechanism and alteration resulting in various types of shock.

Normal mechanism	Pathology	Type of shock
Normally working cardiac pump	Poor pump contractile capacity-*Myocardial infarction*	Cardiogenic
Adequate blood volume to be pumped	Less blood volume-*Hemorrhage, severe dehydration*	Hypovolemic
No obstruction while fluid pump out of the heart	Pump fine but an obstruction to the outflow-*Cardiac tamponade*	Obstructive
Adequately 'resisted peripheral vasculature' and 'protected capillaries'	Vasodilated peripheries leaky capillary basement membranes-*Spinal cord injury, neurogenic shock, septicemia*	Distributive

CLASSIFICATION OF SHOCK

Shock can be broadly classified into four main categories: Hypovolemic, Distributive, Cardiogenic and Obstructive.

A. Hypovolemic Shock

It is primarily caused by decreased intravascular volume.

The two subtypes of hypovolemic shock are:
1. *Hemorrhagic:* It occurs in polytrauma cases with excessive bleeding from open wounds, fractured bones (femur, pelvis) or within any cavity (splenic rupture, pelvic cavity bleeds).

2. *Nonhemorrhagic:* It occurs in severe burns, GI etiologies such as vomiting, diarrhea, or renal pathologies like diuresis.

In this chapter, hypovolemic (hemorrhagic) shock and its management will be discussed.

B. Distributive Shock

The primary pathology in distributive shock is peripheral vasodilatation. The four subtypes are:
1. *Septic shock:* Sepsis causes extensive cytokine release, and the accumulated bacterial toxins cause a cascade of inflammation, coagulation, and fibrinolytic suppression. Further, it can trigger Systemic Inflammatory Response Syndrome **(SIRS)**.
2. *Anaphylactic shock:* A typical IgE-mediated inflammatory response (allergy) due to hypersensitivity to drugs or bugs causing severe bronchospasm and subsequent cardiac collapse.
3. *Neurogenic shock:* Usually seen in trauma to the spinal cord. There may be a decreased sympathetic tone due to interruption of the autonomic nervous system resulting in peripheral vasodilatation causing reduced cardiac output (Starlings law).
4. *Endocrine shock:* Conditions like myxedema or Addisonian crisis can compromise metabolic function and lead to cardiac collapse.

C. Cardiogenic Shock

It usually manifests as a complication of a pre-existing cardiac disease like ischemic heart disease or wall dysfunction.

D. Obstructive Shock

Any obstruction that impedes the blood flow from the cardiac area to the body through the vessels can cause obstructive shock. It has two subtypes:
1. *Pulmonary vascular:* The blood flow from the right ventricle to the left is obstructed, e.g., pulmonary thromboembolism.
2. *Mechanical:* The obstruction leads to inadequate filling of the right side of the heart, e.g., tension pneumothorax, cardiac tamponade.

■ PATHOPHYSIOLOGY OF HYPOVOLEMIC SHOCK

Flowchart 2.1 explain the gross dysfunction in a hypovolemic shock.

As the hemorrhagic shock progresses in severity, many ***systemic responses occurs***, such as:
- Cardiovascular system—tachycardia, peripheral vasoconstriction
- Respiratory system—tachypnea
- Urinary system—decreased urine output, increased Na^+, water retention
- Adrenals—cortisol sensitizes cells to catecholamines.

Flowchart 2.1: Pathophysiology of hemorrhagic shock (in brief).

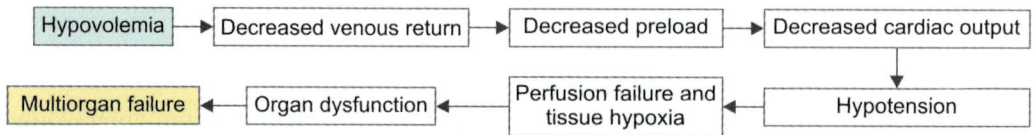

At the cellular level, there is profound *lactic acidosis* and *coagulation system dysfunction* (Flowchart 2.2).

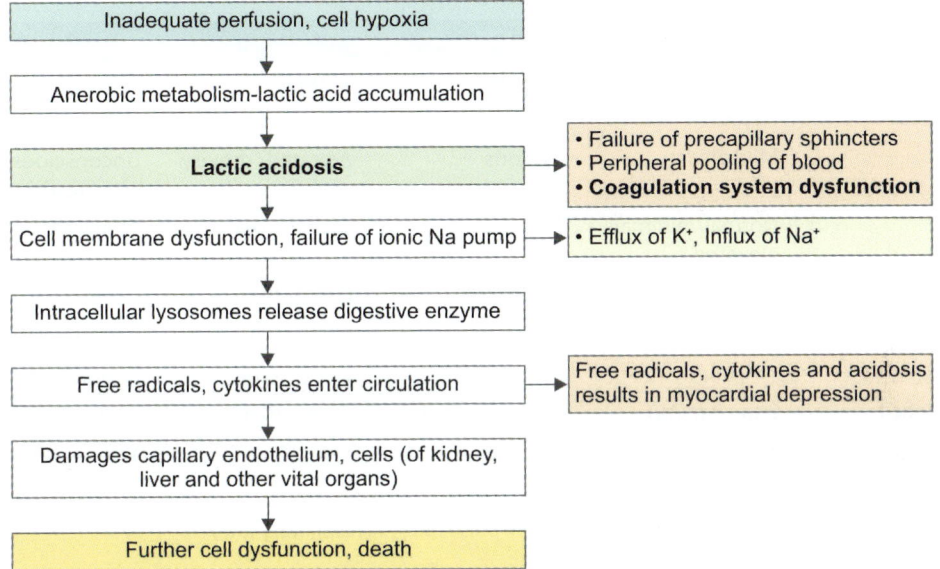

Flowchart 2.2: Cellular level dysfunction in shock (in brief).

■ SEVERITY OF SHOCK

There are 2 phases in shock, compensated and decompensated. Compensated metabolism can be easily reversed, whereas decompensated metabolism is challenging for the physician to reverse and therefore, the prognosis of the patient depends upon the phase of shock.

A. Compensated Shock

Given inadequacy in the circulation, the body compensates by reducing the circulation to non-essential organs such as skin, muscles, and GIT and channeling all the available blood to the vital organs such as kidneys, lungs, and brain. *A loss of up to 15% of circulatory volume can be compensated.* If this condition is prolonged, the patient gradually develops metabolic acidosis and experiences ischemic reperfusion syndrome. There is hypothermia due to blood loss. However, timely intervention can reverse the metabolic changes in the body.

B. Decompensated Shock

The available blood for circulation, although initially shunted to the vital organs, will not suffice for prolonged periods. There is usually more than a 30% loss in the circulatory volume at this stage. During this phase, if the fluid volume is not replaced with blood and there is further loss, the patient's condition will deteriorate. Key factors resulting in decompensated shock are progressing acidosis, hypothermia, and coagulation system dysfunction (lethal triad).

ATLS CLASSIFICATION OF SEVERITY OF SHOCK

The American College of Surgeons-Advanced Trauma Life Support (ACS-ATLS) hemorrhagic shock classification links the amount of blood loss to expected physiologic responses in a healthy 70 kg patient **(Table 2.2)**. Up to class II shock, the urine output remains stable.

Table 2.2: ATLS classification of severity of shock.

Variable	Class I	Class II	Class III	Class IV
Blood loss	<15%	15–30%	30–40%	>40%
CNS	Mild anxiety	Anxious	Agitated/ drowsy	Unconscious/ comatosed
PR	Normal/minimally elevated	Tachycardia	Tachycardia	Tachycardia
BP	Normal	Decreased	Decreased	Decreased
RR	Tachypnea	Tachypnea	30–40/min	>40/min, labored
Urine output	>30 mL/hr	20–30 mL/hr	5–15 mL/hr	Anuric
Base deficit	0 to –2 mEq/L	–2 to –6 mEq/L	–6 to –10 mEq/L	>–10 mEq/L
Need for blood	Monitor	Possible	Yes	Massive blood transfusion

(CNS: central nervous system; BP: blood pressure; PR: pulse rate; RR: respiratory rate)

CLINICAL FEATURES (OF HEMORRHAGIC SHOCK)

Almost all patients with hemorrhagic shock present with a history of trauma with/without fracture, and/or overt bleeding wounds. Sometimes, the source of bleeding could be covert, such as fracture of pelvis and femur, rib fractures with hemothorax, and injury to abdominal organs (liver, spleen) or a vascular injury. A detailed systemic examination along with investigations (FAST scan, CT scan, angiography, or needle aspirations) help diagnose covert bleeds.

The typical clinical features of hemorrhagic shock are:
- **Orientation**—the patient may be normally oriented or drowsy
- Sometimes, patients may have nausea/vomiting due to sympathetic stimulation
- **Cold clammy extremities, loss of skin turgor**
- **Pulse**—tachycardia, low volume (rapid and thready pulse)
- **Blood pressure**—hypotension
- **Respiratory rate**—tachypnea
- **Urine output**—decreased.

MANAGEMENT GUIDELINES OF HYPOVOLEMIC SHOCK

The most common type of shock managed in the trauma center is post-traumatic hypovolemic hemorrhagic shock. It can be managed with specific guidelines, such as:
- **Resuscitate** with ATLS protocol: Airway, breathing, circulation, disability and exposure. A multidisciplinary approach must be in place if there are other injuries.
- Start high-flow **oxygen**

- Secure an **IV line** of 14-16 gauge. Note that a larger bore IV cannula helps to rush greater fluid volumes.
- Withdraw the blood and send it for **baseline investigations** along with Hb, PCV, blood grouping, and typing. Arrange the matched and adequate blood for transfusion.
- Start **IV fluid followed by blood transfusion**: Crystalloids (normal saline, ringer lactate) are the best fluid to start, followed by blood transfusion (packed RBCs). *The role of colloids (dextran) remains controversial as they can hamper with coagulation system.*
  Note: Normal saline contains only NaCl, whereas ringer lactate contains Na, Cl, potassium, calcium, and lactate. The lactate helps tackle metabolic acidosis as it converts into bicarbonate in the liver.
- **Urinary catheterization:** The patient must be catheterized as it helps to monitor urine output. Normal urine output in an adult in 0.5 mL/kg/hour.

  ==Adequate urine output is the most important indicator of restored adequate tissue perfusion, and the 'patient is out of shock.'==

- Perform all necessary investigations to **identify any source of the active bleed, such as** chest X-ray, ultrasound, CT scan (abdomen, pelvis) and CT angiography.
  Once the active bleeder is identified, all measures to control it should be done posthaste (e.g. pelvic packing). Patients may require urgent abdominopelvic exploration or arterial embolization procedures to stop the active bleeding from abdominopelvic organs.
- **Stabilize long bone fracture with appropriate splints**. An unstable pelvis fracture should be immediately stabilized with a **pelvic binder/pelvic sheet** followed by an external fixator. Military antishock trousers (MAST) can also be used in pelvic fractures.
  Note: MAST is applied to the abdomen, pelvis and lower limbs. The underlying physiologic concept of MAST is to apply pressure to the lower extremities to shift the patient's blood volume from the abdomen, pelvis, and lower extremities to the upper body and central circulation. However, MAST garments are rarely used as they can result in lower limb compartment syndrome and ischemia.

  During the resuscitation, the patient must be monitored by checking vital parameters periodically (pulse rate, blood pressure, O_2 saturation), orientation, urine output, lactate levels (normal level is <2.3 mmol/L), and base deficit. Note that a*dequately maintained urine output is the most crucial indicator of restored adequate tissue perfusion, and the 'patient is out of shock.'*

CONCLUSION

The initial symptoms of shock can be detected clinically. Early diagnosis and management would prevent the progression of shock into an irreversible decompensated stage. Further, compensated shock can be easily reversed with minimal residual damage, whereas decompensated shock will progress into multiple metabolic complications. Therefore, the patient's prognosis depends on the time and speed of intervention.

A Note on Massive Blood Transfusion

Definition

Massive blood transfusion requires more than ten units of blood [packed red blood cells (PRBCs)] within 24 hours of the injury.

Patients with moderate to severe blood loss will have specific metabolic deficits such as *lactic acidosis, hypothermia,* and *coagulopathy*. Acidosis and hypothermia further exacerbate hypothermia. The decreased ability to stop bleeding leads to further hypothermia and acidosis, creating a positive feedback loop that results in worsened patient outcomes and therefore, to avoid such metabolic mayhem in severe blood loss, fresh frozen plasma (FFP) and platelets (Pl) must be transfused in addition to PRBCs in a ratio of 1:1:1 (PRBC: FFP: Pl) to avoid the deleterious effects of coagulopathy.

Complications of Massive Blood Transfusion

Metabolic alkalosis, hypokalemia, hypocalcemia, transfusion-related acute lung injury (TRALI-acute respiratory distress within 6 hours of transfusion), and transfusion-associated circulatory overload (TACO).

3 CHAPTER

Soft Tissue Injuries–Part 1

Soft tissue injuries are inherent to any fracture in the body. A fracture is defined as a "**break in the structural and anatomical integrity of the bone associated with a certain degree of soft tissue injury depending on the substantial force it withstood**". However, the mere appearance of an osseous injury often distracts from the presence of the soft tissue injury. It is ubiquitous to sustain such occult injuries without any evident fracture.

This chapter will discuss acute soft tissue injuries commonly seen in orthopaedic practice.

■ TYPES OF SOFT TISSUE INJURY

A. Based on Skin Epidermal Layer Integrity

The skin epidermal layer could be intact or breached/disrupted.

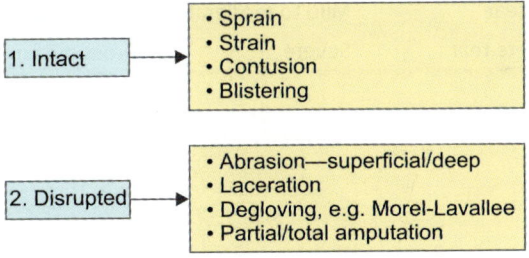

B. Based on Duration

Duration	Type of Force	Injury
Acute	1. Twisting 2. Direct blow	1. Sprain/strain/ligament tear 2. Ligament injury/neurovascular injury/open wound
Chronic	Repetitive stress (resulting in microtrauma)	Tendinitis/tendinopathy/bursitis

The most commonly injured soft tissue structures are muscles and tendons/ligaments. The neurovascular structures (artery and nerves) could also be damaged depending on the velocity of force.

ACUTE INJURIES WITH INTACT EPIDERMAL LAYER

In the acute event of trauma, soft tissues with intact epidermal layer can be injured in three main forms—sprain, strain and contusion.

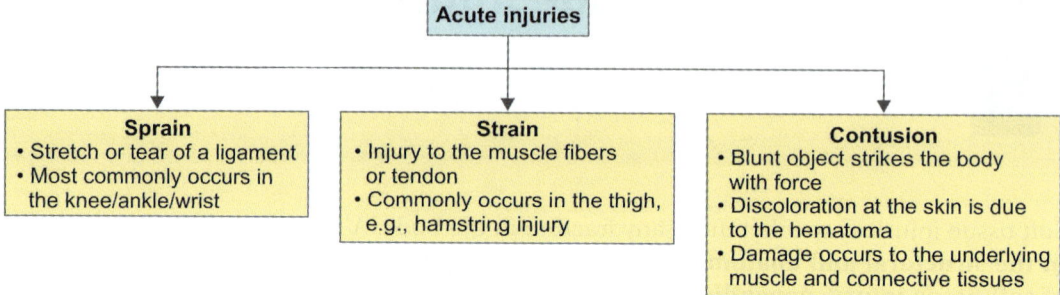

GRADING THE SEVERITY OF INJURY WITH INTACT EPIDERMAL LAYERS

The grading of sprain and strain helps the clinician form a standardized treatment protocol. Further, it helps in prognosticating the injury **(Table 3.1)**. **Figures 3.1 and 3.2** show various grades of ankle ligament sprain and muscle strain, respectively.

Table 3.1: Grading of sprain and strain.

Grade of injury	Structural damage	Instability	Function	Prognosis
1st degree	Few fibers strained	None	Normal	Excellent
2nd degree	Partial tear	Mild to moderate	Mild dysfunction	Good-excellent
3rd degree	Complete tear	Severe	Gross dysfunction	Poor-fair

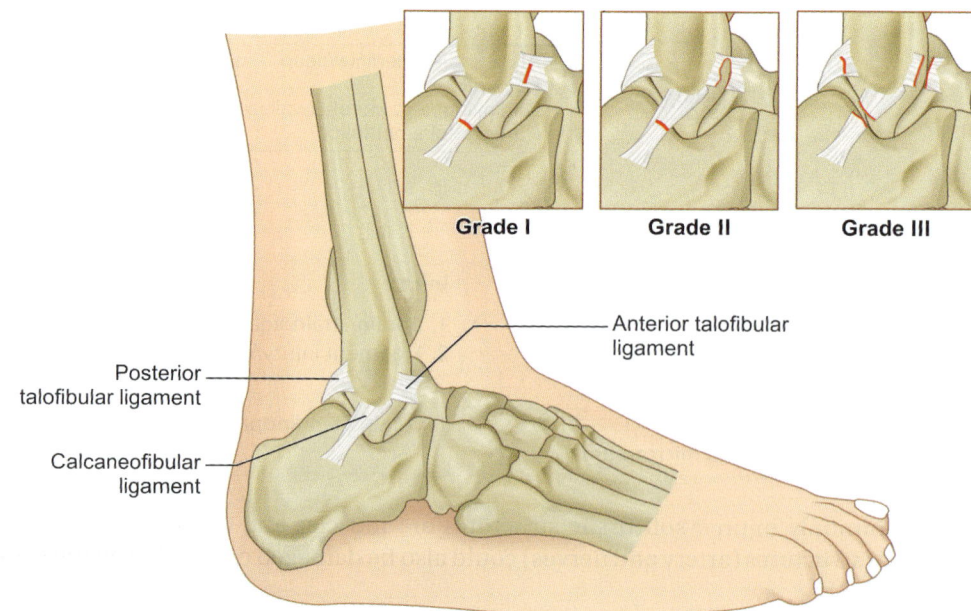

Fig. 3.1: Grade of sprain.

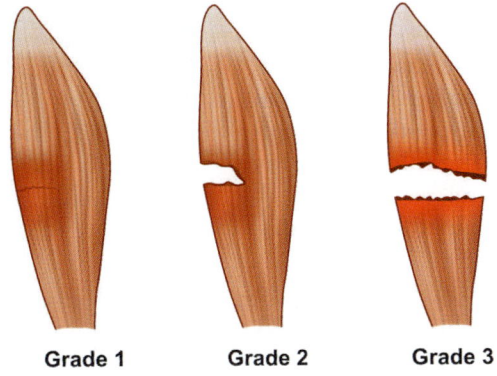

Grade 1   Grade 2   Grade 3

Fig. 3.2: Grade of strain.

CLINICAL FEATURES

The signs and symptoms vary according to the force applied and the mechanism of injury.

Symptoms

Pain, swelling and difficulty using the affected part remain the common complaint. In case of significant soft tissue injury (Grade 3), especially in the lower limb, the patient would be unable to bear weight or may find difficulty in weight bearing.

Signs

- Swelling is noticed over the injured part **(Fig. 3.3)**.
- Ecchymoses/bruising (hematoma in the subcutaneous plane) may be present **(Fig. 3.4)**.
- The patient will be able to point to the area of tenderness—the clinician has to palpate along the area gently.
- Range of motion is often painful and restricted.
- Assess the status of nerve function and limb vascularity.
- Ligament stability test should be performed with care.

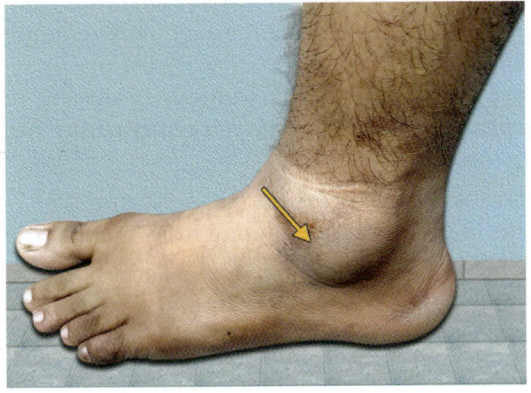

Fig. 3.3: Swelling over the lateral aspect of the ankle around lateral malleolus in ankle sprain (yellow arrow).

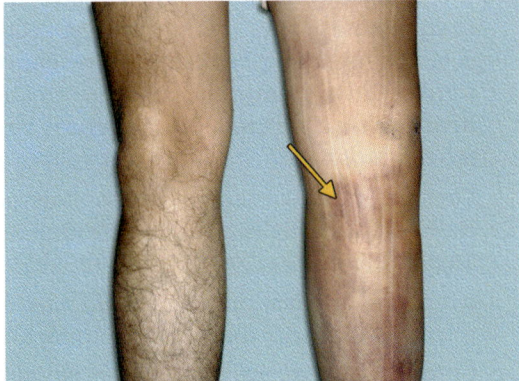

Fig. 3.4: Ecchymoses on medial side of the left knee (yellow arrow) indicating injury to the medial collateral ligament of the knee.

INVESTIGATIONS

1. **Plain radiograph:** In any case of trauma, the first investigation after a thorough examination is always a plain radiograph of the respective part. The role of an X-ray in a soft tissue injury is to:
   a. Rule out any associated fracture/dislocation
   b. Malalignment of the joint due to significant ligament injury **(Figs. 3.5A and B)**.
2. **Stress radiograph:** It is performed to assess the grade of ligament injury **(Fig. 3.6)**. Occasionally, a lower grade (1/2) could be grade 3 while imparting stress to the affected area.
3. **Ultrasonography (USG):** Using ultrasound has proven to be reliable in identifying ligament (especially extraarticular ligament) and tendon injuries in the acute phase.
4. **MRI:** MRI is the *gold standard for identifying soft tissue injuries. It also helps detecting bone contusion and occult fractures.*

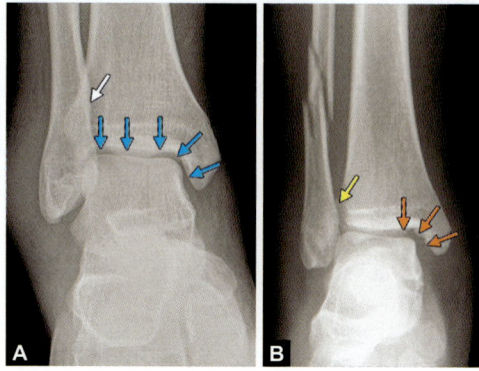

Figs. 3.5A and B: (A) Shows a normally aligned ankle joint space (blue arrows) and normal syndesmotic space (white arrow); (B) Shows malaligned ankle with abnormally increased syndesmotic space (yellow arrow) and medial joint space (orange arrows).

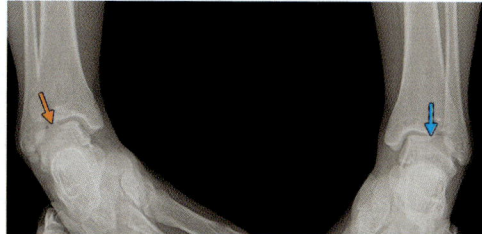

Fig. 3.6: Left ankle inversion stress shows tilted talus (orange arrow), while right ankle shows normally aligned talus (blue arrow).

TREATMENT

The treatment of sprains and strains could be *conservative* or *surgical repair/reconstruction*.

Conservative treatment works effectively for acute grades 1 and 2 soft tissue injuries. The majority of grade 3 injuries also receive conservative therapy. However, some individuals with grade 3 injury may require surgical treatment if the functional recovery is less than optimum.

In some cases of grade 3 injuries, especially in elite athletes or patients with high demand, surgical treatment may be offered **(Flowchart 3.1)**.

1. **Conservative treatment** comprise treatment in acute and delayed phase. Treatment in *acute phase* comprises *RICE protocol, analgesics,* and *splinting.* **Delayed phase** comprises *rehabilitation, bracing* and *return to routine activities and sports.*

   - First line line treatment of acute soft tissue injuries is **RICE protocol (Figs. 3.7 and 3.8)**

   Rest—This is usually done by splinting the affected part and preventing movement at the adjacent joint.

   Ice pack—Application over the affected part induces vasoconstriction, thereby reducing the inflammatory process and helping bring the swelling down.

   Compression—Helps to reduce swelling mechanically.

   Elevation—Limb elevation promotes circulation and prevents gravity-assisted venous pooling.

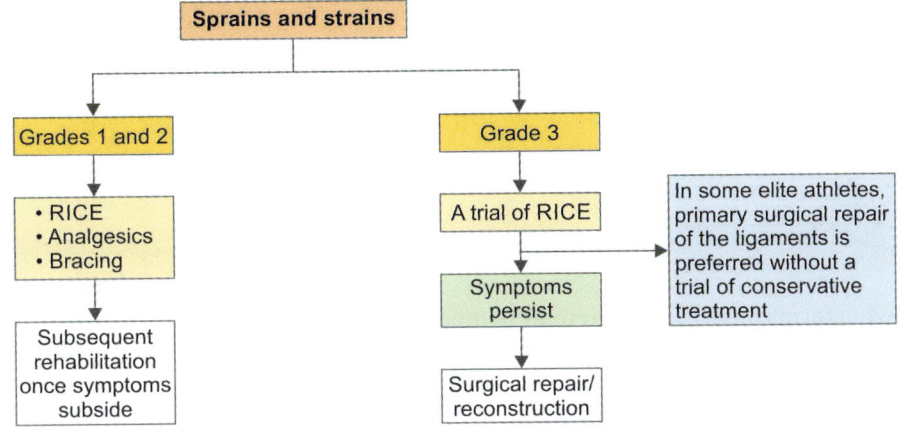

Flowchart 3.1: Treatment algorithm of sprains and strains.

(RICE: Rest, Ice, Compression, Elevation)

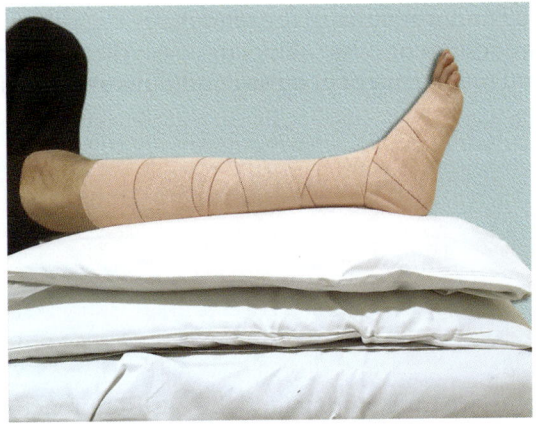

Fig. 3.7: Compression and elevation of ankle.

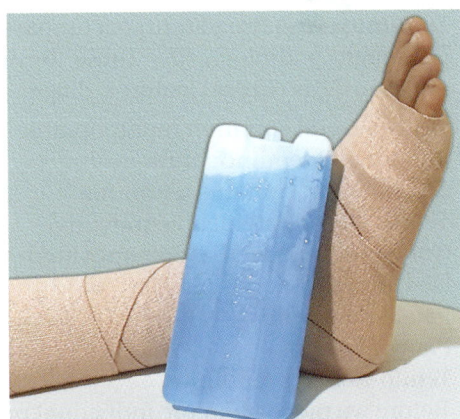

Fig. 3.8: Ice pack over the injured ankle.

- Analgesics and anti-inflammatory medication for 1–2 weeks.
- Rehabilitation is started when the acute phase has subsided and the pain and swelling have improved. If necessary, the injured area might be braced.
- Once the patient regains a pain-free range of motion and sufficient strength, they are permitted to return to their regular activities and sports.

2. **Surgical treatment:** Surgical repair/reconstruction of the injured ligament/muscle is considered if the recovery is suboptimal. Additionally, acute surgical repair is considered in select patient.

■ COMPLICATIONS

The natural history of acute injuries (grades 1 and 2) usually heals uneventfully. However, in grade 3, injuries in some patients may not heal, and patients may experience unresolved symptoms that progress to chronic pain, dysfunction, and/or instability. Occasionally, Complex Regional Pain Syndrome (CRPS) may ensue, prolonging recovery.

CHAPTER 4

Soft Tissue Injuries–Part 2

The following terms have evolved to refer to tendon injury and pain:
- **Tendinitis:** Acute incomplete structural tendon disruption accompanied by inflammation.
- **Paratenonitis:** Inflammation of the outermost layer of the tendon and may be accompanied by synovitis of the tendon sheath.
- **Tendinosis:** Intratendinous degeneration due to chronic overuse with no significant inflammation.
- **Tendinopathy:** Broad term encompassing all abnormalities of the tendon.

Although pathologically, these terms are different, the clinician uses these terms synonymously as clinical features, diagnosis and management of these conditions are similar.

There are several common tendinopathies, such as:
- Rotator cuff tendinopathy
- Calcific supraspinatus tendinitis
- Tennis elbow (lateral epicondylitis)
- Golfer's elbow (medial epicondylitis)
- De Quervain's tenosynovitis
- Patellar tendinitis
- Plantar fasciitis
- Tendo-Achilles tendinitis

Before we move on to the individual problems, we must understand the basic approach to a patient with tendinopathy.

■ FACTS OF TENDON ANATOMY AND FUNCTION

- Tendons are tough fibroelastic structures that connect muscles to bones. The principal function of the tendon is to transmit force across a joint to enable movement.
- The main *constituent of a tendon is Type I collagen*, which is responsible for making the tendon suited to carry loads and maintain tension for long periods.
- The major cellular component comprises tenoblasts and tenocytes, which are responsible for laying down the collagen matrix. Chondrocytes, synovial cells and endothelial cells are also present.
- The physical junction between tendon and bone is called an enthesis, which absorbs and distributes the concentrated load over a broader area of the bone.
- The low metabolic rate and well-developed anaerobic energy generation capacity enable tendons to make movements more efficient.
- However, this hypovascularity and low metabolic rate are responsible for the slow healing following a tendon injury and predispose to hypoxic tendon degeneration.
- Overuse tendon injuries often occur near or at the enthesis.

ETIOLOGY AND RISK FACTORS IN TENDINOPATHY

Usually, a combination of intrinsic and extrinsic factors is responsible for the development of tendinopathy.

A. Extrinsic Factors

Overuse and repetitive use during activities of athletes, heavy manual laborers, carpentry, typing, painting, or any activity that involves repetitive motions.

B. Intrinsic Factors

Primarily attributed to changes in microvascularity and subsequently reduced healing of the tendon.
- **Aging:** It is the *most important intrinsic risk factor* responsible for tendinopathy.
- Diabetes mellitus
- Hypertension
- Increased serum lipids
- Hyperuricemia
- Poor limb biomechanics such as malalignment, etc.

PATHOGENESIS

Stressful activities cause microtears in the tendon, which induces the release of growth factors that promote collagen synthesis, resulting in the healing of the tears. However, following excessive repetitive stress and microtrauma, these lesions do not get adequate time to repair themselves, and the damage rate exceeds the healing rate. The tendon injuries progressively worsen with disorganized macro- and microstructure, resulting in tendinopathy. It causes pain and dysfunction. **Flowchart 4.1** summarize the pathogenesis of tendinopathy.

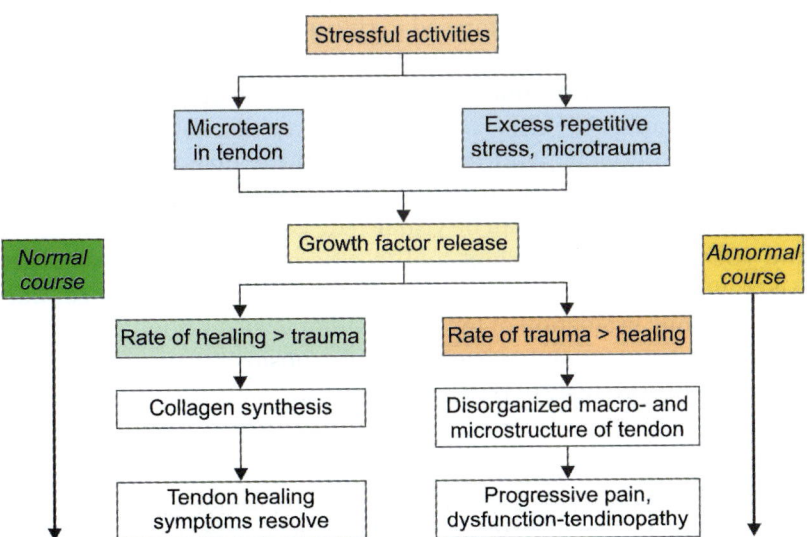

Flowchart 4.1: Pathogenesis of tendinopathy (in brief).

CLINICAL FEATURES

Tendinitis/tendinopathy is common in patients in their 40s to 50s (middle age). There is *history of repetitive stress/overuse/trauma/recent increase in or change in the type of activity may be present.*

Symptoms
- **Pain** at the site of the affected tendon:
    a. Sharply localized in the acute stage and dull aching after a few weeks
    b. Usually, the pain increases with activity
- **Decrease in strength** in the affected area. Occasionally, there can be swelling of the affected structure.

Signs
- Inspection for *muscle atrophy*—gives an idea about the duration of tendinopathy.
- *Local tenderness* is often present at the site of the affected tendon.
- A *palpable crepitus* may be present, and the *range of motion* is often reduced.
- The physical examination must include "**tests that stress or stretch the tendon in question to reproduce pain**" and other tests that load adjacent structures to rule out differentials.

INVESTIGATIONS

In most cases, the tendinopathy is a clinical diagnosis. Initially, two investigations are performed:
1. Plain X-ray of the affected part to rule out tendon calcification or underlying bony pathology.
2. Blood test to rule out metabolic abnormality (DM, thyroid dysfunction). USG or MRI are not routinely performed. They are asked if there is doubt regarding the diagnosis or if the condition is not responding to the conservative treatment.

The details of investigation are discussed below:
- **X-rays:** Usually normal in tendinopathies. Occasionally, calcification is present in the degenerated tendon. It must be performed to rule out underlying bony pathologies.
- **Blood investigations:** Often, tendinopathies are associated with diabetes mellitus, thyroid dysfunction, hyperuricemia, and hyperlipidemia. Therefore, the patient must be investigated for the same.
- **MRI:** Although not routinely performed to confirm the diagnosis, it is the investigation of choice to diagnose various spectrums of tendinopathy. Apart from tendon pathology, ligaments, cartilage, and muscle can be visualized.
- **Ultrasound (USG):** It is an excellent tool to assess various spectrum of tendinopathy. Further, USG offers several advantages over MRI—a more economical alternative, the possibility of dynamic evaluation of tendons, and no claustrophobia. However, it remains an operator-dependent instrument leading to false positive or negative results resulting in lower sensitivity and specificity of USG over MRI.

TREATMENT

Most tendinopathies respond to conservative treatment, while a few may require surgical treatment if the conservative treatment fails for more than 6–8 months.

- **Conservative treatment:** It involves rest to the affected part, pain relief by medications and physiotherapy, promoting tendon healing, and controlling the metabolic factors involved in tendinopathy.
  - *Rest* to the affected part can be achieved by:
    - *Activity reduction and activity modification:* Tendon injuries are primarily due to overuse of a particular muscle group, and if the affected tendon is not allowed to rest and heal, it typically worsens.
    - *Orthotics:* Braces, splints, or slings may be prescribed to reduce movement and allow the tendon to rest.
  - *Pain relief by*
    - *Cold therapy: Ice packs* are recommended for acute tendinopathies
    - *Hot pack:* Chronic tendinopathies often respond to heat therapy
    - *NSAIDs or other analgesics:* Locally as gel and orally to relieve pain.
    - *Local corticosteroids:*
      - Administered locally around the tendon (never in the substance) if primary pain relief measures (rest, NSAIDs, local gels, physiotherapy, braces) fail.
      - Helpful for short-term relief of symptoms. Moreover, postinjection overuse is associated with tendon weakness, rupture, etc.

> Local corticosteroid should be used with caution in Achilles tendinopathies as post-injection rupture of Achilles tendon is not uncommon, and is a disaster.

  - *Physiotherapy*
    - *To relieve pain:* Cold packs, moist heat, shortwave diathermy, laser therapy and others to relieve pain.
    - *To retain and regain movement:* Once pain reduces, mobilization should be started to retain and regain movements.
    - *To regain strength:* Once the pain has reduced and movements are restored, the patient should be taught proper stretching techniques and eccentric muscle strengthening exercises.
  - *Promoting tendon healing by*
    - *Extracorporeal shockwave therapy (ESWT):* It is a non-invasive treatment that uses high-pressure mechanical waves to promote healing and inhibit pain receptors.
    - *Local injection of platelet-rich plasma (PRP):* Recently, many studies have shown promising results of local PRP injection in tendinopathies. PRP is rich in platelets which secrete several growth factors (TGF-ß, FGF, PDGF, epidermal growth factor, VEGF) that promote collagen synthesis and healing. Locally injected PRP can facilitate the healing process of the degenerated tendon.
  - *Controlling the associated metabolic factors,* such as diabetes mellitus (DM), thyroid dysfunction, hyperuricemia and hyperlipidemia.
- **Operative management:** Operative treatment is *reserved for severe tendinopathy not responding to conservative treatment for 6-8 months*: In such cases, the frayed, damaged tendon is debrided, and torn edges are repaired.

The details of various tendinopathies across the body are discussed in Chapter on regional conditions.

CHAPTER 5

Dislocation of Major Joints

INTRODUCTION TO DISLOCATIONS

■ DEFINITION

Dislocation: A joint is said to be dislocated if two articulating surfaces are "no more in contact" with each other **(Fig. 5.1)**.

Subluxation: A joint is said to be subluxated if two articulating surfaces are still in "partial contact" with each other.

A joint that can dislocate or subluxate intermittently, known as *recurrent dislocation* or *subluxation*.

Fracture–dislocation: This term is used when the joint is dislocated, and one or both articulating surfaces are fractured **(Fig. 5.2)**. Some authors also term fracture-dislocation as *'complex dislocation.'*

■ HOW A JOINT REMAINS STABLE?

A joint remains stable due to the **integrity of static** (bone, ligaments, capsule) and **dynamic** (muscle-tendon unit) stabilizers. They can also be considered as **bony (articulating surface**

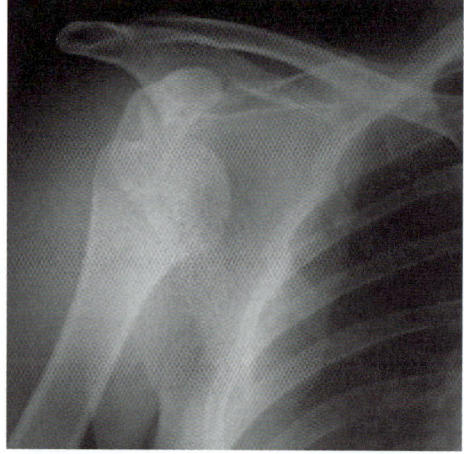

Fig. 5.1: Anterior dislocation of the shoulder showing empty glenoid and humeral head lying inferior to the coracoid process.

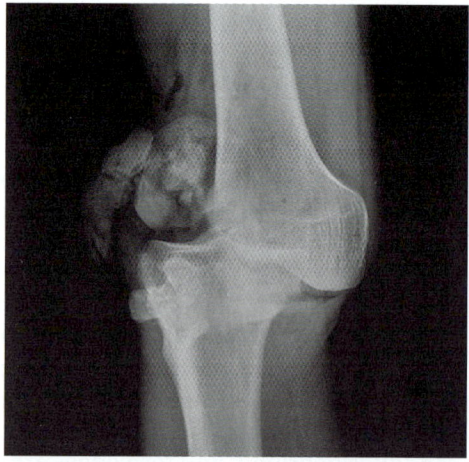

Fig. 5.2: Fracture dislocation of the knee. Note that the contact between tibia and femur is lost and lateral femoral condyle is fractured.

morphology) and ***soft tissue stabilizers***. Apart from these factors, ***negative pressure in the joint*** also contributes for the stability of a joint.

- **The normal bony morphology of the articulating surfaces:** The normal bony morphology of both articulating surfaces is a *static stabilizer of the joint.* Any morphological anomaly, congenital or acquired, of one or both surfaces, could result in dislocation or subluxation of the joint. Several examples are mentioned below:
  - In recurrent patella dislocation, the *shape of the femoral trochlea* (a longitudinal groove between two femoral condyles in which patella descends and ascends during knee flexion and extension, respectively) *is often flat (trochlear dysplasia)*, causing less lateral restraint on the patella resulting in lateral patella dislocation.
  - In developmental dysplasia of the hip, the congenitally abnormal shape of the acetabulum and femoral head results in dislocation or subluxation of the hip.
- **Intact ligaments and capsule:** Ligaments and capsule are *static stabilizers of a joint.* They permit enough flexibility to allow normal movement but prevent abnormal motion of the joint in any one direction. Injury to the ligament or capsule may happen during dislocation. Furthermore, *excess laxity of ligaments/capsule may predispose a joint for recurrent dislocation.*
- **The muscle cover around the joint:** Muscles are *dynamic stabilizers of the joint as they* can contract and relax to provide adequate stability. For example, in the shoulder's abduction–external rotation (ABER) position, the shoulder is not only stabilized anteriorly by labrum and glenohumeral ligaments but also by intact subscapularis muscle, which contracts to support already stretched ligaments. However, in the case of a complete subscapularis tear, the joint may subluxate or dislocate in an extreme abduction-external rotation position as there is no further anterior support to stretched or torn ligament.

CLASSIFICATION OF DISLOCATION

- **Traumatic dislocation:** It occurs after a *significant trauma* in an *"otherwise morphologically normal"* joint. The force causing dislocation is severe enough to overcome the restraint provided by the static and dynamic stabilizers.
- **Atraumatic dislocation:** It occurs after insignificant or no trauma in an *"otherwise morphologically abnormal"* joint. The force causing dislocation or subluxation is minimal as the stability of static or dynamic structures is already compromised. For example, *atraumatic shoulder dislocators often exhibit abnormal generalized soft tissue laxity, faulty muscle patterns of contraction, or bony dysplasia resulting in compromised stability.* Such patients can dislocate their shoulders with ease or sometimes voluntarily. The latter is also called "habitual dislocators."
- **Pathological dislocation:** The joint surfaces and/or static stabilizers are destroyed during an infective or inflammatory process affecting the joint, leading to subluxation or dislocation.
  For example, hip or knee tuberculosis destroys the joint, leading to persistently dislocated joint.
- **Paralytic dislocation:** A joint can dislocate if there is paralysis/spasticity of surrounding supporting muscles. A classic example—poliomyelitis, wherein the joints (hip) dislocate due to paralysis of muscles. It is also observed in the shoulder joint after hemi/quadriplegia due to atony in shoulder muscles. Paralytic dislocations are also seen in cerebral palsy.
- **Congenital:** It is present by birth due to congenital malformation of articulating surfaces and other soft tissues. It is commonly observed in hip and knee.

PATHOANATOMY OF A DISLOCATION

- **Traumatic dislocation or subluxation** cannot happen without damage to the bony or soft tissue (capsule and ligament) restraints.

    During an episode of traumatic dislocation, soft tissue restraints are almost always torn. For example, *in anterior shoulder dislocation,* the anteroinferior labrum is always torn (Bankart lesion), and the posterolateral head of the humerus shows an impaction fracture (Hill-Sachs lesion). *In lateral patella dislocation*, the medial restraint (medial patellofemoral ligament) is often torn. Further, an injury to the medial or lateral facet of the patella may lead to an osteochondral fracture.

    Occasionally, the ligament substance withstands the stress but pulls away along with a bony fragment where the ligament is attached to the bone. For example, bony avulsion of anterior cruciate ligament from tibia.

    The most significant point to remember is that during the traumatic dislocation, the *adjacent neurovascular bundle is always at risk of compression or stretch, and that renders traumatic dislocation an orthopaedic emergency (Table 5.1).*

- **Atraumatic dislocation** may not show any damage as joints dislocate easily due to existing abnormal congenital morphology in bony or soft tissue. Also, there is less or no risk of nerve injury.

Table 5.1: Common joints predisposed for traumatic dislocation with associated nerve injury.

Joint	Type or site of dislocation	Nerve injury
Cervical spine	Common at the cervical spine level	Spinal cord
Dorsolumbar spine	Commonly at the dorsolumbar junction	Spinal cord, conus medullaris, cauda equina
Shoulder	Most commonly, anterior Sometimes, posterior or inferior	Axillary, brachial plexus
Elbow	Posterior	Median
Wrist	Lunate, perilunate	Median
Hip	Posterior (most common), anterior	Sciatic (in posterior dislocation), femoral (in anterior dislocation)
Knee	Posterior, anterior, posteromedial, or posterolateral	Tibial, common peroneal
Patella	Lateral	
Ankle	Anterolateral	Posterior tibial, deep or superficial peroneal at ankle level
Foot	Lisfranc (tarsometatarsal), Chopart (intertarsal)	

CLINICAL FEATURES OF TRAUMATIC DISLOCATION

Symptoms

Pain and swelling around the dislocated joint and inability to use a limb or bear weight (in case of lower limb joint dislocations).

Signs

- ***Often characteristic deformity:*** For example, flexion, adduction, and internal rotation deformity at the hip joint in posterior dislocation of the hip.
- *Loss of contour of the joint* may be observed, especially if the joint is not deep seated.
- *Painfully restricted range of movement*
- *Altered limb length:* Shortening (posterior dislocation of hip, elbow, knee dislocation) or lengthening (pubic type of anterior dislocation of the hip) of the limb.
- ***An accurate neurovascular assessment is mandatory.***
- Occasionally, a dislocation can result in ***compartment syndrome***. For example, there is a high chance of compartment syndrome in knee or elbow dislocation.

■ INVESTIGATIONS

- **Plain X-ray** of the joint—two views are generally required to assess the direction of dislocation **(Figs. 5.3A and B)**.
- **CT scan** is required if there is an associated fracture **(Fig. 5.4)**. Furthermore, bony dysplasia of articular surface can be assessed better on CT scans. For example, trochlear and glenoid dysplasia in patella and shoulder dislocation, respectively.
- **Angiography:** If associated with vascular injury. Usually combined with a CT scan.
- **Magnetic resonance imaging:** Usually, it is acquired after the joint is reduced to assess ligament, capsule, muscle-tendon, or cartilage injuries.

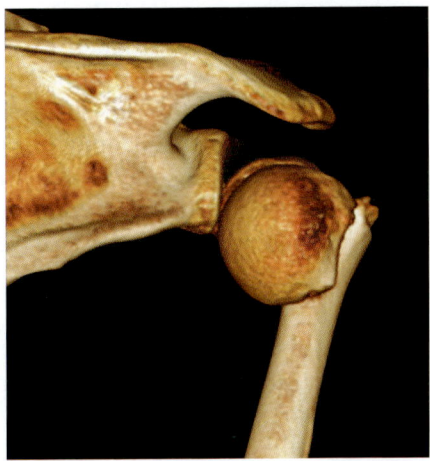

Fig. 5.4: 3D CT scan shows posteriorly dislocated and fracture of the head of the humerus.

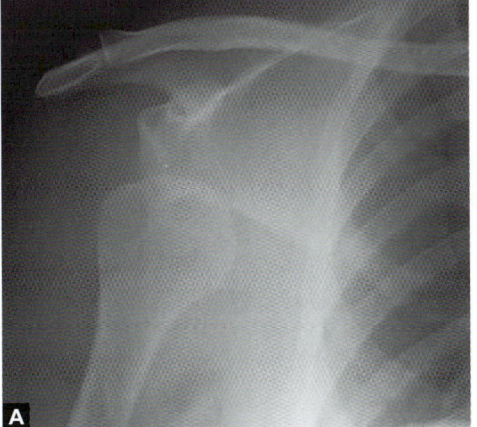
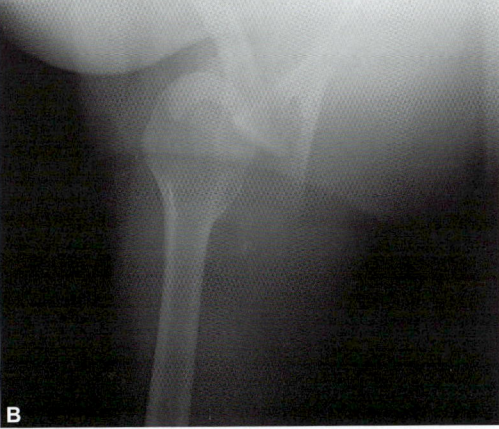

Figs. 5.3A and B: Anterior dislocation of the shoulder. (A) Anteroposterior view; (B) Axillary view showing anteriorly dislocated humeral head.

- **Nerve conduction velocity (NCV) and electromyography (EMG):** In case of associated nerve injury.

TREATMENT

The treatment of acute, chronic neglected and recurrent joint dislocation is different.

A. **Acute traumatic dislocation:** *All acute dislocations are orthopaedic emergencies due to impending/existing pressure over the neurovascular bundle.* Further, the nutrition of articular surface cartilage is compromised for the duration of dislocation, jeopardizing cartilage health.

   The essence of dislocation treatment is "reduction of dislocation" as early as possible. In most cases, closed reduction (CR) can be achieved. However, *if CR attempts fail, one must perform an open reduction of the dislocation.*

   Several reasons for a failed CR of dislocation are—buttonholing of articulating surface through the capsule, entrapped bony fragment or soft tissue between the joint surfaces, or a chronic dislocation presenting after a few days to weeks.
   - After CR of dislocation, **joint is immobilized** *for 2–3 weeks* to let the soft tissues (ligaments, capsule) heal to prevent the recurrence of dislocation.
   - Immobilization is followed by **rehabilitation** through gentle mobilization of joints, progressive usage of limb or weight-bearing, muscle strengthening, and proprioceptive exercises.

B. **Chronic unreduced dislocation**
   - Mostly, it requires open reduction due to fibrosis and contracture of soft tissues.
   - Occasionally, the ligaments may require repair or reconstruction to achieve stability.
   - Immobilization for 2–3 weeks.
   - Rehabilitation.

C. **Chronic recurrent dislocators**: Ligament and bony repair/reconstructive procedures depend upon the existing pathological abnormality (soft tissue/bony/both).

COMPLICATIONS OF TRAUMATIC DISLOCATION

Immediate/Early
- Neurovascular damage
- Compartment syndrome
- Irreducible dislocation
- Associated fracture of articulating surfaces.

Late
- Myositis ossificans
- Stiffness
- Recurrent dislocation
- Avascular necrosis
- Osteoarthritis of the joint.

DISLOCATIONS AROUND THE SHOULDER

SURGICAL ANATOMY

- The true shoulder joint (glenohumeral) is formed between the glenoid and the humerus head **(Fig. 5.5)**.
- The glenoid is lined by fibrocartilagenous 'glenoid labrum.' The labrum acts like a 'chock-block,' deepening the glenoid cavity and thus enhancing the stability of the shoulder.
- Various **static and dynamic restraints** stabilizing the shoulder (glenohumeral joint) are:
  - *Static restraints*: Normal geometry of bony articular surfaces (humeral head and glenoid), joint capsule, glenoid labrum, glenohumeral ligaments (superior, middle, and inferior), and negative intra-articular pressure are static restraints.
  - *Dynamic restraints*: Rotator cuff muscles, various scapular muscles, the long head of the biceps, and the deltoid provide dynamic stability to the joint.

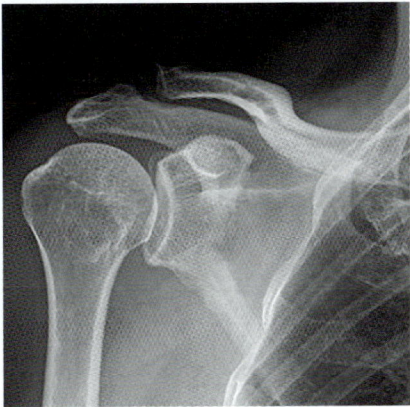

Fig. 5.5: X-ray of normal shoulder showing normal articulation between humeral head and glenoid cavity.

RELEVANT PATHOANATOMY

- During a **traumatic shoulder dislocation (anterior or posterior)**, the labrum and/or capsule are torn. Also, there is an impaction fracture of the humeral head. Sometimes, it is accompanied by a glenoid rim fracture. Rarely, there could be a tear of the rotator cuff, especially in an older person. These pathological entities, if do not heal, result in a recurrently unstable shoulder.
- **Atraumatic shoulder dislocation** is generally due to *pathological laxity of the joint capsule,* or abnormal muscle patterning, which may result in instability. It is often multidirectional (2 or more directions—anterior, posterior and inferior).
- In cases of **posterior dislocation**, it is often accompanied by *glenoid dysplasia*.

TYPES OF SHOULDER DISLOCATIONS

The *shoulder is most commonly dislocated among all the joints*, accounting for up to 46% of all dislocations. The shoulder dislocates in three directions—anterior, posterior, and inferior, with respect to the glenoid.
1. **Anterior dislocation:** It is the *most common type (96%)*, wherein the head of the humerus lies anterior to the glenoid **(Fig. 5.6)**. There are three subtypes—subglenoid, subcoracoid, and subclavicular.

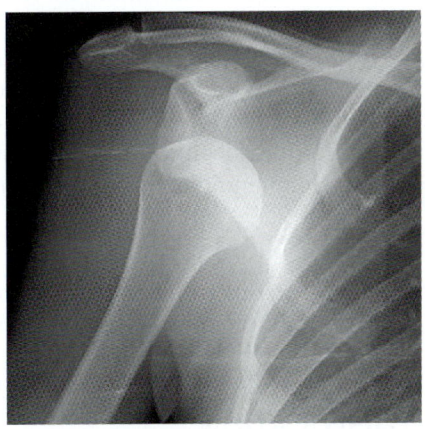

Fig. 5.6: X-ray right shoulder showing anterior shoulder dislocation (of humeral head) and empty glenoid.

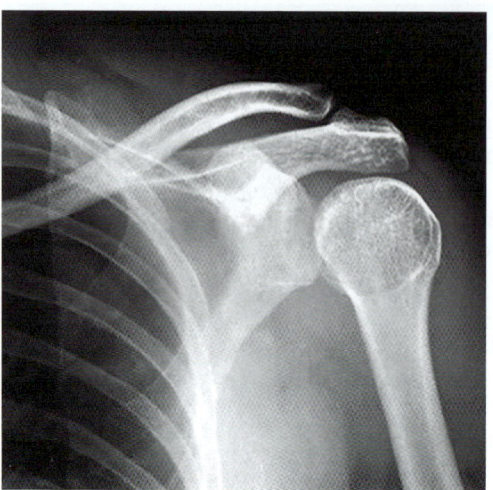

Fig. 5.7: X-ray of left shoulder showing posterior dislocation.

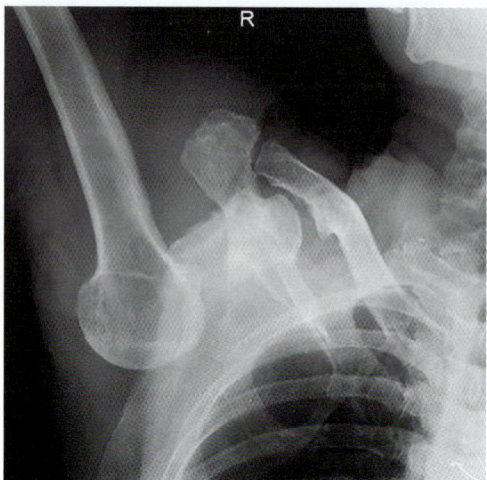

Fig. 5.8: X-ray of right shoulder showing luxatio erecta.

2. **Posterior dislocation:** In this less common type of dislocation (2–4%), the head of the humerus lies posterior to the glenoid **(Fig. 5.7)**.
3. **Inferior dislocation**: It is the rarest form of dislocation (0.5%), also known as *luxatio erecta,* wherein the head of the humerus lies inferior to the glenoid with a hyperabducted arm **(Fig. 5.8)**.

ACUTE ANTERIOR DISLOCATION OF THE SHOULDER JOINT

■ PATHOANATOMY

Anterior dislocation is the most common type of shoulder dislocation (96%). In the traumatic anterior shoulder dislocation, there are **two essential lesions** present on the glenoid (Bankart lesion) and humeral head (Hill-Sachs lesion).
1. **Bankart lesion:** It is the detachment of anteroinferior labrum from the glenoid margin. Sometimes, the labrum avulses along with a bony glenoid margin known as "Bony Bankart."
2. **Hill-Sachs lesion:** It is an impaction fracture on the posterolateral aspect of the head of the humerus. It occurs while the posterolateral part of the head humerus hitches against the anterior glenoid margin during anterior dislocation.

■ MECHANISM OF INJURY

1. Fall on an outstretched hand with arm in abduction and external rotation
2. Anterior directed force on the shoulder from behind.

■ CLINICAL FEATURES OF ACUTE TRAUMATIC ANTERIOR SHOULDER DISLOCATION

Symptoms

There is pain and swelling over the affected shoulder and an inability to move the shoulder.

Signs
1. The **shoulder contour is lost** with **fullness in front of the axilla (Fig. 5.9)**.
2. Typically, the *arm is held in slight abduction and external rotation* with an *inability to internally rotate and touch the opposite shoulder*. Even passively, internal rotation cannot be performed *(c.f., posterior dislocation of shoulder where external rotation is impossible)*.

Specific Signs in an Acute Shoulder Dislocation (Fig. 5.9)

A: **A**xillary concavity is reduced due to inferiorly dislocated humeral head
B: **B**ryant's test: Anterior axillary fold is at a lower level when compared to the normal side
C: **C**allaway's test: Increased anteroposterior diameter of the axilla
C: **C**ontour of the shoulder lost due to flattening
D: **D**uga's test: Inability to touch the opposite shoulder (as patient cannot internally rotate shoulder)
H: **H**amilton ruler test: A ruler placed on the lateral aspect of the arm touches the acromion (ruler fails to touch the acromion on the normal side)
H: **H**ollow posterior aspect of the shoulder
I: **I**ncreased length of arm compared to normal side
R: **R**egimental badge sign: Loss/decrease in sensation over axillary nerve distribution area over the upper lateral aspect of the arm.

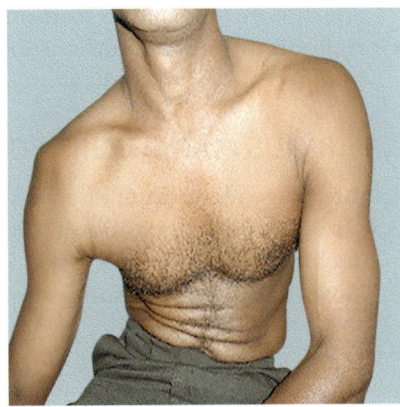

Fig. 5.9: Loss of right shoulder contour due to anterior dislocation.

■ INVESTIGATIONS

1. **Plain X-ray of the shoulder:** AP and axillary view **(Figs. 5.10A and B)**. *Note: the axillary view is usually required to confirm anterior/posterior direction of dislocation of humeral head with respect to the glenoid.*

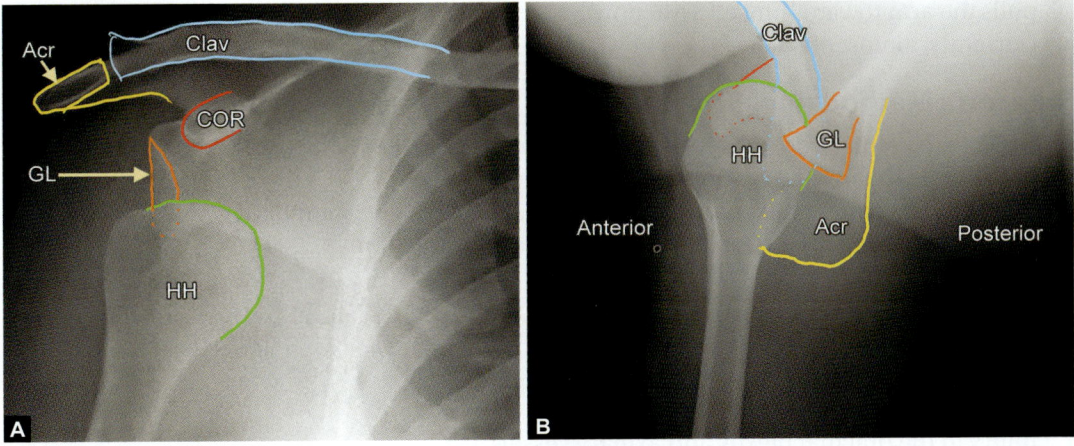

Figs. 5.10A and B: Anterior dislocation of the shoulder: (A) Anteroposterior view; (B) Axillary view shows that humeral head is lying anterior to the glenoid.
(HH: humeral head; GL: glenoid cavity; Acr: acromion; Clav: clavicle; Cor: coracoid process; Ant: anterior; Post: posterior)

2. **MRI:** It is the *confirmatory investigation to detect Bankart and Hill-Sachs lesion.* It is important to note that MRI is performed after the reduction of the shoulder.
3. **CT scan:** It is performed if there is an associated fracture of the glenoid, head of the humerus, or greater tuberosity (GT) avulsion.

TREATMENT OF ACUTE ANTERIOR DISLOCATION

- The **reduction of dislocation must be performed as early as possible** in sedation/general anesthesia, followed by **immobilization** of the shoulder in an arm sling for 3 weeks.
- **Rehabilitation:** Shoulder mobilization and muscle strengthening exercises must be initiated once immobilization is over to regain movement and power of the shoulder.

VARIOUS MANEUVERS FOR REDUCTION OF ANTERIOR DISLOCATION

1. **Leverage technique:** Kocher's method, Milch method
2. **Traction-countertraction technique:** Hippocratic method, Stimson method, Matsen technique
3. **Scapular manipulation**.

Kocher's Method

- Quite popular
- **Method:** With the patient sitting/lying supine, the elbow is bent to 90 degrees, the arm adducted, and gradually externally rotated till the forearm lies in the coronal plane of the body. Then, internally rotate the arm. Once the shoulder is reduced, the patient will be able to touch the tip of the opposite shoulder.
- **Disadvantage:** Excess rotational stress over the arm could result in a spiral fracture of the humerus and tear of subscapularis tendon.

Hippocratic Method (Fig. 5.11)

- **Method:** The examiner pushes his leg into the axilla (counter traction) of the patient and pulls the arm toward himself (traction).
- Currently, almost obsolete.

Stimson's Method (Fig. 5.12)

- Used in patients who present with *old unreduced anterior dislocation of the shoulder* between 3 weeks and 6 weeks
- **Method:** The patient lies prone on the couch, and a weight is applied over his wrist, which acts like traction. The edge of the bed is like countertraction.

COMPLICATIONS OF ACUTE ANTERIOR DISLOCATION SHOULDER

Acute

- *Axillary nerve palsy*
- Injury to the brachial plexus and axillary vessels
- Associated fracture of the greater tuberosity or anterior glenoid rim
- Possibility of associated rotator cuff tear in older patients (>45–50 years).

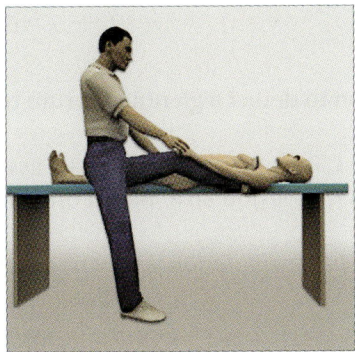

Fig. 5.11: Hippocratic method.

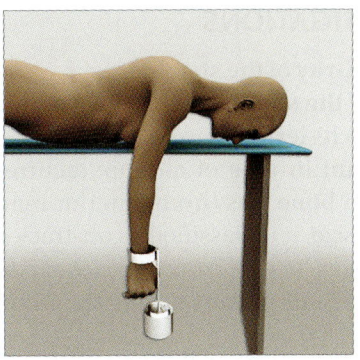

Fig. 5.12: Stimson's method.

Chronic

- Shoulder stiffness (secondary frozen shoulder)
- ***Recurrent dislocation:*** Among all, it is *one of most common complications.*

RECURRENT ANTERIOR DISLOCATION OF SHOULDER

Recurrent anterior dislocation of the shoulder is quite frequent. The younger the patient (<20–25 years) at the time of the first dislocation, the higher the chance of re-dislocation.

■ PATHOANATOMY

1. **Bankart lesion:** Presence of anteroinferior glenoid labrum tear (Bankart lesion) or bony Bankart lesion.
2. **Hill-Sachs lesion:** It is an impaction fracture on the posterolateral aspect of the head of the humerus, which occurs when the head of the humerus impacts against the anterior glenoid margin.
3. **Erosion of anterior glenoid margin:** Often, the anterior margin of the glenoid suffers bony erosion due to repeated dislocation, wherein repeated head engagement with anterior glenoid margin results in glenoid bony erosion.

■ CLINICAL FEATURES

The patient may come with an acutely dislocated shoulder or may have a history of repeated dislocations which might be self-reduced or reduced by the doctor.

In a reduced shoulder, several other signs are positive such as:
1. **Apprehension test**
2. **Relocation-release test**
3. *Always examine for generalized ligament laxity by assessing the Beighton score,* which may predispose to recurrent dislocation.

> **Box 5.1:** Beighton score.
>
> It is a **9-point clinical scoring system** to assess **soft tissue laxity and hypermobility**. **Five clinical parameters**—little finger passive dorsiflexion >90°, thumb passive dorsiflexion to the flexor aspect of forearm, elbow passive hyperextension >10°, knee passive hyperextension >10°, and ability to touch the floor by flat palms while bending forward and keeping knee straight. Each parameters gets score 0 or 1 on each side, while bending forward gets 0 or 1. **Score of 4 or higher hyperlaxity.**

INVESTIGATIONS

1. **Plain X-ray** of the shoulder
2. **MRI of the shoulder:** It is the diagnostic investigation to detect a glenoid labrum tear and Hill-Sachs lesion.
3. **CT scan:** In case of chronic recurrent dislocation, CT scan is performed to assess the glenoid bone loss (from anterior margin) and Hill-Sachs lesion size. Based on Hill-Sachs lesion size, it is classified as on-track or off-track.

   Currently, two parameters-glenoid bone loss and Hill-Sachs lesion size are essential in surgical decision-making during the treatment.

TREATMENT OF RECURRENT ANTERIOR DISLOCATION

Currently, the treatment of recurrent dislocation of the shoulder depends upon the amount of glenoid bone loss [more or less than 25% of anteroposterior (AP) diameter of the glenoid] and Hill-Sachs lesion characteristics.

1. **Arthroscopic/open Bankart repair:** It is performed when the AP glenoid bone loss is <20–25% (compared to the normal side). The torn anteroinferior labrum is resutured onto the glenoid margin by arthroscopic or open method using suture anchors.
2. **Latarjet procedure:** It is performed when the anteroposterior diameter of the glenoid is eroded >20–25%. *In such a situation, the chance of lone arthroscopic labral repair failure increases due to high bone loss, and mere soft tissue repair cannot restore anterior stability.*

   In the Latarjet procedure, the tip of the coracoid (2 cm) is osteotomized along with the attachment of the coracobrachialis and the short head of the biceps. The osteotomized coracoid is then fixed onto the anterior glenoid margin with two screws **(Fig. 5.13)**. Once the bony coracoid is fixed to the anterior glenoid margin, it covers the anterior glenoid bony deficiency and provides enhanced anterior bony support. Furthermore, the attached coracobrachialis tendon over the tip of coracoid and inferior subscapularis fibers provide a sling effect to prevent anterior dislocation during abduction.
3. **Remplissage** is performed for large or an off-track Hill-Sachs lesion. It is performed in addition to Bankart repair. It is a procedure wherein the infraspinatus tendon is sutured over the Hill-Sachs defect to prevent the engagement of the Hill-Sachs lesion with the glenoid margin in external rotation of the shoulder.

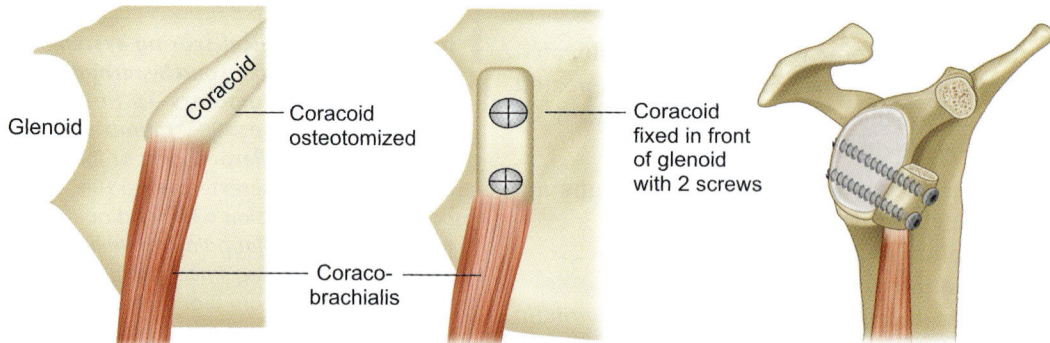

Fig. 5.13: Latarjet procedure.

> **Procedures of historical importance**
> 1. **Putti-Platt procedure:** In this procedure, the subscapularis is divided vertically and sutured by double breasting it resulting in limited external rotation of the shoulder. Hence, Putti-Platt procedure prevents anterior dislocation of shoulder by limiting external rotation, as shoulder dislocates anteriorly in external rotation.
> 2. **Bristow's procedure:** Biomechanically, Bristow procedure is similar to Latarjet. However, in Bristow procedure the tip of coracoid process is fixed with single screw over glenoid margin (cf. Latarjet wherein two screws are used). Currently, Latarjet is preferred over Bristow's for better biomechanic performance.

POSTERIOR DISLOCATION OF THE SHOULDER JOINT

- In comparison to anterior dislocation, posterior dislocation of the shoulder is rare. Note that posterior dislocation is *often missed due to subtle clinical and radiological signs.*
- Apart from trauma, posterior dislocation typically occurs after ***Epilepsy, Electric shock/Electrocution, Ethanol intoxication, and Electroconvulsive therapy (4Es)***.

MECHANISM OF INJURY

1. **Indirect trauma** results in posterior shoulder dislocation when the shoulder is in a position of *flexion, adduction, and internal rotation*. Electric shock may cause posterior dislocation owing to greater muscular force of internal rotators (latissimus dorsi, pec major, and subscapularis) than external rotators (infraspinatus and teres minor)
2. **Direct trauma:** This results from posteriorly directed force applied to the anterior part of the shoulder, resulting in posterior dislocation.

PATHOANATOMY

- **Posterior labral tear with or without posterior glenoid margin erosion/fracture (Reverse Bankart lesion).** Some patients may have ***glenoid dysplasia*** with increased retroversion of the glenoid.
- **Reverse Hill-Sachs lesion:** Impaction fracture over the *anteromedial aspect of the humeral head.*

CLINICAL FEATURES

Symptoms
Pain and swelling of the shoulder with difficulty or inability to move the shoulder.

Signs
These patients present with an attitude of ***adduction and internal rotation*** at the shoulder with an inability to ***externally rotate the shoulder*** (active and passive). (*cf., anterior dislocation, wherein the patient cannot perform internal rotation at the shoulder*).
- There is posterior fullness and anterior emptiness with loss of shoulder contour
- Examination of neurovascular structure is a must, especially axillary nerve.

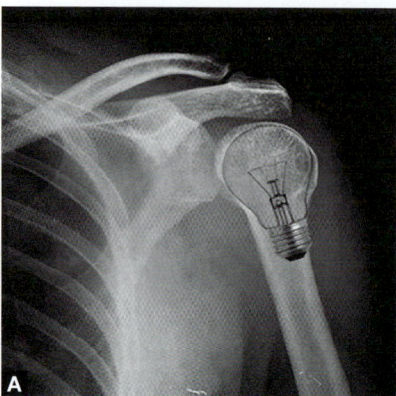 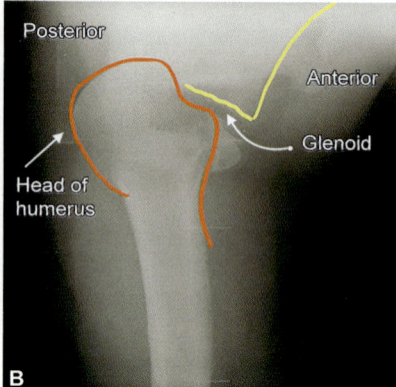

Figs. 5.14A and B: (A) Anteroposterior view of the shoulder showing light bulb sign; (B) Axillary view with posteriorly dislocated head humerus with respect to glenoid.

INVESTIGATIONS

1. **Anteroposterior view of X-ray of the shoulder:**
    - Typical radiological feature: *"Light bulb sign"* (head of the humerus on the same axis as the shaft producing a lightbulb shape) **(Fig. 5.14A)**
    - Vacant glenoid
    - *Rim sign*: Wide glenohumeral space
2. **Axillary view of the shoulder:** Posteriorly dislocated head of the humerus **(Fig. 5.14B)**.
3. **CT and MRI scan of the shoulder:**
    - To look for glenoid bony erosion, glenoid dysplasia
    - Labral tear, reverse Hill-Sachs lesion

TREATMENT

- **Acute:** Reduction of dislocation under sedation/general anesthesia *(Depalma method)* as early as possible, followed by immobilization in a neutral or slight external rotation brace for three weeks and rehabilitation.
- **Chronic persistent posteriorly dislocated shoulder** is generally treated by open reduction and **modified McLaughlin procedure**. In the modified *McLaughlin procedure*, the subscapularis tendon and lesser tuberosity are transferred medially into reverse Hill-Sachs defect and fixed with suture anchors or screws.

In cases where the head is more than 50% damaged, either humeral head is reconstructed with allograft or hemireplacement of shoulder is performed.

COMPLICATIONS OF POSTERIOR DISLOCATION SHOULDER

- Shoulder stiffness
- Nerve injury: Axillary nerve, suprascapular nerve
- Recurrent dislocation and chronic pain
- Osteonecrosis of the head of the humerus
- Post-traumatic arthritis.

Table 5.2 shows the difference between various shoulder dislocations.

Depalma method
The affected arm is first adducted and internally rotated, with caudal traction applied. Then, maintaining traction and internal rotation, the medial aspect of the upper arm is pushed laterally, disengaging the humeral head from the glenoid fossa.

Table 5.2: Differences between various dislocations of the shoulder.

	Anterior	Posterior	Luxatio erecta
Frequency	Most common	Rare and quite commonly missed	Quite rare
Mode of injury	Traumatic and atraumatic	Epilepsy, electric shock, and electroconvulsive therapy	Holding an object while vertical fall
Mechanism of injury	Hyperabduction and external rotation	Flexion, adduction and internal rotation	Hyperabduction with vertical fall
Position of head	Head is anterior to glenoid	Head is posterior to glenoid	Head is inferior to glenoid near chest wall
Attitude at shoulder	Abduction and external rotation	Internal rotation and adduction	Hyperabduction
Pathology	• Bankart lesion • Hill-Sachs lesion	• Posterior labral tear • Reverse Hill-Sachs lesion	• Anteroinferior labral tear • Often rotator cuff tear

ACROMIOCLAVICULAR JOINT DISLOCATION

X-rays of normal and dislocated acromioclavicular joints are shown in **Figures 5.15** and **5.16**, respectively.

SURGICAL ANATOMY OF ACROMIOCLAVICULAR (AC) JOINT

- The AC joint is formed between the acromion and lateral end of the clavicle
- The AC joint is stabilized by two important structures, AC joint capsule and coracoclavicular ligaments **(Fig. 5.17)**.
    1. **Acromioclavicular joint capsule (ACJC):** It is responsible for the horizontal stability of the AC joint.
    2. **Coracoclavicular ligament (CCL):** CCL has two components, *conoid* (medial) **and** *trapezoid* (lateral), which are responsible for the vertical stability of AC joint.
    In AC joint injury **(Fig. 5.18)**, there is a variable degree of damage to the AC joint capsule and CC ligaments. A complete rupture of the ACJ capsule and CCL results in complete ACJ dislocation.

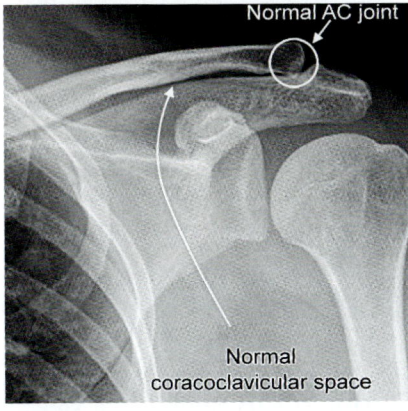

Fig. 5.15: X-ray of normal acromioclavicular (AC) joint.

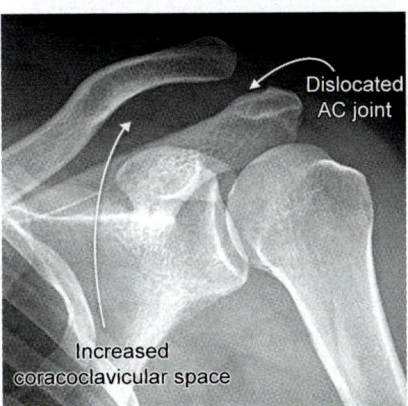

Fig. 5.16: X-ray of dislocated acromioclavicular (AC) joint with increased coracoclavicular space.

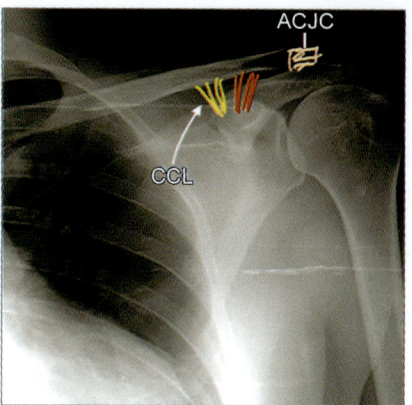
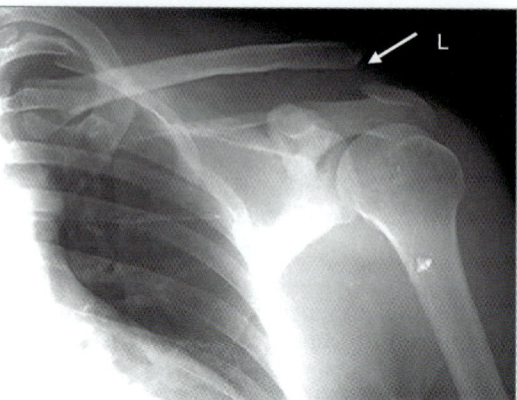

Fig. 5.17: Stable AC joint by ACJC and CC ligaments. (ACJC: acromioclavicular joint capsule; CCL: coracoclavicular ligament)

Fig. 5.18: In ACJ dislocation, the ACJ capsule and CC ligaments are partially or wholly damaged, leading to varying degrees of ACJ dislocation.

MECHANISM OF INJURY

Mostly seen in young adults after
- Road traffic accident
- Fall over the tip of the shoulder.

CLASSIFICATION (ROCKWOOD)

Rockwood classified ACJ dislocation into six types (I–VI). Type III onwards are high-grade dislocations and usually require "surgical" treatment. Further classification details are out of scope for undergraduates.

CLINICAL FEATURES

Symptoms

The patient complaints of pain and swelling over the shoulder and inability/difficulty to elevate the arm.

Signs

- The lateral end of the clavicle is prominent due to dislocation **(Fig. 5.19)**
- Bony tenderness is present over the lateral end of the clavicle
- One must always rule out injury to neurovascular structures, especially brachial plexus injury.

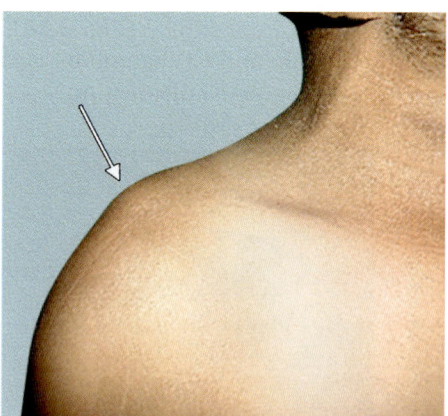

Fig. 5.19: Prominent lateral end clavicle (white arrow).

INVESTIGATION

Plain X-ray of the shoulder: Anteroposterior **(Fig. 5.18)**, axillary, and Zanca view. *(Zanca view is a special AP view performed by tilting the X-ray beam 10–15° cephalad).*

Chapter 5: Dislocation of Major Joints

TREATMENT OF ACUTE ACJ DISLOCATION

Minimally displaced AC joint dislocations (Rockwood Type I, II) are managed conservatively, while grossly dislocated ones (Type III-VI) may require surgical intervention.
1. **Minimally displaced ACJ dislocation (Types I and II):** Arm sling support for 2–3 weeks
2. **Displaced ACJ dislocation (Types III-VI):** Many options are described in literature for management of high grade ACJ dislocation, such as:
    - Figure of four bandage—usually unsuccessful in keeping the joint reduced **(Fig. 5.20)**.
    - Reduction of dislocation and fixation with hook plate **(Fig. 5.21)**, K-wires, suture anchors.
    - Arthroscopic dog button fixation with suture tapes **(Fig. 5.22)**.
    - AC joint reconstruction using auto/allograft.

TREATMENT OF SYMPTOMATIC CHRONIC ACJ DISLOCATION

It is treated by acromioclavicular joint reconstruction using semitendinosus graft.

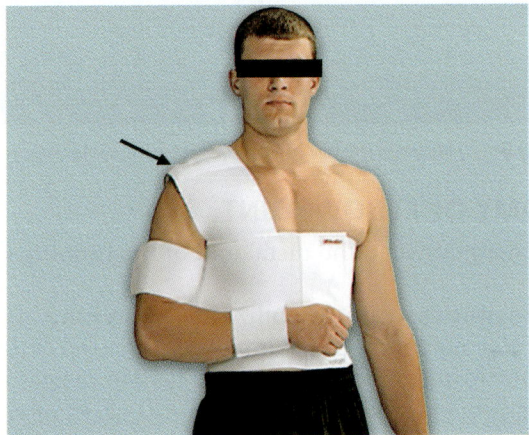

Fig. 5.20: Figure of four bandage in the treatment of acromioclavicular joint dislocation.

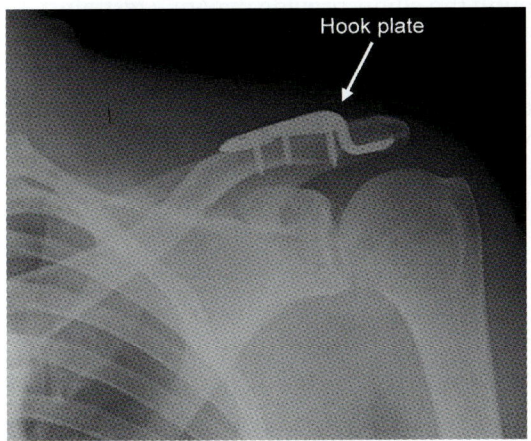

Fig. 5.21: Hook plate stabilization of ACJ dislocation.

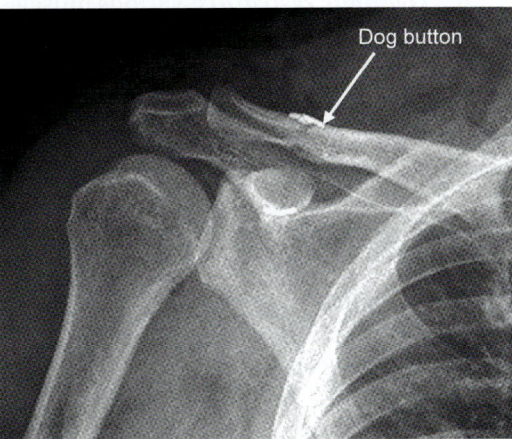

Fig. 5.22: Dog button stabilization of ACJ dislocation with suture tapes.

ELBOW DISLOCATIONS

Elbow dislocation is the most common joint dislocation in children (cf, shoulder dislocation, which is the most common in adults). **Figures 5.23A and B** shows a plain lateral radiograph of a normal elbow and posteriorly dislocated elbow, respectively.

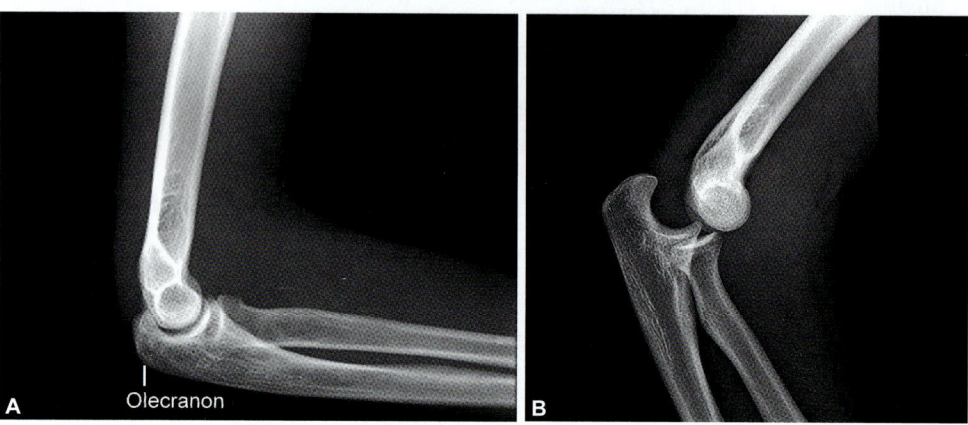

Figs. 5.23A and B: (A) Normal elbow joint; (B) Posterior dislocation of elbow joint.

SURGICAL ANATOMY OF ELBOW JOINT
- The elbow joint is formed between the distal end of the humerus, upper end of the ulna, and the radial head.
- Various **static and dynamic restraints** stabilize the elbow joint.
  A. *Static restraints:* Normal geometry of bony articular surfaces (distal humerus, ulna, and radial head), joint capsule, medial and lateral collateral ligament, and negative intra-articular pressure provide static restraint. In most cases of elbow dislocation, *lateral ulnar collateral ligament (LUCL) is torn.* Note that *coronoid process* and *ulnohumeral bony articulation* are most important bony supports for the elbow stability.
  B. *Dynamic restraints:* Various muscles around the elbow provide dynamic restraint.

RELEVANT PATHOANATOMY
During a traumatic elbow dislocation, the collateral ligaments and capsule are torn. In most cases, the lateral collateral ligament (LCL), especially, LUCL, is injured, followed by the medial ligament complex. In several cases, the coronoid process is fractured rendering elbow quite unstable. Further, there is a risk of injury to the brachial artery and median or ulnar nerve as they get entrapped between the two articulating surfaces.

MECHANISM OF INJURY
- Fall on the outstretched hand
- Road traffic accidents.

TYPES OF ELBOW DISLOCATIONS
It is classified into five types as per the position of the ulna with respect to the distal humerus **(Fig. 5.24)**.

1. **Posterior dislocation:** It is the *most common (80%) type of elbow dislocation*, wherein the ulna moves posteriorly with respect to the distal humerus **(Fig. 5.24)**. Further, it can be posteromedial or posterolateral.
2. **Anterior dislocation:** It is rare compared to the posterior type, wherein ulna moves anterior to the distal humerus.
3, 4 **Lateral or medial dislocation:** In this type, ulna and radius move laterally or medially.
5. **Divergent dislocation:** In this rare type, ulna and radius diverge medially and laterally, respectively.

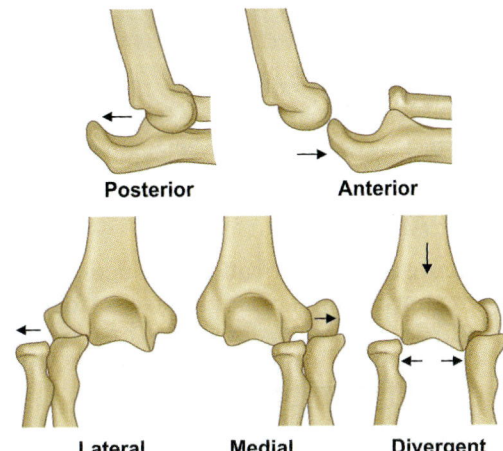

Fig. 5.24: Types of elbow dislocation.

CLINICAL FEATURES

Symptoms
- History of trauma
- Pain, swelling, and deformity of the elbow
- Inability to move the elbow joint.

Signs
- Prominent olecranon at the back of the elbow **(Fig. 5.25)**
- Supraolecranon hollowing **(Fig. 5.25)**
- *Three bony point* (medial epicondyle, lateral epicondyle and tip of olecranon) *relationship is disturbed*
- The neurovascular assessment is essential as there is a risk of injury to the *brachial artery, median and ulnar nerve*.
- Always *rule out compartment syndrome*.

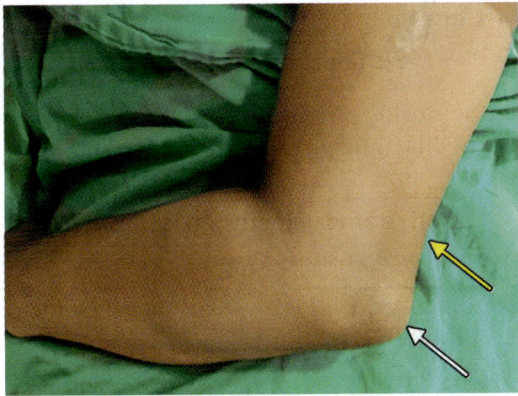

Fig. 5.25: Posterior dislocation elbow showing prominent olecranon tip (white arrow) and supra-olecranon hollowing (yellow arrow).

INVESTIGATIONS
- **Plain X-ray of the elbow:** AP and lateral view **(Fig. 5.26)**. Classic features are:
  - Empty olecranon fossa.
  - A line drawn through the long axis of the radius shaft does not pass through the center of the capitellum.
- **CT scan:** If there is an associated fracture
- **MRI of the elbow:** It is performed after the reduction of the elbow to assess injuries to collateral ligaments.

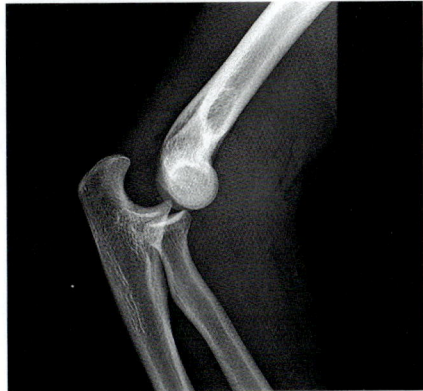

Fig. 5.26: Lateral view of the elbow showing posterior dislocation of the elbow joint.

Terrible triad of elbow dislocation: Fracture of coronoid tip, fracture of radial head and LCL injury. *Note that the terrible triad of elbow always require operative intervention.*

TREATMENT

- **Acute elbow dislocation:** Reduction of dislocation as early as possible and immobilization in above elbow slab for 2–3 weeks followed by mobilization and rehabilitation.
- **Chronic elbow dislocation:** Open reduction of dislocation and ligament reconstruction

COMPLICATIONS

- **Acute**
    - Injury to brachial artery, median and ulnar nerve
    - Compartment syndrome.
- **Chronic**
    - ***Stiffness:*** It can occur due to soft tissue contracture. ***Myositis ossificans*** is a major cause of stiffness, especially if there have been a history of massage or forcible mobilization during phase of rehabilitation.
    - Instability (due to torn ligament)
    - Elbow osteoarthritis.

COMMON DISLOCATIONS AROUND THE WRIST

Common dislocations around the wrist are:
A. **Lunate dislocation:**
   - Lunate dislocates out of the rest of the carpus. It is common after high-velocity injury.
   - **Clinical features:** Patient presents with pain and swelling of the wrist an inability to move the wrist joint. There is tenderness present over the lunate fossa. *Injury to the median nerve is common in lunate dislocation.*
   - **Investigations:** Wrist PA and lateral views X-ray shows two important signs:
     - *Piece of pie sign:* In the PA view of the wrist, the lunate appears triangular in shape, simulating a slice of pie **(Fig. 5.27A)**.
     - *Spilled teapot sign:* In a lateral wrist X-ray, the lunate is rotated and no more articulates with the rest of the carpus **(Fig. 5.27B)**.
   - **Management:** Closed/open reduction of dislocation. It may also require stabilization with K wires and ligament repair.
   - **Complication:**
     - Median nerve compression
     - Avascular necrosis of lunate.
B. **Perilunate dislocation:** Lunate stays in its place, whereas other carpal bones dislocate.
C. **Trans-scaphoid perilunate dislocation:** Perilunate dislocation in association with a scaphoid fracture.
D. **Distal radio-ulnar joint dislocation:** It is commonly seen in association with Galeazzi fracture-dislocation.

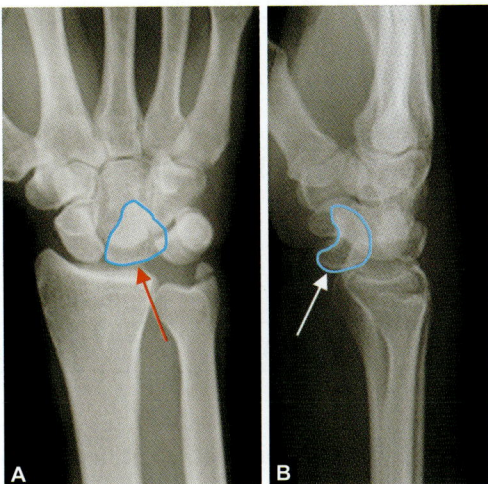

Figs. 5.27A and B: Lunate dislocation: (A) PA view of the wrist showing piece of pie sign (red arrow); (B) Lateral view of the wrist showing spilled teapot sign (white arrow).

HIP DISLOCATION

SURGICAL ANATOMY OF THE HIP JOINT

- The hip joint is formed between the **femoral head** and the **acetabular socket**. The deep acetabular socket is lined by the acetabular labrum and inferiorly lined by a transverse ligament.
- **Strong muscles all around the hip joint**
  - *Hip flexor*: Iliopsoas
  - *Hip extensor*: Gluteus maximus
  - *Hip external rotators*: Obturator internus, gemelli (superior, inferior) and piriformis
  - *Hip internal rotators*: Tensor fascia lata and anterior fibers of the gluteus medius
  - *Hip abductors*: Gluteus medius and gluteus minimus
  - *Hip adductors*: Adductors (longus and magnus).
- **Capsule and ligaments:** A strong capsule envelopes the hip joint. There are three important ligaments:
  1. *Anterior:* Bigelow's ligament/iliofemoral (strongest ligament of the body)
  2. *Medial:* Pubofemoral
  3. *Posterior:* Ischiofemoral.

  The deep acetabular socket, strong capsule, multiple muscles, and various ligaments render the hip joint quite stable.

  Hence, the degree of trauma must be severe to dislocate a hip joint; therefore, hip dislocations occur in high-velocity injuries such as road traffic accidents.
- **Important structures anterior and posterior to the hip joint**
  - *Anteriorly:* The femoral nerve and artery are anterior to the hip joint and hence, prone to injury in anterior dislocation of the hip joint.
  - *Posteriorly:* The sciatic nerve, superior and inferior gluteal vessels are posterior to the hip joint and hence, prone to injury in posterior dislocation of the hip joint.

- **Vascularity of the femoral head:** Femoral head vascular supply is via medial and lateral circumflex femoral vessels and partly by foveal vessels. These vessels are prone to injury during hip dislocation. *(Read Chapter 18 on fracture neck femur for vascular supply to head femur).*

Type of Hip Dislocation: Anatomic Classification
- Posterior: Most common, 90%
- Anterior
- Central.

POSTERIOR DISLOCATION OF THE HIP JOINT

DEFINITION
In posterior dislocation of the hip, the femoral head is dislocated posterior to the acetabulum **(Figs. 5.28A)**.

MECHANISM OF INJURY
Hip dislocations typically result from high-velocity injuries such as road traffic accidents. A classic example of RTA causing posterior dislocation is *dashboard injury* during a vehicular head-on collision **(Fig. 5.28B)**. A brief mechanism of dashboard injury is mentioned in **Flowchart 5.1**.

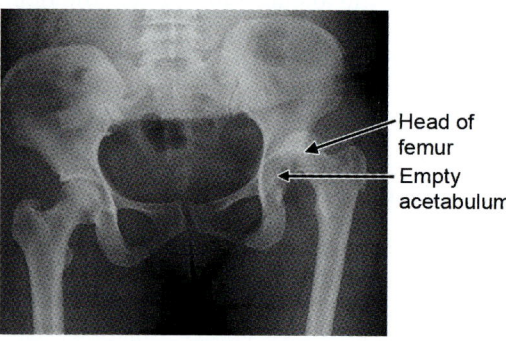

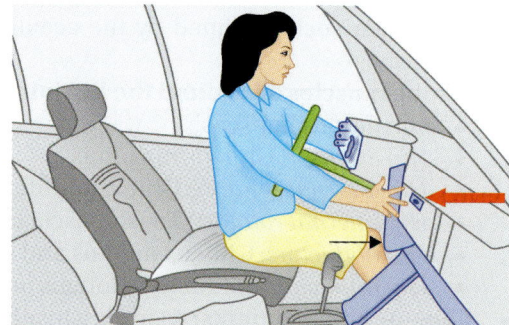

Fig. 5.28A: X-ray of the pelvis with both hips showing normal right hip joint and dislocated left hip joint.

Fig. 5.28B: Dashboard injury. Red arrow depicts the force of oncoming vehicle during head-on collision, while black arrow depicts knee or leg hitting the dashboard.

Flowchart 5.1: Steps for the mechanism of dashboard injury.

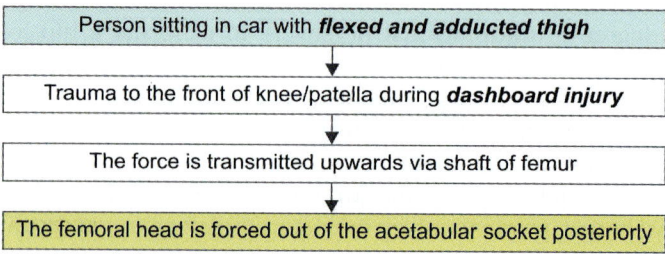

Chapter 5: Dislocation of Major Joints

While femoral head is forced out of the acetabulum posteriorly, two mechanical complications may happen:
1. While head femur is being forced out of the acetabulum, it may hit against the posterior wall of acetabulum, resulting in acetabular wall fracture. Posteriorly directed dashboard injury to the knee could also result in patella fracture or knee ligament injuries, especially posterior cruciate and lateral collateral, while upward transmitted force via shaft could result in femoral shaft or femoral neck fracture.
2. A posteriorly dislocated head femur may compress the sciatic nerve (which is just posterior to the acetabulum) leading to foot drop.

CLINICAL FEATURES

Hip dislocations always occur in a **high-velocity injuries**, such as road traffic accidents.

Symptoms

Pain and swelling around the hip and inability to bear weight.

Signs

- The typical attitude of the lower limb is (**Fig. 5.29**)
    - *Flexed* at the hip
    - *Adducted* at the hip
    - *Internally rotated* at the hip

  Note: If the limb is in external rotation, always suspect associated fracture shaft of the femur/fracture neck femur.
- The femoral head is palpable in the gluteal region.
- *Vascular sign of Narath is positive*: The femoral artery pulse is not palpable in the inguinal region to the absence of the femoral head from the acetabulum.
- *Shortening of the lower limb*
- Observe for the features of sciatic nerve injury that results in foot drop.
- After the reduction of the hip, examine the knee for knee ligament injuries or fractures that could occur due to direct impact.

INVESTIGATIONS

- **Plain X-ray of the pelvis with both hips:** AP and lateral view (**Fig. 5.30**)
  Radiological findings are:
    - Femoral head out of the acetabular socket
    - The lesser trochanter is less prominent

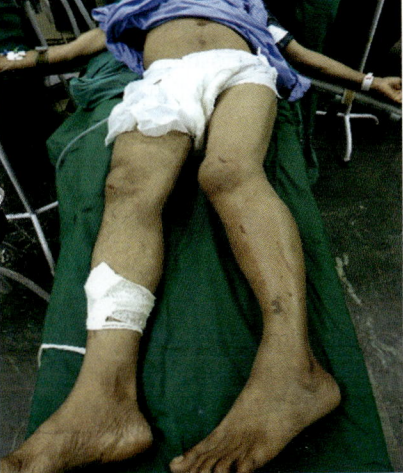

Fig. 5.29: Attitude of the left lower limb in posterior dislocation hip-flexed, adducted and internally rotated at the hip joint.

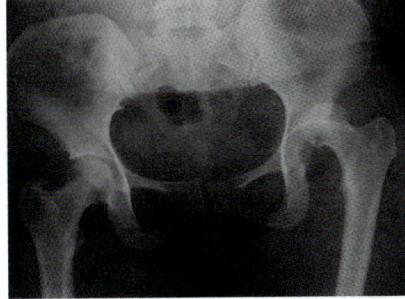

Fig. 5.30: AP view of the pelvis showing left posterior hip dislocation showing empty acetabulum, broken Shenton line, superiorly migrated femoral head, and adducted shaft femur.

- Shenton's line is broken
- Femoral shaft is adducted
- **CT scan:** It is *almost always performed after the reduction of dislocation* in cases where:
  - If there is a fracture of the acetabulum or femoral head
  - Loose body (fracture fragments) in the hip joint, resulting in a widened joint space.

TREATMENT

Since hip dislocations results from high-velocity injury, there can be associated injury to the head, chest, abdomen, pelvis, and other fractures. Appropriate assessment and treatment of other conditions are necessary per ATLS protocol. Regarding hip dislocation:

- **Closed reduction of the dislocation** must be performed preferably under general anesthesia **and at the earliest**. There are various methods of reducing dislocation, which is mentioned in **Box 5.2**.
  - After closed reduction, the lower limb should be immobilized in Thomas knee splint with below-knee skin traction or upper tibial skeletal traction for three weeks.
  - Later, partial followed by full weight-bearing, is allowed.
- **If closed reduction fails, open reduction of dislocation** must be performed. Closed reduction may fail due to soft tissue interposition or button-holing of femoral head through the capsule.

Box 5.2: Methods of closed reduction.
- Bigelow
- Allis
- Stimson

COMPLICATIONS

Acute

- *Injury to the sciatic nerve and superior gluteal vessels.* The sciatic nerve injury results in foot drop, while superior gluteal vessel rupture may result in bleeding.
- *Associated fractures* of the acetabulum, femoral head/neck, femoral shaft, and patella.
- *Knee ligament injury*: Due to direct posterior force over the knee, there is a high risk of injury to the posterior cruciate ligament and posterolateral corner of the knee (lateral collateral ligament, popliteus tendon, popliteofibular ligament, posterolateral capsule).

Chronic

1. *Avascular necrosis (AVN) of femur head:* It occurs due to disrupted vascularity of the femoral head.
2. *Secondary osteoarthritis* of the hip following AVN or femoral head fracture or cartilage injury.
3. *Heterotrophic ossificans*
4. *Recurrent dislocation:* It is rare as the acetabular socket is quite deep.

1. **Sciatic nerve injury** results in foot drop
   - Usually neuropraxia/axonotmesis type of nerve injury
   - Often, only the common peroneal component is affected
   - Mostly managed conservatively. Gradually recovers over 3–18 months

2. **Associated fracture of acetabulum** could result in
   – Unstable reduction of hip due to lack of support from posterior wall of the acetabulum. This may require ORIF of posterior wall for stable reduction, and restoration of hip joint congruity
   – The fragments from the acetabulum or femoral head fracture can migrate into the joint and lead to nonconcentric reduction of hip. This may require removal of loose body (open/arthroscopic).
3. **Avascular necrosis** of head femur
   Later, it results in 2° osteoarthritis of hip joint.
4. **Myositis ossificans**
   Often seen after open reduction of hip/fracture fixation of acetabulum.

ANTERIOR DISLOCATION OF HIP JOINT

Anterior hip dislocation is uncommon as compared to posterior dislocation. It ***results after high-velocity injury***.

TYPES OF ANTERIOR DISLOCATION

There are two types: **Obturator** (inferior) and **pubic** (superior).

CLINICAL FEATURES

Symptoms

Pain and swelling of the index hip and inability to bear weight.

Signs

Tenderness is present over the hip joint.

Attitude of the limb (Fig. 5.31): It varies according to the type of dislocation.
- *Obturator type:* Flexed, abducted, and externally rotated hip
- *Pubic type:* Extended, abducted, and externally rotated hip

Limb length discrepancy:
- *Pubic type:* Limb lengthening
- *Obturator type:* Limb shortening

Neurovascular examination: Assessment of femoral nerve and femoral artery is essential in anterior dislocation of the hip joint.

INVESTIGATIONS

X-ray of pelvis with both hips AP **(Fig. 5.32)** and affected hip lateral view. CT scan, if associated fracture of acetabulum/femoral head.

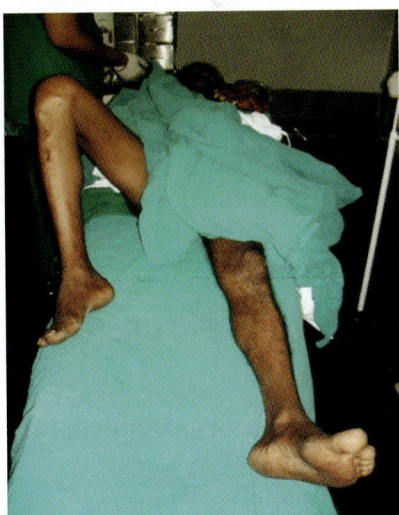

Fig. 5.31: Attitude of lower limb in the anterior dislocation of the right hip—flexed, abducted and externally rotated.

■ TREATMENT

Closed reduction should be performed at the earliest *(Reverse Bigelow method)* followed by immobilization in Thomas splint/above knee traction for 3 weeks. Then, the patient is mobilized, and rehabilitation is initiated.

■ COMPLICATIONS

Acute

- *Injury to the femoral nerve and vessels*
- Associated acetabular fracture, femoral shaft fracture, patella fracture
- Knee ligament injury.

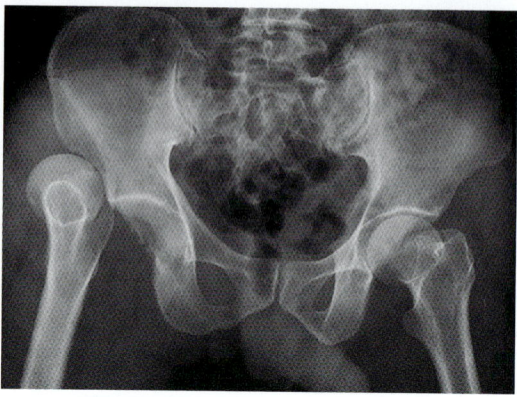

Fig. 5.32: X-ray of pelvis with both hips showing anterior dislocation of the right hip joint.

Chronic

- Avascular necrosis: It can lead to secondary osteoarthritis of the hip
- Heterotrophic ossificans
- Recurrent dislocation: Very rare.

CENTRAL FRACTURE DISLOCATION OF THE HIP

A central fracture dislocation of the hip is one wherein the femoral head is pushed medially due to fracture of floor of the acetabulum.

■ MECHANISM OF INJURY

The central fracture-dislocations occur after **high-velocity injury** (RTA, fall from a height on the side of the hip). Fall over the lateral aspect of the thigh results in centripetal force over the greater trochanter, which forces the femoral head into the floor of the acetabulum and fractures the acetabular floor causing central fracture-dislocation **(Fig. 5.33)**.

■ CLINICAL FEATURES

Symptoms

Pain and swelling around the hip and inability to bear weight.

Signs

- Tenderness over the hip joint is present
- Active leg raising is not possible

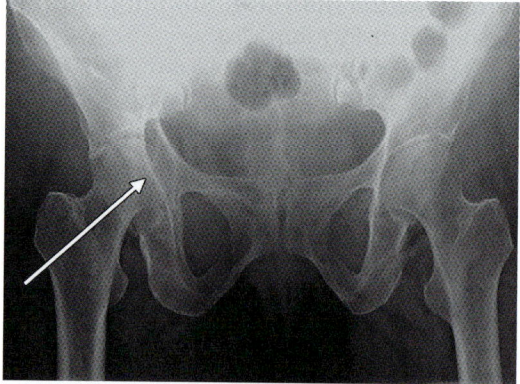

Fig. 5.33: X-ray of the pelvis shows central fracture-dislocation (white arrow), wherein the floor of acetabulum is broken and femoral head has migrated medially.

- Restricted and painful movements
- Shortening of the lower limb

INVESTIGATION
- **X-ray of pelvis:** Anteroposterior view **(Fig. 5.33)**, iliac and obturator views
- **CT scan of the hip with 3D reconstruction.**

TREATMENT
- Closed reduction followed by lateral traction over the hip for a few weeks.
- Open reduction and internal fixation by plates and screws restore the acetabulum's articular congruity.

COMPLICATIONS
- Secondary osteoarthritis of the hip joint: Due to incongruous acetabulum/AVN hip/both
- Avascular necrosis: Due to disrupted femoral head vascularity
- Heterotrophic ossification

DISLOCATION AROUND THE KNEE

KNEE DISLOCATION

DEFINITION
A dislocated knee implies that the femoral condyles and tibial plateau are no more in contact with each other **(Fig. 5.34)**. **Figure 5.35** show knee fracture dislocation wherein the tibial plateau is dislocated posteriorly and tibial plateau is also fractured.

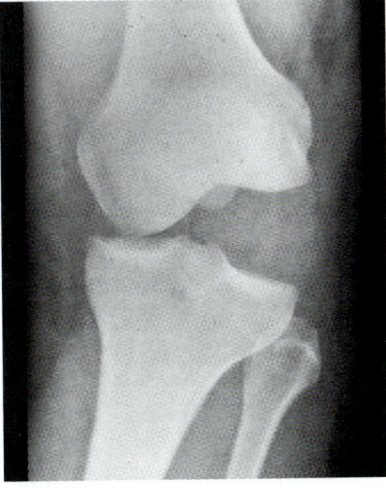

Fig. 5.34: X-ray of knee (AP view) showing dislocated knee.

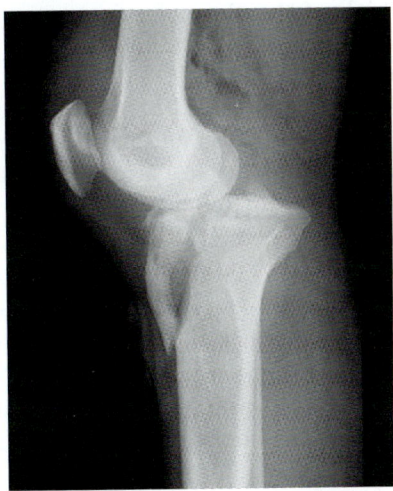

Fig. 5.35: Lateral X-ray showing posterior fracture-dislocation of the knee.

SURGICAL ANATOMY AND PATHOANATOMY

- The knee remains stable and mobile due to *normal bony morphology of articulating bones, various intact functional ligaments (cruciates and collaterals), joint capsules, and muscles* around the knee.
- In knee dislocation, there is a **significant injury to the stabilizing structures of the knee**. Usually, two or more ligaments are injured.
- Further, a dislocated knee can **injure popliteal vessels and nerves** (tibial/common peroneal/both). The popliteal vessel is injured due to compression, laceration, or transection. Sometimes, there can be acute post-traumatic thrombus formation inside the vessel after compression or minor laceration leading to vascular insufficiency of the limb. The nerve injury is predominantly axonotmesis or neuropraxia. Rarely, it could be neurotmesis.

MECHANISM OF INJURY

Typically, knee dislocations result from **high-velocity injuries**, such as road traffic accidents or fall from height. Rarely, subluxation of the knee can also occur in an obese person with minor trauma.

CLINICAL FEATURES

Symptoms

Pain, swelling, and deformity of the knee and inability to bear weight.

Signs

- A deformity may be present around the knee.
- Soft tissue and/or bony tenderness is present over the knee depending upon which structure (ligament, capsule, bone) is damaged.
- **A meticulous neurovascular examination** is necessary as there is a high risk of associated neurovascular injury to the tibial nerve, common peroneal nerve, and popliteal vessels. Always palpate the vessels (dorsalis pedis, posterior tibial) at the time of primary examination and then serially to rule out any delayed thrombosis in the popliteal vessel.
- **Compartment syndrome** should be ruled out.
- Knee examination under sedation or anesthesia would reveal instability in various planes due to damage to ligaments and joint capsule.

INVESTIGATIONS

- **X-ray:** AP and lateral view of the knee **(Fig. 5.34)**. It confirms dislocation and also helps in ruling out associated fractures.
- **Computed tomography (CT) scan:** It is required if there is an associated fracture of articulating bones.
- **Angiography:** It is required to rule out vascular injury, especially if distal pulses are not palpable/feeble. It can be combined with a CT scan **(Fig. 5.36)**.

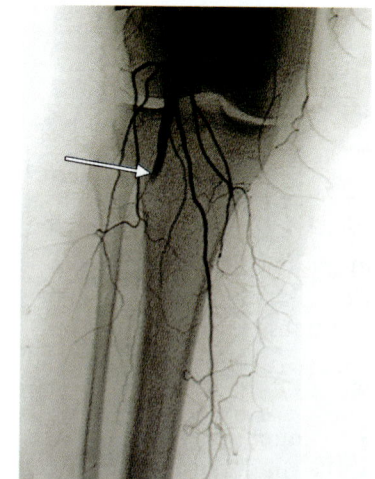

Fig. 5.36: Angiography of the leg showing a cutoff in the popliteal artery (white arrow).

- **Magnetic resonance imaging (MRI):** It is performed to confirm the extent of injury to various ligaments, capsule, menisci, and bone contusions.
- **Nerve conduction velocity (NCV):** It is performed if there is a nerve injury. *Note that NCV is performed after three weeks of injury.*

TREATMENT

Acute Treatment

- *Immediate or urgent reduction of dislocation is a priority.* Once the knee is reduced, it must be stabilized in a long leg knee brace or external fixator for three weeks to allow healing of periarticular soft tissues and capsules.
  Following the reduction, *serial pulse examination is mandatory* to rule out delayed popliteal artery thrombosis.
    - *If there is an associated vascular injury:* Exploration and vascular repair and external fixator application.
    - *If associated nerve injury:* Most nerve injuries in a knee dislocation are neuropraxia or axonotmesis type of injury, requiring a conservative approach and allowing the nerve to recover spontaneously. In case there is no/poor recovery, exploration and repair of the nerve can be taken up after a few months. Sometimes, tendon transfers are required.

Later (After Few Days to Few Weeks)

- Ligament repair/reconstruction
- Rehabilitation: Knee mobilization, muscle strengthening exercises, proprioceptive exercises.

COMPLICATIONS

- Compartment syndrome
- Acute neurovascular injury: Injury to periarticular nerves (Tibial, common peroneal) and popliteal artery.
- Chronic instability of the knee due to ligamentous insufficiency.
- Knee stiffness
- 2° osteoarthritis.

PATELLA DISLOCATION

Primary patella dislocation is not uncommon. It is one of the frequent causes of knee instability in young individuals, especially women. *Most commonly, the patella dislocates laterally.* Occasionally, it may dislocate medially.

In this section, we will discuss lateral patella dislocation.

ETIOLOGY

- Traumatic
- During sports or other episodes of twisting injury to the knee
- Others: Congenital, habitual
  Note: Details of congenital and habitual dislocation of the patella is out of scope for undergraduates.

SURGICAL ANATOMY AND RELEVANT PATHOANATOMY

The primary anatomic stabilizers of the patella in the trochlear groove are
A. **Bony factors**
   - Trochlear and patella morphology
   - Q angle
   - Femoral torsion and anteversion
B. **Soft tissue factors**
   - *Medial patellofemoral ligament (MPFL):* It is the *most important soft tissue stabilizer of the patella* in the trochlear groove. MPFL is a thin ligament that is medially attached to the medial border of the patella and laterally between the medial epicondyle and adductor tubercle.
   - The balance between vastus medialis and lateralis.

Pathology

Disruption of MPFL is the most common pathology in traumatic lateral patella dislocation. Furthermore, during an acute dislocation (medial/lateral), the patellar rubbing against the femoral condyle could result in an osteochondral (OC) fracture of either patella or femoral condyle.

Other significant pathological process contributing to patella dislocation are trochlear dysplasia, increased Q angle, patella alta (high-riding patella), or increased femoral anteversion.

CLINICAL FEATURES

The clinical presentation could be acute or recurrent patella dislocation; the latter presentation is more common.
- **Acute patella dislocation:** The patient presents with an acutely dislocated patella, wherein the patella is displaced laterally **(Fig. 5.37)**. There is pain and swelling over the knee, and the patient cannot bear weight. There is tenderness over the patella and femoral condyles. Knee movements are painful and restricted.
- **Recurrent patella dislocation:** These patients report a recurrent feeling of giving away in their knee.
   - *Patellar apprehension sign is positive.* The patella is gently pushed laterally by the clinician, and the patient's face is watched for any apprehension.
   - *Assess features of ligament laxity* indicated by increased Beighton score.
   - Increased "Q" angle may be present
   - Others could be increased femoral anteversion, external tibial torsion.

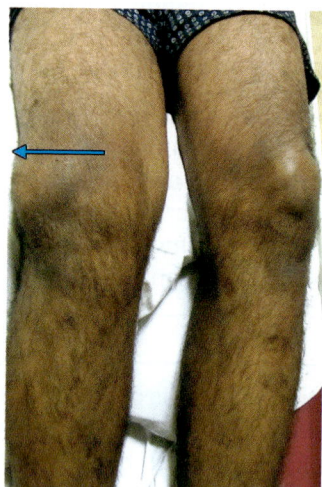

Fig. 5.37: Right knee lateral patella dislocation (blue arrow).

INVESTIGATIONS

- **X-ray of the knee; AP, lateral and skyline view:** Look for patella Alta (Insall-Salvati ratio >1.2), patella tilt, dislocation/subluxation, and features of trochlear dysplasia (crossing sign).

- **MRI of the knee:** It is useful to detect *MPFL tear, loose body* (broken osteochondral fragment from patella or femoral condyle during patella dislocation), and *trochlear dysplasia*.
  Note: Dejour has classified into four types—type A to D. A and B are low grade dysplasia, whereas C and D are high grade dysplasias. Further details are not required for undergraduates.

TREATMENT

1. **Primary patella dislocation**
   - Reduce the dislocation. Following the reduction, the knee is immobilized in a knee brace for three weeks. After three weeks, the knee is rehabilitated by mobilization, muscle strengthening, and proprioceptive exercises.
   - A large loose body from the patella may require arthroscopic removal/fixation.
   - Primary MPFL repair is can be performed in high demand athletes.
2. **Recurrent patella dislocation**
   The procedure(s) will depend on existing abnormalities, soft tissue, and bony. Almost all cases have a defunct MPFL. Therefore, MPFL reconstruction is almost always performed. Other bony procedures are performed case to case basis.
   i. ***Soft tissue reconstruction:*** MPFL reconstruction
   ii. **Correction of bony factors**
      a. *High-grade trochlear dysplasia*: Trochleoplasty
      b. *High Q angle:* Medialization of the tibial tuberosity
      c. *Patella alta*: Distalization of the patella
      d. *Excess femoral anteversion*: Corrective osteotomy of the femur.

Orthopaedic Emergencies
- Acute dislocations
- Compartment syndrome
- Septic arthritis
- Open fractures presenting within eight hours
- Neurovascular injuries with/without amputation
- Traumatic amputation of the limb/digits (clean cuts) for re-implantation in patients who present within 8 hours of injury
- Fracture neck femur in young adult who present with 8–12 hours where fixation of fracture is possible

Notes

SECTION 2

Fractures and Ligament Injuries

SECTION OUTLINE

6. Basics of Orthopaedics
7. Introduction to Fractures
8. Fractures in Children and Physeal Injuries
9. Fracture Clavicle
10. Fracture around the Shoulder
    - Fracture of Proximal Humerus, Greater Tuberosity and Scapula
11. Relief of Joint Pain
12. Fracture Shaft Humerus, Supracondylar Humerus and Other Fractures around Elbow
13. Fracture of Forearm Bone, Galeazzi and Monteggia Fracture
14. Fractures around the Wrist and Hand
    - Distal Radius (Colles, Smith, Barton, Chauffer), Carpal Bones (Scaphoid), Metacarpals and Phalangeal Fractures
15. Fracture Pelvis
16. Injuries of the Spine and Spinal Cord
17. Fracture Acetabulum
18. Fracture Femur Neck and Intertrochanteric Femur
19. Fracture around Knee—Patella, Distal Femur and Proximal Tibia
20. Fracture Shaft Femur and Subtrochanteric Femur
21. Fractures of Both Bone Leg, Tibial Plafond, Calcaneum and Small Bones of Foot
22. Fracture of the Ankle
23. Complications of Fracture
24. Open Fracture
25. Ligament Injury of Knee, Ankle and Other Sports Injuries

CHAPTER 6

Basics of Orthopaedics

■ COMMON TERMINOLOGIES IN ORTHOPAEDICS

Fracture (#): It is defined as a discontinuity in the anatomical integrity of the bone **(Fig. 6.1)**.

Dislocation: When two articular surfaces of the *joint* are *no more in contact* with each other **(Fig. 6.2)**.

Subluxation: When two articular surfaces of the joint are *partially in contact* with each other.

> It is essential to note that the *fracture occurs in a bone*, whereas *dislocations occur at the joint*.
> For example, radius/ulna/femur/vertebra fracture, while hip joint/knee joint/shoulder joint dislocate!
> Hence, avoid saying "knee joint is fractured or femur is dislocated."

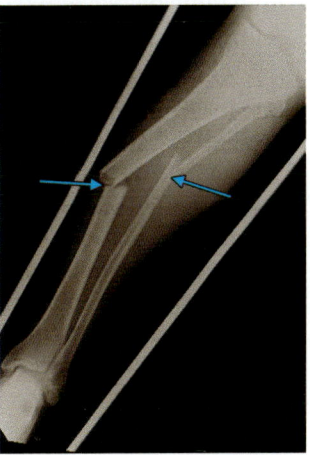

Fig. 6.1: Fracture of tibia and fibula (blue arrows).

Fracture–dislocation: However, a term fracture-dislocation is often spelled together. It implies that the joint is dislocated/subluxated and there is a fracture in one/both articulating bones **(Fig. 6.3)**. Some authors also term fracture-dislocation as *'complex dislocation'*.

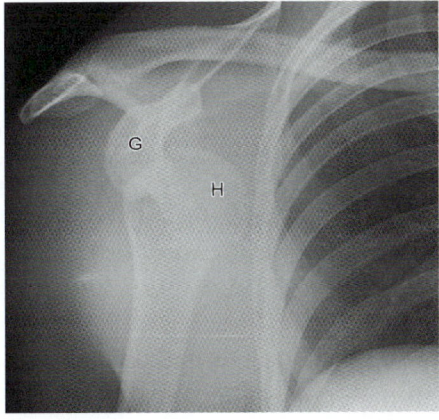

Fig. 6.2: Anterior dislocation of the right shoulder. Note that the humeral head (H) is no more contact with the glenoid (G).

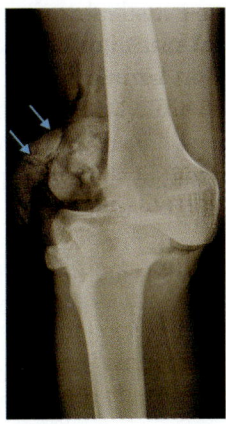

Fig. 6.3: Fracture dislocation of the right knee. Knee dislocated whereas lateral femoral condyle is fractured (blue arrows).

For example, during the posterior dislocation of the hip, the head of the femur or acetabulum is often fractured. The term used to explain such a condition is *posterior fracture-dislocation of the hip joint.*

Displacement: It is a term used to define the *location of the distal fragment* of *fracture or distal articular surface* with respect to the proximal fragment in a three-dimensional orientation.

Sprain: Sprain implies injury to the ligament.

Strain: Strain implies injury to the muscle.

■ MACROANATOMY AND FUNCTION OF THE BONE

A long bone has several parts **(Fig. 6.4)**

1. **Epiphysis:** It is present at the end of a long bone, which is filled with cancellous bone while outer layer is a compact bone. The surface is covered with cartilage. In kids, it is the growing end of the bone.
2. **Physis/growth plate:** It is open in growing kids while appears as a thin line between epi- and metaphysis
3. **Metaphysis:** The part of bone, which is in between epiphysis and diaphysis, and flares above the diaphysis.
4. **Diaphysis:** It is the shaft of the bone, which consists of cortical bone. It provides structural strength to the bone.
5. **Apophysis:** An apophysis is a normal developmental outgrowth of a bone which arises from a separate ossification center, and fuses to the bone later in development. However, unlike epiphysis, it does not contribute to the longitudinal growth of the bone. Furthermore, an apophysis usually does not form a direct articulation with another bone at a joint, but often forms an important insertion point for a tendon or ligament. Several examples of apophysis are greater trochanter (attachment of gluteus medius and minimus), tibial tuberosity (attachment of patellar tendon), and calcaneal tuberosity (attachment of tendoachilles).

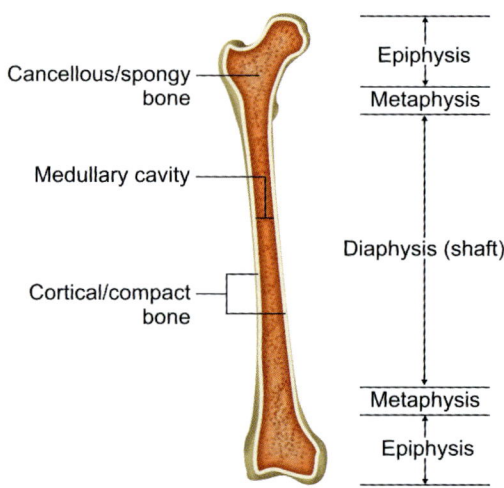

Fig. 6.4: Parts of a long bone.

Practical implication of apophysis

When unfused, apophysis can easily be mistaken for fractures. A prolonged traction injury to apophysis, especially in adolescent kids involved in vigorous sports activity, may result in apophysitis, e.g., Sever's disease (calcaneal tuberosity apophysitis), Osgood-Schlatter disease (tibial tuberosity apophysitis).

- The ends of a long bone are often capped with cartilage (hyaline/fibro) to form a joint.
- The outer aspect of the bone is covered with the periosteum, while the endosteum lines the medullary cavity. The deepest layer of the periosteum (cambium layer) has excellent potential to form new bone.

Structurally, a bone could be cortical or cancellous type.
A. Compact (cortical) bone:
- It is the outer wall of all bones, especially long bones and subchondral bone.
- It consists of compact units known as osteons/haversian system.

B. Cancellous (trabecular) bone:
- It is like a honeycomb meshwork and is more porous than compact bone.
- It is present at the end of long bones, vertebral body, pelvis, ribs, short bones and flat bones.
- The interconnected meshwork of the honeycombed structure adds to the strength of the bone and adds up the surface area.
- The space between the meshwork is filled with marrow.

Function of the bone: Bone provides framework to the body, attachment to various structures (muscle, tendon, and ligaments), leverage to multiple joints, and protection to the viscera. Also, bone is a metabolically active structure, which acts as a reservoir for calcium and provides space and structural support for the hematopoietic cells in the marrow.

■ STRUCTURAL COMPOSITION OF BONE (FLOWCHART 6.1)

A bone is composed of cells and matrix. Typically, there are three major bone cells: Osteoblast, osteoclast, and osteocyte. The matrix of the bone has inorganic and organic components. **Flowchart 6.1** briefly describes the composition of the bone.

■ BONE MATRIX

- The bone matrix is predominantly composed of *type 1 collagen*, which are produced by the osteoblasts. Other substances are also part of the matrix such as proteoglycans (glycosaminoglycan-protein complex), matrix proteins (osteocalcin, osteonectin, and osteopontin), and growth factors. The matrix collagen is ***responsible for the tensile strength of bone***. Proteoglycans are responsible for ***compressive strength***, while matrix protein play role in ***mineralization and bone formation***.
- The matrix also acts as a ***scaffold for hydroxyapatite crystals***. About 50% of bone is minerals wherein calcium and phosphorus together form hydroxyapatite crystals. Minerals impart ***compressive strength to bone***. An unmineralized matrix is known as an "osteoid."

Note: During demineralization of bone (osteoporosis), both matrix and mineral are resorbed.

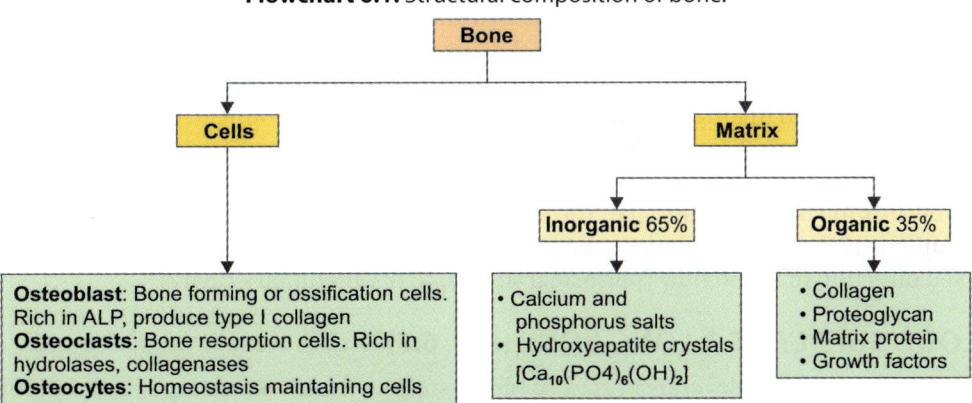

Flowchart 6.1: Structural composition of bone.

Osteoblast: Bone forming or ossification cells. Rich in ALP, produce type I collagen
Osteoclasts: Bone resorption cells. Rich in hydrolases, collagenases
Osteocytes: Homeostasis maintaining cells

- Calcium and phosphorus salts
- Hydroxyapatite crystals $[Ca_{10}(PO4)_6(OH)_2]$

- Collagen
- Proteoglycan
- Matrix protein
- Growth factors

(ALP: alkaline phosphatase)

BONE CELLS

1. **Osteoblast**
    - Osteoblasts are *'bone-forming cells,'* which are 4–6% of total bone cells.
    - **Derivation:** Bone marrow has mesenchymal stem cells, which secrete bone morphogenic protein (BMP). BMP converts osteoprogenitor cells into osteoblasts.
    - **Function:** Osteoblasts stay close to the haversian system and lay down Type 1 collagen and other noncollagenous protein for osteoid formation.
    Along with parathyroid hormone (PTH), osteoblasts play an *essential role in the initiation and control of osteoclast.* Osteoblasts secrete RANK ligand (RANKL), which binds to the RANK receptor on pre-osteoclasts and thus induces their differentiation. Osteoblasts also secrete osteoprotegerin (OPG), which prevents RANK/RANKL interaction by binding to RANKL; this prevents osteoclast differentiation. Thus, the balance between RANKL and OPG sysnthesis by osteoblasts determines osteoclast concentration and activity.
    - Later, osteoblast gets converted into osteocytes.
2. **Osteoclast**
    - Osteoclasts are multinucleated cells, which are *'bone resorptive cells.'*
    - **Derivation:** Osteoclasts develop from mononuclear precursors in marrow under the influence of osteoblast.
    - **Function:** Osteoclasts are bone resorptive cells. Osteoclasts have extended cytoplasmic process into matrix, which cause matrix acidification by releasing H^+ ions resulting in bone resorption.
3. **Osteocyte**
    - Osteocytes are most abundant (90%) and long lived (25 years) cells of the bone responsible for *mineral homeostasis* and *mechanoreception.*
    - **Derivation:** They are derived from osteoblasts differentiation.
    - **Function:** Osteocytes play an essential role in *mineral homeostasis,* especially phosphate. Osteocytes also play a role in *mechanosensation.* Osteocytes connect with each other via their cytoplasmic process and helps assessing the stress and deformation in bone, and therefore, help bone remodeling.

MICROSCOPIC STRUCTURE OF THE BONE

The basic microscopic unit of a lamellar bone is known as the *osteon* **(Fig. 6.5)**. Osteons are a series of concentric lamellae surrounding the Haversian canals (central longitudinal canal). Haversian canals are connected to other Haversians by horizontal Volkmann's canal **(Fig. 6.6)**. The blood vessels run in longitudinal Haversian canals. They are connected with the endosteal and periosteal surface through Volkmann canals providing an extensive network of vessels across the bone **(Fig. 6.6)**. Usually, the blood flows 'centrifugally,' i.e., from the medullary cavity towards the periosteal surface. The cortical surface is also supplied by periosteal vessels. In disrupted medullary circulation, the periosteal vessels take over the circulation with the reversed direction of blood flow (periosteal surface to the medullary cavity).

BLOOD SUPPLY OF A LONG BONE (FIG. 6.7)

A typical long bone has several sources of blood supply—nutrient, metaphyseal, epiphyseal and periosteal vessels.

Chapter 6: Basics of Orthopaedics

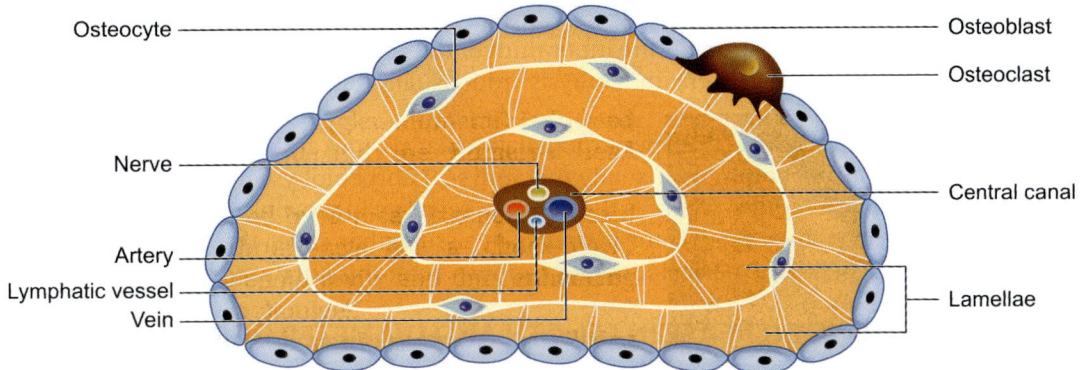

Fig. 6.5: Unit of bone—osteon.

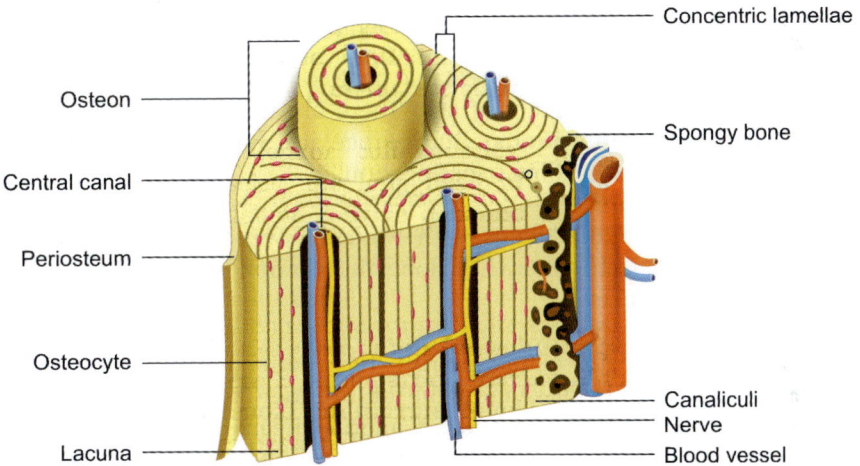

Fig. 6.6: Bone canal system.

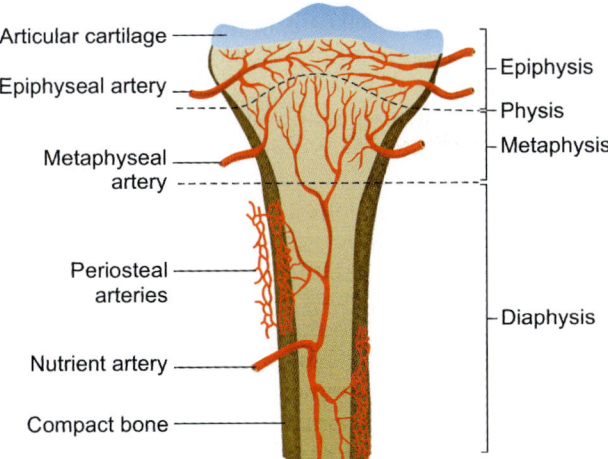

Fig. 6.7: Blood supply of bone.

- **Nutrient artery:** It enters the bone via the nutrient foramen and divides into ascending and descending branches. It supplies the inner third of the cortex.
- **Metaphyseal artery:** It enters metaphysis and usually, anastomoses with epiphyseal vessels.
- **Epiphyseal artery:** Derived from periarticular vascular arcades and enter epiphysis through small opening in the epiphysis. Usually metaphyseal and epiphyseal vessels anastomose near growth plate in adults, whereas they remain separate in growing kids.
- **Periosteal artery:** They arise from various soft tissues that cover the bone. It forms an anastomoses beneath the periosteum and supplies outer third of the cortex.

HOW DOES BONE INCREASE IN LENGTH AND DIAMETER DURING GROWTH?

1. **Length or longitudinal growth** (interstitial growth): By *physeal growth*
2. **Width/thickness** (appositional growth): By *periosteal apposition* of bone.

BONE OSSIFICATION

Bone ossification is a bone formation process that begins around the 6–8th week of embryonic development and ends at 24–25 years of age. There are two types of bone ossification—**endochondral** and **intramembranous**. Both processes start with mesenchymal tissue precursor but further change according to ossification.

A. **Endochondral ossification:**
- Endochondral ossification begins with mesenchymal tissue transforming into cartilage, later replaced by bone. All long/tubular bones, except the clavicle, develop by endochondral ossification.
- In endochondral ossification, *mesenchymal cells transform into chondrocytes*. Chondrocytes secrete extracellular matrix to form perichondrium and a cartilage model for bone, which resembles the shape of the future bone. Chondrocytes in the center of the model secrete collagen X and fibronectin, altering the matrix allowing mineralization.
- The mineralization traps the chondrocyte causing the latter's apoptosis. Apoptosis of chondrocytes create a void that allows blood vessels to invade hollow spaces. The space gradually enlarges, forming a medullary cavity. The blood vessels also carry osteogenic cells that help convert perichondrial cells into periosteum.
- Osteoblasts create a thick compact bone in diaphysis (periosteal collar), which forms *primary ossification center*.
- While bone continues to form in diaphysis, the chondrocytes at the end of bone continue to proliferate giving length to the bone. These end of bone gradually become epiphysis and physis
  After birth, the entire process of diaphyseal ossification repeats in the epiphysis where secondary ossification center forms. The process in epiphysis continues till adulthood.

B. **Intramembranous ossification:**
- Intramembranous ossification directly converts the mesenchymal tissue to bone and forms the flat bones of the skull and clavicle.
- Mesenchymal cells differentiate into osteoblasts and group to form ossification centers. Osteoblast starts forming osteoid (uncalcified collagen-proteoglycan matrix). Gradually, calcium-phosphate starts binding to osteoid resulting in bone formation. The osteoid surrounds blood vessels, which forms spongy/cancellous bone. These vessels will eventually form bone marrow.

Flowchart 6.2: Intramembranous and endochondral ossification (in brief).

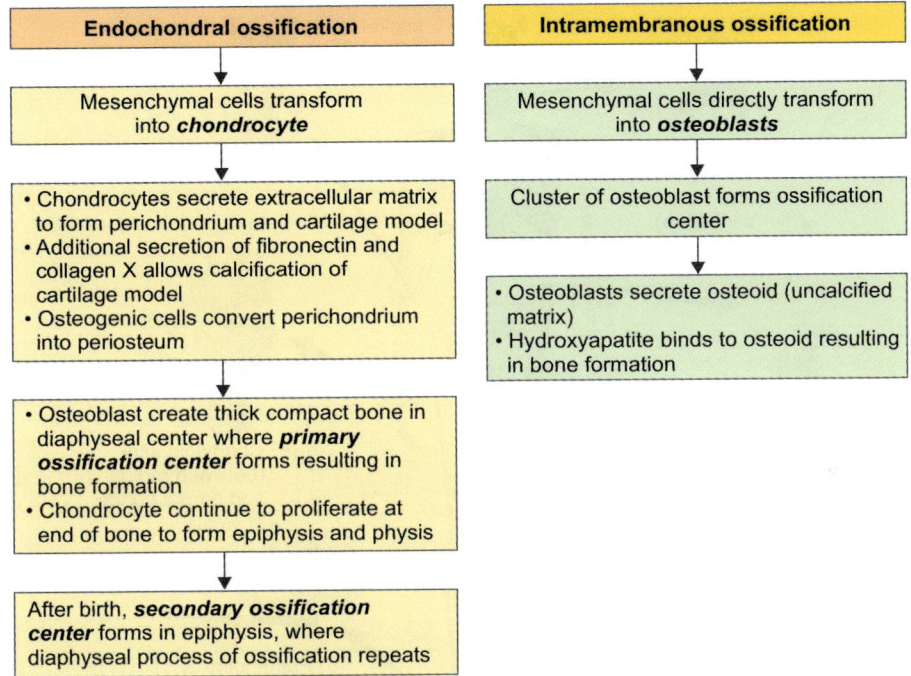

- Apart from the bony ossification of flat bones, ==intramembranous ossification is also responsible for bone width increase==, wherein the new bone is laid by the deepest layer of periosteum forming cortical/compact bone, and old bone is removed from endosteal osteoclasts.

Flowchart 6.2 summarizes the steps of endochondral and intramembranous ossification.

■ TYPES OF JOINTS

The various type of bone joints are mentioned in **Flowchart 6.3** and shown in **Figure 6.8**.

Flowchart 6.3: Types of joints.

Joints

- **Fibrous/synarthrosis** (immobile joints)
  - **Syndesmosis:** Distal tibiofibular joint
  - **Sutures:** Skull sutures
  - **Gomphosis:** Tooth sockets

- **Cartilaginous** (slight movement)
  - **Synchondrosis:** Hyaline cartilage is interposed, e.g., rib-sternum
  - **Symphysis:** Fibrocartilage is interposed, e.g., symphysis pubis

- **Synovial** (movement possible)
  - **Hinge joint:** Elbow, knee, ankle
  - **Pivot joint:** Atlantoaxial, radioulnar
  - **Ball-and-socket joint:** Hip, shoulder
  - **Saddle joint:** 1st carpometacarpal
  - **Gliding joint:** Intercarpal, acromioclavicular, sternoclavicular
  - **Ellipsoid/condyloid joint:** Radiocarpal, metacarpophalangeal

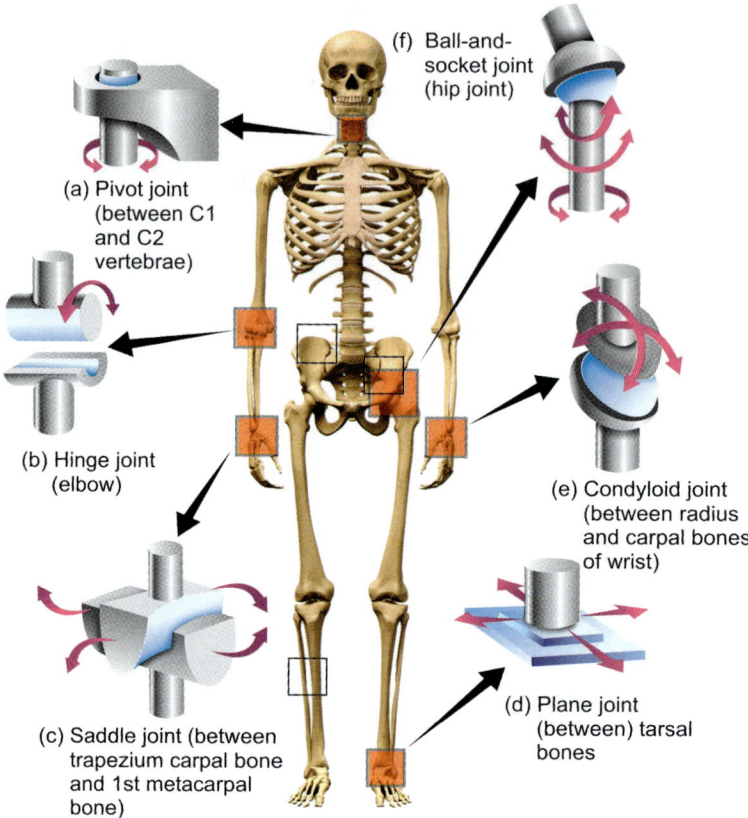

Fig. 6.8: Various joints of the body.

Notes

CHAPTER 7

Introduction to Fractures

DEFINITION

A fracture is defined as a partial or complete break in the anatomical continuity of the bone.

CLASSIFICATION OF FRACTURE

A fracture can be classified in several ways **(Box 7.1)**. These classifications help determine the etiopathology, treatment, and prognosis. Hence, the idea of these classifications is essential.

> **Box 7.1:** Fracture classification.
>
> A. *Clinical type:* Closed/open
> B. *Etiological:* Traumatic/pathological/stress
> C. *Radiological:* Pattern of fracture
> D. *Mechanism of injury:* Direct/indirect
> E. *Extent of fracture:* Complete/incomplete
> F. *According to displacement:* Displaced/undisplaced
> G. *Joint involvement:* Intra-articular/extra-articular

A. Clinical type of fracture: Closed and open

1. ***Closed fracture***: When a fracture and/or its hematoma do not communicate with the external environment via any wound, it is called a closed fracture.
2. ***Open fracture***: When a fracture or its hematoma or both communicate with the external environment via a wound, it is called an open fracture **(Fig. 7.1)**.

B. Etiological: Traumatic, pathological and stress

1. ***Traumatic fracture***: When a frank history of trauma results in a fracture in an otherwise normal bone.
2. ***Pathological fracture***: If the bone is already weakened due to an underlying disease (infection/tumor/osteoporosis), the fracture can occur with minimal or no trauma as the force required to cause the fracture is minimal.
3. ***Stress fracture***: Repeated cyclic microtrauma can cause a fracture in an otherwise normal bone. The following are common sites for stress fracture:
   i. Metatarsal: Second metatarsal neck fracture seen in new army/police recruits after prolonged unaccustomed marches is known as the '*march fracture.*'
   ii. Upper third fibula: *Jumping fracture*
   iii. Lower third fibula: *Runners' fracture*
   iv. Neck femur

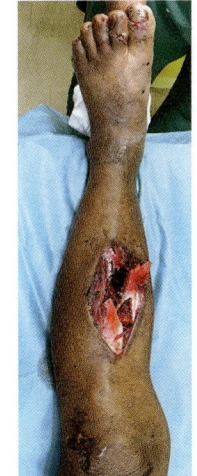

Fig. 7.1: Open fracture of the tibia.

v. Ulna shaft: During excess push-ups.
vi. Posteromedial tibia: Unaccostomed excess running/jogging/skipping could result in stress fracture of posteromedial lower third tibia, which is known as *'shin splint'*.

C. Radiological

It explains fracture personality based on the mechanism of injury **(Fig. 7.2)**:
1. ***Transverse #:*** The fracture line is perpendicular to the the long axis of the bone.
2. ***Oblique #:*** The fracture line makes an angle with respect to the long axis of the bone.
3. ***Spiral #:*** The fracture line runs in two planes.
4. ***Comminuted #:*** Where there are more than two fragments at the same level of the bone.
5. ***Segmental #:*** When there is a fracture at two different levels of the bone.
6. ***Avulsion fracture:*** Sudden forceful contraction of muscle leads to the avulsion of muscle/ligament from its bony attachment. For example, supraspinatus and infraspinatus can avulse along with greater tuberosity, triceps along with tip of olecranon, patellar tendon with lower pole of patella and anterior or posterior cruciate ligament with a part of tibial plateau.

D. According to mechanism of injury: Direct and indirect (Table 7.1)
1. ***Direct injury:*** It occurs due to direct impact/force on the bone. It often results in comminuted or segmental #.
2. ***Indirect injury:*** Indirect injury results in a fracture away from the site of impact due to transmitted force. Such fractures are transverse, spiral, or avulsion #. Other examples of indirect # are burst fracture of a vertebra after falling from a height, twisting injury to the ankle resulting in spiral fracture of the tibia or fibula, and transverse fracture of the patella due to eccentric contraction of quadriceps against the flexed knee.

E. According to the extent of the fracture
1. ***Complete fracture***: When the fracture line involves both cortices of bone.
2. ***Incomplete fracture***: When the fracture line does not involve other cortex or some part of cortex. Examples of incomplete fractures are Greenstick fracture, Torus fracture, and plastic deformation.
    i. *Greenstick fracture:* It is observed in children where bones are soft. The bone may bend with or without fracture. Usually, one cortex (convex) is completely fractured, and the other cortex (concave) is bent **(Fig. 7.3)**.

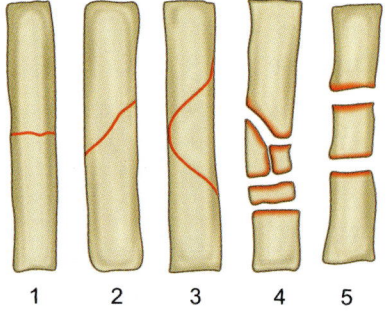

Fig. 7.2: Radiological classification of fractures. 1. Transverse; 2. Oblique; 3. Spiral; 4. Comminuted; 5. Segmental.

Table 7.1: Various fractures and mechanism of injury.	
Type of fractures	**Mechanism of injury/force involved**
Transverse	Indirect bending force (equal on both ends)
Oblique	Indirect bending forces (unequal on both ends)
Spiral	Indirect twisting force at the ends of bone
Comminuted	Direct force over the bone
Segmental	Direct force over the bone
Avulsion	Violent contraction of muscle

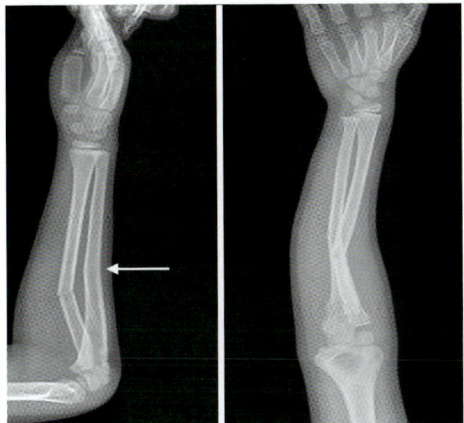

Fig. 7.3: Plain radiograph of forearm showing greenstick fracture of ulna (white arrow).

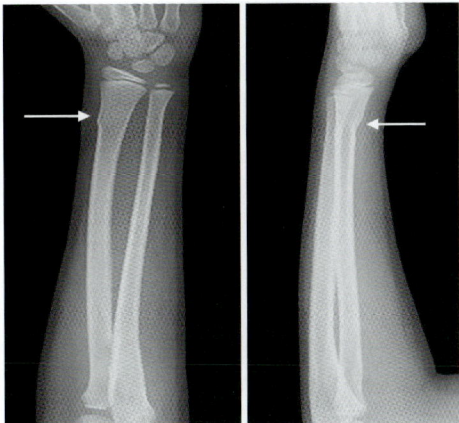

Fig. 7.4: Plain radiograph of forearm showing torus fracture of radius (white arrows indicate cortical buckling).

ii. *Torus fracture:* It also occurs in children wherein one or both cortices are buckled due to vertical compression force but remain undisplaced **(Fig. 7.4)**.

iii. *Plastic deformity:* Another type of incomplete fracture is a plastic deformity, wherein the bone appears to be bent (bowed) without any obvious fracture line on a radiograph.

F. **According to the displacement of the fracture (Figs. 7.5 to 7.7)**
1. *Undisplaced* #: Where # does not result in separation of the proximal and distal fragments **(Figs. 7.5 and 7.6)**.
2. *Displaced* #: Where # results in separating the proximal and distal fragments **(Fig. 7.7)**.

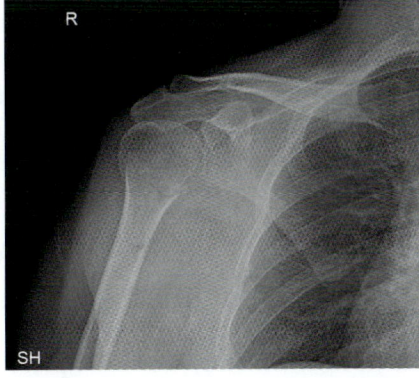

Fig. 7.5: X-ray (AP view) of the shoulder showing undisplaced fracture of surgical neck of humerus.

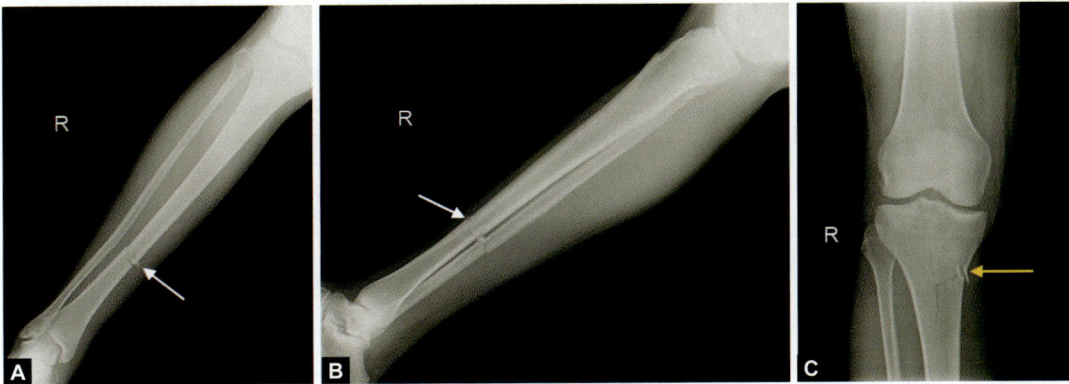

Figs. 7.6A to C: X-rays of leg showing minimally displaced fracture: (A and B) Tibia shaft transverse undisplaced fracture in both AP and lateral views (white arrows); (C) Upper end of tibia undisplaced # (yellow arrow).

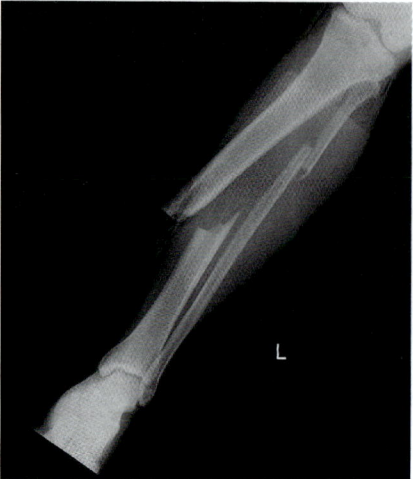

Fig. 7.7: Displaced tibia-fibula fracture where proximal and distal fragments of the tibial and fibular shaft are not in contact.

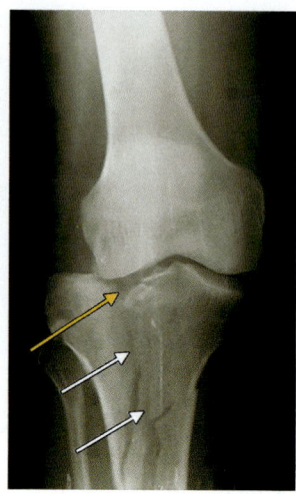

Fig. 7.8: Intra-articular fracture of right tibia. Note that white arrows indicate extra-articular line of fracture which enters joint at yellow arrow level.

G. According to the involvement of joint
1. *Extra-articular* #: Where # line does not enter into the joint.
2. *Intra-articular* #: Where # line enters into the joint **(Fig. 7.8)**.
   (Read: A note on intra-articular # at the end of this chapter on page 81).

■ CLINICAL FEATURES OF FRACTURE

Symptoms: Due to fracture, the patient complains of pain, swelling, and inability or difficulty using the limb. In case of undisplaced or impacted fractures, the patient may still use the limb, albeit with difficulty. For example; in a displaced fracture of the neck femur, the patient will be unable to bear weight, whereas they will be able to bear weight in case of an undisplaced or impacted fracture neck femur.

Signs: Clinical examination reveals *swelling, deformity,* and *limb shortening.* Palpation reveals *bony tenderness* at the fracture site, which is one of the most significant clinical signs of a fracture.

Other clinical signs are *bony crepitus* and *abnormal mobility at the fracture site* (between the proximal and distal ends of the bone). Another sign is *loss of transmitted movement,* wherein lifting the distal part of the limb does not cause any movement of the proximal end due to fracture.

However, in clinical practice, bony crepitus, abnormal mobility at the fracture site, and loss of transmitted movement in not intentionally tested as they may aggravate pain and can also damage surrounding soft tissue and neurovascular structures. Nevertheless, loss of transmitted movement can be tested indirectly in upper and lower limbs by asking the patient to elevate the limb actively. Any inability in elevating the limb may indicate a fracture.

Neurovascular assessment of the limb: In a limb with fracture/dislocation, neurological and vascular assessment must be done immediately. Any deviations from normal must be recorded, and repeat examinations should be performed at the serial interval.

A. **Vascular assessment:** A limb with normal vascularity would be *pink* (look), *warm* (feel), *adequate capillary refill in the nail bed (within 2 seconds),* pinprick over finger/toe pads would result in the immediate appearance of blood at the tip, and vessels will be palpable. Any deviations from normal should be investigated further with arterial doppler or CT angiogram.
B. **Neurological assessment:** A thorough *sensory and motor examination* of the limb is warranted. However, sometimes, due to pain and fracture (broken lever arm), the motor power appears less, even if there is no neurological injury. If one is unsure about neurological injury, one must reassess motor power after the pain is less or the fracture has been stabilized.

Symptoms of fracture	Signs of fracture
▪ Pain ▪ Swelling ▪ Inability or difficulty in using the limb	▪ Deformity, shortening ▪ Bony tenderness ▪ Bony crepitus ▪ Abnormal mobility at the fracture site ▪ Loss of transmitted movement

■ INVESTIGATIONS

Typically, each patient with a suspected fracture is assessed with **plain radiographs,** which should have a minimum of two views if possible. Further evaluation may require a **CT scan,** especially if the fracture is intra- or periarticular or in an area where the anatomy is complex (pelvis/spine/scapula). **Vascular Doppler scan or CT angiogram** helps assess vascular injury to the limb. **MRI** scan is required to assess the soft tissue injury (ligaments, tendons, and muscles). **A bone scan** (for fracture) is rarely performed in current scenarios.

1. **Plain radiograph:** It is an essential investigation to diagnose a fracture. One must follow the *"rule of two's"* while taking a radiograph (two views, two joints, and two occasions).
    ♦ *Two views:* A minimum of two views are required to confirm the fracture, as a single view can miss a fracture or severity of the displacement **(Fig. 7.9)**.

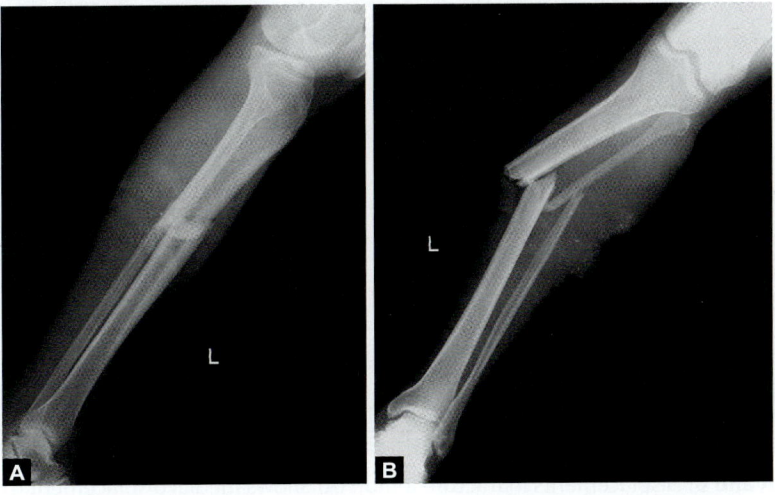

Figs. 7.9A and B: X-rays of leg: (A) Shows minimally displaced tibial fibula shaft fracture in lateral view while; (B) Shows same fracture completely displaced in AP view.

- *Two joints:* One joint above and another one below should be included in the X-ray as the forces causing fracture can be transmitted to the neighboring joints too.
- *On two occasions:* X-rays should be repeated before and after the management.

A good radiograph should reveal the following characteristics of a fracture.

- *Displacement, overriding, angulation,* and *rotation.*
- Displacement means abnormal position or spatial orientation (anterior-posterior, medial-lateral) of the distal fracture fragment with respect to the proximal, e.g., in **Figure 7.10**, the distal fragment of the femur is medially and posteriorly displaced with overriding.

> The displacement of the fracture fragment mentioned is always of the 'distal fragment' as the proximal fragment is considered stable due to its fixity to the torso. However, in spine injuries, the displacement mentioned is of the superior vertebra, as the distal vertebra is considered fixed to the torso.

2. **Computed tomography (CT scan):** A CT scan is generally indicated in two situations:
   a. A fracture is suspected clinically. However, it is not visible on a plain X-ray.
   b. To assess *intra- and periarticular fractures* and *fractures in areas of complex anatomy* like the pelvis, spine, elbow, proximal humerus, scapula, distal femur, foot, and ankle. A mere plain X-ray may not reveal the complexity of fractures (intra- or periarticular fracture), displacement, and comminution in such regions due to complex and overlapping anatomy **(Fig. 7.11)**. Further, three-dimensional CT scan (3D CT scan) reconstruction helps understand these fracture configuration in a better fashion.
3. **Magnetic resonance imaging (MRI):** It is performed in case of *suspected soft tissue injuries (ligament, muscle-tendon, and cartilage)* **(Fig. 7.12)**.

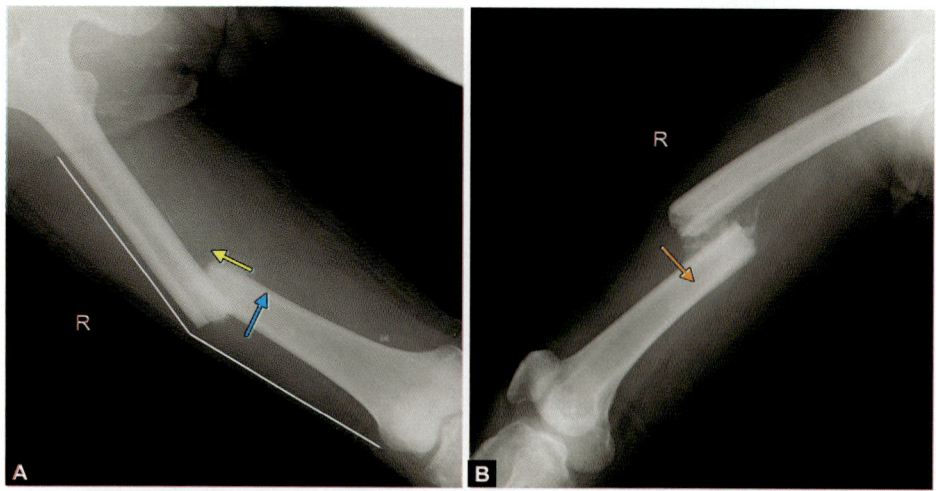

Figs. 7.10A and B: Displacements in fracture femur: (A) Shows medial displacement (blue arrow), overiding (yellow arrow) and lateral angulation (white line); (B) Posterior displacement (orange arrow).

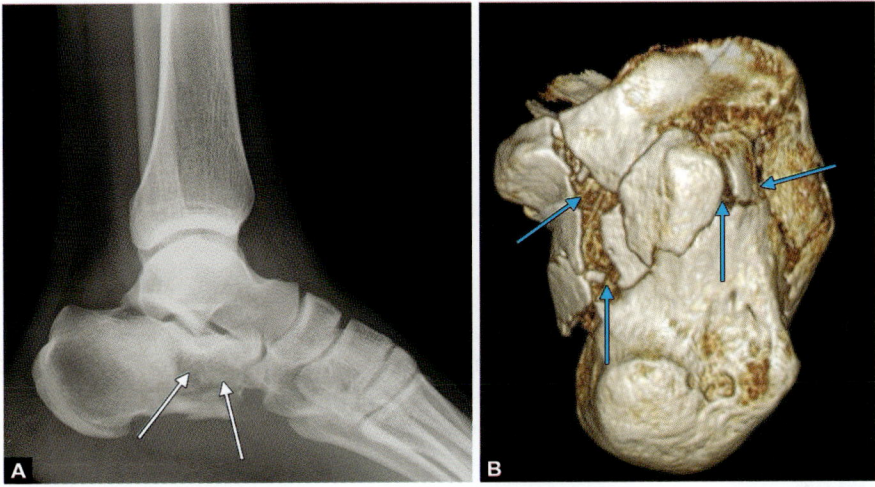

Figs. 7.11A and B: (A) Plain X-ray lateral view of fracture calcaneum (white arrows); (B) CT scan of same calcaneum fracture with gross comminution (blue arrows).

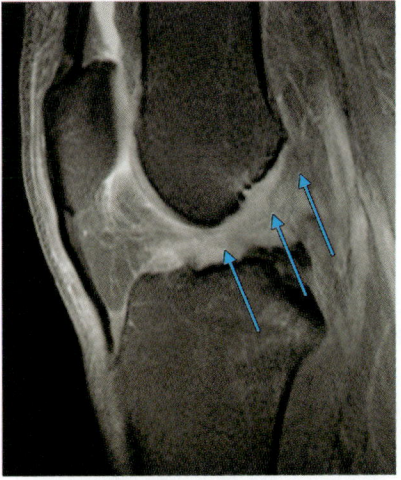

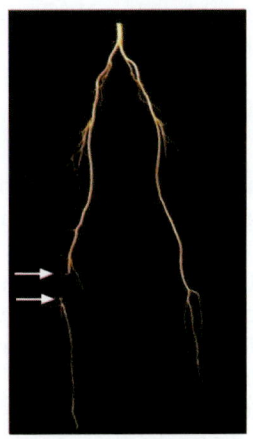

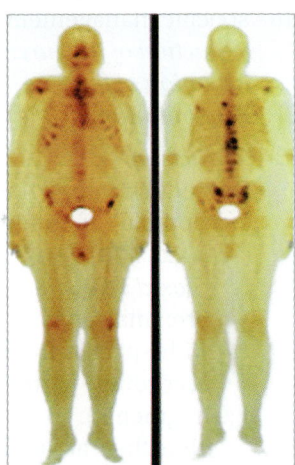

Fig. 7.12: MRI of the knee showing torn anterior cruciate ligament (blue arrows).

Fig. 7.13: Arteriogram of lower limb vessels showing flow cutoff (white arrows) in right popliteal artery.

Fig. 7.14: Bone scan showing multiple hot spots in vertebrae, pelvis and humerus.

Sometimes, MRI scan is the investigation of choice for undisplaced fractures such as fracture scaphoid waist, which is not apparent on a plain X-ray.

4. **Angiogram (plain or CT scan or MRI):** It is performed to assess the *arterial status* of the limb **(Fig. 7.13)**.
5. **Doppler scan:** It is performed to assess the *venous or arterial* status (blockage, kinking of vessel) of the the limb.
6. **Bone scan (Fig. 7.14)**: In the current scenario, with the availability of CT and MRI, a bone scan is not routinely performed to assess fractures **(Fig. 7.14)**. They are more useful in assessment of bony metastasis. *[For details of bone scan, Refer Chapter 50]*.

MANAGEMENT OF FRACTURES

The management of fracture involves general management of the patient and specific management of the fracture.

A. General management: The general management of patient must involve *assessment as per ATLS protocol*.
1. Airway
2. Bleeding
3. Circulation
4. Disability and exposure
   All above parameters must be assessed and managed on standard principles.
5. Further, one must assess other systemic injuries to head, chest, and abdomen-pelvis organs, which must be treated as interdisciplinary approach.
6. Management of hemorrhagic shock/blood loss
7. Appropriate splintage of the limb
8. Analgesics
9. Tetanus toxoid and gas gangrene prophylaxis.

B. Specific principles of fracture management:
The specific management of fracture involves three "R"s:
1. *Reduction of fracture:* Closed/open
2. *Retention of fracture*
3. *Rehabilitation*.

a. **Reduction**
   The reduction of a fracture aims to align the "displaced fracture ends" to the "normal" or "acceptable" anatomical alignment. The reduction can be achieved by the *closed* or *open method*.
   1. *Closed reduction (CR):* Traction and countertraction are applied over the distal and proximal ends of a fracture, respectively, *without opening the fracture site,* along with specific manipulation and maneuvers over the fragments (proximal and distal according to the displacements of fragments) to reduce the fracture. Thus the fracture is brought back into normal alignment. Often, CR is done under an image intensifier to confirm the adequateness of reduction **(Fig. 7.15)**.
   2. *Open reduction (OR):* The *fracture site is opened surgically,* and the fracture ends are aligned manually to achieve anatomical alignment **(Fig. 7.16)**.

b. **Retention**
   Once the fracture ends are aligned in anatomical orientation by closed or open reduction, they are "retained in the anatomical position" by various methods

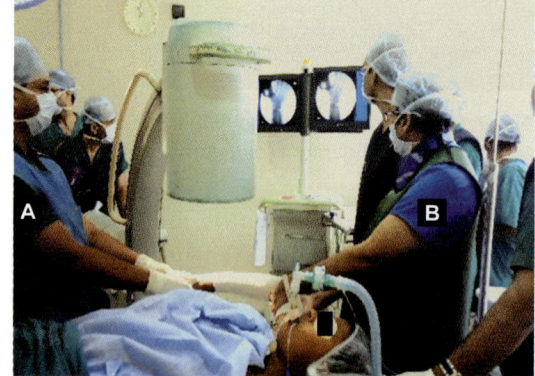

Fig. 7.15: Closed reduction of distal radius fracture under image intensifier. To align the fracture, Surgeons A and B are giving traction and countertraction, respectively.

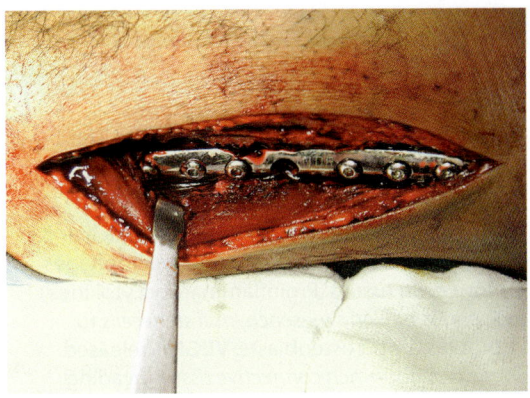

Fig. 7.16: Open reduction of fibula and internal fixation by a plate.

Table 7.2: Examples of method of reduction and type of retention for various fractures.

Reduction method	Retention type	Examples
Closed	Plaster of Paris	Colles' fracture
Closed	Traction/POP	Fracture femur in children
Open/closed	External fixator	Open fracture
Closed/open	Internal fixation by nail	Fracture femur in adult
Open	Internal fixation by plate	Fracture humerus shaft in adult

for the fracture to heal over the next few weeks-months. These methods include splints, slings, other orthoses, casts, plates, nails, screws, or wires, which are selected according to the age of the patient, site and type of fracture **(Table 7.2)**.

c. **Rehabilitation**
WHO's definition of rehabilitation is *"a set of interventions designed to optimize functioning and reduce disability in individuals with health conditions in interaction with their environment."*
During rehabilitation, the patient's functional status is restored to the original functional activity level by gradual joint mobilization, muscle strengthening, and weight-bearing. Rehabilitation aims to prevent joint stiffness, muscle wasting, and disuse osteoporosis.

STAGES OF FRACTURE HEALING

Fracture healing involves a set of complex biological events to restore bone and fracture ends to the pre-injury status. It comprises several stages:
- Stage of **hematoma**: Soft tissue and bone injury results in bleeding at the fracture site resulting in a hematoma.
- Stage of **inflammation and cellular proliferation**.
- Stage of **callus formation**.
- Stage of **remodeling**.

These stages are described in **Table 7.3**.

TYPES OF FRACTURE HEALING

There are two types of fracture healing—primary and secondary.
1. **Primary # healing**: It occurs during *"rigid/absolute stability (immobilization)"* of the fracture, where barely any callus formation is seen radiologically around the fracture site. Typically, *primary healing is seen after a plate fixation of a long bone*, which is a rigid form of a internal fixation **(Fig. 7.17)**.

Table 7.3: Stages of fracture healing.

Stages of healing	Duration	Cardinal features
Stage of hematoma	<1 week	Bleeding from fracture ends and adjacent soft tissue forms **hematoma**, which acts as a framework for callus formation. The fracture ends undergo **necrosis**.
Stage of inflammation and granulation tissue	1–2 weeks	*An acute aseptic inflammatory response characterizes this stage* wherein there is a release of **proinflammatory cytokines** such as ILs, TNF and BMPs, which help stimulate neutrophils and macrophages at the site, helping *remove dead tissues*. Proinflammatory cytokines also *sensitize endosteal, periosteal, and mesenchymal stem cells* to form chondrocytes, fibroblasts, and osteoblasts. **VEGF** is released to promote *angiogenesis and fibrin-rich connective tissue* invading hematoma to form a mesh of granulation tissue.
Stage of a soft callus	2–4 weeks	*Growth of the soft callus characterizes this stage.* ***Away from the # site 'circumferentially'***: Osteoblasts from the cambium layer form a **'woven bone' periosteally**. ***At the # site***: The mesenchymal progenitor cells differentiate into fibroblasts and chondrocytes, producing an extracellular matrix of fibrocartilaginous framework replacing hematoma.
Stage of hard callus	4–16 weeks	Gradually, the **soft callus gets converted into a hard callus** (woven bone) from the *periphery to the center* due to the deposition of hydroxyapatite crystals.
Stage of remodeling	Many years	Gradually over the months and years, the **hard callus gets re-shaped according to the stress and strain over bone and callus (Wolff's law),** and fracture becomes indistinguishable from the parent bone. The medullary canal is restored, and the **woven bone is completely converted into organized lamellar bone**.

(ILs: interleukins; TNF: tumor necrosis factor; BMP: bone morphogenetic protein; VEGF: vascular endothelial growth factor)

Note that fractures of cancellous bones (calcaneum, ends of a long bone) heal with primary # healing.

The mechanism of primary healing involves the **'cutting cone mechanism'** (osteoclast in front of cone removes necrotic bone, followed by trailing osteoblast that lays down new bone).

2. **Secondary # healing**: It occurs during **"relative stability (immobilization)"** of the fracture, where a fair amount of callus is present around the fracture site. Typically, *secondary healing of a long bone fracture is observed in fracture managed by cast/traction/intramedullary nail fixation* **(Fig. 7.18)**. A secondary # healing undergoes five typical stages of # healing **(Table 7.3)**.

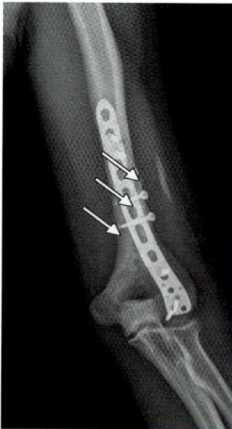

Fig. 7.17: Direct fracture healing with no callus seen at the distal humerus fracture site (white arrows) fixed with a plate.

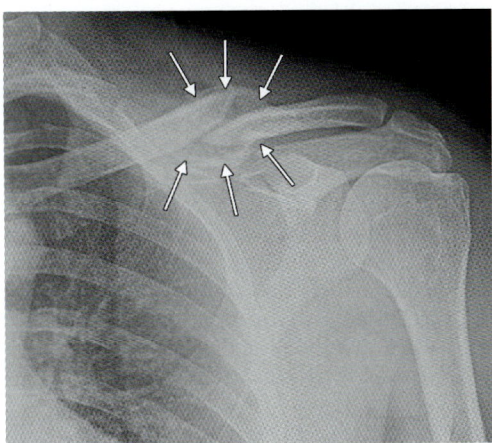

Fig. 7.18: Indirect or secondary fracture healing of a clavicle fracture managed with sling (multiple white arrows around callus).

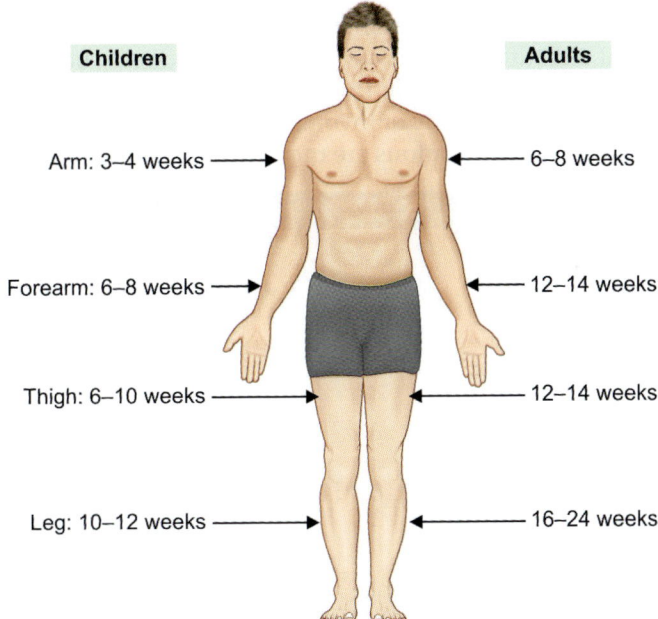

Fig. 7.19: "Average time required" for fracture union in children and adults in upper and lower extremities.

TIME REQUIRED FOR FRACTURE HEALING

The average time required for fracture healing in children and adults is shown in **Figure 7.19**.

FACTORS AFFECTING THE FRACTURE HEALING

The factors affecting fracture healing (stimulate or retard) can be divided into local and systemic factors. Closed fracture, stable fracture (post management), adequate vascularity at

site, young age, good health, and absence of co-morbidities stimulate healing. The factors influencing fracture healing are mentioned in **Table 7.4**.

Table 7.4: The local and systemic factors affecting the fracture union.

Local	Systemic
Retards	**Retards**
• Type of #- comminuted • Open #, soft tissue loss, infection • Bone loss • Poor vascularity • Unstable fixation • Radiation at the # site	• Old age • Diabetes, nicotine in any form • Systemic diseases: Anemia, jaundice • Poor nutritional state, low vitamin D, calcium • Systemic drugs: Steroids, bisphosphonates, quinolones, NSAIDs • Poor immune state: HIV • Poor tissue quality: Ehler-Danlos syndrome
Stimulates	**Stimulates**
Cancellous bone	Head injury (? Due to high serum calcitonin levels)

COMPLICATIONS OF FRACTURE

After a fracture, there can be local and systemic complications. The **local complication** involve local tissues (skin and subcutaneous tissue, nerve, artery, vein, bone, joint, muscle) and usually does not have any systemic effect. In contrast, **general/systemic complications** can affect the functioning of the entire body or involve various systems of body such as CNS, CVS, respiratory, etc. The fracture complications are mentioned in **Table 7.5**.

Table 7.5: Complications after a fracture.

	Local	General/systemic
Acute	• Skin injury • Nerve injury • Vascular injury • Muscle-tendon injury • Physeal injury • Local visceral injury	• Hemorrhagic shock • Crush syndrome • Injury to chest, abdomen, and other organs like eye, face, ear, etc.
Early	• Skin necrosis • Fracture blisters • Gas gangrene • Gangrene • Volkmann ischemia/compartment syndrome • Venous thrombosis	• Fat embolism • Pulmonary thromboembolism • Pneumonia • Tetanus • Delirium tremens • Acute respiratory distress syndrome (ARDS) • Septicemia
Delayed/late	• *Nerve*: Tardy ulnar nerve palsy • *Muscle*: Myositis ossificans, Volkmann ischemic contracture, Sudeck's dystrophy • *Bone/fracture*: Malunion, nonunion, delayed union, growth disturbance (causing deformity, limb length discrepancy), cross union, chronic osteomyelitis • *Joint*: Stiffness, 2° osteoarthritis	• Post-traumatic stress disorder • Renal calculi • Disuse osteopenia • Bedsore

These local/systemic complications can occur in acute, early, and chronic phase:
- **Acute/immediate:** Within 24 hours
- **Early:** Develop between 24 hours to two weeks
- **Delayed/chronic:** After a few weeks to months.

The details of these complications are discussed in Chapter 23 and other respective sections.

A NOTE ON INTRA-ARTICULAR FRACTURE

Definition: A fracture where the fracture line runs into the joint or disrupts the joint surface **(Fig. 7.20)**.

Pathoanatomy: Since the # line runs into the joint, it disrupts the articular surface lined by hyaline cartilage. *An incongruent joint surface could result in secondary osteoarthritis of the joint if the fracture and articular surface are not restored anatomically.* Further, the involvement of the joint could result in joint stiffness.

Clinical features: The clinical features of an intraarticular fracture are similar to extra-articular fractures. However, in addition to the typical findings, there is *hemarthrosis as fracture opens in to the joint resulting in swelling of the joint. The joint movements are not possible due to severe pain.*

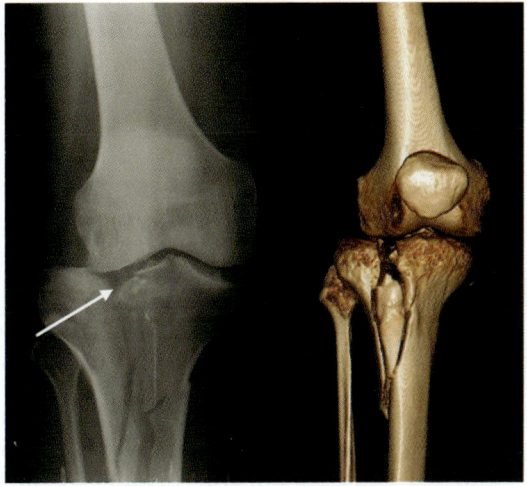

Fig. 7.20: X-ray of the right knee (left image) showing intra-articular fracture of the proximal tibia (white arrow). The right image shows the corresponding 3D CT scan.

Investigation:
1. *X-ray:* AP and lateral views **(Fig. 7.20)**
2. *CT scan* **(Fig. 7.20)**: It is the *single most important investigation for diagnosing and assessing intra-articular fractures.* It is required for preoperative planning. Furthermore, it may also be done postoperatively to confirm the reduction achieved during surgery.

Treatment: *Accurate restoration of the joint surface congruity by closed or open reduction is paramount,* followed by rigid internal/external fixation.

Complications:
1. Secondary degenerative arthritis
2. Deformity and stiffness of the joint
3. Joint instability (due to altered articular bony morphology).

A NOTE ON PATHOLOGICAL FRACTURE

Definition: Pathological fracture is defined as a *fracture in a diseased bone due to local or systemic cause with trivial trauma.*

Etiology: The underlying cause for a pathological fracture could be:
- *Metabolic:* Osteoporosis, osteomalacia, hyperparathyroidism
- *Neoplastic:* Primary or metastatic tumors

- **Developmental:** Osteogenesis imperfecta
- **Infection:** Osteomyelitis

Clinical features: Patients give a history of trivial trauma. Furthermore, there may be pain at the fracture site even before the fracture due to the underlying disease (infection/tumor).
- Present clinical features are of a fracture—pain, swelling and difficulty in using the affected part.
- There is deformity and shortening. Bony tenderness is present at the fracture site.
- There may be systemic or local features of a pre-existing disease or underlying pathology.

Investigations: A plain X-ray of the bone is the first investigation **(Fig. 7.21)**. Radiologically, the *fracture pattern is often unusual*. It may show evidence of underlying disease.
- Depending upon the etiology, other investigations required are CT scan, bone scan, PET scan and MRI.
- Blood tests may be required—ESR, CRP, calcium, phosphorus, alkaline phosphatase, etc.
- The rest of the investigations are as per etiology.

Treatment: It comprises treatment of the underlying cause and stabilization of the fracture. Further, the type of stabilization method (nail/external fixator) depends upon the underlying etiology.
- The pathological fracture of a long bone, especially metastatic bone disease, is mainly stabilized by the intramedullary nail **(Fig. 7.22)**.
  Occasionally, a diseased long bone without fracture, especially a *proven metastatic bone disease*, can be prophylactically stabilized based on **Mirel's score**. Mirel proposed a scoring system based on four characteristics: (1) site of the lesion; (2) nature of the lesion; (3) size of the lesion; and (4) pain. All the features are assigned progressive scores ranging from 1 to 3. *If Mirels score > 8, it needs a prophylactic fixation.*
- In the presence of infection in a long bone, an external fixator application is a more suitable choice.
- Vertebral pathological fractures due to tumor/infection can be stabilized with plates and rods. Osteoporotic vertebral fractures may require kyphoplasty/vertebroplasty.

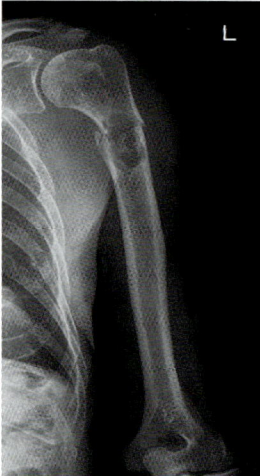

Fig. 7.21: Pathological fracture of left humerus due to a metastatic lesion (from renal cell carcinoma).

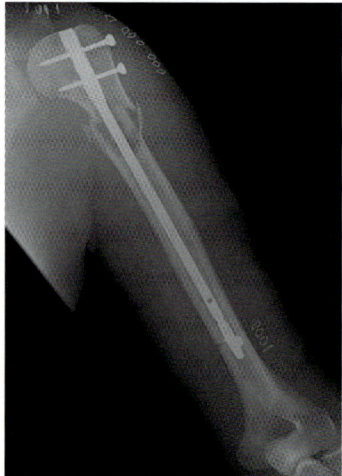

Fig. 7.22: Intramedullary nail fixation of pathological fracture.

CHAPTER 8

Fracture in Children and Physeal Injuries

PECULIARITIES OF BONE AND FRACTURES IN CHILDREN

1. Bones in children are more resilient and can endure more energy. Hence, it can get *deformed before it is fractured*. This deformation can give rise to unique types of fractures, such as Greenstick fracture, Torus fracture, and plastic deformation (Refer Chapter 6 for details). Most fractures in adult bone can also occur in a child's bone. However, there are some fractures which are common in children **(Box 8.1)**.

Box 8.1: Common fractures in children.
- Fracture supracondylar humerus
- Fracture lateral condyle humerus (lateral epicondyle + capitellum + lateral half of trochlea)
- Fracture both bones forearm
- Greenstick # of forearm bones
- Torus fracture/plastic deformity of forearm bones
- Spiral # tibia
- Physeal injuries

2. There can be **associated injury to the physis**. Later, this could result in **shortening and deformity** of the limb.
3. The *periosteum in a child's bone is thick and loose* compared to an adult bone. Periosteum of child's bone is also more active than the adult periosteum. Hence, pediatric fractures (#s) heal more rapidly than adult #s.
4. **The remodeling potential** of pediatric fracture is superior in the case of:
    - Younger patient
    - If the fracture is closer to the joint
    - The bony deformity in the direction of the plane of the joint movement remodels better compared to the deformity perpendicular to the plane of motion. For example, an anteroposterior angular deformity in the lower end tibia is better remodeled compared to mediolateral deformity as the former is in the same plane in which ankle dorsiflexion-plantar flexion occurs.

   Note: There is no remodeling of rotational malalignment.

PHYSEAL INJURIES

DEFINITION

Physis is the growing end of the bone in children and adolescents **(Fig. 8.1)**. After completing growth at skeletal maturity, the physis is replaced by a physeal line.

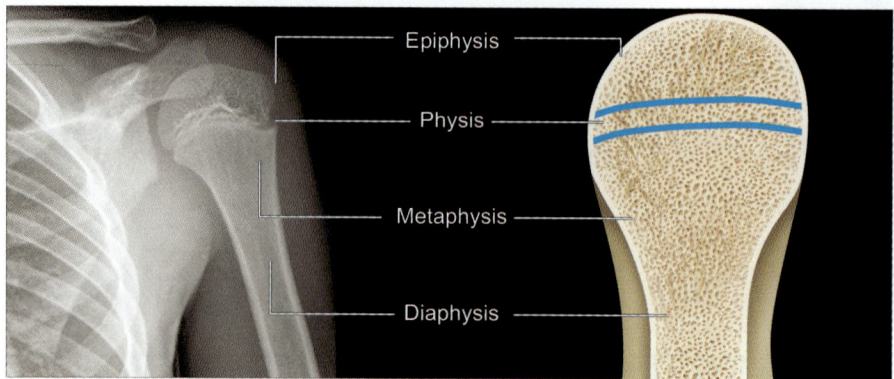

Fig. 8.1: X-ray of the upper end humerus and a representative bone image showing various parts of bone including physis.

SURGICAL ANATOMY OF PHYSIS

Physis is present at either end of a long bone in children for longitudinal growth.
- ***Histologically, it has four layers:*** Resting (germinal), proliferative, hypertrophic, and zone of calcification. The proliferative zone is characterized by *rapidly multiplying chondrocytes* and it is the *metabolically most active zone*. The *hypertrophic zone is the 'weakest'* as it lacks collagen and calcified tissue. Most physeal separation occurs through hypertrophic layer because it cannot resist shearing stress.

FUNCTION OF PHYSIS

It is responsible for **longitudinal growth of the bone** during the growing phase of a child.

INJURY TO THE PHYSIS RESULTS IN

- ***Longitudinal growth affected:*** Limb length discrepancy (shortening).
- ***Asymmetric growth disturbance:*** Angular deformity of the limb.

PHYSEAL INJURY CLASSIFICATION: SALTER-HARRIS CLASSIFICATION (FIGS. 8.2 AND 8.3)

Type 1: Complete transverse physeal separation. It results in epiphyseal separation from the metaphysis.
Type 2: Fracture crosses physis transversely and exits obliquely through the metaphysis. It is the *most common type (75%) of physeal injury*. Small triangular metaphyseal fragment is also known as ***Thurston-Holland sign*** (Fig. 8.2).
Type 3: Fracture crosses physis transversely and exits epiphysis obliquely/vertically. These fractures can result in physical bars.
Type 4: Fracture crosses physis transversely and exits epiphysis and metaphysis obliquely/vertically.
Type 5: Crush injury to the physis.

CLINICAL FEATURES

The cinical features are similar to a fracture of bone, such as:

Chapter 8: Fracture in Children and Physeal Injuries

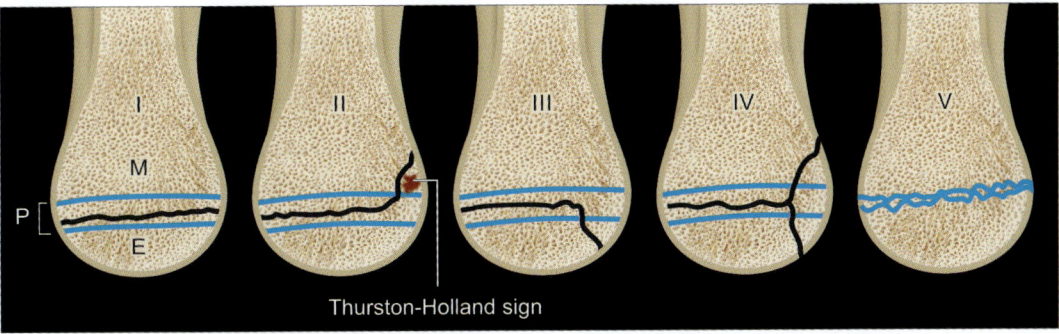

Fig. 8.2: Diagrammatic representation of physeal injuries (Types I–V)
(The area between blue lines represents physis, whereas black line represents fracture line).
(P: Physis; E: Epiphysis; M: Metaphysis)

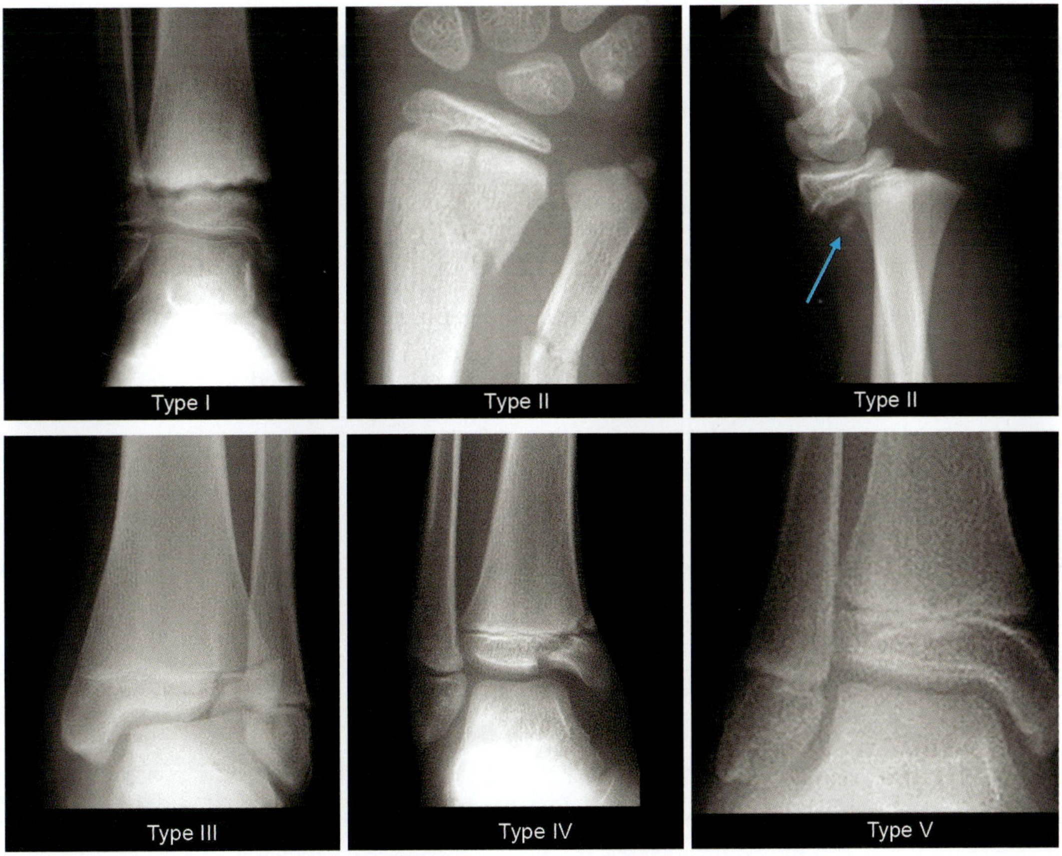

Fig. 8.3: X-ray of various types of Salter-Harris physeal injuries. Blue arrow in right most upper image indicates small metaphyseal fragment—Thurston-Holland sign.

- Pain, swelling, and deformity of the limb
- Inability or difficulty to bear weight or use the limb
- Bony tenderness is present over the site of injury
- Deformity
- Limited and painful range of motion at the joint.

Pnemonic to remember SALTER's physeal injury classification by acronym **SALTR**
- Type 1-**S: S**plit (split between epiphysis and metaphysis)
- Type 2-**A: A**bove (through metaphysis)
- Type 3-**L: L**ower (through epiphysis)
- Type 4-**T: T**hrough and through (epi- and metaphysis)
- Type 5-**R: R**uined/crushed physis

■ INVESTIGATIONS

Plain X-ray: Anteroposterior (AP) and lateral view. Occasionally, normal side radiographs are needed to compare injuries.

CT or MRI: Rarely needed to confirm injuries if X-rays appear normal.

■ TREATMENT

The principle of treatment of displaced physeal injuries is *"accurate reduction of the physis."* To avoid complications, such as growth disturbance/deformity, displaced physeal injuries should be treated as early as possible.
- **Undisplaced injury:** Plaster of Paris (POP) cast
- **Displaced physeal injury:** Closed reduction and cast application *or* closed reduction and internal fixation with screws/wires/plates.

■ COMPLICATIONS OF PHYSEAL INJURY

- Longitudinal growth disturbance leading to shortening of the limb
- Angular deformity of the limb
- Arthritis of the joint, especially if epiphysis is involved and damaged
- Nonunion
- Bony/physeal bar formation: Especially in case of epiphyseal injury.

Notes

CHAPTER 9

Fracture Clavicle

SURGICAL ANATOMY OF CLAVICLE

It is a 'S' shape bone (when seen from top) which articulates medially with sternum and laterally with acromion forming sternoclavicular and acromioclavicular (AC) joint, respectively. It is also connected to coracoid by coracoclavicular ligament, which has two parts—conoid (medial) and trapezoid (lateral). The AC joint capsule and coracoclavicular ligaments stabilize the lateral end of clavicle.

The clavicle connects upper limb (scapula) with trunk sternum. **Figures 9.1 and 9.2** show normal clavicle and fracture clavicle.

Peculiarities of clavicle

- It is the first bone to start ossification in fetus (5–6 weeks). However, medial (sternal end) is the last long bone epiphysis to fuse at 22–25 years of age.
- Only long bone with 'two' primary ossification center (all other long bones have single ossification center).
- Only long bone to largely undergo intramembranous ossification (cf. other long bones ossify by endochondral ossification). However, lateral end of clavicle ossifies in endochondral ossification.
- Only long bone which lies horizontally.
- Only long bone which does not have medullary canal.

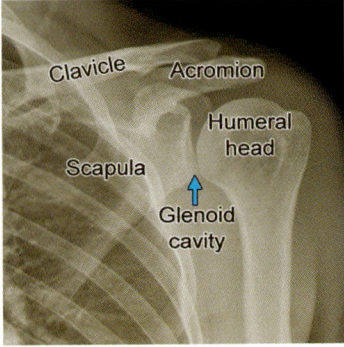

Fig. 9.1: X-ray of a normal clavicle.

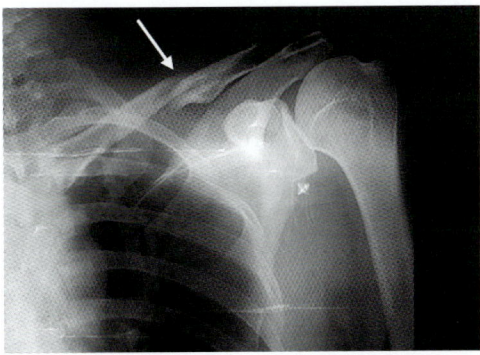

Fig. 9.2: X-ray of a fracture clavicle (white arrow).

COMMON SITE OF FRACTURE

Allman classification: Clavicle fractures in middle one-third, lateral one-third or medial one-third.
- **Group I**—*middle one-third shaft fracture (80%):* It is the *most common location of clavicle fracture* as clavicle is weakest in the middle third according to sectional geometry, section modulus and proportions of rigidity. Further, fracture occurs commonly over the medial two-third and lateral one-third junction due to sudden change in the cross-sectional geometry (tubular central third to flat lateral third).
- **Group II**—*lateral one-third fracture (15%):* Lateral end clavicle fractures are often associated to injury to AC joint, and are prone to nonunion (cf. middle third which are prone to malunion)
- **Group III**—*medial one-third fracture (5%).*

MECHANISM OF INJURY

1. Fall on the affected shoulder (87%): *Most common mechanism of injury*
2. Direct blow on to the shoulder (7%)
3. Fall on outstretched hand (6%).

FRACTURE CLAVICLE MID-SHAFT

The most common site of fracture clavicle is at the medial two-third and lateral one-third junction with classic displacement as described below **(Fig. 9.3)**.
- **Medial fragment is displaced superiorly:** Due to upward pull of sternocleidomastoid.
- **Lateral fragment is displaced inferiorly:** Due to downward drag by gravity and weight of arm.

CLINICAL FEATURES

Symptoms: Pain and swelling over the clavicle and inability/difficulty to elevate or move arm at the shoulder joint.

Signs:
- Swelling is present over the clavicle.
- Bony tenderness is present over the clavicle shaft.
- Painfully, restricted ROM of the shoulder.
- Examination of neurovascular structures of the upper limb is a must to rule out injury to brachial plexus and subclavian artery, which lie below the clavicle.

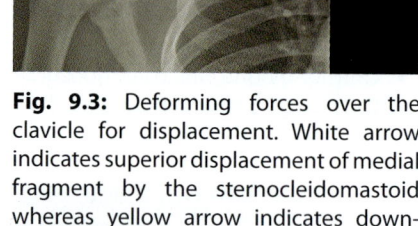

Fig. 9.3: Deforming forces over the clavicle for displacement. White arrow indicates superior displacement of medial fragment by the sternocleidomastoid whereas yellow arrow indicates downward displacement of the distal fragment due to the weight of arm.

INVESTIGATION

Plain X-ray of the clavicle—AP view **(Fig. 9.2)**, 30° cephalic view.

TREATMENT

There are two ways of manging a mid-shaft clavicle fracture, conservative and operative **(Flowchart 9.1)**.

Flowchart 9.1: Treatment algorithm for mid-shaft clavicle fractures.

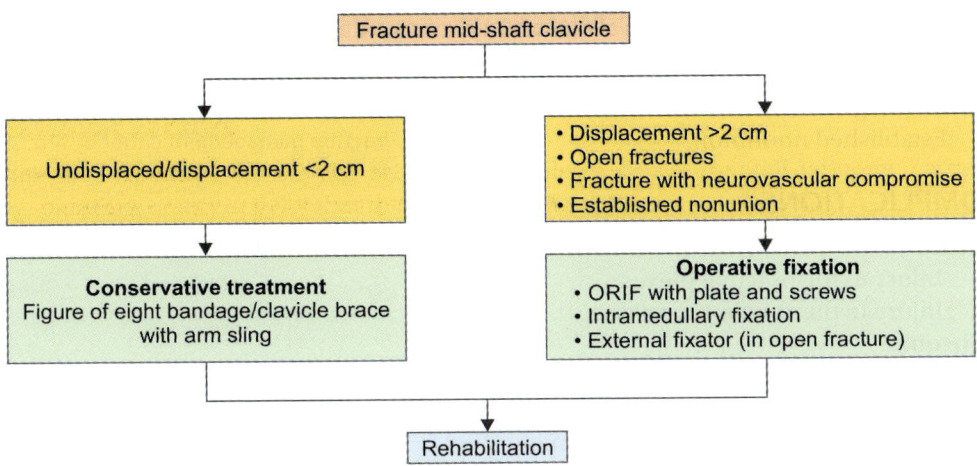

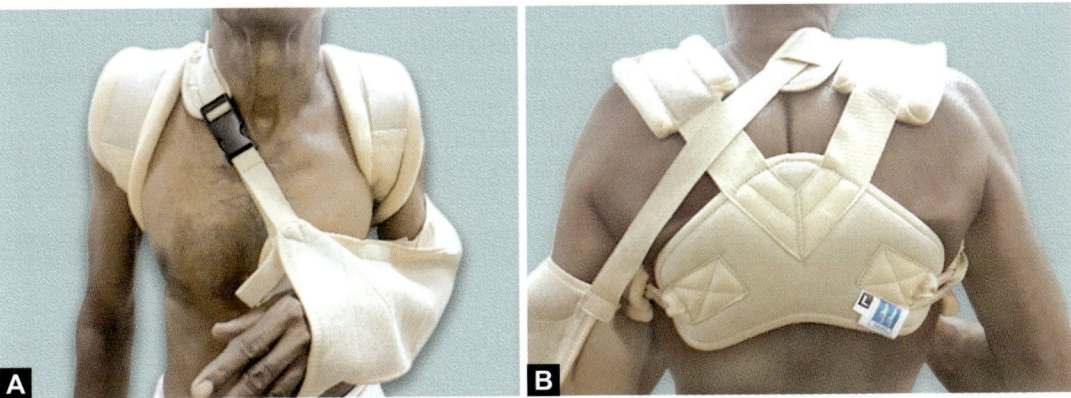

Figs. 9.4A and B: Clavicle brace with arm sling.

1. **Conservative treatment:** Since a large majority of mid-shaft clavicle fractures unite naturally without any intervention, most of the *middle third clavicle* fractures are managed conservatively by *clavicular brace or figure of eight bandage with cuff and collar sling* for 6–8 weeks **(Figs. 9.4A and B).**

   (*Note*: Clavicular brace aims to push the medial fragment downwards, while arm sling lifts the distal fragment upward to counter the weight of arm displacing fragment downward).

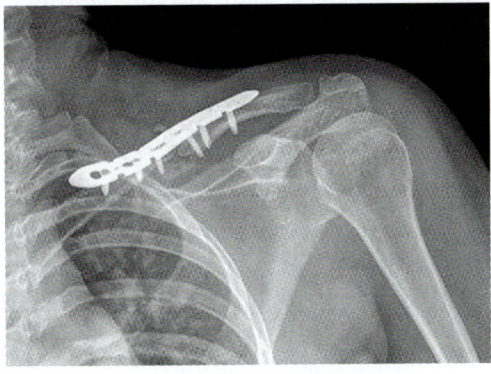

Fig. 9.5: ORIF of clavicle with plate.

2. **Operative management:** *Open reduction and internal fixation by plate* **(Fig. 9.5)**/*intramedullary device* is performed with certain criteria mentioned below:

- Displaced fracture (if there is >2 cm overlap between medial and lateral ends)
- Open fracture of the clavicle
- Associated with neurovascular deficit
- Floating shoulder
- Established nonunion.

Note: Current evidence does not show any difference between the results of clavicle fracture management either by arm sling or arm sling with figure of eight strapping.

COMPLICATIONS

1. **Acute**
   - Injury to the brachial plexus
   - Injury to the subclavian vessels.
2. **Chronic**
   - *Malunion:* Malunion is the most common complication of a conservatively managed middle-shaft clavicle fracture. However, it rarely poses any functional problem, and only a bony bump is seen at the malunited fracture site, which might occasionally be cosmetically annoying. Therefore, a *malunited clavicle without any major functional impairment does not require any treatment.* A functionally impairing malunion would require osteotomy of malunion and internal fixation.
   - *Stiffness of the shoulder:* It can happen due to immobilization with brace. However, almost everyone recovers with physiotherapy.
   - *Nonunion of fracture:* It is uncommon. If it occurs, it can be managed on standard principles of nonunion treatment.

LATERAL THIRD CLAVICLE FRACTURE

- It is less common (12–15%) than middle third clavicle fractures.
- Lateral third clavicle fracture may be associated with acromioclavicular joint dislocation or injury to coracoclavicular ligaments.

Mechanism of injury: It happens during RTA/fall over the tip of the shoulder.

Clinical features: Pain, swelling and deformity over the lateral end of the clavicle and patient may find difficult to move shoulder. Examination reveals bony tenderness over the lateral end of clavicle.

Diagnosis: X-ray of clavicle AP view **(Fig. 9.6)**.

Treatment
- *Undisplaced fracture:* It is managed conservatively with an arm sling for 4 weeks followed by mobilization of shoulder **(Fig. 9.7)**. A figure of four bandage is also described to manage lateral end clavicle fracture **(Fig. 9.8)**.
- *Displaced fracture or associated AC joint dislocation:* ORIF with plate and screws. AC joint stabilization might be required.

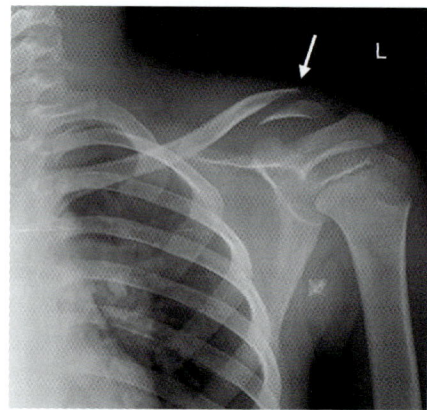

Fig. 9.6: Lateral third clavicle fracture (white arrow).

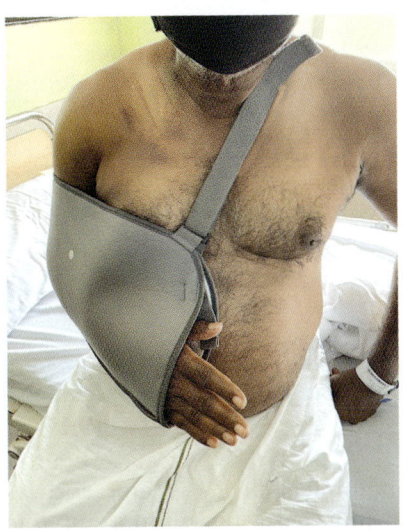 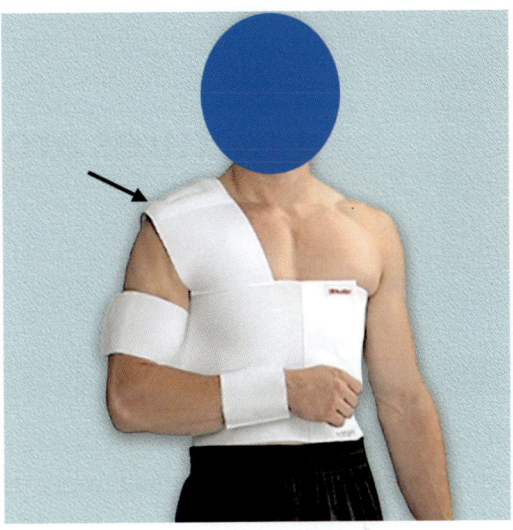

Fig. 9.7: Arm pouch or arm sling used for fracture lateral end clavicle.

Fig. 9.8: Figure of four bandage or splint used for lateral end clavicle fracture. Black arrow over strap over clavicle indicates pressure over the lateral end clavicle for reduction.

Complication

Nonunion: Unlike middle third fracture which are prone for malunion, lateral third fractures are prone for nonunion.

MEDIAL THIRD CLAVICLE FRACTURE

- Rare
- Usually occurs after RTA. There may be associated injury to the chest
- Most fractures can be managed conservatively by a sling.

Notes

CHAPTER 10

Fractures around the Shoulder

FRACTURE PROXIMAL HUMERUS

SURGICAL ANATOMY OF PROXIMAL HUMERUS

Proximal humerus consists of four parts: Humeral anatomical head, greater and lesser tuberosity and surgical neck neck **(Fig. 10.1A)**. These four parts play important role in understanding the fractures of proximal humerus (Neer's classification). Further, the greater tuberosity houses attachment of supraspinatus, infraspinatus and teres minor tendons from anterior to posterior. The lesser tuberosity houses attachment of subscapularis. These muscle attachments are responsible for displacement of tuberosities following the fracture of proximal humerus. The blood supply to proximal humerus is derived from anterior and posterior circumflex vessels. The surgical neck of humerus is closely related to axillary nerve which might get injured in fractures of proximal humerus and dislocation of shoulder. Also, the medial aspect of shoulder is closely related to brachial plexus and axillary vessels which also might get damaged in injuries of proximal humerus. X-ray of normal proximal humerus and fracture proximal humerus are shown in **Figures 10.1A and 10.1B. Figure 10.1A** also depicts various 'four' parts of proximal humerus, which are considered in Neer's classification.

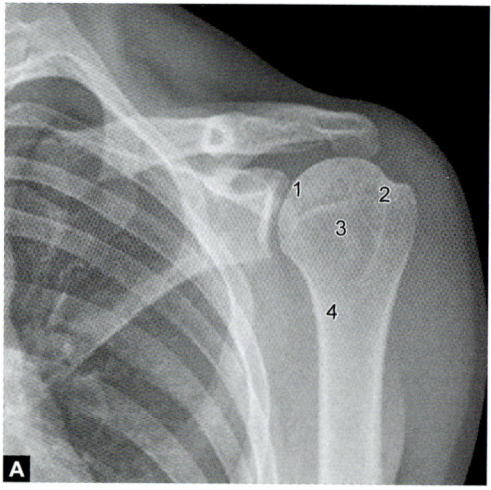 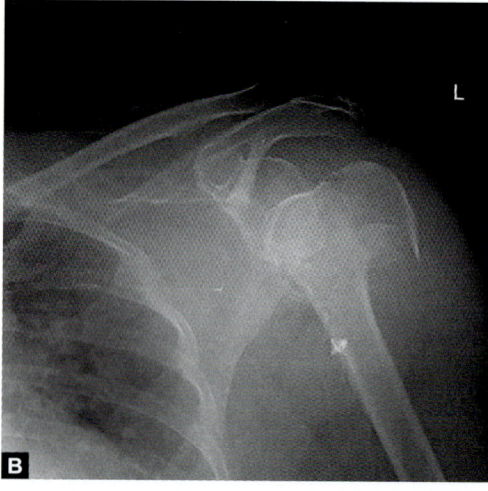

Figs. 10.1A and B: (A) Normal X-ray of left proximal humerus with *normal "four parts"*. 1. head of the humerus, 2. greater tuberosity, 3. lesser tuberosity, 4. shaft of the humerus; (B) X-ray of displaced proximal humerus #.

MECHANISM OF INJURY

The fracture of proximal humerus (PH) are observed both in young adults as well as elderly. The mechanism of injury in variable in both populations.
- **Young adult:** High velocity injury—road traffic accident (RTA), fall from height.
- **Elderly:** The PH fracture is quite common in elderly population and occurs due to fall on ground. It is often due to associated osteoporosis.

Associated injuries: They are common in high velocity injury.
- Axillary nerve injury, brachial plexus injury.
- Rarely, axillary artery injury.

CLASSIFICATION OF PROXIMAL HUMERUS FRACTURE

Neer's "Part" Classification

Neer considered various parts of the proximal humerus (head of the humerus, greater tuberosity, lesser tuberosity, and neck humerus) as a ***separate or displaced part into his classification only if the # lines running between or through these areas separated them apart either by 1 cm displacement or 45° angulation or both.***

Note: *Mere presence of fracture lines between these areas does not constitute a separate part. They need to be displaced or angulated.*

It is classified as **(Fig. 10.2)**
- One-part
- Two-part
- Three-part
- Four-part
- Fracture dislocation.

CLINICAL FEATURES

Symptoms: Pain and swelling over the shoulder and inability to move the shoulder.

Signs:
- Often, there is ecchymosis over the shoulder and arm.
- Bony tenderness is present over the proximal humerus.

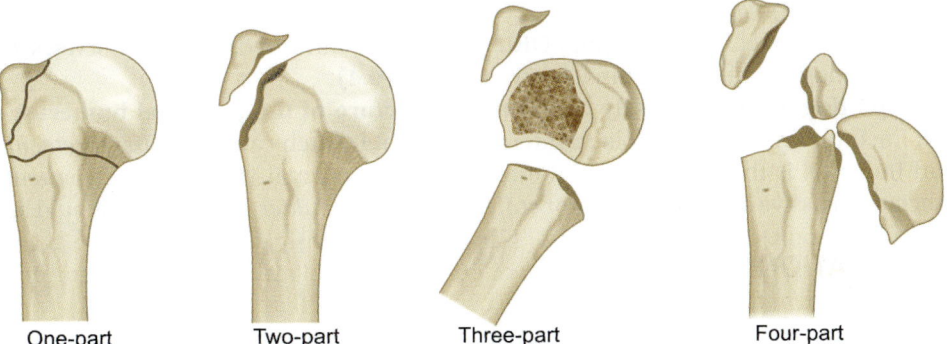

Fig. 10.2: Neer's part classification of proximal humerus fracture.

- Any attempted movements at the shoulder joint are painful.
- The neurovascular examination of the upper extremity is must to rule out injury to brachial plexus/axillary nerve or vascular injury (axillary artery injury).

INVESTIGATIONS

- **Plain X-ray of shoulder:** Various views performed are AP **(Fig. 10.3A)**, axillary and scapular-Y views. . However, axillary view might be difficult to perform in acute trauma.
- **Computed tomography (CT) scan with 3D reconstruction (Figs. 10.3B and C):** Due to the complex geometry of the proximal humerus, it is often difficult to understand the fracture pattern of the proximal humerus with a mere plain X-ray. Hence, a CT scan with 3D reconstruction is quite helpful in understanding the fracture pattern and displacement, which is further required to decide the plan of management.

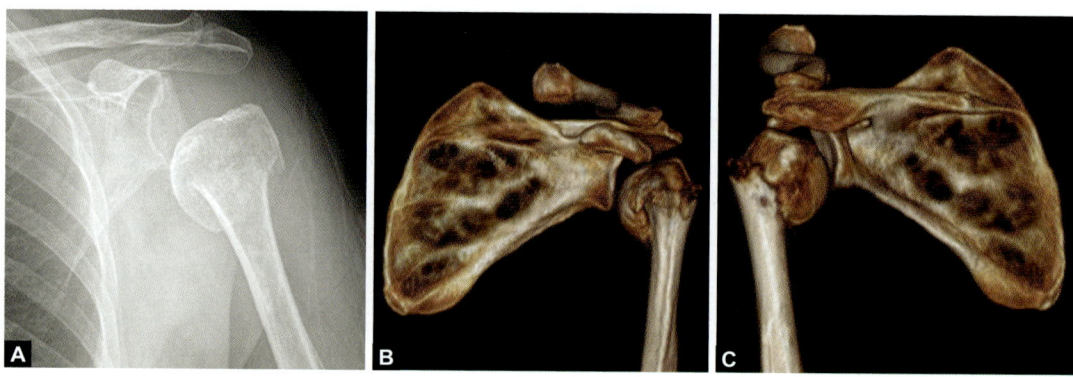

Figs. 10.3A to C: Plain X-ray and 3D CT scan of left shoulder showing comminuted fracture of the proximal humerus.

TREATMENT

The undisplaced/minimally displaced fractures can be managed conservatively, whereas displaced ones may require surgical intervention.
- **Undisplaced/minimally displaced fracture of the proximal humerus:** They are managed conservatively in an arm sling for 2–3 weeks, followed by gentle mobilization **(Flowchart 10.1)**.
- **Displaced fracture**: It often require ORIF with plates/intramedullary nail/screws/K-wires to restore anatomy of the proximal humerus **(Fig. 10.4)**.
- **Head splitting fracture/grossly comminuted fracture of the proximal humerus:** Often, such fractures are not amenable to internal fixation. In such cases, *hemireplacement* of the head humerus is the alternative if the rotator cuff is normal **(Fig. 10.5)**. In patients with associated massive irreparable rotator cuff tear, *reverse shoulder replacement* should be done.

COMPLICATIONS

- **Acute**
    - Neurovascular injury to axillary artery/axillary nerve/brachial plexus.
    - Rotator cuff tear.

Chapter 10: Fractures around the Shoulder

Flowchart 10.1: Treatment of fracture proximal humerus.

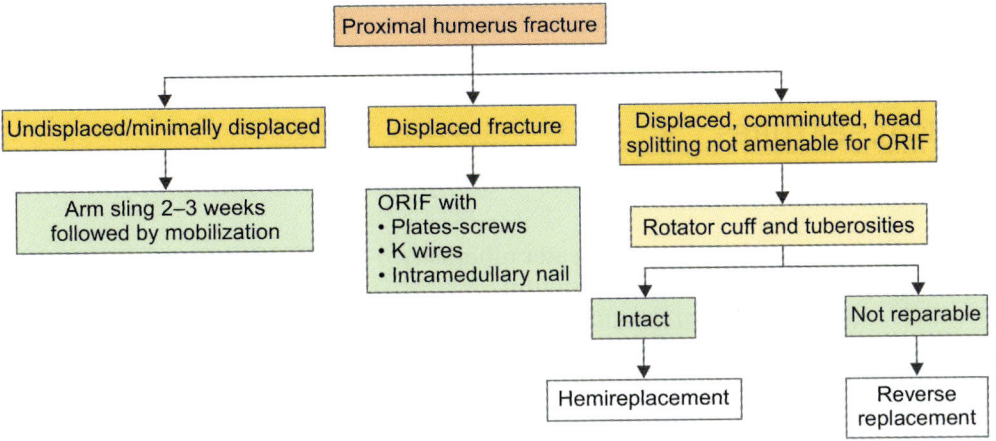

(ORIF: open reduction internal fixation)

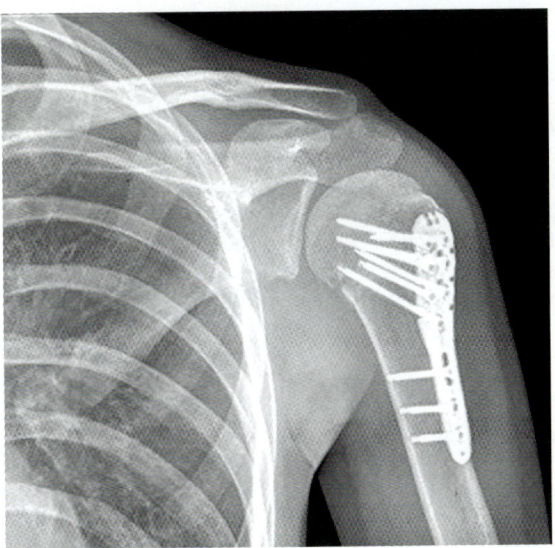

Fig. 10.4: Open reduction internal fixation of proximal humerus fracture with plate.

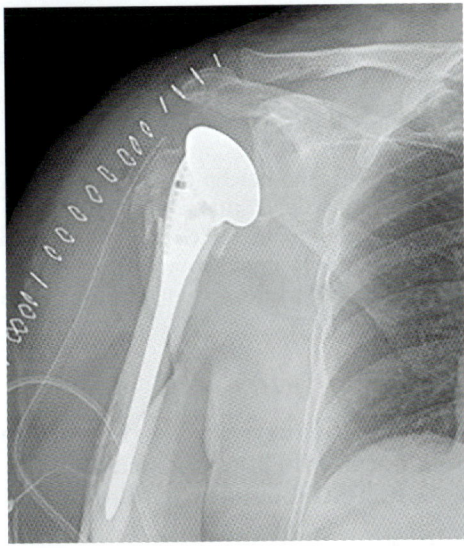

Fig. 10.5: Hemireplacement of the shoulder.

- **Chronic**
    - Malunion
    - Nonunion
    - Stiffness of shoulder
    - *Avascular necrosis of the head of the humerus*: It is a rare possibility, especially in fracture dislocations, humeral head splitting or comminuted displaced fractures of PH fracture, jeopardizing the vascularity of the head of the humerus.
    - Secondary osteoarthritis of the shoulder joint. It occurs after avascular necrosis or injury to the articular cartilage of the humerus in head split fractures.

FRACTURE GREATER TUBEROSITY OF THE HUMERUS

MECHANISM OF INJURY
Fall over the tip of shoulder/outstretched arm.

CLINICAL FEATURES
Symptoms: Pain and swelling over the shoulder and inability/difficulty to move the shoulder.

Signs:
- There is bony tenderness over the greater tuberosity.
- The movements at the shoulder are painful.
- Patient is unable to perform shoulder abduction and external rotation.
- Occasionally, greater tuberosity (GT) fracture is associated with anterior dislocation of the shoulder; hence, the symptoms and signs could be of anterior dislocation of the shoulder.
- Check neurovascular integrity of the upper limb—rule out injury to axillary nerve/brachial plexus and axillary artery.

Surgical anatomy of greater tuberosity

The greater tuberosity (GT) houses the attachment of supraspinatus, infraspinatus and teres minor from anterior to posterior, respectively, which provide abduction and external rotation to the shoulder, respectively.

Because of the attachment of these tendons over the GT, a fracture of GT could result in posterosuperior displacements of GT due to the pull of these tendons and that could result in malunion or nonunion of GT. A mal- or nonunited GT fragment would result in poor function of the shoulder in terms of loss of abduction and external rotation.

Hence, GT fractures cannot be taken for granted just being a small fragment and appropriate treatment must be planned.

INVESTIGATIONS
- **X-ray shoulder:** AP view **(Fig. 10.6)** and axillary view.
- **CT scan with 3D reconstruction**.
- **MRI/USG shoulder:** To rule out associated rotator cuff tear.

TREATMENT
The undisplaced/minimally displaced fractures can be managed conservatively, whereas displaced ones may require surgical intervention.
- **Undisplaced:** Arm sling for 3–4 weeks followed by gradual mobilization of the shoulder.
- **Displaced >5 mm or tilted/rotated >45 degrees:** Open or arthroscopic fixation of the greater tuberosity with screws **(Fig. 10.7)** or suture anchors.

COMPLICATIONS
- **Shoulder stiffness or secondary frozen shoulder**
- **Nonunion of GT:** It results in weakness in abduction and external rotation strength of the shoulder, along with loss of movements at the shoulder. It may require open reduction and internal fixation to restore the function of the shoulder.

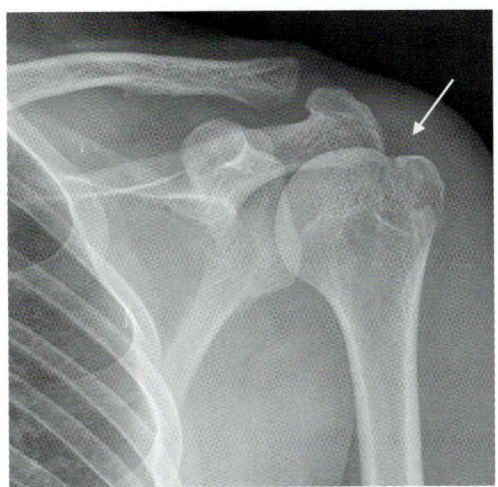 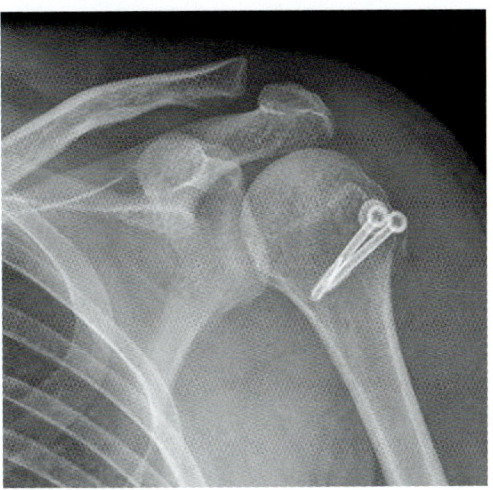

Fig. 10.6: Fracture greater tuberosity of humerus (white arrow).

Fig. 10.7: Open reduction and internal fixation of greater tuberosity with cancellous screws.

- **Malunion of GT:** It may result in painful arc syndrome, decreased shoulder strength in the abduction and external rotation, and limited movements. If the function is poor, osteotomy of malunited fragment followed by fixation in anatomic position would be required to restore function.

FRACTURE SCAPULA

Surgical anatomy: It is a flat triangular bone, which connects the upper extremity to thorax. The glenoid cavity of the scapula articulates with the head of humerus forming the glenohumeral joint. It also provides attachment to various muscle of shoulder.

Mechanism of injury: Usually fractured in *RTA/other high velocity injuries*.

Due to high velocity injury and proximity to chest, humerus and clavicle, it can result in **associated injuries** to proximal humerus, AC joint, ribs and chest. One must always rule out *brachial plexus injury and vascular injury to the axillary or subclavian vessels.*

Fracture of scapula can occur in neck of scapula, body of scapula, glenoid and other areas such as spine, acromion process and coracoid.

CLINICAL FEATURES
- Pain and swelling around shoulder and difficulty in moving shoulder.
- Bony tenderness is present over the fractured part of the scapula.
- The movements at shoulder are painful and restricted.
- *Always rule out injury to chest, spine, brachial plexus and subclavian vessels.*

INVESTIGATIONS
- **Plain X-ray of shoulder:** AP **(Fig. 10.8)**, scapular Y view.
- **CT scan with 3D reconstruction.**

Section 2: Fractures and Ligament Injuries

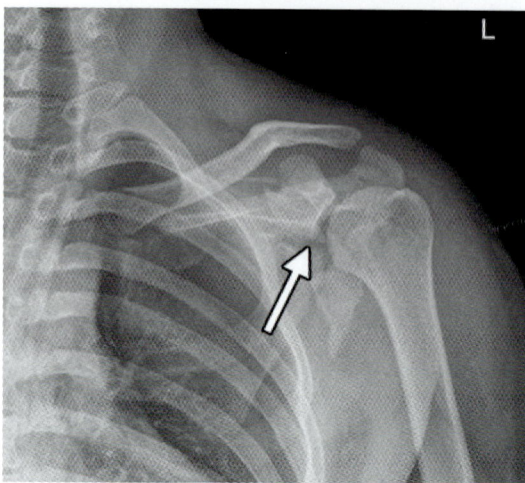

Fig. 10.8: Fracture glenoid extending into the body of scapula (white arrow).

▪ TREATMENT

The undisplaced/minimally displaced fractures can be managed conservatively, whereas displaced ones may require surgical intervention.
- **Undisplaced fracture:** Arm sling for 3 weeks, followed by shoulder mobilization and rehabilitation.
- **Displaced fracture:** ORIF with screws and plates.

Notes

CHAPTER 11

Relief of Joint Pain

▪ INTRODUCTION

Pain is one of the most common complaints in musculoskeletal disorders. Pain may arise from bone, joint, capsule, ligament, muscle, tendon or fascia.

A variety of conditions could result in joint pains, namely:
- **Traumatic:** Injury to musculoskeletal structures—fractures, dislocation, sprain, strain
- **Infective:** Pyogenic, tubercular
- **Inflammatory:** Rheumatoid, systemic lupus erythematosus (SLE), ankylosing spondylitis
- **Metabolic:** Crystal-induced arthritis—gout, pseudogout (CPPD)
- **Degenerative:** Osteoarthritis, tendinopathy, bursitis
- **Neuralgic conditions:** Nerve compression.

PATHOGENESIS OF JOINT PAIN

Stimulating the so-called 'silent nociceptors' is one-way pain is produced in joints. In healthy joints, these afferent nerve fibers are dormant. However, after tissue damage or the introduction of inflammation, these nociceptors become active and begin to transmit nociceptive information to the brain. This additional input from the periphery by the 'silent nociceptors' is one of the contributing factors responsible for the generation of arthritis pain. A different process that initiates arthritis pain is peripheral sensitization, wherein the activation threshold of joint nociceptors is reduced, and afferent nerves become hyper-responsive to both normal and noxious types of movement. Both processes come into play in chronic conditions such as osteoarthritis and rheumatoid arthritis.

▪ MANAGEMENT

The management of the pain depends upon several factors—diagnosis, duration (acute/chronic) and severity of pain. Relevant history, examination and investigations help arrive at the diagnosis.
- Treating the etiology for pain by appropriate medications, such as disease-modifying antirheumatoid drugs (DMARDs), and antitubercular therapy (ATT), itself can decrease pain.
- A pain of inflammatory/infective/traumatic origin requires analgesics with anti-inflammatory effects. In such cases, mere paracetamol may not work effectively.
- Mild moderate pain can be managed with milder analgesics (paracetamol, COX-2 inhibitors), whereas severe pain may require other NSAIDs or opioids.

As mentioned, there is a multiplicity of factors causing joint paint; hence the approach should also be multifaceted. Apart from treating etiology, the following ways can approach the management of joint pains:
- Education and lifestyle modification
- Pharmacological therapies
- Adjuvant modalities.

EDUCATION AND LIFESTYLE MODIFICATION

Patient education and lifestyle modification are the fundamental elements for relieving musculoskeletal pain.
- **Aerobic and strengthening exercises** have clear benefits with regard to both pain reduction and improved function in people with knee and hip osteoarthritis.
- **Weight loss** also reduces osteoarthritic knee pain in overweight individuals by reducing the forces that act on the joint.
- **Braces and orthotics** are also effective when used in conjunction with aerobic exercises.
- A small proportion of individuals may need **psychological/cognitive-behavioral therapies** as part of a multidisciplinary strategy.

PHARMACOLOGICAL THERAPIES

Two major drugs are used to relieve joint pain—NSAIDs and opioids.

Non-steroidal Anti-inflammatory Drugs (NSAIDs)

Unless there is a contraindication, NSAIDs remain the primary drug for relieving joint pain. Depending upon pain and/or inflammation symptoms, a wide variety of NSAIDs are used to relieve pain.

Mechanism of action—NSAIDs' primary anti-inflammatory and antinociceptive effects are due to an inhibitory effect on cyclo-oxygenase (COX) enzymes and a subsequent decrease in inflammatory prostaglandins such as PGE2 and prostacyclin.

COX enzyme has two recognised isoforms—Cyclooxygenase-1 (COX-1) and COX-2. The COX-1 enzyme controls many cellular functions, such as platelet aggregation, kidney afferent arteriole vasodilation, and acid defence of the stomach mucosa, whereas COX-2 is an enzyme produced during inflammation. The inhibition of COX-2 is the cause of the analgesic and anti-inflammatory effects of conventional NSAIDs, whereas the inhibition of COX-1 is the cause of the adverse ulcerogenic impact of NSAIDs.

Classification of NSAIDs

- **Non-selective COX inhibitor:** Aspirin, indomethacin, piroxicam, ibuprofen, naproxen and mefenamic acid.
  - All of them have potent anti-inflammatory and analgesic effects. However, side effects are prominent.
- **Preferential COX-2 inhibitor:** Diclofenac, aceclofenac, meloxicam, nimesulide.
  - These drugs have great anti-inflammatory effect.
- **Selective COX-2 inhibitor:** Celecoxib, etoricoxib.
  - They are used for mild-moderate pain and inflammation.

- **Analgesic antipyretic with poor anti-inflammatory action:** Paracetamol (acetaminophen).
  - All age groups and degenerative musculoskeletal (MSK) disorders respond well to paracetamol. The tolerance profile and overall safety record of paracetamol are generally favorable. However, it is not a great choice for inflammatory-origin pain, where NSAIDs work better.

Use: Despite all the adverse effects, NSAIDs continue to be one of the main pharmacological treatments for acute and chronic MSK pain, especially the pain due to increased inflammation (inflammatory, infective arthritis). However, their use in the long-term (>3–4 weeks) is associated with major side effects.

Adverse effects: Gastrointestinal events, including perforation, ulceration and bleeding, are a few well-documented complications. Other recognized problems include edema and renal failure.

Contraindication: History of peptic ulcer disease, gastrointestinal bleeding, renal disease, liver disease, and bleeding disorders.

Opioids

Opioids are useful when pain does not respond to NSAIDs, or the latter is contraindicated.

Classification

- **Natural:** Morphine, codiene.
- **Semi-synthetic:** Diacetylmorphine (heroin), pholcodine.
- **Synthetic:** Pethidine, pentazocine, tramadol, fentanyl, and dextropropoxyphene.

Indication: The main indication for administering opioids is individuals in whom NSAIDs is contraindicated or pain is severe and not responding to NSAIDs. Recent developments in transdermal sustained-release formulations (fentanyl, buprenorphine) have increased the safety and utility of strong opioid therapy. Transdermal fentanyl has been shown to reduce pain and improve function. However, their use should be kept limited to conditions where NSAIDs fail or cannot be used.

Adverse effects: The most common opioid side effects are constipation, nausea, vomiting, and somnolence. Addiction is reported on long-term use.

Antidepressants

Antidepressants' antinociceptive impact is independent of their antidepressant effect and occurs at lower doses and for a shorter time of treatment. Although various effects have been noted, tricyclic antidepressants (amitriptyline, nortriptyline) act to block serotonin and noradrenaline absorption and have the best antinociceptive efficacy.

Tricyclic antidepressants have positive effects in people with fibromyalgia and back pain, although their primary antinociceptive justification for use in neuropathic pain. In most musculoskeletal problems, these medications are nevertheless beneficial as adjuvant therapy and are not regarded as front-line analgesics.

ADJUVANT MODALITIES

- **Topical medications:** Topical NSAIDs have a proven efficacy across joint pains with fewer side effects than oral therapy. However, the effects are short-lived and useful for mild pain.

- **Intra-articular injections:** Currently, two intra-articular therapies are used, steroid and viscosupplementation (hyaluronic acid injection).

  Intra-articular steroid injections are widely used to control pain due to inflammation in rheumatoid arthritis (RA) and occasionally in osteoarthrosis (OA).

  Intra-articular hyaluronic acid (viscosupplementation) is a high-molecular-weight polysaccharide with myriad biological actions that has gained favor for symptomatic therapy in OA-related joint pain.
- **Transcutaneous electrical nerve stimulation (TENS):** TENS has an established general role in treating chronic pain. It is a non-invasive peripheral stimulation technique used to relieve pain. During TENS, pulsed electrical currents are delivered across the intact surface of the skin to activate underlying nerves. TENS reduces spinal stimulatory neurotransmitters (glutamate and aspartate) and, at the same time, activates modulatory opioid, serotonin and/or muscarinic receptors to reduce pain behaviors. The underlying mechanisms of action remain unclear.
- **Cryotherapy:** It works by shocking the body into controlled hypothermia. This stimulates a semi-hypothermic response. This reduces the inflammatory response of the body.
- **RICE therapy for acute joint pain:** Rest, Ice, Compression and Elevation works well for acute joint pain, especially one of a traumatic origin.

Notes

CHAPTER 12

Fracture Shaft Humerus, Supracondylar Humerus and Other Fractures around Elbow

FRACTURE SHAFT HUMERUS

■ INTRODUCTION

Humeral shaft fractures represent 3–5% of all fractures. The *fracture in mid-shaft is most common (60%) of all*. It has a bimodal distribution with a peak in third decade in men and seventh-eighth decade in women due to osteoporosis.

■ SURGICAL ANATOMY AND CLINICAL SIGNIFICANCE

The humerus shaft houses muscular attachments of many muscles such as pectoralis major, teres major, latissimus dorsi, brachialis, etc. However, clinically most significant relation lies with **radial nerve which courses posterior aspect of humerus shaft in the spiral groove**. *The radial nerve is at highest risk for injury in the spiral groove due to mid-shaft fracture humerus*. After leaving spiral groove from lateral side, the radial nerve penetrates the lateral intermuscular septum and lies in front of the septum. Coursing distally, radial nerve supplies brachioradialis and extensor carpi radialis longus. At this point, the radial nerve is quite close to the lateral aspect of lower third of shaft humerus and *is at risk of injury in lower third shaft fractures especially if latter is oblique or spiral in nature* (Holstein-Lewis fracture, Refer to page 106).

■ MECHANISM OF INJURY

The shaft of humerus fracture occurs due to direct or indirect injuries:
- **Direct trauma:**
  - Direct blow to the arm or road traffic accident (RTA).
  - Direct trauma results in comminuted fracture.
- **Indirect trauma:**
  - Fall on outstretched hand with/without rotational force to the upper limb, arm wrestling.
  - Indirect trauma results in spiral fracture, transverse/oblique fracture.

■ CLINICAL FEATURES

Symptoms
Patient complaints of pain, swelling, and deformity over the arm and inability to use upper limb.

Signs
- Gross swelling over the arm.
- Bony tenderness is present over the fracture site.
- *Always look for injury to neurovascular structures especially to radial nerve and brachial artery.* In case of radial nerve injury, the patient will have inability to dorsiflex the wrist and thumb-finger (wrist drop), and sensory loss over the dorsum of first webspace.

INVESTIGATIONS
Plain X-ray of the arm: AP, lateral view **(Fig. 12.1)**.

TREATMENT
A large majority of fracture shaft humerus can be managed conservatively due to excellent union rates. Nevertheless, lower third spiral or oblique fractures (Holstein-Lewis fracture) are almost always managed surgically due to risk of radial nerve injury during attempts of closed reduction **(Flowchart 12.1)**.
- **Conservative treatment:** More than 90% shaft humerus # can be managed conservatively by closed reduction and hanging cast or "U-slab" application **(Fig. 12.2)**.
  - *Hanging cast*: It is applied for *middle third shaft fractures which are long oblique/spiral type*. This cast is a typically an above elbow cast but *extends 1 inch above the fracture site. Since, gravity* acts as reduction and maintenance force for fracture in hanging cast, the upright or semi-upright position of patient during the treatment is must.
    (*Note:* Hanging cast is not applied in transverse fracture due to potential distraction during management).
  - *U-slab or coaptation splint:* It extends from axilla to the elbow and then extends upward up to the tip of the shoulder. It *acts by dependency traction and hydrostatic pressure* but greater stabilization and less distraction than hanging cast.
    Both the casts are removed after 2–4 weeks and it is changed to *functional arm brace* for another 6–8 weeks. During this period, elbow, wrist and shoulder mobilization is initiated.

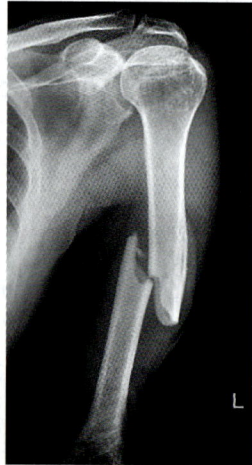

Fig. 12.1: X-ray showing fracture midshaft humerus.

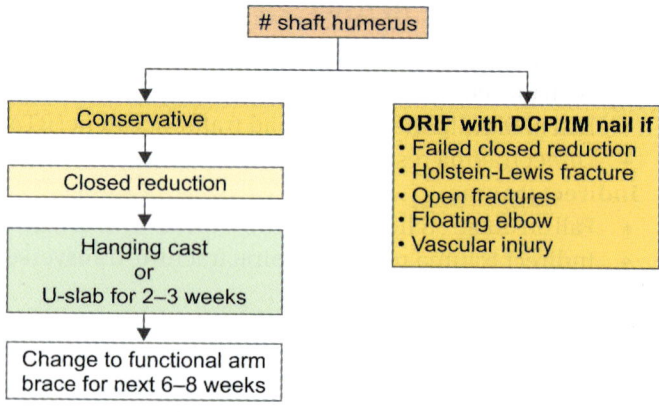

Flowchart 12.1: Treatment algorithm for fracture shaft humerus.

(ORIF: open reduction and internal fixation; DCP: dynamic compression plate; IM: intramedullary)

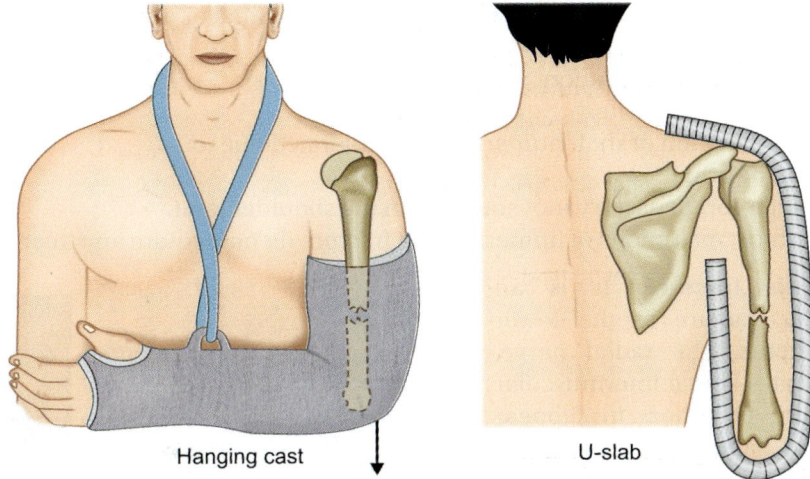

Fig. 12.2: Above elbow hanging cast (left image) and U-slab (right image) for fracture midshaft humerus. Arrow indicates gravity and weight of the arm helping reduce the fracture.

- **Operative management:** *Open reduction internal fixation (ORIF) by dynamic compression plate (DCP) or closed/open reduction and internal fixation (CRIF) by intramedullary nail.* ORIF by DCP is the most common fixation method of # humerus shaft **(Fig. 12.3)**.

COMPLICATIONS

1. **Radial nerve injury:** It is most frequently observed after mid-shaft fracture in spiral groove and lower third fracture, which is also known as Holstein-Lewis fracture (Refer **Fig. 12.4**).

    Clinical features of radial nerve palsy:
    - *Motor features:* Typically, it results in *wrist drop* wherein the patient has inability to extend *wrist joint, thumb* [at carpometacarpal (CMC), metacarpophalangeal (MCP) and interphalangeal (IP) joint] and *fingers* at MCP joints.
    - *Sensory features:* There is loss of sensation over dorsum of the first web space, which is the autonomous zone for radial nerve.

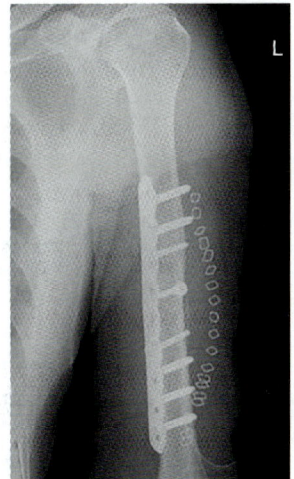

Fig. 12.3: ORIF by DCP.

MANAGEMENT

A large majority of radial nerve injury in closed fracture shaft humerus are of **neuropraxia or axonotmesis** type of nerve injury. Hence, spontaneous improvement is expected. Therefore, most patients are managed conservatively.

In cases of no or poor recovery of radial nerve after 3–4 months injury, *exploration and repair of the radial nerve (neurorrhaphy) with or without grafting* should be attempted. If repair fails or patient presents after 9 months, *modified Jones tendon transfer* should be performed (*Refer Chapter 41, page 489; Chapter 42, page 502*).

2. **Injury to the brachial artery:** More common with proximal or distal third fractures.
3. **Delayed and nonunion:** Due to
   a. Inadequate immobilization
   b. Distraction at the # site.
4. **Malunion**: Malunion of shaft humerus is well tolerated due to:
   a. Bulk of the arm
   b. Adequate compensatory movement from the shoulder joint.

   Therefore, most malunions of humerus shaft fracture do not require any treatment.

Holstein-Lewis fracture: It is an oblique/spiral fracture at the lower end of humerus. The radial nerve, which penetrates lateral intermuscular septum from posterior to appear anteriorly on lateral aspect of the humerus, is in close proximity to the tip of the distal fracture fragment or the fracture gap **(Fig. 12.4)**. Therefore, radial nerve often gets entrapped in the fracture site or might get lacerated, especially when closed reduction is attempted in such a fracture. Hence, Holstein–Lewis fracture is one such fracture of humerus which is an absolute indication for operative management by ORIF with plate as risk of radial nerve injury during closed reduction and cast application is quite high.

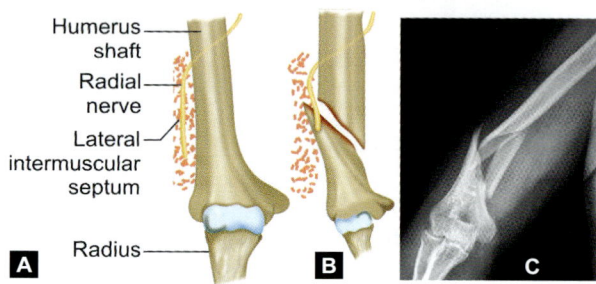

Figs. 12.4A to C: (A) Close relation of radial nerve to the lower lateral shaft of humerus; (B) Radial nerve getting trapped between two fragments of the Holstein-Lewis fracture; (C) X-ray of Holstein-Lewis fracture humerus.

FRACTURE SUPRACONDYLAR HUMERUS

INTRODUCTION

Supracondylar fracture of the elbow is the *most common fracture around elbow in children*. It accounts for more than 80% of all elbow injuries. Mostly, it occurs in children between 5–8 years old.

There are six ossification center around the elbow; four in the lower end (capitellum, trochlea, two epicondyles), one each in radial head and olecranon **(Fig. 12.5)**. **Box 12.1** mentions the age of appearance of these growth centers. The knowledge of these ossification centers are important to understand the growth pattern of the elbow and not to mistake the growth centers as a fracture.

DEFINITION

A fracture of the distal end humerus where the *fracture line runs just above the coronoid and radial fossa transversely sparing the epicondyles* **(Fig. 12.6)**.

CLASSIFICATION

There are two methods of classifying a supracondylar #, which are based upon direction of the fracture line and displacement.

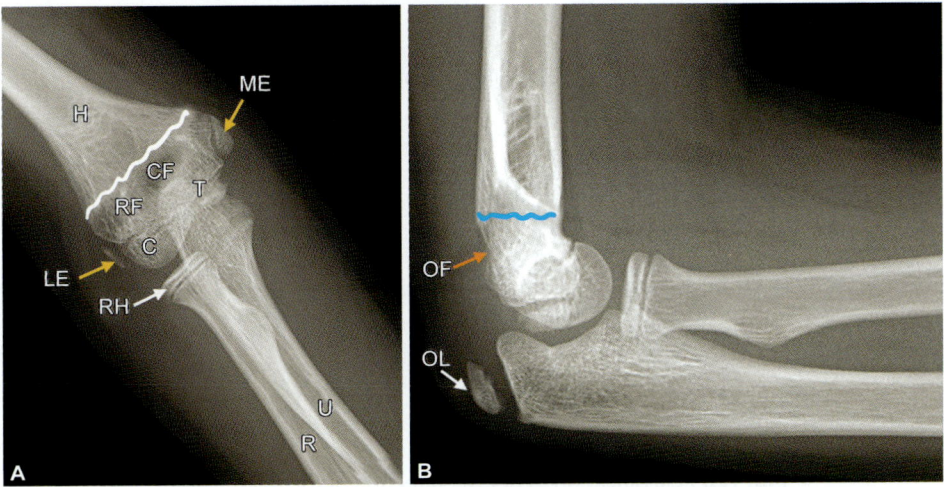

Figs. 12.5A and B: Ossification centers around the elbow. White line (AP view) and blue line (lateral view) represents area where supracondylar fracture occurs.
(LE: lateral epicondyle; ME: medial epicondyle; RH: radial head; T: trochlea; C: capitellum; RF: radial fossa; CF: coronoid fossa; OF: olecranon fossa; OL: olecranon; R: radius; U: Ulna; H: humerus)

Box 12.1: Appearance of different ossification centers (in years)—
CRITOL.

Capitulum (1); **H**ead **R**adius (3); **M**edial or **I**nternal epicondyle (5); **T**rochlea (7); **O**lecranon (9); **L**ateral epicondyle (11)

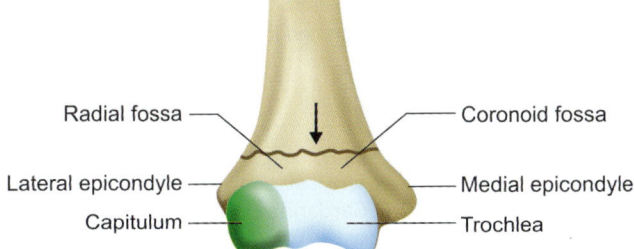

Fig. 12.6: Fracture line (black arrow) in supracondylar humerus.

A. **According to the direction of the fracture line (Fig. 12.7)**
   1. Extension type: It is the most common type (98%).
   2. Flexion type: It is quite a rare type (2%).
   Extension type: # Line runs superior to inferior and from posterior to anterior.
   Flexion type: # Line runs inferior to superior from posterior to anterior.

B. **According to the displacement of fracture: Gartland's classification (Fig. 12.8)**
   1. **Type I:** Undisplaced fracture
   2. **Type II:** Partially displaced # with intact posterior hinge
   3. **Type III:** Completely displaced fracture
   4. **Type IV:** Completely displaced fracture with instability in both flexion and extension.
      (*Note: Type IV has been recently added to the original classification*).

MECHANISM OF INJURY

Fall on the outstretched hand.

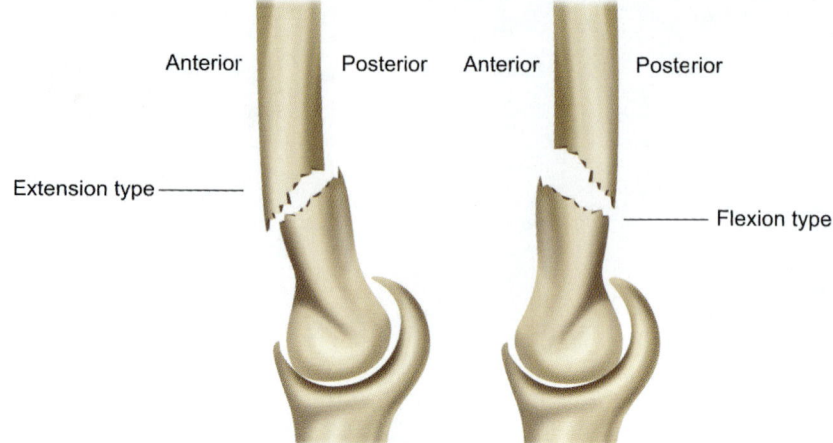

Fig. 12.7: Classification as per the direction of the fracture line.

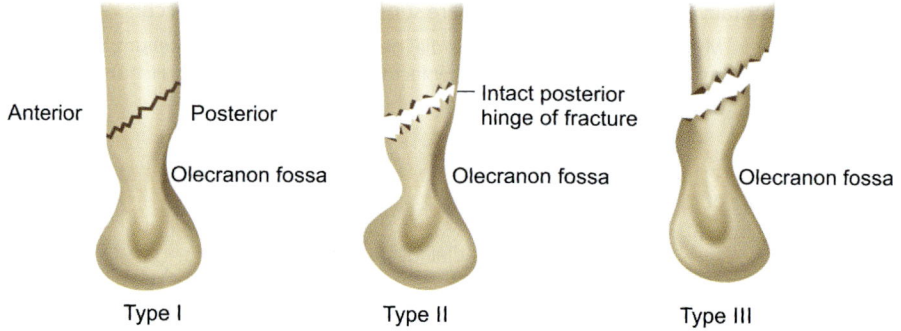

Fig. 12.8: Gartland's classification for supracondylar fracture of humerus.
Note: Type IV is not shown in the figure.

■ CLINICAL FEATURES

Symptoms

- Pain, swelling and deformity around the elbow
- Inability to use the upper limb and move the elbow.

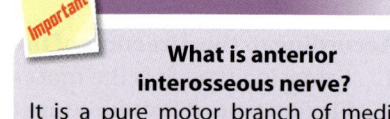

What is anterior interosseous nerve?
It is a pure motor branch of median nerve supplying flexor pollicis longus, pronator quadratus and radial two tendons of flexor digitorum profundus.

Signs

- Bony tenderness over the supracondylar region of the humerus.
- Three bony points relation is intact.
- Neurovascular examination is important as ***neurovascular deficit is not uncommon***.
    - Palpate radial and ulnar arteries.
    - Rule out any neurological injury. The common type of associated nerve injuries are mentioned below.
        - ***Extension type #:*** Anterior interosseous nerve, radial nerve.
        - ***Flexion type #:*** Ulnar nerve injury.
    - ***Always rule out compartment syndrome***.

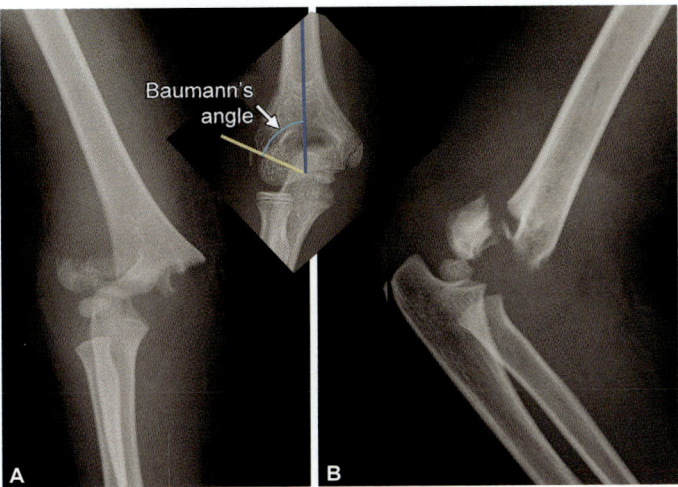

Fig. 12.9: (A) Anteroposterior and (B) lateral view of elbow X-ray showing displaced Gartland type III supracondylar fracture. Inset picture shows Baumann's angle measurement.

INVESTIGATIONS

Plain X-ray of the elbow: AP, lateral view **(Fig. 12.9)**. The classic displacement of distal fragment of the extension type supracondylar fracture are:
1. Posterior shift
2. Posterior tilt
3. Medial shift
4. Medial tilt
5. Internal rotation
6. *Altered Baumann's angle*.

Arterial Doppler of brachial vessels: If there is vascular compromise.

Baumann's angle or humeral-capitellar angle is an *angle between the humeral shaft axis and lateral condyle physis in the AP view of the elbow. The normal Baumann's angle is 65-80°.*
 Due to significant variation between two individuals, *a difference of more than 5° between the two sides is considered abnormal.*
 An increased Bauman's angle indicates malreduction of supracondylar fracture, which results in residual varus and internal rotation deformities.

TREATMENT (FLOWCHART 12.2)

The treatment of supracondylar # depends upon *two* major factors:
1. Displacement of # (according to *Gartland* classification)
2. Injury to the brachial artery/compartment syndrome.

A. **In a normal vascular limb (normal pulse, pink and warm hand), the factor in deciding treatment is "displacement."**

Flowchart 12.2: Treatment algorithm for managing a supracondylar fracture with/without vascular deficit.

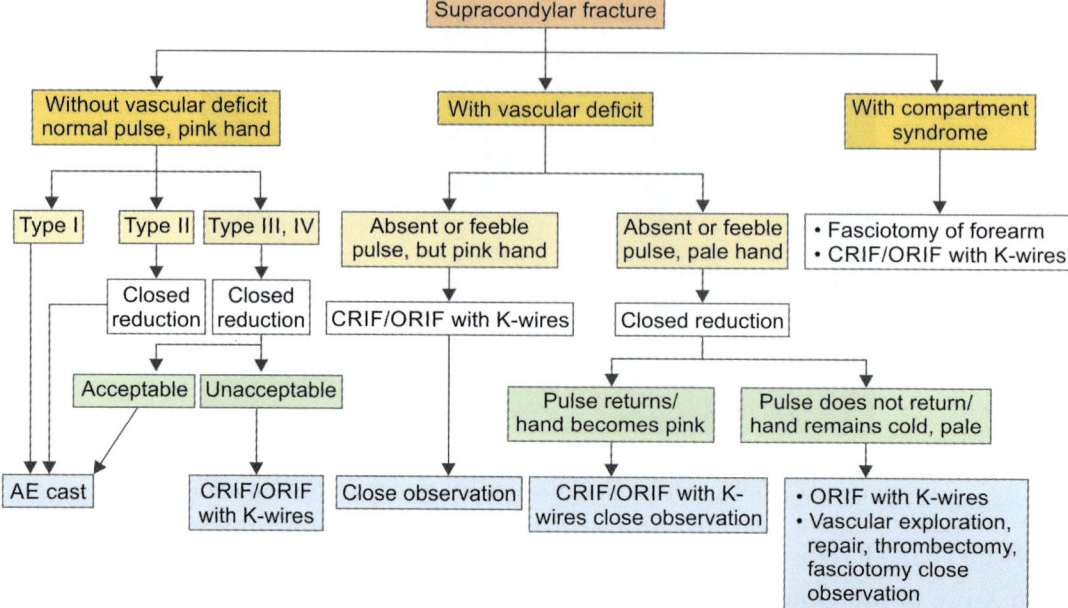

(CRIF: closed reduction and internal fixation; ORIF: open reduction and internal fixation; AE: above elbow)

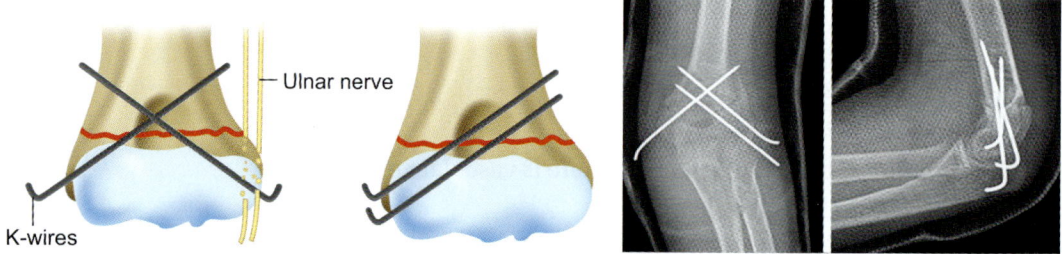

Fig. 12.10: Illustrative technique (cross K-wire from both epicondyles or only from lateral side) and X-ray showing K-wire fixation of supracondylar humerus.

- ***Gartland type 1:*** Above elbow slab application with elbow in 90° flexion for 3 weeks.
- ***Gartland type 2:*** Above elbow slab application for 3 weeks with the elbow in 100°–110° flexion (increased flexion closes the anterior opening of the fracture)
- ***Gartland type 3:*** *Closed reduction under GA and above elbow cast application*

  or

  Closed reduction under GA with K-wire fixation and above elbow slab application **(Fig. 12.10)**.
- ***Gartland type 4:*** CRIF/ORIF with K-wires

B. **Limb with an absent or feeble pulse, but with pink hand:** Immediate gentle closed reduction of fracture must be performed, followed by K-wire fixation and above elbow slab application. A pink, warm hand with adequate capillary filling, even without radial pulse indicates that the elbow collaterals are adequate, providing adequate circulation of the distal part of the limb, and therefore, there is no need for any vascular exploration. However, close observation of vascularity (capillary filling under the nail bed, color and hand temperature) must continue for several days.

C. **Limb with absent or feeble pulse with pale hand:** Immediate gentle closed reduction of fracture must be done. If hand becomes warm with adequate capillary filling, it indicates that the fracture end was kinking the vessel, jeopardizing the circulation, which has now been relieved. Then, fix the fracture with K-wires. Keep the limb under observation for several days. However, no change in distal vascularity after a gentle closed reduction, indicates that either the brachial artery is transected or thrombosed. In such a situation, the fracture site is immediately explored and managed with ORIF with K-wires. Further, the brachial artery is explored. A transected vessel is repaired, while a thrombectomy is performed for a thrombosed vessel.

Note that vascular repair is always followed by fasciotomy of the forearm to avoid reperfusion injury-induced compartment syndrome.

D. **In a limb with associated compartment syndrome:** It requires fasciotomy of forearm, ORIF of fracture with K-wires. After few days, the wound closure can be done with secondary suturing/skin graft.

Rehabilitation: After cast removal (at 3 weeks), gentle active elbow mobilization is started. Massage or forcible passive mobilization should be avoided to prevent myositis ossificans.

Special tractions required for several days old irreducible supracondylar fracture for gradual reduction

In case of SC fracture which are few days old with gross swelling, it may not be easy to perform closed reduction under GA due to swelling. Hence, occasionally traction is required to gradually reduce the fracture.
- **Dunlop traction:** Skin traction via forearm needed for gradual reduction of supracondylar fracture.
- **Smith's traction:** Olecranon pin traction needed for gradual reduction of supracondylar fracture.

However, currently, these tractions are not commonly practised.

COMPLICATIONS (BOX 12.2)

Acute Complications

- **Nerve injury**
  - *In extension type supracondylar fracture,* the chance of injury to various nerves are in order of anterior interosseous nerve > radial nerve > ulnar nerve.
  - *In flexion type supracondylar fracture,* ulnar nerve injury is more common.
- Most of the time, nerve injuries are neuropraxia or axonotmesis
- Nerve injury could also be *iatrogenic* during K-wire fixation, especially if K-wire is inserted from the ulnar side, injuring the ulnar nerve (*see* **Fig. 12.10**).

Box 12.2: Complications of supracondylar fracture humerus.

Acute
- Nerve injury
- Brachial artery injury
- Compartment syndrome

Chronic
- Volkmann ischemic contracture
- Malunion (cubitus varus deformity)
- Myositis ossificans
- Elbow stiffness
- Cubitus valgus (rare)

- **Vascular injury:** Injury to the brachial artery is not infrequent due to the sharp end of displaced fracture **(Fig. 12.11)**. Due to the displaced # fragment, the brachial artery may injured in following ways.
    - Kinking, compression or vasospasm, laceration, or transection.
    - Intimal tear followed by thrombosis.
- **Compartment syndrome/Volkmann ischemia:** It is a known complication of supracondylar fracture. *For further details, refer Chapter 23.*

Chronic Complications

A. Volkmann's ischemic contracture (VIC): It is a sequel to Volkmann's ischemia or compartment syndrome.

Pathology

Due to the ischemia of muscles and nerves during compartment syndrome, there is severe injury to the muscle mass and nerves. Mostly, *Volkmann ischemia involves deep followed by superficial volar compartment of the forearm affecting the flexor group of muscles.* In severe cases, the extensor compartment is also involved. During the recovery phase, there is *fibrosis and contracture of muscles* and *perineurial fibrosis* of the nerves. Neuromuscular affection of the forearm compartment results in major dysfunction.

Clinical features

Inspection:
- There is marked atrophy of forearm and hand muscles **(Fig. 12.12)**. Forearm skin is dry and scaly with atrophic nails.
- There may be scars around elbow and forearm of previous surgery (repair of vessel/fasciotomy).
- Flexion deformity of wrist and fingers **(Fig. 12.12)**.

Palpation:
- Features of healed supracondylar fracture, such as distal humerus bony irregularity or malunion of the fracture.
- Flexor tendons in hand-forearm are cord-like/fibrotic.
- ***Volkmann's sign positive:*** Fingers at MCP and IP joints can be extended only if the wrist is flexed due to constant length or bowstringing phenomena.

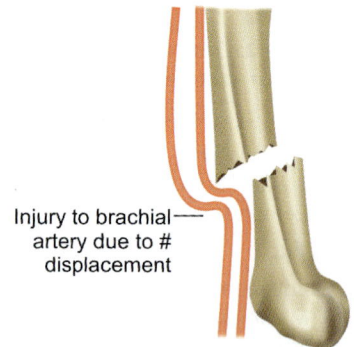

Fig. 12.11: Kinking of brachial artery due to # displacement.

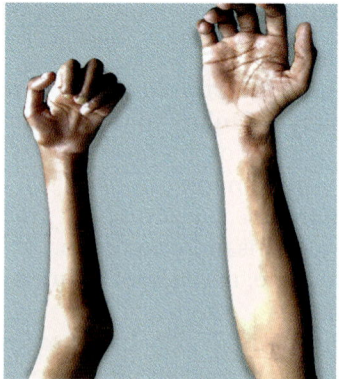

Fig. 12.12: Left forearm shows gross forearm atrophy and flexed fingers due to VIC.

Movements: The wrist and finger joints are stiff.

Neurovascular examination: Varying sensory deficit over wrist and hand due to ischemic injury to the nerves (median, ulnar). There is motor weakness in forearm and hand muscles due to damage to the median and ulnar nerve.

Investigations
- X-ray of the affected part.
- Nerve conduction velocity (NCV) of upper limb nerves.

Treatment
The treatment of VIC depends on severity of the deformity; mild, moderate or severe.
- **Mild deformity:** It is characterized by *involvement of flexor digitorum profundus and flexor pollicis longus*, which is managed by:

  Initially, conservative treatment is tried with
    - Passive stretching of contracted muscles
    - Splintage in a functional position

  However, If there is no response to conservative treatment, surgical treatment is opted
    - *Maxpage 'flexor-pronator muscle slide' surgery* can be performed, wherein flexor-pronator muscles are released from the medial epicondyle and slid distally resulting in improved finger-wrist extension.
    - Neurolysis of the nerves
- **Moderate deformity:** It is characterized by *involvement of entire flexor compartment and nerve damage*, which requires:
    - Maxpage soft tissue sliding surgery
    - Excision of the scarred tendons, neurolysis of involved nerves
    - Tendon transfers
    - Rarely; bone shortening, proximal row carpectomy.
- **Severe deformity:** This stage is characterized by gross damage to the muscles of both extensor and flexor compartment and nerves, which requires multiple-stage reconstruction in the form of:
    - Free muscle transfer
    - Nerve grafting and reconstruction
    - Flap coverage of skin.

B. Malunion of supracondylar fracture: Most frequently, malunited supracondylar humerus # results in **cubitus varus/gunstock deformity**. Rarely it can result in cubitus valgus deformity.

Clinical features of cubitus varus
- Cubitus varus deformity with decreased carrying angle. It is also known as *gunstock deformity* **(Fig. 12.13)**
- Three bony points (two epicondyles and tip of olecranon) relationship is normal.
- The elbow range of motion is full. There is slight hyperextension at the elbow compared to the normal elbow
- *In most cases, patients are functionally asymptomatic.* However, the deformity is *cosmetically unwanted.*

Diagnosis
X-ray of the elbow with arm and forearm: AP and lateral view.

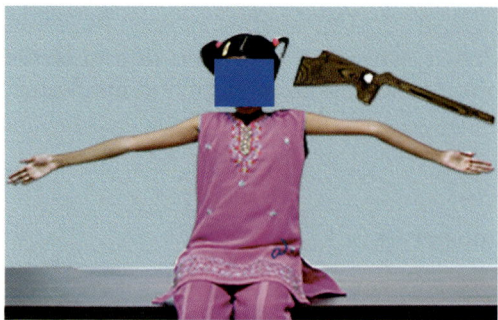

Fig. 12.13: Cubitus varus/gunstock deformity of the left elbow. Inset picture shows a barrel gun with gunstock. *Note: Gunstock is the wooden stock or support to which the barrel of a gun is attached usually at an angle.*

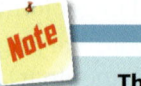

Three bony points relationship and clinical relevance

The three bony points (medial and lateral epicondyle and tip of olecranon) of the elbow form a triangle in a 90° flexed elbow, whereas they fall in a straight line in an extended elbow. Injuries, such as posterior dislocation of the elbow, displaced olecranon #, intercondylar #, and epicondylar #, disturb the relation, whereas the relationship is preserved in supracondylar #.

Treatment

- Milder deformities can be left alone
- Cosmetically unacceptable cubitus varus requires *modified French lateral closed wedge osteotomy* to correct the varus deformity.

C. Cubitus valgus deformity: Rarely malunion of fracture supracondylar humerus cause cubitus valgus deformity. The deformity per se may not be troublesome.
- However, in a progressive cubitus valgus deformity, there can be tardy ulnar nerve (TUN) palsy which may present with high ulnar nerve palsy (*refer Chapter 42*).
- The deformity per se may not require correction, but TUN palsy would require anterior ulnar nerve transposition.
- A gross valgus deformity can be corrected with corrective osteotomy.

D. Myositis ossification: *For details of myositis ossificans, refer Chapter 23.*

■ DIFFERENTIAL DIAGNOSIS

Other common injuries around the elbow, such as posterior dislocation of the elbow, lateral condyle fracture, and epicondyle fracture could be a differential diagnosis.

Table 12.1 shows the clinical difference between a supracondylar fracture and posterior dislocation of the elbow.

Table 12.1: Clinical differences between a supracondylar fracture and posterior dislocation of the elbow.		
Features	**Supracondylar fractures**	**Posterior dislocation of the elbow**
Age	Children	Usually adults
Swelling	Gross swelling around the elbow	The posterior prominence of the olecranon is observed. Minimal swelling
Bony crepitus and abnormal mobility	Felt at lower end of humerus	None
Three bony points relation	Intact	Disturbed
Shortening of	Arm	Forearm

INTERCONDYLAR FRACTURE OF HUMERUS

It is an *intra-articular fracture of the distal humerus*, wherein the fracture line involves the articulating surface of the distal humerus (capitellum/trochlea). **Figure 12.14** shows standard AP, lateral view of the elbow, and AP view of fracture intercondylar humerus.

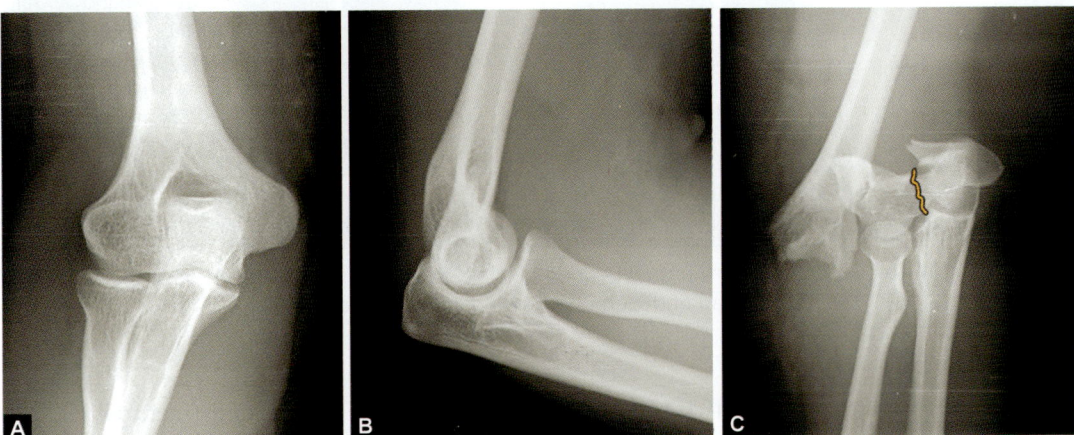

Figs. 12.14A to C: Normal elbow joint: (A) AP view; (B) Lateral view; (C) AP view showing supracondylar fracture with intercondylar extension (yellow line).

■ MECHANISM OF INJURY

Intercondylar fracture of the humerus is common in two settings—high and low-velocity injuries.
- **High-velocity injury:** It is common in young individuals after *road traffic accidents* or *fall from height*.
- **Low-velocity injury:** It is common in *older persons with osteoporosis* after a fall over the tip of the elbow.

■ CLINICAL FEATURES

Symptoms
- Pain and swelling over the elbow
- Difficulty in moving the elbow joint.

Signs
- Bony tenderness over the distal humerus
- Crepitus can be felt while moving the elbow
- In patients with high-velocity injury, there is a chance of *neurovascular injury* due to the proximity of the brachial artery, median nerve, ulnar nerve, or radial nerve with fracture fragments. Further, there is a chance of *compartment syndrome*. Therefore, a careful neurovascular examination is mandatory.

■ INVESTIGATIONS

- **X-rays of the elbow** AP and lateral view **(Figs. 12.15A and B)**
- **CT scan:** It helps understand the fracture's configuration **(Fig. 12.15C)**.

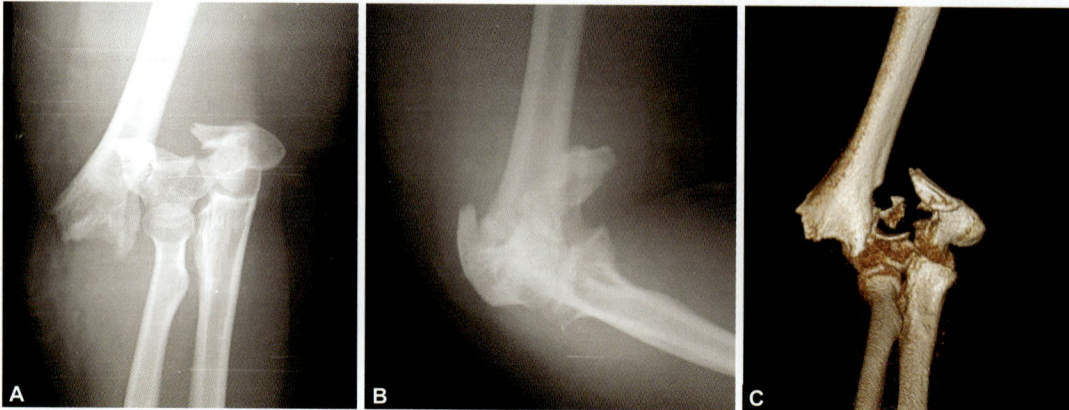

Figs. 12.15A to C: Intercondylar fracture: (A and B) Plain X-rays of AP and lateral views of the elbow; (C) 3D CT scan of the elbow showing intercondylar fracture.

TREATMENT

- **Non-operative:** Non-operative treatment is indicated for undisplaced fractures, elderly patients with displaced fractures and severe osteopenia and comminution where the fracture is not fixable, or patients with significant comorbid conditions where surgery is not possible. In such a case:
    - *Above elbow cast* is applied for six weeks, followed by rehabilitation.
    - *"Bag of bones":* It is attempted in grossly comminuted fracture, wherein after attempted reduction, the arm is placed in a collar and cuff with as much flexion as possible. The idea is to obtain a painless "pseudarthrosis," which allows motion.
- **Operative:** Like all intra-articular fractures, intercondylar fractures of the humerus should also be treated on the same principles with the restoration of the articular surface to attain a congruous joint along with rigid internal fixation.
    - ORIF with plates and screws **(Fig. 12.16)**
    - Total elbow arthroplasty: Rarely, this may be considered in markedly comminuted fractures and with fractures in osteoporotic bone.

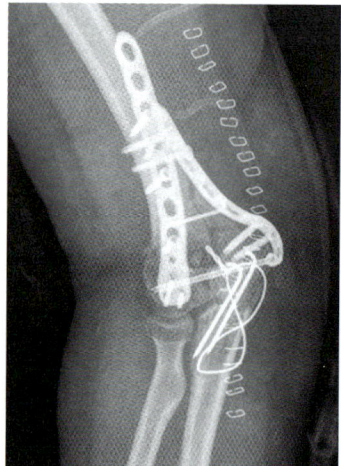

Fig.12.16: ORIF with plates and screws.

COMPLICATIONS

- **Acute**
    - Neurovascular injury
    - Compartment syndrome.
- **Chronic**
    - Stiffness (loss of motion)
    - Post-traumatic arthritis
    - Myositis ossificans.

LATERAL CONDYLE FRACTURE

Lateral condyle fractures are observed in children and is the second most common fracture of the elbow in children. It is one of the injuries, which can be *commonly missed on the plain X-ray.* Due to the pull of common extensor muscle group attachment on lateral epicondyle, *the lateral condyle fragment is often rotated and displaced.* Therefore, most lateral condyle # require surgical treatment due to tendency to rotate and displace.

■ WHAT IS A LATERAL CONDYLE?

The lateral condyle is a combination of:
- Lateral epicondyle
- Capitellum
- The lateral half of the trochlea.

■ MECHANISM OF INJURY

Fall on the outstretched hand with *varus* angulation.

■ CLASSIFICATION: 'MILCH'

It is classified into two types by Milch **(Fig. 12.17)**.
- **Milch type I:** # line is lateral to trochlear groove. It is a *type IV Salter-Harris injury.*
- **Milch type II:** # line extends into the apex of trochlear groove. It is a *type II Salter-Harris injury.*

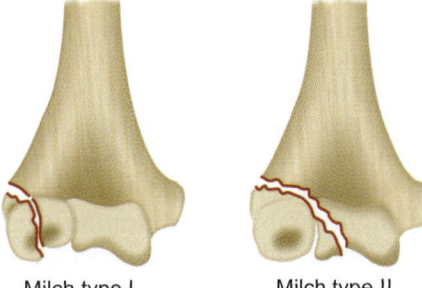

Milch type I   Milch type II

Fig. 12.17: Milch classification.

■ CLINICAL FEATURES

Symptoms
- Pain, swelling, and deformity around the elbow
- Difficulty in moving elbow.

Signs
- Tenderness present over the lateral condyle of the elbow
- Altered three bony points relation
- Painful elbow range of motion (ROM).

■ INVESTIGATIONS

Plain X-ray elbow—AP and lateral view **(Fig. 12.18)**.

■ TREATMENT

Accurate reduction of lateral condyle is a must for the symmetric growth of the elbow. Even though undisplaced fracture is managed with above elbow cast application, it tends to displace in the cast. Hence, a weekly X-ray should be performed to

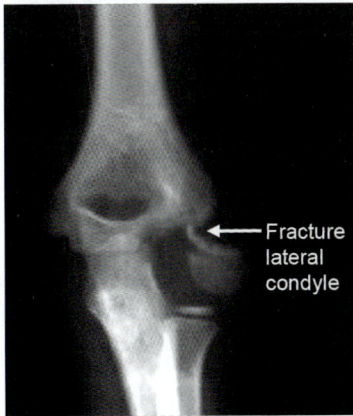

Fig. 12.18: Fracture lateral condyle.

Section 2: Fractures and Ligament Injuries

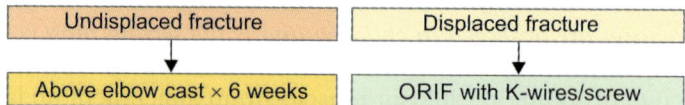

Flowchart 12.3: Lateral condyle fracture.

confirm the reduction. In case of displacement in cast or a primarily displaced fractures, it should be internally fixed. **Flowchart 12.3** summarized the treatment of the lateral condyle.

COMPLICATIONS

- **Nonunion:** It is quite common, especially in a displaced fracture of the lateral condyle. *Furthermore, nonunion may result in cubitus valgus and tardy ulnar nerve palsy.* A nonunion of the lateral condyle can be treated with open reduction and internal fixation with/without bone graft.
- **Avascular necrosis (AVN):** It can occur after surgical fixation due to disruption in blood supply. AVN can result in cubitus varus.
- Malunion
- Osteoarthritis of the elbow in late-stage if # remained malunited/nonunion/avascular necrosis (AVN). Since the lateral condyle is a part of the elbow joint, any of the above complications (malunion/nonunion/AVN) would result in elbow joint incongruity causing elbow osteoarthritis.

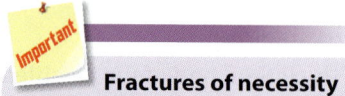

Fractures of necessity

Those fractures (#), which mostly need operative management:
- # lateral condyle (in children)
- Galeazzi and Monteggia # dislocations (in adult)
- Displaced # neck of femur

Cubitus Valgus

- *Nonunion of the lateral condyle remains the most common cause of cubitus valgus* (Fig. 12.19). Due to the nonunion of the lateral condyle, the medial side continues to develop (grow) longitudinally while the lateral growth area (lateral condyle) no longer develops longitudinally. Hence, normal medial growth and inadequate lateral growth pushes the forearm into the valgus.
- Valgus deformity per se may not be troublesome. However, a progressive cubitus valgus may result in **tardy ulnar nerve palsy**.
- The valgus deformity can be left alone if no primary cosmetic concern exists. However, a gross deformity may need medial closing wedge osteotomy to correct the deformity.

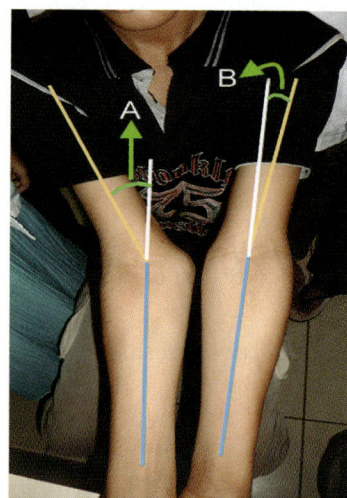

Fig. 12.19: Cubitus valgus of the right elbow. The yellow and blue lines represent arm and forearm axis, respectively whereas white line indicates the extension of forearm axis superiorly. The angle between white and yellow line indicates carrying angle, which is increased on right side (A>B).

Tardy Ulnar Nerve Palsy

Tardy ulnar nerve palsy implies "late-onset ulnar nerve palsy."

Etiology

It is most commonly associated with cubitus valgus. Occasionally, it is due to entrapment in the callus in # around the elbow.

Pathophysiology of tardy ulnar nerve palsy (TUNP) in cubitus valgus depicted in **Flowchart 12.4**.

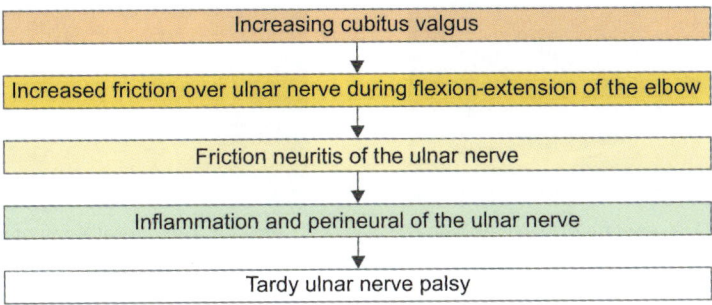

Flowchart 12.4: Pathophysiology of tardy ulnar nerve palsy.

Clinical Features

- Frequently, TUNP is associated with cubitus valgus deformity.
- Features of **high ulnar nerve weakness in the wrist and hand** are present—decreased sensation over the medial aspect of the hand, wasting of hypothenar eminence, weakness of flexor carpi ulnaris, medial two flexor digitorum profundus, interossei, medial two lumbricals, adductor pollicis, and abductor digiti minimi. Book test (Froment's sign) and card test are positive.

Investigations

- **X-ray** of the elbow (AP, lateral)
- **Nerve conduction study of the upper limb** to assess degree of damage to the ulnar nerve.

Treatment

The treatment of tardy ulnar nerve palsy is the **anterior transposition of the ulnar nerve**, i.e., ulnar nerve is translocated anterior to the medial epicondyle to avoid friction induced injury behind the medial epicondyle **(Fig. 12.20)**.

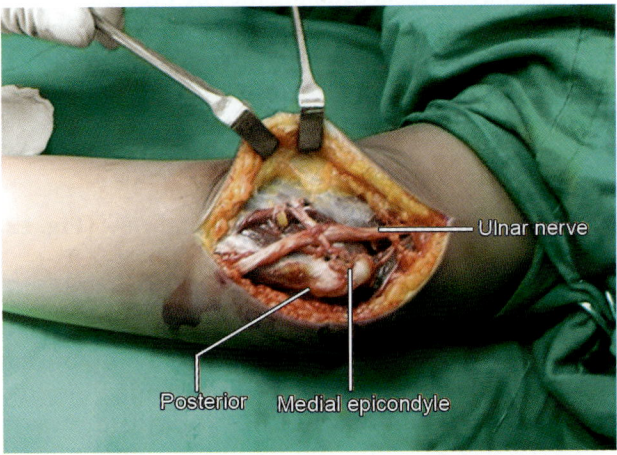

Fig. 12.20: Anterior transposition of the ulnar nerve.

FRACTURE OLECRANON

Olecranon is a curved, thick superior part of the ulna, which projects behind the elbow and houses the attachment of the triceps tendon. X-rays of a normal olecranon and fracture olecranon are shown in **Figures 12.21** and **12.22**.

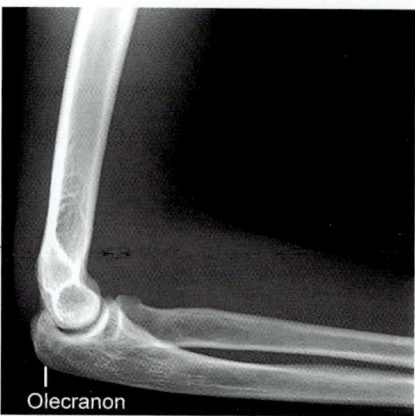

Fig. 12.21: X-ray of a normal elbow showing normal olecranon.

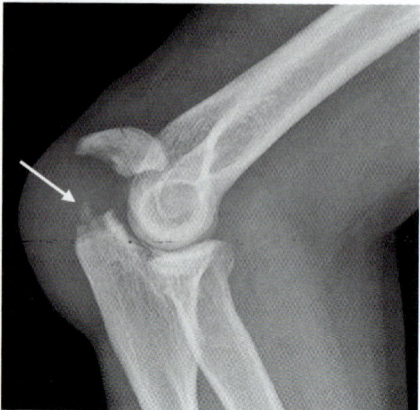

Fig. 12.22: Lateral X-ray of an elbow showing fracture olecranon.

MECHANISM OF INJURY

Fall onto the point of the elbow.

CLINICAL FEATURES

Symptoms
- Pain and swelling over the elbow
- Inability/difficulty in bending elbow.

Signs
- Swelling and local bruising may be present
- Bony tenderness is present over the olecranon
- *A gap is a palpable over the fractured olecranon*
- *Extension of the elbow against gravity is difficult*
- *Three bony points relation is altered.*

INVESTIGATION

Plain X-ray of the elbow: AP and lateral view **(Fig. 12.22)**.

TREATMENT (FLOWCHART 12.5)

Olecranon fracture is an intra-articular #. An undisplaced # is managed conservatively, whereas displaced ones require accurate open reduction and internal fixation to restore articular surface in order to avoid secondary osteoarthritis of the elbow joint. ORIF can be done by tension band wiring (TBW) or a plate.

Flowchart 12.5: Treatment of fracture olecranon.

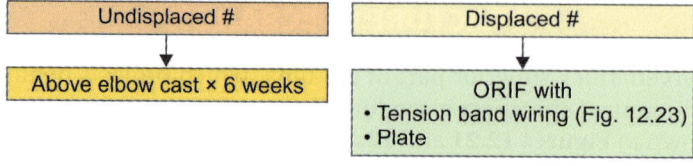

Chapter 12: Fracture Shaft Humerus, Supracondylar Humerus and Other Fractures around Elbow

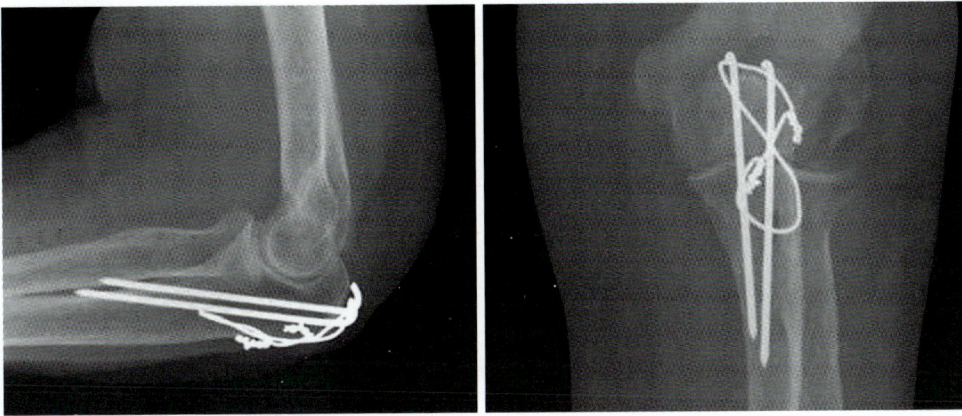

Fig. 12.23: Postoperative radiograph of the elbow showing tension band wiring of fracture olecranon.

COMPLICATIONS OF OLECRANON FRACTURE

- Loss of movement, especially active extension
- Nonunion
- Elbow stiffness
- Secondary osteoarthritis of the elbow joint.

> **What is the principle of Tension band wiring?**
> In tension band wiring, the distractive forces at the fracture site are converted into compressive forces, especially when movement is initiated.

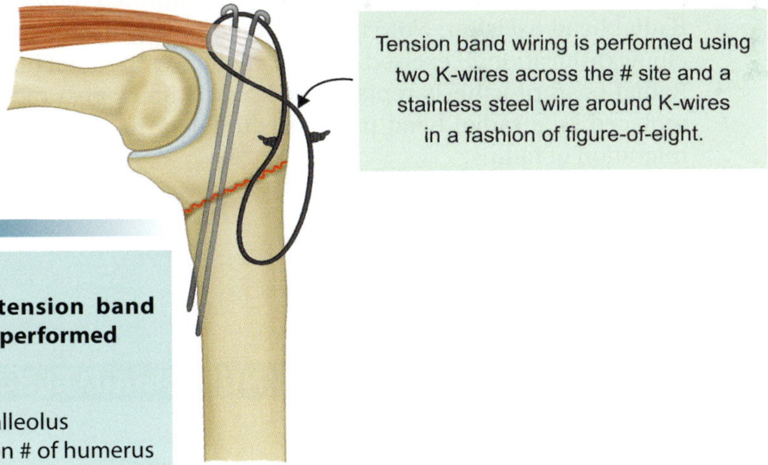

Tension band wiring is performed using two K-wires across the # site and a stainless steel wire around K-wires in a fashion of figure-of-eight.

Note

Fractures (#) for which tension band wiring (TBW) is commonly performed
- Transverse # of olecranon
- Transverse # of patella
- Transverse # of medial malleolus
- Greater tuberosity avulsion # of humerus

Fig. 12.24: Tension band wiring.

RADIAL HEAD FRACTURE

Radial head fracture can occur in isolation or during elbow. The injury can occur due to fall on the outstretched hand or road traffic accident.

CLASSIFICATION

Mason's classification
- Type 1: Undisplaced
- Type 2: Minimally displaced
- Type 3: Comminuted
- Type 4: Associated with elbow dislocation and often ulnar collateral ligament injury.

CLINICAL FEATURES

Pain, swelling and difficulty in moving elbow. There will be *bony tenderness over the radial head* and *pronation-supination is painful*.

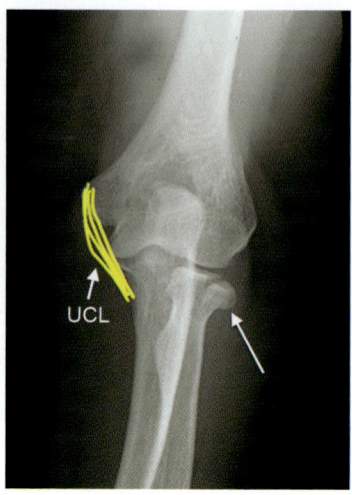

Fig. 12.25: X-ray of the elbow showing radial head fracture (white arrow).
(UCL: ulnar collateral ligament)

DIAGNOSIS

- **X-ray of the elbow:** AP, lateral **(Fig. 12.25)**
- **CT scan of the elbow:** To assess displacement and comminution.

TREATMENT

It depends upon age of patient, degree of angulation, and number of fragments and displacement.
- **Minimally displaced/angulated:** Above elbow slab × 3 weeks
- **Displaced/angulated:** ORIF with Herbert screw
- **Comminuted:** There are two options for a comminuted radial head #—
  - Radial head excision: Note that it should be avoided in acute phase in a patient with elbow dislocation. If excised acutely, replace with radial head prosthesis.
  - Radial head prosthesis replacement: Sometimes, post radial head excision, it can be replaced by a radial head prosthesis to keep the elbow stable and prevent proximal migration of radius.

COMPLICATIONS

- Elbow stiffness
- Myositis ossificans.

PULLED ELBOW (NURSEMAID ELBOW)

DEFINITION

It is a traumatic subluxation of the radial head in children between 2 and 6 years.

ETIOLOGY

It occurs when a *child is pulled with a jerk while holding the distal end of the forearm or wrist with the elbow in extension* **(Fig. 12.26)**—the radial head subluxes out of the annular ligament.

Chapter 12: Fracture Shaft Humerus, Supracondylar Humerus and Other Fractures around Elbow

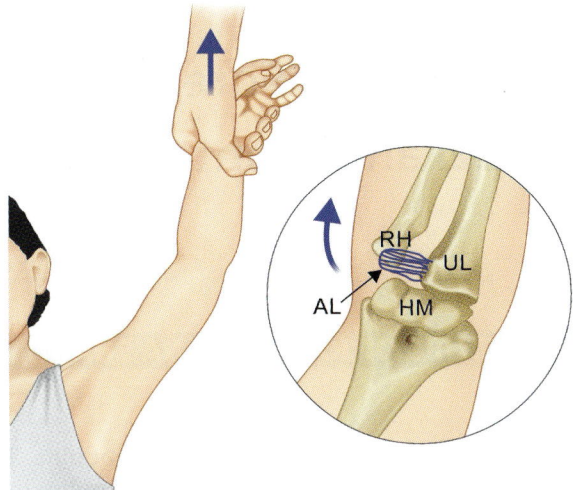

Fig. 12.26: Nursemaid or pulled elbow showing subluxation of radial head from annular ligament.
(AL: Annular ligament; RH: Radial head; UL: ulna; HM: Humerus)

CLINICAL FEATURES

The child cries incessantly and does not allow anyone to touch the upper limb. They hold the elbow in slight flexion and the forearm in pronation.

INVESTIGATION

X-ray of the elbow *almost always appears normal.*

TREATMENT

While holding the arm and elbow in one hand, the forearm is supinated with a jerk, which reduces the radial head, and the child stops crying. Sometimes, an above-elbow slab may be applied for 1–2 weeks to stabilize the radial head.

Notes

CHAPTER 13

Fracture of Forearm Bone, Galeazzi and Monteggia Fracture

FRACTURE OF RADIUS ULNA SHAFT

■ INTRODUCTION

There are two forearm bones, curved radius and almost straight ulna. Three radioulnar joint (superior, middle and inferior) join these two bones. Middle radioulnar joint is formed by interosseous membrane. Typically pronation-supination at radioulnar joints. **Figure 13.1** shows a normal forearm bone and **Figure 13.2** shows a fracture of both forearm bones. *The most worrying acute complication of forearm bone fracture is compartment syndrome.*

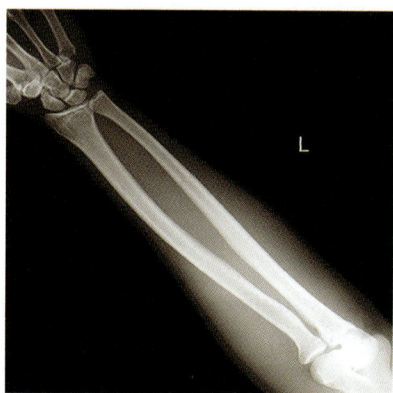

Fig. 13.1: X-ray of normal forearm bones.

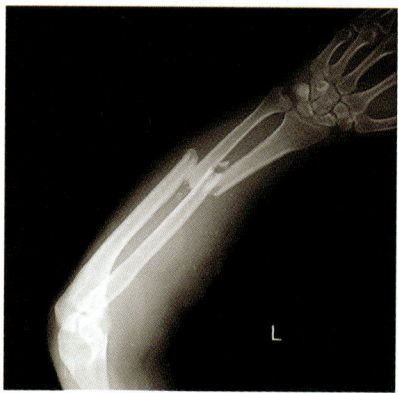

Fig. 13.2: X-ray of fracture both bones forearm.

■ MODE OF TRAUMA
- Road traffic accident (RTA)
- Fall on the ground.

■ MECHANISM OF INJURY
- Direct injury
- Fall on an outstretched hand
- Twisting injury.

■ CLINICAL FEATURES

Symptoms: Pain, swelling, and deformity in the forearm and inability to use the upper limb.

Signs
- Bony tenderness over the radius and ulna
- Loss of transmitted movement
- Neurovascular examination must be performed
- *Always watch for compartment syndrome.*

DIAGNOSIS

Plain X-ray forearm: AP and lateral view **(Fig. 13.2)**.

TREATMENT (FLOWCHART 13.1)

A. **Undisplaced #:** Above elbow cast for 10–12 weeks
B. **Displaced #:**
   - Conservative: Closed reduction is and above elbow cast application for 12 weeks if the alignment is satisfactory.
   - Operative: If alignment after closed reduction is not acceptable, plan for open reduction and internal fixation (ORIF) with dynamic compression plate (DCP).

Flowchart 13.1: Treatment algorithm for fracture both bones forearm.

(GA: general anesthesia; ORIF: open reduction and internal fixation; DCP: dynamic compression plate)

COMPLICATIONS

Acute
Compartment syndrome. It is the most significant complication of the forearm # and must be ruled out.

Chronic
- *Malunion*: It results in decreased pronation and supination
- *Cross union*: No pronation/supination
- Nonunion.

Important facts about forearm fracture management are shown in Boxes 13.1 and 13.2.

> **Box 13.1:** Points of interest while performing closed reduction of fracture both bone forearm.
>
> - While performing the closed reduction of forearm fracture, the maintenance of interosseous space is must to retain the radial bow and ulnar alignment. A maintained interosseous space helps in retaining the forearm rotational movement. Also, it prevents cross union.
> - The position of immobilization in the cast after forearm fracture reduction is in:
>   - *Supination:* For upper one-third forearm fractures
>   - *Midprone:* For middle one-third forearm fractures
>   - *Pronation:* For lower one-third forearm fractures
>
> Specific position in various areas is to negate the supinator and pronator forces of proximal and distal thirds.

> **Box 13.2:** Indication for ORIF in forearm fractures (#).
>
> - Monteggia and Galeazzi #
> - All displaced # in adults, which are unstable on closed reduction
> - All isolated displaced # radius
> - Ulnar # with angulation >10°

MONTEGGIA FRACTURE DISLOCATION

DEFINITION

Fracture of the upper third of shaft ulna with dislocation of the superior radioulnar joint (SRUJ). **Figure 13.3** shows a normal upper third forearm with elbow joint X-ray and normal SRUJ relation, while **Figure 13.4** shows an X-ray of Monteggia fracture dislocation (MFD).

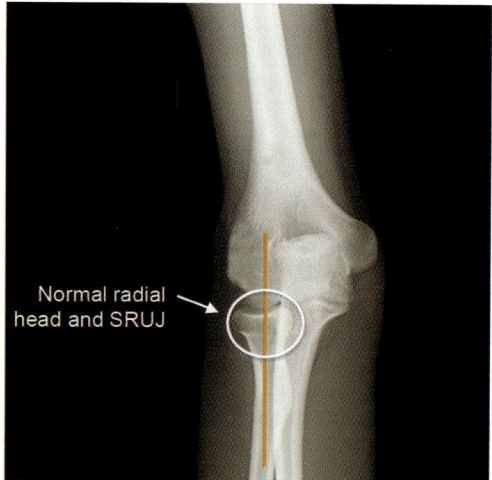

Fig. 13.3: AP view X-ray of normal upper third forearm with elbow X-ray. The brown 'radiocapitellar' line passing through radial shaft-head axis intersecting capitellum.

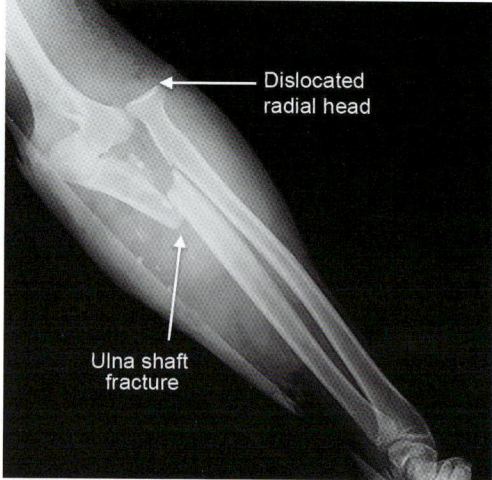

Fig. 13.4: X-ray showing Monteggia # dislocation. The radial axis line is not intersecting capitellum.

> Normal anatomical relationship between head radius and capitellum is defined by a line (brown radiocapitellar line of **Figure 13.3**), which passes via the center of shaft radius through the center of capitellum. This relation does not change in any view of X-ray. In MFD, the line does not pass through the center of capitellum indicating radial head dislocation.

■ MECHANISM OF INJURY

Fall on the outstretched hand *with forearm fully pronated.*

■ CLINICAL FEATURES

Symptoms: Pain, swelling, and deformity of the forearm and inability or difficulty in using forearm.

Signs
- Bony tenderness over the proximal ulna shaft. A fracture gap may be felt over the ulnar shaft.
- Tenderness over the radial head is present, and the radial head is dislocated.
- *Always rule out compartment syndrome*
- *Always look for posterior interosseous nerve (PIN) palsy*: PIN palsy is characterized by the inability to extend the thumb and finger metacarpophalangeal (MCP) joints.

Note: *As PIN winds around the neck of the radius, it is prone to palsy in MFD as it gets stretched due to the dislocation of the radial head* (**Fig. 13.5**).

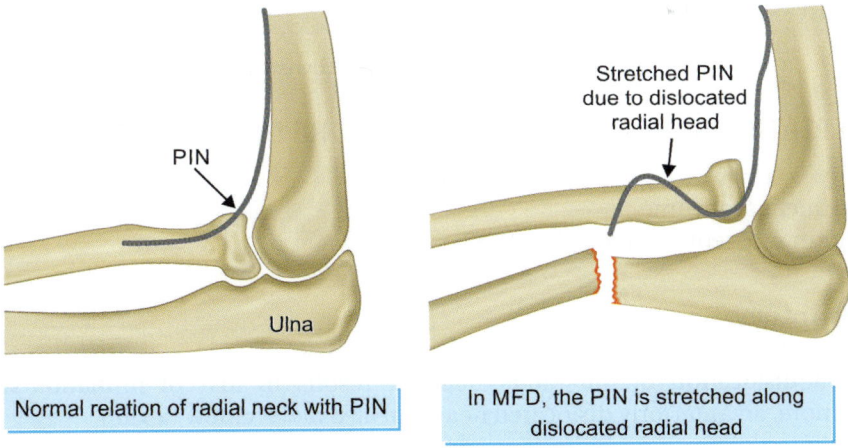

Fig. 13.5: Relation of the PIN with proximal radius, wherein PIN winds around the radial neck.
(MFD: Monteggia fracture dislocation; PIN: posterior interosseous nerve)

■ CLASSIFICATION OF MONTEGGIA FRACTURE DISLOCATION

Bado classification, which is based upon radiological finding, is used to classify Monteggia fracture-dislocation (MFD).

Bado's classification has four types, which are based on the "direction of radial head dislocation."
- Type 1: Anterior
- Type 2: Posterior
- Type 3: Lateral
- Type 4: Associated radial shaft fracture.

INVESTIGATIONS

Plain X-ray of forearm including elbow: AP, lateral view (*see* **Fig. 13.4**).

TREATMENT

The essential aspect of the treatment of MFD is restoration of ulnar shaft length. Once the length of the ulna is restored, it promptly reduces the head of the radius into the SRUJ. The MFD can be managed conservatively in children (<10 years) by closed reduction and cast application, whereas it needs ORIF in >10 years **(Flowchart 13.2)**.

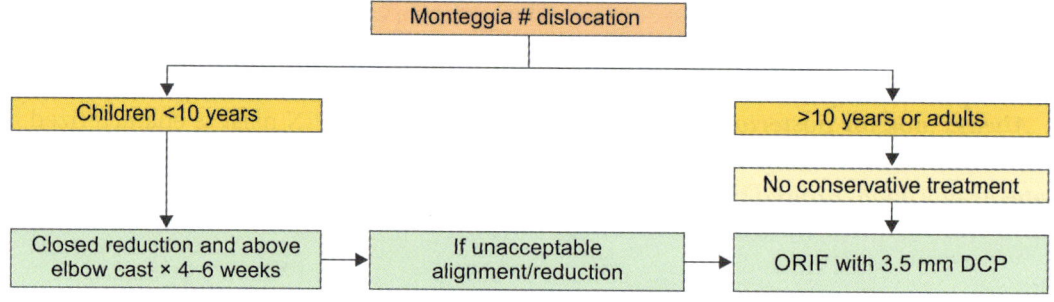

Flowchart 13.2: Algorithm to treat Monteggia fracture-dislocation.

(ORIF: open reduction and internal fixation; DCP: dynamic compression plate)

COMPLICATIONS OF MONTEGGIA FRACTURE DISLOCATION

Acute
- Compartment syndrome
- Posterior interosseous nerve palsy (PIN).

Chronic
- Malunion of ulna
- Nonunion of ulna
- Persistent dislocation of the radial head. It results in loss of pronation-supination. Furthermore, an anteriorly dislocated head can also block elbow flexion
- Elbow stiffness.

GALEAZZI FRACTURE DISLOCATION (PIEDMONT'S FRACTURE)

DEFINITION

Fracture at the junction of middle/lower one-third of radius shaft with dislocation of distal radioulnar joint (DRUJ) **(Figs. 13.6A to C)**.

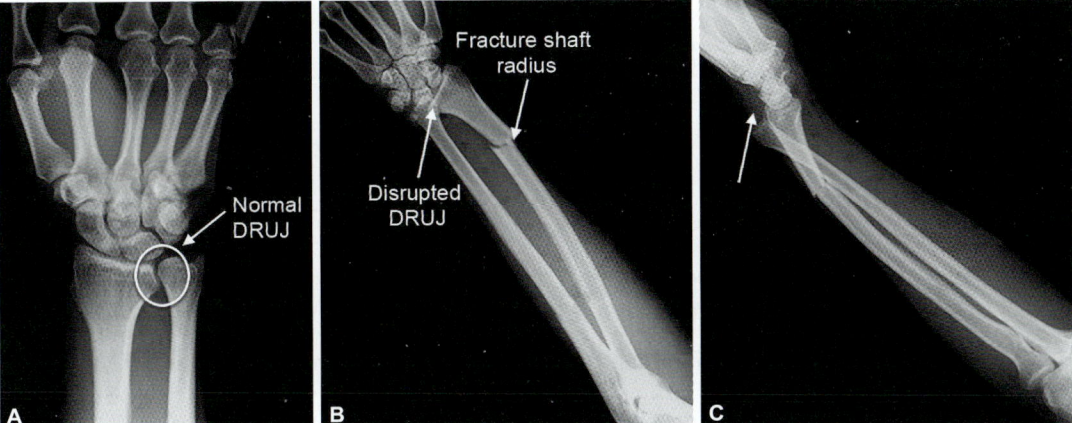

Figs. 13.6A to C: (A) Posteroanterior view of X-ray of distal forearm with wrist showing normal distal radioulnar joint (DRUJ) relation; (B and C) Showing Galeazzi fracture-dislocation in PA and lateral view (white arrow in lateral view shows dislocated DRUJ).

MECHANISM OF INJURY

Fall on the outstretched hand *with full supination* (cf MFD which occurs in pronation).

CLINICAL FEATURES

Symptoms
Pain, swelling, and deformity of the forearm and inability to use the upper limb.

Signs
- Bony tenderness is present over the distal one-third shaft radius
- Prominent distal ulna (due to dislocated DRUJ) with tenderness present over DRUJ
- Attempted movements of the wrist (dorsiflexion, palmarflexion) and forearm (pronation, supination) are painful
- Dislocated DRUJ shows a positive piano-key sign (ballottement of distal ulna). However, eliciting piano-key sign could be very painful in acute cases.

INVESTIGATIONS

Plain X-ray of forearm including wrist: PA and lateral view **(Fig. 13.6)**.

TREATMENT (FLOWCHART 13.3)

- **Patients <10 years of age:** The Galeazzi fracture-dislocation (GFD) can be managed conservatively with CR and above elbow cast application for six weeks.
- **Patients >10 years of age:** GFD should always be managed with ORIF with 3.5 mm DCP.

COMPLICATIONS

- Malunion of radius: Restricted pronation-supination
- Nonunion of radius

Section 2: Fractures and Ligament Injuries

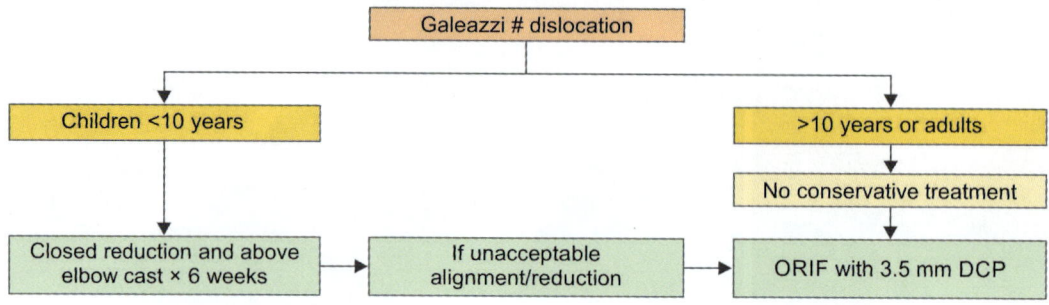

Flowchart 13.3: Algorithm to treat Galeazzi fracture-dislocation.

(ORIF: open reduction and internal fixation; DCP: dynamic compression plate)

- Persistent dislocation of DRUJ: It results in restricted and painful pronation-supination. Piano key sign is positive (the distal ulna can be balloted in anteroposterior plane with respect to the distal radius).
- Wrist pain and stiffness
- Distal radioulnar joint arthritis: It results in wrist pain and stiffness. There will be tenderness over DRUJ, and there might be crepitus during elicitation of piano key sign.

Notes

CHAPTER 14

Fractures around the Wrist and Hand

COLLES' FRACTURE

X-ray of a normal wrist and a Colles' fracture is shown in **Figures 14.1** and **14.2**.

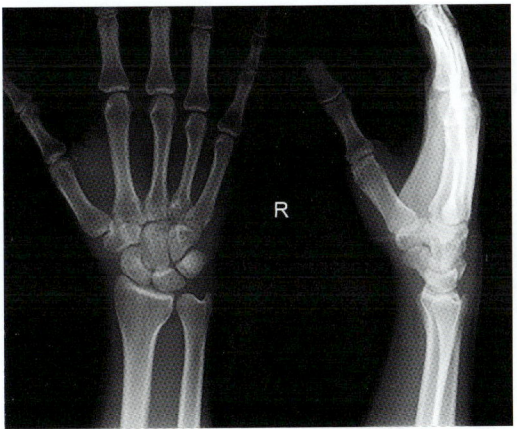

Fig. 14.1: X-ray of a normal wrist—posteroanterior (PA) and lateral view.

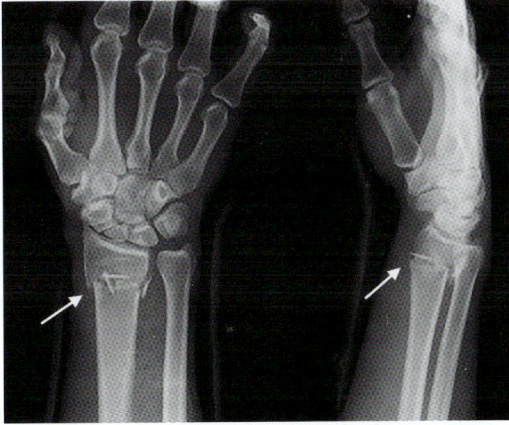

Fig. 14.2: X-ray showing Colles' fracture. Left image shows fracture in PA view (white arrow), while right image shows fracture in lateral view.

DEFINITION

Fracture of the distal end of radius, 2 cm proximal to the articular cartilage margin at corticocancellous junction, characterized by the following displacements **(Fig. 14.3)**:
- Dorsal displacement
- Dorsal tilt
- Lateral displacement
- Lateral tilt
- Supination
- Impaction.

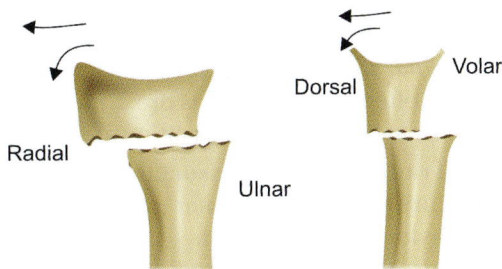

Fig. 14.3: Illustrative image showing lateral tilt and lateral displacement (left image), dorsal tilt and dorsal displacement (right image) in Colles' fracture.

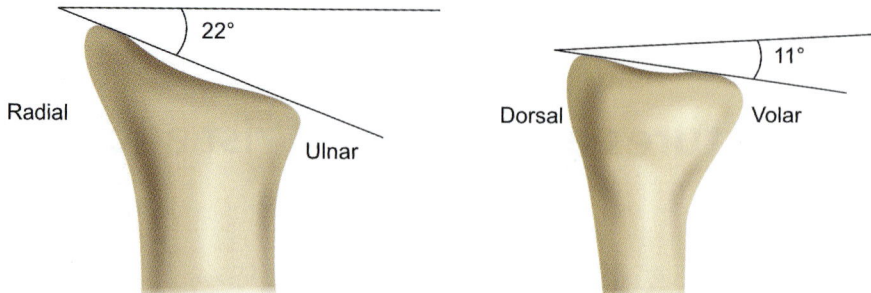

Fig. 14.4: Illustrative image showing normal angulations of the lower-end radius. Left image shows radial tilt, whereas right image shows volar tilt.

The intact distal radius has a normal volar tilt of 11° and radial tilt of 22° **(Fig. 14.4)**, which is altered after distal radius fracture. Assessment of these two angles on PA and lateral view of the wrist after the reduction of fracture helps assess accuracy of reduction.

CLINICAL FEATURES

- Colles' # is common in the *elderly* and *osteoporotic individuals*, especially females. There is a history of fall on an outstretched hand.
- Pain and swelling over the wrist, difficulty in wrist movements.

Signs
- *Dinner fork deformity* **(Fig. 14.5)**
- Bony tenderness over the distal radius
- The *relationship between the radial and ulnar styloid processes is disturbed*. Typically, *the radial styloid process is 8–14 mm distal to the ulnar styloid process*. In distal radius #, the distance between two styloid processes decreases, and often radial styloid is proximal to the ulnar styloid process.
- Although uncommon, examine for median nerve injury.

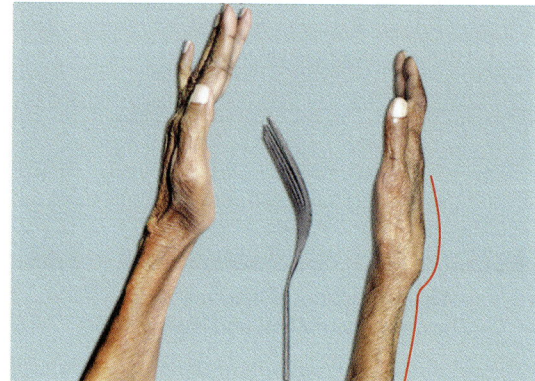

Fig. 14.5: Dinner fork deformity of right wrist; left side is normal.

Distal radius # is often associated with:
- Injury to distal radioulnar joint (DRUJ)
- # styloid process of ulna
- Injury to triangular fibrocartilage complex (TFCC) of the ulna.

INVESTIGATIONS

- **Plain X-ray:** Posteroanterior and lateral view of the wrist **(Fig. 14.2)**
- **CT scan of the wrist** can be performed in case of comminuted fracture with intra-articular extension.

TREATMENT

A large majority of Colles' fracture can be managed conservatively with closed reduction and below elbow cast application. *The typical position of below elbow Colles's cast is known as 'handshake position'* **(Fig. 14.6A)**. Few patient may require operative intervention in form of closed reduction and internal fixation (CRIF) with K-wires/ORIF with plate/external fixation **(Figs. 14.6B and C)**.

Both conservative and operative treatments for Colles' # are discussed in **Flowchart 14.1**.

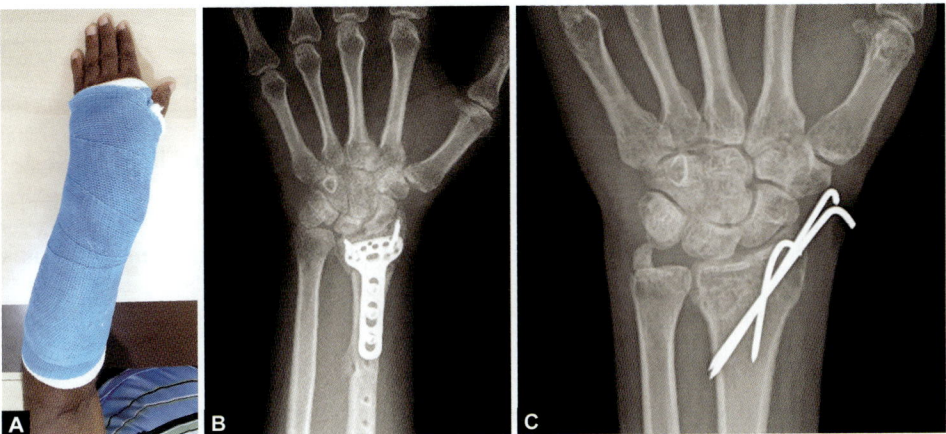

Figs. 14.6A to C: Colles' fracture: (A) Below elbow cast in handshake position; (B) ORIF and plate fixation; (C) CRIF and K-wire fixation.
(ORIF: open reduction and internal fixation; CRIF: closed reduction internal fixation)

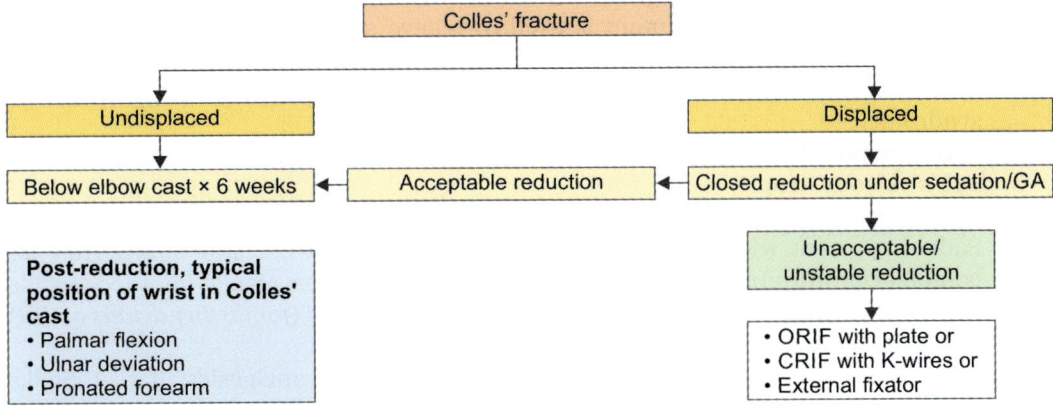

Flowchart 14.1: Algorithm to treat Colles' fracture.

(GA: general anesthesia; ORIF: open reduction and internal fixation; CRIF: closed reduction internal fixation)

Why is Colles' cast applied in a specific position?

1. Palmar flexion to counter dorsal tilt and dorsal displacement
2. Ulnar deviation to counter radial tilt and radial displacement
3. Pronated forearm to counter supination of the fragment.

Typical below elbow Colles' cast position—*handshake position*

COMPLICATIONS
- Stiffness of wrist and hand
- Malunion leading to manus valgus deformity
- Radiocarpal osteoarthritis
- Carpal tunnel syndrome
- Complex regional pain syndrome/Reflex sympathetic dystrophy/Sudeck's dystrophy
- Rupture of extensor pollicis longus tendon
- Shoulder hand syndrome
- Subluxation of distal radioulnar joint (DRUJ).

DESCRIPTION OF COMPLICATIONS OF COLLES' FRACTURE
- **Wrist and finger stiffness**
  - *Prevention:* Active movement of the fingers should be encouraged in the cast
  - *Treatment*: Physiotherapy.
- **Malunion**
  - One of the most frequent complications of Colles' #, resulting in "manus valgus deformity."
  - *Cause of malunion:* Displaced untreated fracture, poor reduction, or re-displacement after reduction.
  - *Treatment*
    - If the deformity is 'functionally asymptomatic', it may not require surgical treatment apart from physiotherapy to regain acceptable function.
    - If the deformity is causing functional deficit, [pain/decreased range of motion (ROM)], it requires a corrective osteotomy.
- **Carpal tunnel syndrome (CTS)**
  - A malunited fragment can encroach the carpal tunnel, thereby reducing space available for the median nerve causing CTS.
  - Initially, conservative treatment is tried to relieve symptoms of CTS. If there is no response, it may need carpal tunnel release by dividing flexor retinaculum. Occasionally, distal radius corrective osteotomy is required to correct malunion causing carpal tunnel syndrome.
- **Complex regional pain syndrome (CRPS)/reflex sympathetic dystrophy (RSD)/Sudeck's osteodystrophy**
  - It is observed few weeks after the treatment of the Colles (conservative or operative). Patients present with increasing pain and stiffness in wrist and hand. They also complain of burning or paresthesia in hand. Examination reveals mottled, swollen hand with painful and decreased movements of wrist-hand (*for further details of CRPS, refer Chapter 23*).
  - The treatment of CRPS is intensive physiotherapy and analgesics. Rarely, Stellate ganglion block may be tried.

  The extended form of Sudeck's dystrophy is known as shoulder hand syndrome, wherein even the shoulder becomes stiff along with stiffness of the wrist and hand.
- **Subluxation of distal radioulnar joint**
  - A subluxed DRUJ results in a decrease in ulnar deviation and forearm rotations.
  - *Treatment*: If pronation-supination is painful and decreased, *Darrach's resection* of the lower end of the ulna (2.5 cm) is performed.

- **Triangular fibrocartilage complex (TFCC) injury**
  - It results in ulnar-sided wrist pain along with weak grip strength
  - The foveal sign is positive, and ulnar deviation is painful
  - MRI is diagnostic
  - Treatment ranges from physiotherapy, wrist brace, and analgesics to surgical debridement and repair of TFCC.
- **Extensor pollicis longus (EPL) tendon rupture**
  - EPL rupture causing '*thumb drop*' is observed as a chronic complication of Colles' fracture. During the wrist movement, the dorsal callus of fracture/irregularity at the fracture site results in chronic irritation and attrition of EPL tendon resulting in EPL rupture.
  - *It is more common in "undisplaced # of the distal radius."*
  - *Treatment*: Tendon transfer "extensor indicis to EPL."
- **Radiocarpal osteoarthritis**
  - Observed after intra-articular distal radius fracture.
  - Results in painful and limited wrist ROM.

SMITH'S FRACTURE (REVERSE COLLES')

DEFINITION

Fracture of distal end radius (1" proximal to the articular surface) with lateral tilt and lateral displacement but there is ***ventral tilt and ventral displacement***, which is reverse of Colles' # (Figs. 14.7A and B).

MECHANISM OF INJURY

- Fall on the dorsum of the wrist, with the wrist in palmar flexion
- Fall on the palm with the forearm in supination with the weight of the falling body, causing the upper limb to pronate with the hand relatively fixed to the ground.

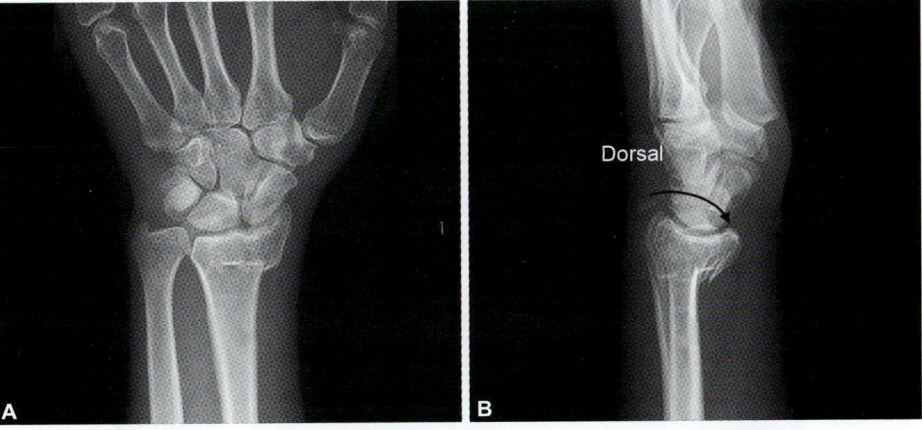

Figs. 14.7A and B: PA X-ray of the wrist: (A) Shows radial displacement, lateral X-ray; (B) Shows volar tilt and displacement. (Curved black arrow shows the ventral tilt of the distal fragment).

CLINICAL FEATURES

- Pain, swelling and deformity of the wrist
- *Reverse dinner fork deformity*
- Tenderness is present over the distal radius. *Radial and ulnar styloid process relation is altered*
- *Higher risk of median nerve compression (due to volar ward displacement of the fragment).*

INVESTIGATIONS

X-ray wrist—PA, lateral view. PA view shows lateral displacement and tilt similar to Colles' fracture **(Fig. 14.7A)**. However, lateral view shows volar tilt and volar displacement **(Fig. 14.7B)**. **CT scan** can be done in comminuted fracture with intra-articular extension.

TREATMENT

Closed reduction and below elbow cast application can be tried. If reduction is satisfactory and stable, the cast can be continued for 6–8 weeks. However, many Smith's fracture are unstable and require **ORIF with plate and screws**.

BARTON FRACTURE

DEFINITION

It is a **vertical, marginal (dorsal/volar) intra-articular** # of the distal radius in the *coronal plane* with the *displacement of entire carpal bones* along with distal fragment.

CLASSIFICATION

- **Dorsal Barton:** Fracture along the dorsal margin of the distal radius **(Fig. 14.8A)**.
- **Volar Barton:** Fracture along the volar margin of the distal radius **(Fig. 14.8B)**. *Note that Volar Barton # is more common!*

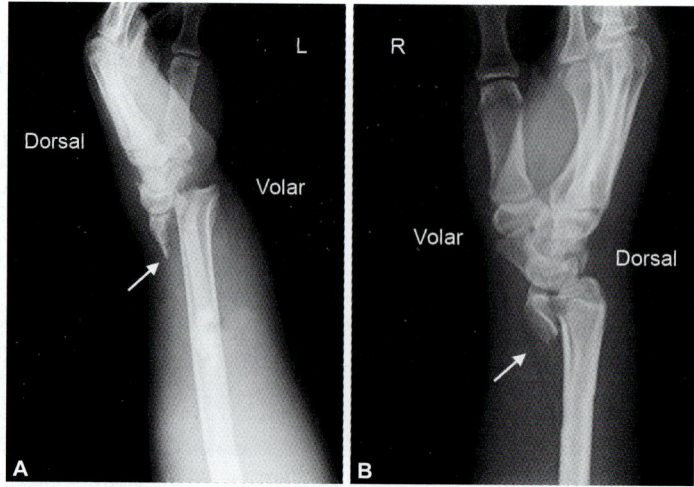

Figs. 14.8A and B: Lateral X-ray wrist showing: (A) Dorsal Barton #; (B) Volar Barton #.

MECHANISM OF INJURY
Fall on the outstretched hand.

CLINICAL FEATURES
Symptoms: Pain, swelling, and deformity around the wrist and inability to use wrist-hand.

Signs
- Bony tenderness is present over the distal radius.
- Radial and ulnar styloid process relation is altered.
- Volar Barton variant may show signs of ***median nerve compression*** as volarly displaced fragment compresses the median nerve in the carpal tunnel.

INVESTIGATIONS
X-ray of the wrist (PA and lateral view). **CT scan** is performed in case of comminuted fracture.

TREATMENT
Usually, conservative treatment is less preferred for Barton fracture in modern orthopaedics as accurate reduction and maintenance of retention in the cast is difficult and the chance of redisplacement is high. Hence, ***ORIF with plate and screws is the treatment of choice***.

CHAUFFEUR'S FRACTURE/HUTCHINSON FRACTURE/BACKFIRE FRACTURE

DEFINITION
It is an **intra-articular oblique fracture of radial styloid**. They are commonly seen in the elderly.

MECHANISM OF INJURY
Historically, it has been described to happen in situations when the *car backfired while the chauffeur was hand-cranking the car to start*. The backfire forced the crank to rapidly spin backwards out of driver's grasp and strike the back of the wrist **(Fig. 14.9)**.

It is also seen after the *fall on the outstretched hand*.

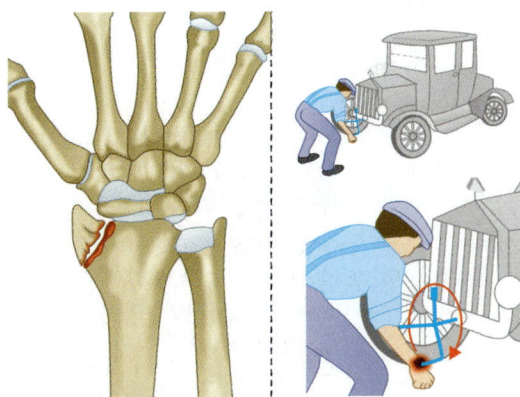

Fig. 14.9: Chauffeur fracture.

CLINICAL FEATURE AND INVESTIGATION
Pain and swelling over the wrist. Tenderness is present over the radial styloid process and wrist movements are painful. X-rays (PA and lateral view) are diagnostic.

TREATMENT
- For stable fractures—Colles' cast for six weeks.
- Unstable, displaced fracture—internal fixation with a screw.

SCAPHOID FRACTURE

Among all carpals, the scaphoid is most prone to fractures (60-70%). Before fracture scaphoid is discussed, it is important to understand blood supply of scaphoid, which has a bearing in complication of scaphoid fracture.

■ BLOOD SUPPLY TO THE SCAPHOID AND ITS APPLIED ANATOMY

The blood supply to the scaphoid is by the radial artery branches—dorsal carpal and superficial palmar. The *'dorsal carpal artery' supplies 80% of the scaphoid,* while *'superficial palmar artery' supplies 20% of the scaphoid* (Fig. 14.10).

The primary vascular supply is from the dorsal carpal branch in a ***retrograde fashion*** (distal to proximal).

Clinical significance: Since the vessels of the scaphoid enter from distal to proximal (retrograde fashion), it may get disrupted at # site, especially in waist #, which jeopardises the proximal fragment's vascularity. *Vascular compromise due to waist # may result in nonunion of waist # or avascular necrosis of proximal fragment.*

■ MECHANISM OF INJURY

Fall on the outstretched hand.

■ COMMON SITES OF FRACTURE (FIG. 14.11)

- **Proximal pole:** 20%
- **Waist:** 70%—commonest location
- **Distal pole:** 10%.

■ CLINICAL FEATURES

Symptoms
- History of fall on the outstretched hand. It is important to note that *undisplaced scaphoid # is often missed as a sprained wrist.*
- Pain and swelling over the radial aspect of the wrist and difficulty moving the wrist.

Signs
- Bony tenderness is present over the scaphoid in the anatomical snuff box
- Axial pressure along the thumb results in tenderness over the anatomical snuff box

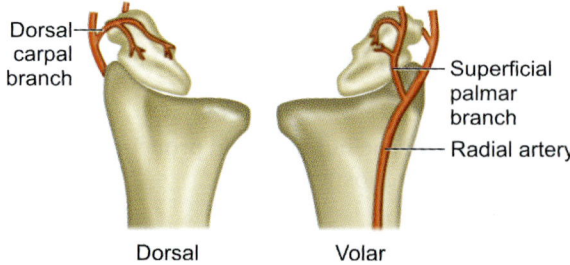

Fig. 14.10: Blood supply of the scaphoid. *Note that blood supply to the scaphoid is from distal to the proximal.*

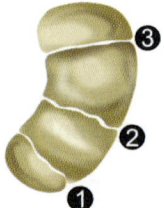

Fig. 14.11: Site of scaphoid fracture (1, proximal pole; 2, waist; 3, distal pole).

- Ulnar deviation of the wrist is painful
- Wrist movements are painful.

INVESTIGATIONS

- **X-ray wrist:** PA, lateral, oblique, ulnar deviation, and clench fist view **(Fig. 14.12)**.
- **MRI scan:** It is the most *sensitive investigation for occult fractures of scaphoid!*
- **CT scan:** It is the best modality to evaluate fracture location, angulation, displacement, and progression of nonunion or union after surgery.

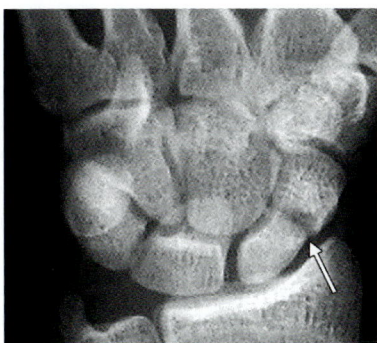

Fig. 14.12: X-ray PA view of the wrist showing scaphoid fracture (white arrow indicates fracture of scaphoid waist).

TREATMENTS

- **Undisplaced #:** Below elbow POP cast with thumb spica cast in *"glass holding position"* for 12–16 weeks **(Figs. 14.13A and B)**.
- **Displaced #:** CRIF/ORIF by *Herbert screw* (headless screw) **(Fig. 14.13C)**.

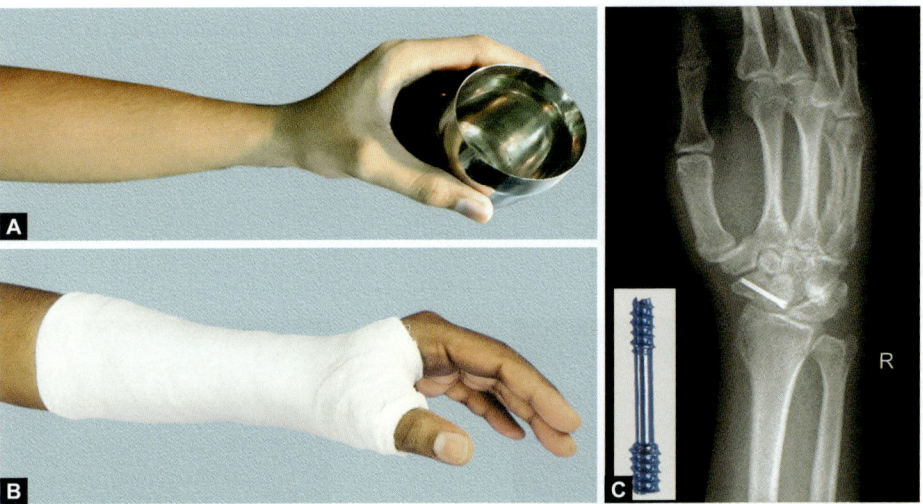

Figs. 14.13A to C: (A) Glass holding position; (B) Scaphoid cast in glass holding position; (C) Internal fixation of scaphoid fracture with Herbert screw. Inset picture shows headless Herbert screw.
(*Courtesy:* Dr Gopinath Bhandari, Consultant Hand Surgeon, Hyderabad)

COMPLICATIONS

- **Avascular necrosis:** Scaphoid #, especially at the waist may result in *avascular necrosis of the proximal fragment*. Later, osteoarthrosis of the wrist joint can ensue.
- **Nonunion or delayed union:** The nonunion or delayed union in scaphoid # is common in waist # due to peculiar blood supply (vide supra). It may require bone grafting (vascularized or non-vascularized) and internal fixation with Herbert screw.
- **Wrist osteoarthritis:** Patient presents with pain in the wrist with decreased movements and grip strength.

Section 2: Fractures and Ligament Injuries

METACARPAL AND PHALANGEAL FRACTURES

BENNETT'S FRACTURE

- **Definition:** *Oblique intra-articular fracture-dislocation of the base of the first metacarpal.*
- **Mechanism:** Usually due to axial loading while punching with flexed and adducted thumb
- **Displacement:** The *distal diaphyseal fragment is pulled laterally, proximally, and dorsally* by abductor pollicis longus, extensor pollicis longus and brevis, and adductor pollicis **(Fig. 14.14)**. The proximal fragment is held in place by ligament connecting it with trapezium.
- **Treatment:** In case of minimal displacement, CR and cast application suffice.
  However, Bennet's # remains unstable in most cases and requires CR/OR and IF with K-wire and cast application for six weeks.
- **Complications:** Osteoarthritis of the 1st CMC joint.

RONALDO'S FRACTURE

- **Definition:** *Comminuted T-shaped intra-articular fracture through the base of the first metacarpal*
- Deforming forces are similar to Bennett's #, *but diaphyseal displacement is not observed* **(Fig. 14.15)**.
- **Treatment:** Cast application or CRIF and K-wire fixation.
- **Complications:** Osteoarthritis of first CMC joint.

MALLET FINGER (BASEBALL FINGER)

- **Definition:** Finger flexion deformity caused by disruption of the terminal extensor tendon distal to the DIP joint.

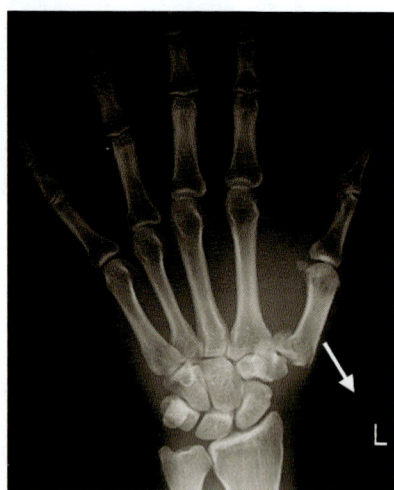

Fig. 14.14: Bennett's fracture of 1st metacarpal. White arrow shows pull of abductor pollicis longus over 1st metacarpal displacing it radially.

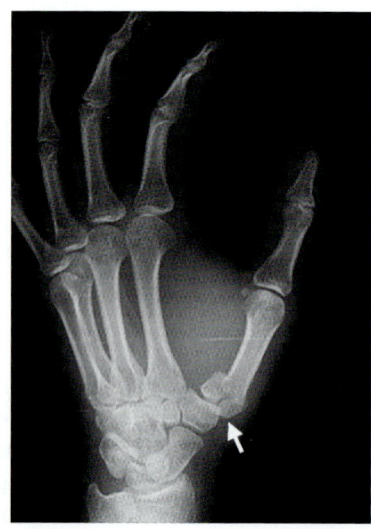

Fig. 14.15: Ronaldo's fracture T-shaped intra-articular fracture of the base.

- **Mechanism of injury:** Sudden forcible flexion of DIP on an extended finger ruptures the extensor tendon at the base of the distal phalanx.
  Sometimes, laceration over the dorsum of DIP could result in Mallet finger.
- **Types:**
  - *Bony*: Extensor tendon avulses with a piece of bone from the base of the distal phalanx.
  - *Tendinous*: Avulsion of the only extensor tendon from the base of distal phalanx.
- **Clinical features:**
  - Flexed finger deformity at DIP joint.
  - Inability to actively dorsiflex at DIP joint.
- **Investigations:** Lateral X-ray of the finger may show bony avulsion at the base of the distal phalanx **(Fig. 14.16)**.
- **Treatment:** Extension mallet splint or surgical pinning of the fragment.
- **Complications:** Stiffness and persistent flexion deformity of DIP joint.

BOXER'S FRACTURE (FIG. 14.17)

- **Definition:** *Transverse or short oblique fracture of the neck of the fifth metacarpal*
- **Mechanism:** While punching an opponent
- **Treatment:** CR and cast application/K-wire fixation.

OTHER METACARPAL FRACTURE (FIG. 14.18)

- Usually, due to road traffic accident (RTA)
- Single or multiple metacarpal #
- Multiple # could result in hand compartment syndrome
- **Treatment:** Cast application/K-wire fixation/mini plate fixation
- **Complication:** Stiffness and Sudeck's dystrophy are most common.

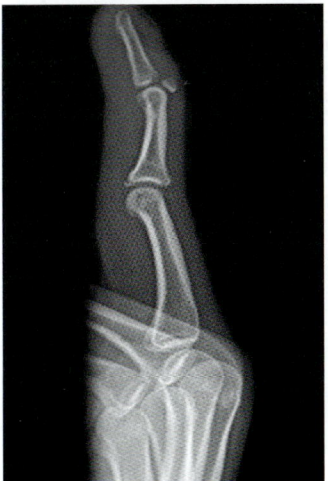

Fig. 14.16: Mallet finger.

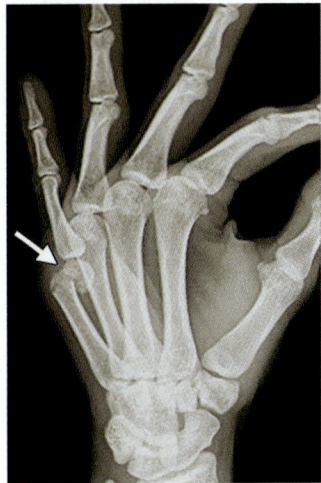

Fig. 14.17: Boxer's fracture.

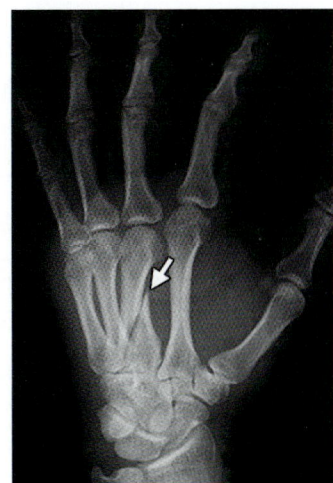

Fig. 14.18: X-ray of a metacarpal fracture.

JERSEY FINGER

- *Avulsion of flexor digitorum profundus (FDP) from the base of the distal phalanx* due to forcible hyperextension of a flexed distal phalanx
- **Treatment:** Surgical repair of FDP.

PHALANGEAL FRACTURE (FIG. 14.19)

- Usually, due to RTA/crush injury
- Single or multiple phalanx #
- **Treatment:** It can be managed in various ways, such as splintage, Buddy strapping wherein adjacent normal finger is strapped together with injured finger to provide support **(Fig. 14.20)**, or K-wire fixation.
- **Complications:** Stiffness, deformity, and malunion.

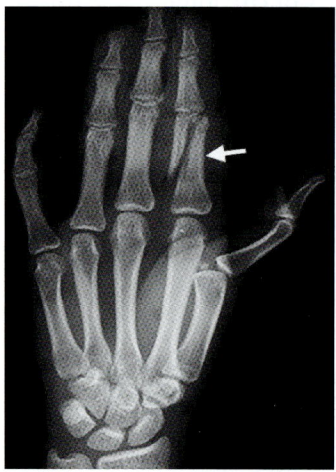

Fig. 14.19: X-ray hand showing oblique fracture of proximal phalanx of Index finger.

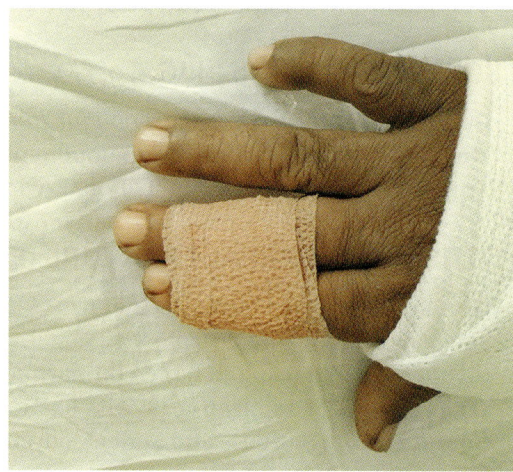

Fig. 14.20: Buddy strapping of index and middle finger.

Notes

CHAPTER 15

Fracture Pelvis

SURGICAL ANATOMY OF THE PELVIS

- **Pelvis** is formed by **two innominate bones** (each formed by ilium, ischium and pubis) and a **sacrum** form the pelvis. These bones form a "ring" along with the ligaments **(Fig. 15.1)**. The innominate bones form the pubic symphysis anteriorly and the sacroiliac joint posteriorly.
- **Pelvic girdle formed by** 5th lumbar vertebra, ilium, ischium, pubis, sacrum, and coccyx bound by capsule and ligaments.
- **The pelvic ring is formed by**—anterior and posterior arch:
    - *Anterior arch*: Pubic symphysis, pubic rami and obturator foraminae.
    - *Posterior arch*: Sacrum, two iliac wings, and two acetabula with strong sacroiliac (anterior, interosseous, and posterior) and iliolumbar ligaments.
- **Major ligaments which stabilize the pelvis are:**
    - *Anterior*: Symphyseal ligament (one each on superior, inferior, anterior and posterior aspect of pubic symphysis) resists external rotation.
    - *Pelvic floor:*
        - *Sacrospinous ligament:* Extends between ischial spine and sacrum. It resists external rotation

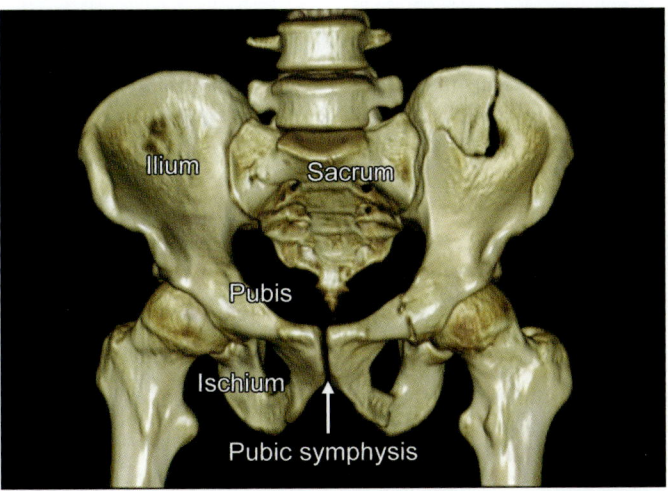

Fig. 15.1: 3D CT scan of the pelvis showing normal bones on right hemipelvis, whereas left hemipelvis shows fracture of left iliac wing and superior pubic ramus.

- *Sacrotuberous ligament:* It extends between sacrum, posterior superior iliac spine and ischial tuberosity. It resists shear and flexion.
- **Posterior sacroiliac ligament complex** comprise anterior and posterior sacroiliac ligaments, interosseous ligaments, and iliolumbar ligament. These ligaments resist external rotation, caudad-cephalad and anteroposterior shear.
- Pelvis houses many **visceral organs** from the urogenital and excretory system, **blood vessels** and **nerves**.
  - Urinary bladder, urethra, prostrate, uterus, vagina (anteriorly)
  - Rectum (posteriorly)
  - Vessels: Internal iliac vessels, superior rectal artery, gonadal vessels
  - Nerves: Lumbar plexus, sacral plexus, coccygeal plexus, and splanchnic nerves.

Hence, injury to visceral organs, vessels and nerves is frequent in the pelvis #.

MODE OF TRAUMA

Most pelvic fractures result from **high-velocity injuries** such as RTA and fall from height.

CLASSIFICATION OF PELVIS FRACTURE

There are two classifications prevalent for pelvis fracture based upon stability **(Tile's)** and mechanism of injury **(Young and Burgess)**.

1. **Tile's classification** is *based on stability of the pelvis*, which in turn is based upon the injury to the posterior arch of the pelvis resulting into a rotationally (horizontal) and vertically stable/unstable pelvis **(Table 15.1)**.
2. **Young and Burgess classification** is *based upon the mechanism of injury* **(Fig. 15.5)**. The various types of injuries are:
   - Lateral compression
   - Anteroposterior compression
   - Vertical shear
   - Combined injury.

Table 15.1: Tile's classification of fracture pelvis.

Type A (posterior arch intact)	**Stable # (rotationally and vertically)** (single break in the ring/# outside the ring) **(Fig. 15.2)**	A1	# *Not* involving the ring: Avulsions of ASIS, AIIS, and IT
		A2	Stable # of the ring
		A3	Transverse # involving sacrum/coccyx
Type B (incomplete disruption of the posterior arch)	**Rotationally unstable, vertically stable (Fig. 15.3)**	B1	External rotation instability: open book type (pubic diastasis)
		B2	Lateral compression injury Ipsilateral injury
		B3	Lateral compression injury bilateral injury
Type C (complete disruption of the posterior arch)	**Rotationally and vertically unstable (Fig. 15.4)**	C1	Unilateral injury
		C2	Bilateral injury
		C3	Associated acetabular #

(#: fracture; ASIS: anterior superior iliac spine; AIIS: anterior inferior iliac spine; IT: ischial tuberosity)

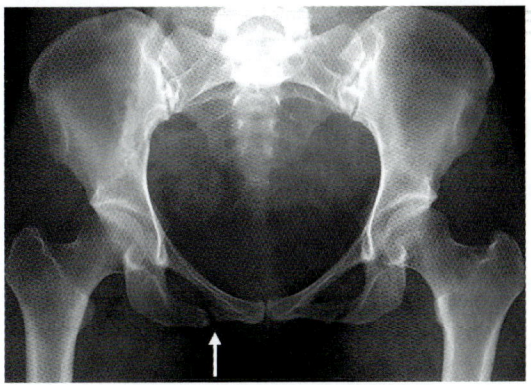

Fig. 15.2: Plain X-ray of the pelvis showing isolated inferior pubic ramus # (stable type).

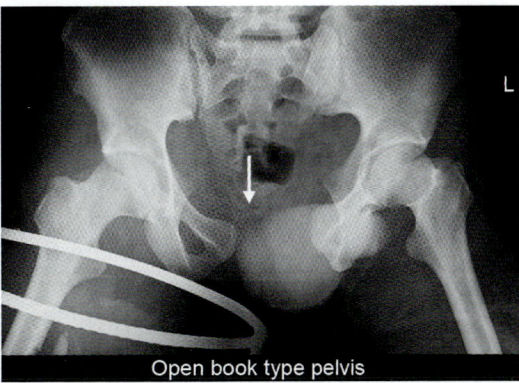

Fig. 15.3: X-ray pelvis showing open book type fracture pelvis with pubic diastasis (white arrow), which is horizontally/rotationally unstable type pelvis #.

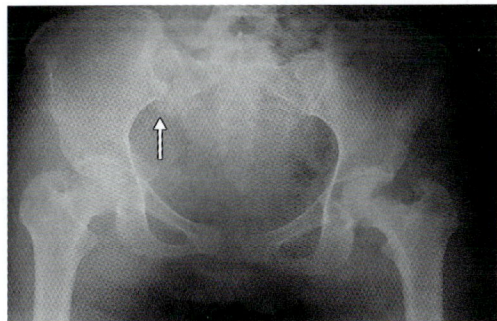

Fig. 15.4: X-ray pelvis showing horizontally and vertically unstable pelvis # (white arrow showing the superior migration of right iliac wing at SI joint indicating vertically unstable pelvis).

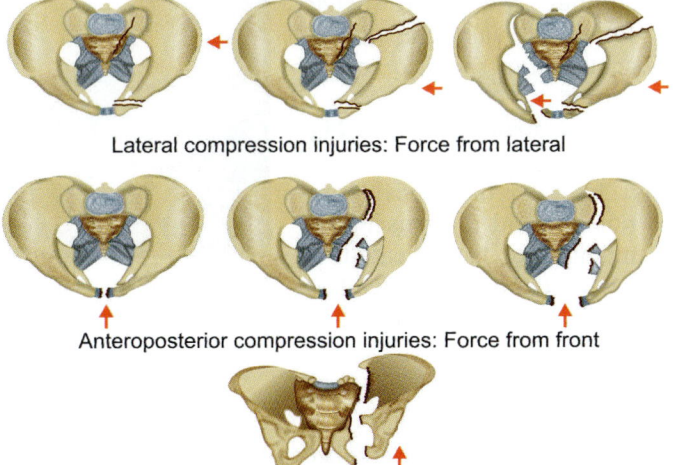

Fig. 15.5: Young and Burgess classification of fracture pelvis showing various mechanisms of injuries. Red arrows points the direction of the force.

CLINICAL FEATURES

The most significant clinical feature of a pelvis fracture is ***hemorrhagic shock and injury to the local viscera***.
- **Features pertaining systemic effect of pelvis fracture and injury to the pelvic organs**
    - *Hemorrhagic shock* is one of the most serious complications of pelvis fracture
    - *Often associated injuries* to the head, chest, spine, abdomen, and limbs as pelvis injuries are a result of high-velocity trauma
    - *Injury to visceral organs* housed in the pelvis (bladder, urethra, rectum, vagina, and uterus)
    - Abdominal distension due to pelvic bleeding, injury to abdominal or pelvis organs, or urinary extravasation
    - Blood at the tip of urethral meatus (in case of urethral injury)
    - Urine extravasation due to ruptured bladder/urethra.
- **Local features arising out of fracture of pelvis bone**
    - Swelling and tenderness over the pelvic bones
    - Inability to bear weight or perform straight leg raise
    - Pelvis compression-distraction test positive
    - Limb length discrepancy in vertically unstable fracture of the pelvis
    - Neurological examination of the lower limb is a must, as there can be damage to the femoral nerve or lumbosacral plexus in pelvic fractures.

> **Why pelvic fractures bleed and result in hypotension?**
>
> **Common source of bleeding**
> - Bleeding from posterior thin-walled venous plexus (80%)
> - Bleeding cancellous bone
>
> **Uncommon source of bleeding**
> Arterial injury (10–20%): Superior gluteal, pudendal or obturator vessels

INVESTIGATIONS

- **Plain X-ray of the pelvis:** AP view **(Fig. 15.6)**.
- **Special 'pelvis series' X-rays** of the pelvis: Inlet, outlet and obturator view. The pelvis series X-ray examines the main pelvic ring, obturator foramina, sacroiliac joints, symphysis pubis, acetabulum, sacral foramina, and the proximal femur.
- **CT scan with 3D reconstruction** (*Refer* **Fig. 15.1**).
- **CT angiography:** In case of hypovolemic shock that does not respond to resuscitative measures, CT angiography is indicated to localize the source of continuous bleeding from pelvic vessels, which could be then embolized in the same setting.

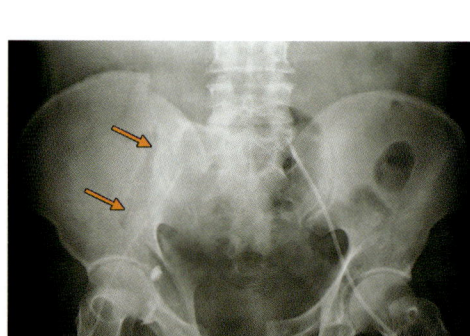

Fig. 15.6: AP view of pelvis X-ray shows pubic diastasis (blue arrows) and right ilium fracture (orange arrows).

TREATMENT

The treatment of pelvis involves primary and secondary aim. **Primary treatment** of fracture pelvis involves thorough assessment of patient, temporary stabilization of pelvis, urinary catheterization, and management of hemorragic shock. **Definitive treatment** involves managing fracture pelvis either conservatively or operatively.

Primary Treatment

- ***Assessment according to advanced trauma life support (ATLS) protocol and multidisciplinary approach:*** Since pelvis fractures result from high-velocity trauma, a thorough assessment of the patient is mandatory. Often, these patients suffer from head, chest, abdomen, and pelvic organ injuries, which require an interdisciplinary approach to manage the injured patient. Unnecessary movement of the patient should be avoided as movements may cause a further bleed in the pelvis due to disturbance of the pelvic hematoma.
- ***Pelvic sheet or pelvic binder:*** After confirmation of diagnosis, a pelvic sheet is applied over the pelvis to 'temporarily' stabilize the pelvic # **(Fig. 15.7)**. Alternatively, a pelvic binder can also be used **(Fig. 15.8)**. The temporary pelvis stability results in less movement of the pelvis, which results in stable hematoma formation over bleeding vessels and cancellous bone. Stable hematoma creates a tamponade effect over the bleeding vessels and bone, causing decreased bleeding and restoration of blood pressure.
- ***IV crystalloids and urinary catheterization:*** After a preliminary assessment of the patient is over, IV crystalloids (normal saline/ringer lactate) must be started through a wide-bore cannula to prevent/manage hypotension. If there is no contraindication for an indwelling catheter, a Foley catheter must be placed to monitor urinary output. In case of urethral rupture (contraindication for Foley), a suprapubic cystostomy should be performed.
  A hemodynamically stable patient with stable and undisplaced/minimally displaced # may not require a blood transfusion. However, those with hypovolemic shock need treatment of the same.
- ***Hypovolemic shock:*** Moderate to severe blood loss, which may result in significant morbidity and mortality, remains a significant concern after pelvic #. It is managed in various ways depending on the severity of hypotension and the cause of bleeding.
  - ***Transfusion of packed red blood cells (PRBCs), fresh frozen plasma (FFP), and platelets*** are transfused in a ratio of 1:1:1 to help counter the harmful effect of massive blood transfusion. Timely and appropriate blood transfusion is essential to control hypotension and its deleterious effects.
  - ***External fixator application over the pelvis:*** Sometimes, urgent external fixator application over the pelvis restores pelvic stability resulting in lesser bleeding, causing quicker improvement in vital parameters of the patient **(Fig. 15.9)**.

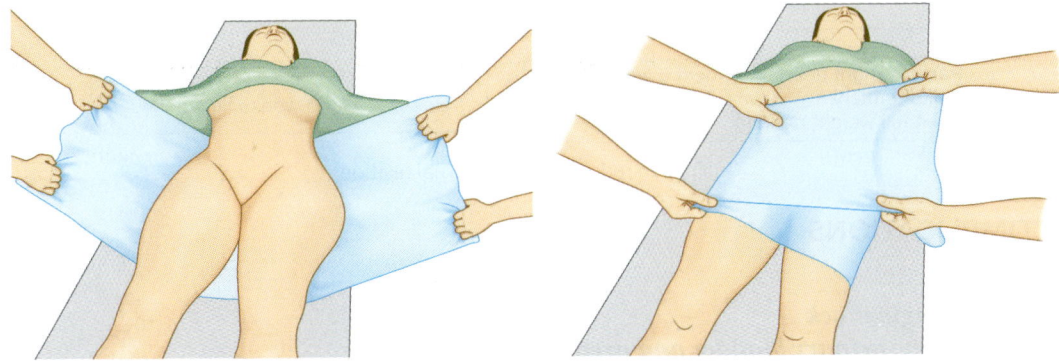

Fig. 15.7: Pelvic sheet application in patients with pelvis fracture.

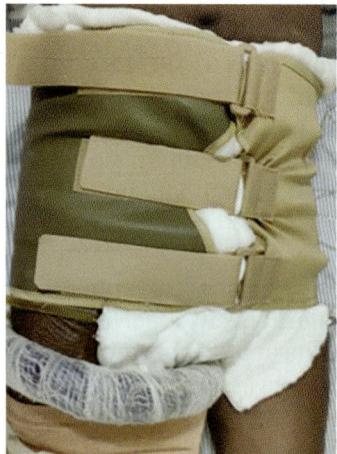

Fig. 15.8: Pelvic binder application for pelvis fracture.

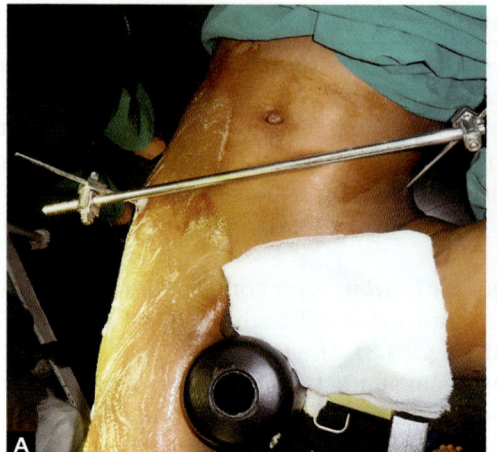

Figs. 15.9A and B: (A) Pelvis external fixator (over the iliac wing); (B) Patient is later ambulated with walker over the pelvis.

- ***CT guided selective embolization of vessels*** is very useful in controlling uncontrolled pelvic arterial bleeding and preventing hypotension.
- ***Exploratory laparotomy*** may be required to control bleeding from abdominal/pelvic organs/bleeders.

Definitive Management of Pelvic

Usually, stable pelvis fractures are managed conservatively, whereas unstable ones require operative fixation electively **(Flowchart 15.1)**. Both external fixators **(Fig. 15.9)** and ORIF with plate **(Fig. 15.10)** is used to stabilize the pelvis fracture.

Flowchart 15.1: Treatment algorithm of the pelvis fractures.

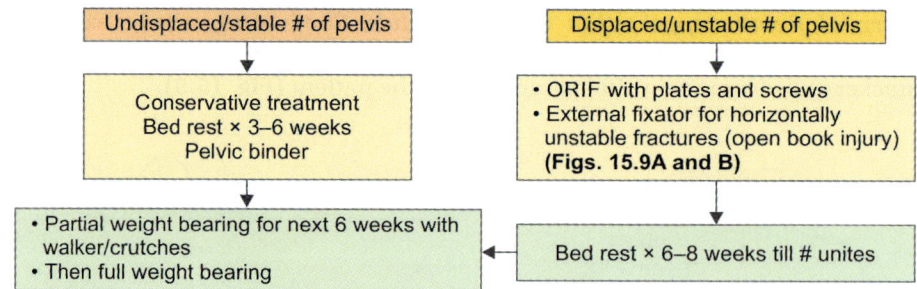

(ORIF: open reduction and internal fixation)

■ COMPLICATIONS

Acute
- ***Hemorrhagic shock***
- ***Injury to the urinary bladder and urethra***
- *Injury to other pelvic viscera*—rectum, vagina, and uterus.

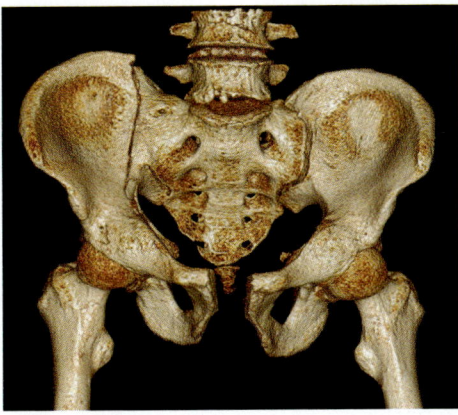 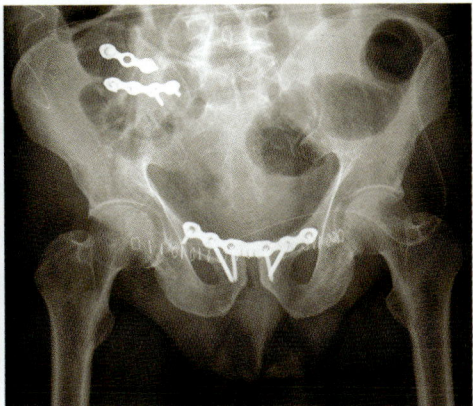

Fig. 15.10: Left image shows 3D recon image of a vertically unstable fracture pelvis (iliac wing fracture) with horizontal instability (pubic diastasis). Right image of pelvis X-ray shows open reduction and internal fixation of both vertically and horizontally unstable pelvis fracture with plates and screws.

- *Injury to neurovascular structures*—sciatic nerve, lumbosacral plexus, pudendal nerve, internal iliac vessels.
- **Morel-Lavallée lesion**: It is a closed internal degloving injury occurring deep to the subcutaneous plane due to disruption of capillaries leading to subcutaneous hemolymph and necrotic fat collection **(Fig. 15.11)**. Smaller lesions are managed conservatively, whereas larger ones require surgical debridement.

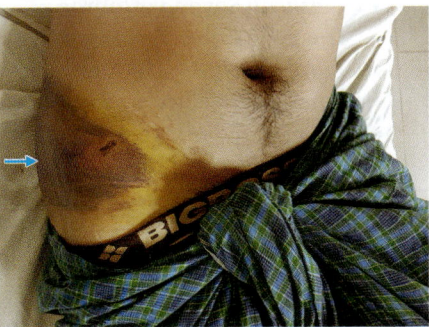

Fig. 15.11: Morel-Lavallée lesion after pelvis fracture (blue arrow).

Subacute/Chronic

- *Complications of recumbence*: Bedsore, respiratory tract infection (RTI), urinary tract infection (UTI) (due to prolonged catheterization), and deep vein thrombosis, and pulmonary thromboembolism.
- *Nonunion or malunion of fractures* may result in limb length discrepancy, especially in vertically unstable #. A malunited pelvis # may also result in obstructed labor.
- *Arthritis of the sacroiliac and hip joint if the said joints* are involved in fracture.
- *Sexual dysfunction* may occur due to injury to pelvic nerves and other associated structures.

Eponyms for fracture pelvis

- **Straddle #:** Bilateral superior and inferior pubic rami #.
- **Open book #:** Due to anterior-posterior compression injury, the pubic symphysis and SI joint is disrupted, and pelvis opens like a book.
- **Malgaigne's #:** Due to lateral compression injury, ipsilateral pubic ramus and SI joint/ilium #.
- **Bucket handle #:** Due to lateral compression injury, pubic ramus # on one side and SI joint/ilium on contralateral side.
- **Jumpers #:** Transverse # of sacrum due to fall from height in suicidal attempt.

16 CHAPTER

Injuries of the Spine and Spinal Cord

■ SURGICAL ANATOMY OF THE SPINE: RELEVANT FACTS

The anatomy of the spine can be discussed in two parts:
1. Vertebral column
2. Spinal cord.

- **The vertebral column has a total of 33 vertebrae (Fig. 16.1):**
  - *Cervical*: Seven vertebrae
  - *Dorsal*: Twelve vertebrae
  - *Lumbar*: Five vertebrae
  - *Sacral*: Five vertebrae
  - *Coccygeal*: Four vertebrae.

  A typical vertebra has several parts; body, pedicle, transverse process, lamina, and spinous process **(Fig. 16.2)**. The key anatomical features of vertebrae of various regions are mentioned in **Table 16.1**.

- **Normal curvature of spine:** The vertebral column is a curved structure in the sagittal plane with *lordosis in the cervical and lumbar region*, whereas *kyphosis in the dorsal and sacral region* **(Fig. 16.1)**. The dorsal and sacral kyphosis are primary curves

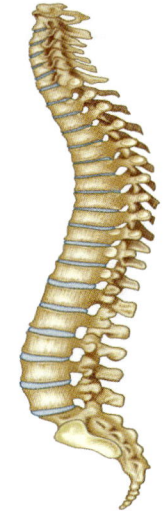

Fig. 16.1: The vertebral column.

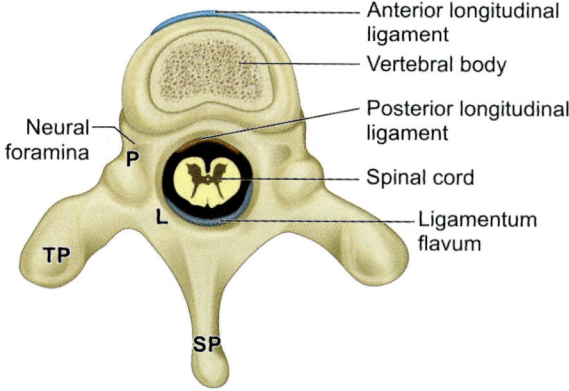

Fig. 16.2: Parts of a typical vertebra with spinal cord in the central canal.
(P: pedicle; TP: transverse process; L: lamina; SP: spinous process)

Table 16.1: Key feature of a typical vertebra.	
Region	**Key feature**
Cervical	Foramen transversarium (vertebral artery and vein passes through it)
Dorsal	Facet for rib (costal facets)
Lumbar	▪ Mammillary process (adjacent to the superior articular facet) ▪ Accessory process (at the base of the transverse process)

(present at birth). In contrast, lordosis of the cervical and lumbar regions are secondary curves, which develop as the child starts extending the neck (achieving head control) and standing without support. Various affections, such as osteoporosis, tuberculosis or trauma, result in change (accentuation/attenuation) in curvature.
- **The stability of the vertebral column** is imparted by bony integrity, facet joint and its capsule, intervertebral disc and various ligaments such as:
  - Anterior and posterior longitudinal ligament
  - Ligamentum flavum
  - Interspinous and supraspinous ligament

  Further, the stability of the spine after trauma can be understood by the 'three column concept' proposed by Denis.

  "Denis" three columns concept of the vertebral column (Fig. 16.3)
  1. **Anterior column:** The anterior longitudinal ligament + anterior half of the vertebral body + anterior half of intervertebral disc
  2. **Middle column:** The posterior longitudinal ligament + posterior half of the vertebral body + posterior half of intervertebral disc
  3. **Posterior column:** Pedicle, lamina, transverse process, ligamentum flavum, spinous process and the inter and supraspinous ligament.

  It is important to understand that injury to two or more columns renders a spine unstable.

- **Functional spinal unit:** Two adjacent vertebrae, intervening intervertebral and all ligaments comprise a functional spinal unit. It is the smallest physiological unit to exhibit the biomechanical characteristics similar to that of the rest of the spine.

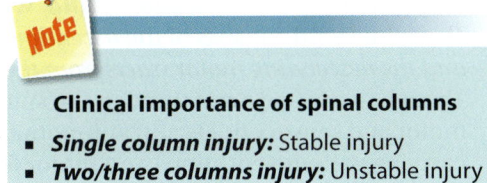

Clinical importance of spinal columns
- **Single column injury:** Stable injury
- **Two/three columns injury:** Unstable injury

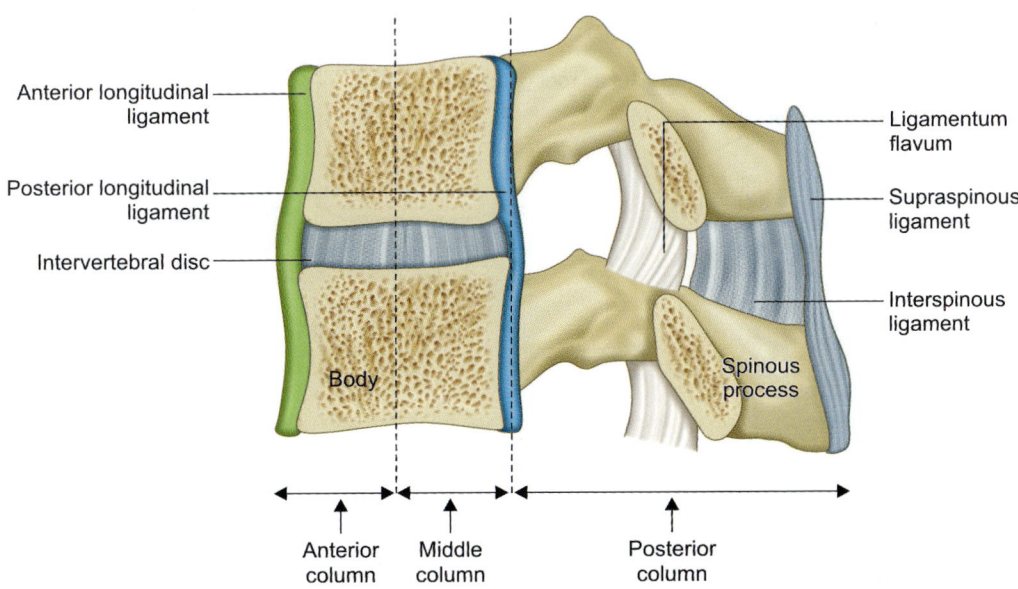

Fig. 16.3: Columns of the spine.

- **Functions of the spinal/vertebral column**
  - The essential function of the vertebral column is to protect the "spinal cord", which runs vertically downward in the spinal canal. Hence, any injury to the vertebral column puts the spinal cord at risk of the damage.
  - Vertebral column also provides attachments to various muscles, ligaments, movements and provide mobility.

SURGICAL ANATOMY OF THE SPINAL CORD

- In adults, the spinal cord runs from the foramen magnum to the lower border of the L1 vertebra or upper edge of the L2 vertebra.
- The spinal cord is made up of **31 spinal segments: 8 cervical, 12 thoracic, 5 lumbar, 5 sacral** and **1 coccygeal**. A spinal segment or myelomere is the transverse division of the spinal cord, and a pair of spinal nerves that leave each segment of the spinal cord **(Fig. 16.4)**. Note that the spinal segment does not match the vertebral level.
- The spinal cord's distal end is bulbous and known as **conus medullaris,** which lies in front of the L1 vertebra. Conus medullaris contains sacral (S2–S5) and coccygeal spinal segments and nerves that controls leg, genitals, bladder and bowel. Superiorly, it is continuous with epiconus comprising L4–S1 segments.
- The terminal L2-L5, S1-S5, and single coccygeal nerve roots form a *'horse tail configuration'* called **cauda equina,** which descends to exit from neural foramina.
- The spinal cord consists of the *ascending sensory tracts comprising fibers from the periphery and the descending motor tracts from the brain.*
  Though many tracts run through the spinal cord, this chapter would discuss only the major motor and sensory tracts and autonomic systems for ease of understanding. Multiple tracts carrying various sensations and motor functions are mentioned in **Table 16.2**.
- **Motor system:** It comprises descending motor tracts—*lateral corticospinal tract (LCST)* and **anterior corticospinal tract (ACST).** These tracts start from the motor cortex of the

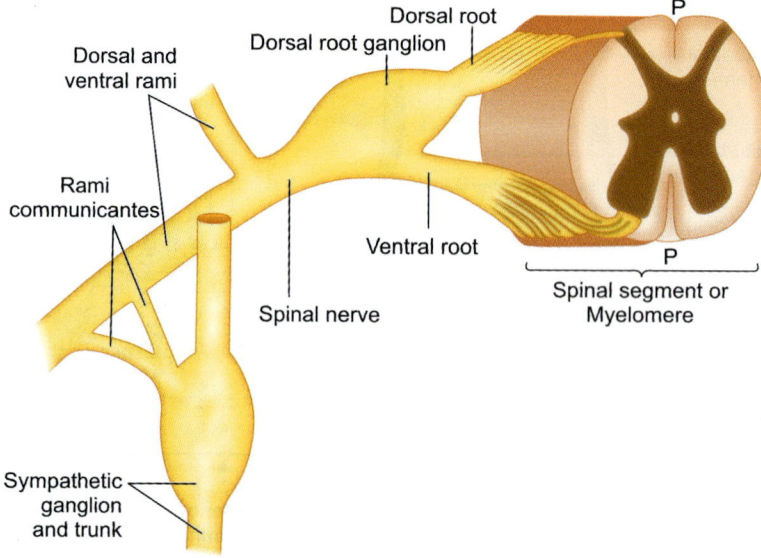

Fig. 16.4: Illustration of a spinal segment.

Chapter 16: Injuries of the Spine and Spinal Cord

Table 16.2: The major sensory-motor tracts of spinal cord and their function.

Tract type	Tract	Function
Sensory (ascending)	Posterior column (FG, FC)	Proprioception, joint and position sense, two-point discrimination, tactile localization, vibration, fine touch and stereognosis
	Anterior spinothalamic	Crude touch and pressure
	Lateral spinothalamic	Pain and temperature
Motor (descending)	Lateral corticospinal	Controls voluntary movement of the extremities
	Anterior corticospinal	Controls the central axial and girdle muscles

(FG: fasciculus gracilis; FC: fasciculus cuneatus)

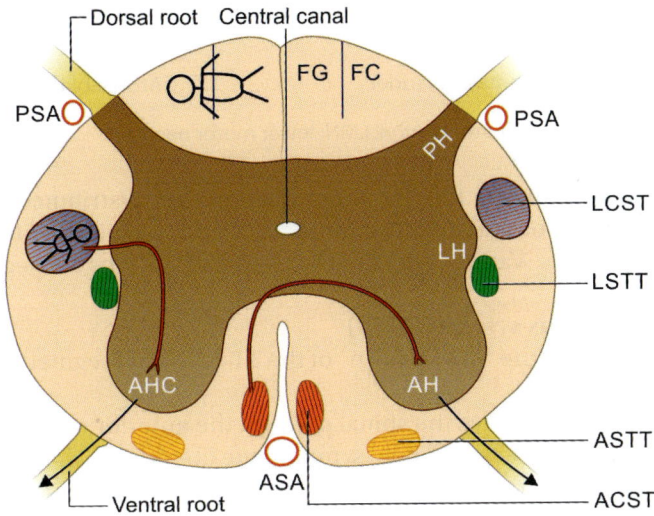

Fig. 16.5: The cross-section of the spinal cord. *Note body homunculus orientation in posterior column and LCST.*
(FG: fasciculus gracilis; FC: fasciculus cuneatus; LCST: lateral corticospinal tract; LSST: lateral spinothalamic tract; ASST: anterior spinothalamic tract; ACST: anterior corticospinal tract; AH: anterior horn; LH: lateral horn; PH: posterior horn; AHC: anterior horn cell; ASA: anterior spinal artery; PSA: posterior spinal artery)

brain and end on the anterior horn cell (AHC). The LCST and ACST comprise 'crossed motor fibers' and 'uncrossed motor fibers', respectively, at the level of pyramids. The LCST fibers end over the AHC of the same side, whereas ACST fibers cross and end over the AHC of the opposite side **(Fig. 16.5)**. *The brain and fibers of descending motor tracts are known as the upper motor neuron (UMN), whereas the AHC which further forms the spinal nerve till the neuromuscular junction is known as the lower motor neuron (LMN).* The difference between UMN and LMN are listed in **Table 16.3**, which is essential for understanding the level of neurological injuries. The peripheral motor system of the body originates from the anterior horn (AH) of the spinal cord and exits the spinal cord via the ventral root. Cranial nerves are also the part of peripheral nervous system.
- **Sensory system:** It comprises various ascending tracts—*posterior column, anterior and lateral spinothalamic tracts*. The sensory input from the body in the form of various sensations is picked up from the dermatomes and ends up in the posterior horn (PH) of

Table 16.3: Differences between UMN and LMN.

	UMN injury	LMN injury
Lesion	Injury to the brain/spinal cord/ motor tracts just before AHC	Injury to the AHC/spinal nerve
Other signs of brainstem/ cortical injury	Present	Absent
Weakness	Often symmetric weakness on one/ both side of the body	Asymmetric weakness or only a group of muscle involvement
Muscle tone	Hypertonia	Hypotonia
Deep tendon reflex	Exaggerated	Decreased/absent
Plantar response	Plantar response: Babinski's	Absent
Clonus	Sustained	Absent
Bladder status	Automatic bladder	Atonic bladder

(AHC: anterior horn cell; UMN: upper motor neuron; LMN: lower motor neuron)

the spinal cord. After entering the PH, the sensations are distributed to various tracts—posterior column, anterior and lateral spinothalamic tract, which is further relayed to the brain as ascending tracts. Various sensory tracts and sensations carried are mentioned in **Table 16.2**.

- **The sympathetic nervous system (SYNS)**
    - SYNS originates from the "lateral horn" of the T1-L2 spinal segment as "thoracolumbar outflow."
    - The sympathetic fibers leave the spinal cord via the anterior root and enter the prevertebral ganglion via white rami. Then, sympathetic fibers leave the prevertebral ganglion via the gray rami and are distributed to the rest of the body via sympathetic chains.
    - *Major function of SYNS* is to supply heart, blood vessels, and sweat glands. The function of SYNS pertinent to spinal cord injury management is effect of SYNS on **blood pressure and heart rate**. The SYNS controls systolic blood pressure by increasing the heart rate through the sinoatrial node and controls diastolic blood pressure by causing vasoconstriction at the level of the arterioles and by the release of catecholamines via adrenals.

Surgical relevance of level of spinal cord injury and blood pressure control

In case of injury to the spinal cord at the level of cervical spine, the entire SYNS via thoracolumbar outflow is temporarily paralysed (neurogenic shock) leading to a drop in the blood pressure due to lower heart rate and vasodilation (bradycardia and hypotension). It recovers in few days. However, this effect is not seen in injuries below the upper dorsal spine injury enabling the maintenance of blood pressure and heart rate as SYNS outflow is well maintained.

- **The parasympathetic nervous system (PSNS)** originates from the craniosacral outflow. The cranial flow is via the vagus nerve and supplies the upper body to the right two-thirds of the transverse colon. The sacral outflow is via the S2, 3, 4 segment, which supplies the rest of the abdominopelvic organs and the lower body.

BLOOD SUPPLY OF THE SPINAL CORD

A brief knowledge of blood supply to the spinal cord is essential to understand the pathology of various spinal cord syndromes, which occur due to a lack of blood supply to the arteries supplying the spinal cord **(Fig. 16.6)**.

The spinal cord is supplied by single anterior and two posterior spinal artery. The anterior spinal artery (ASA) is a branch of vertebral artery, while posterior spinal artery is either branched from vertebral or posterior inferior cerebellar artery. ASA overlies anterior median fissure, whereas PSA lies lateral to the posterior median fissure. These three vertical vessels get segmental reinforcement vessels every 4–6 segments from intercostal and lumbar arteries. One such significant segmental reinforcement is by the arteria magna of Adamkiewicz, which arises between T8-L2 vertebral level on left side of the descending aorta. Of note, the *artery of Adamkiewicz delivers vascular supply a large area of the thoracolumbar region and thus is considered a watershed area*. The area of the spinal cord supplied by these vessels is mentioned in **Table 16.4**.

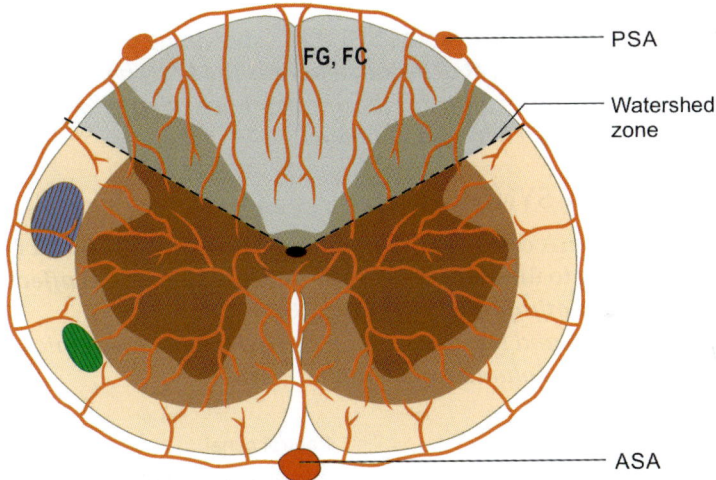

Fig. 16.6: Arterial supply of the spinal cord.
(ASA: anterior spinal artery; PSA: posterior spinal artery; FG: fasciculus gracilis; FC: fasciculus cuneatus)

Table 16.4: Blood supply of the spinal cord.

Main artery	Branch	Supplies
Vertebral artery	"Single" anterior spinal artery (ASA)	Anterior two-thirds of the spinal cord
	"Paired" posterior spinal artery (PSA)	Posterior one-third of the cord

ACUTE SPINAL CORD INJURY

HOW DOES SPINAL CORD INJURY (SCI) OCCURS?

A fracture and/or dislocation of the spine at or above the level of the L1 vertebra can result in acute SCI. The fractured or dislocated vertebra causes injury to the spinal cord by compression, laceration or transection, resulting in:

- Acute sensory loss below the level of the lesion
- Acute motor flaccid paralysis below the level of the lesion
- If the SCI is at the cervical spine level, the autonomic disturbance is noted in the form of a fall in blood pressure and decreased heart rate.
- Loss of control over bladder and bowel.

SPINAL SHOCK AND TYPE OF SCI

Immediately after the acute SCI, there is a complete cessation of all sensory, motor and autonomic activity below the level of the lesion, known as "**spinal shock**." Usually, the spinal shock recovers within 48–72 hours and is characterized by the return of the bulbocavernosus reflex (Osinski reflex).

SCI could be *complete or incomplete type*:
- **Complete SCI:** No sensory or motor sparing below the level of the lesion.
- **Incomplete SCI:** At least some sensory or motor function is preserved below the level of injury.

After the recovery from spinal shock, the SCI starts showing a pattern of **UMN type injury and recovery pattern below the level of lesion, whereas the LMN type of lesion and recovery at the level of the lesion.** Note—an injury to the anterior horn cells at the lesion level results in a LMN type of recovery at the injured level myelomere.

SPINAL CORD INJURY SYNDROMES

- **Anterior cord syndrome:** A condition of the spinal cord due to the **block in ASA**, leading to the disrupted circulation to the anterior two-thirds of the spinal cord *affecting the function of motor tracts and spinothalamic tract* (Fig. 16.7).

This results in motor palsy and loss of sensation carried by spinothalamic tracts, whereas the functioning of the posterior column tract remains normal.

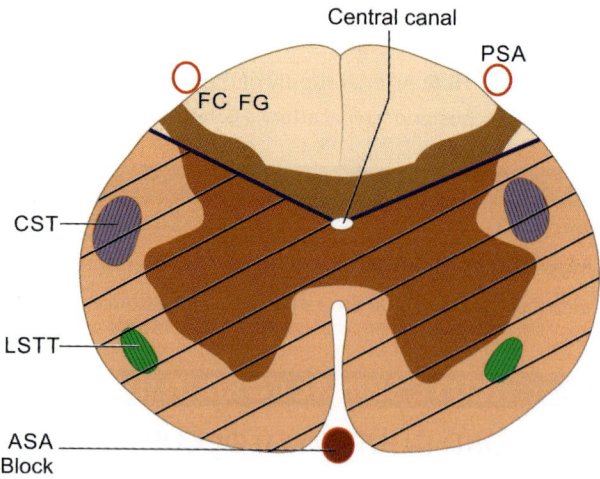

Fig. 16.7: Anterior cord syndrome (obliquely hashed area shows affected zone).
(FC: fasciculus cuneatus; FG: fasciculus gracilis; PSA: posterior spinal artery; CST: corticospinal tract; LSTT: lateral spinothalamic tract; ASA: anterior spinal artery)

- **Posterior cord syndrome:** A spinal cord condition due to the **block in PSA**, leading to the disrupted circulation to the posterior one-third of the spinal cord **affecting the function of posterior column tracts** (Fig. 16.8). It could be uni- or bilateral.
  This results in a loss of sensation carried by the posterior column tract, whereas corticospinal and spinothalamic tract function remains normal.
- **Central cord syndrome:** A syndrome due to *injury to the central part of the SC resulting in more weakness in the upper limb than the lower limb, bladder dysfunction, and variable sensory loss* (Fig. 16.9).

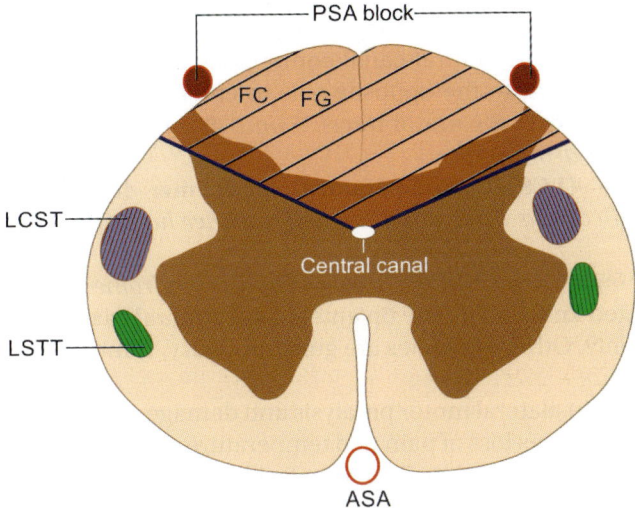

Fig. 16.8: Posterior cord syndrome (obliquely hashed area shows affected zone).
(FC: fasciculus cuneatus; FG: fasciculus gracilis; PSA: posterior spinal artery; LCST: lateral corticospinal tract; LSTT: lateral spinothalamic tract; ASA: anterior spinal artery)

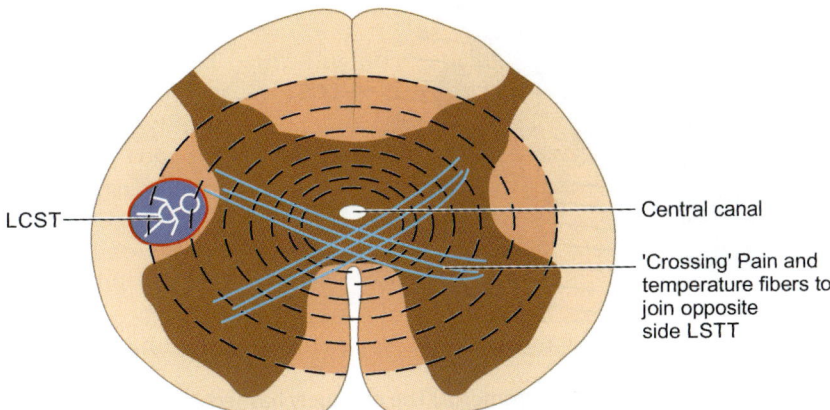

Fig. 16.9: Central cord syndrome. The circular hashed lines represent the expanding edema/pressure around the central canal. *Keep in mind that the motor homunculus in the LCST depicts the cervical region more medially than the sacral area. As a result, people with central cord syndrome typically have more upper than lower limb weakness.*
(LCST: lateral corticospinal tract; LSTT, lateral spinothalamic tract)

Section 2: Fractures and Ligament Injuries

- The *most common cause of central cord syndrome is hyperextension injury in a spondylotic cervical spine due to "pincer grasp" type of mechanism of injury to the spinal cord.*
- In traumatic central cord syndrome, there is more edema in the central part of the spinal cord compared to the periphery. Since the cervical and thoracic motor fibers in the lateral corticospinal tract are located more toward the central canal **(Fig. 16.9)**, it affects the motor power of the upper limb more than the lower limb.
- It also *affects the fibers carrying pain and temperature fibers* which cross the midline adjacent to the central canal to crossover to the contralateral side to join the spinothalamic tract leading to loss of pain and temperature sensation in the extremity.
- Central cord syndrome is also observed in "syringomyelia", wherein the central canal dilates gradually. The dilating central canal compresses upon the adjacent 'crossing pain and temperature fibers' to the opposite side to enter LSTT. Further, the dilating canal may exert pressure over the motor tracts. *A limb devoid of pain and temperature could result in Charcot's arthropathy.*

- **Lateral cord syndrome (LCS)/Brown-Séquard syndrome:** It is also known as *hemisection of the spinal cord as a result of damage to either half side of the spinal cord* **(Figs. 16.10A and B)**.
    - The *classic mode of injury described for Brown-Séquard syndrome is a "stab injury"* to the back with a pointed knife where the tip enters the vertebral canal and damages the cord from one side only. Other etiologies are gunshot injury, tumor in the spinal canal or infection.
    - LCS is characterized by ipsilateral motor paralysis and damage to the PC tract below the level of the lesion (1), whereas loss of pain and temperature occurs on the opposite side, beginning one or two segments below the lesion level (2).

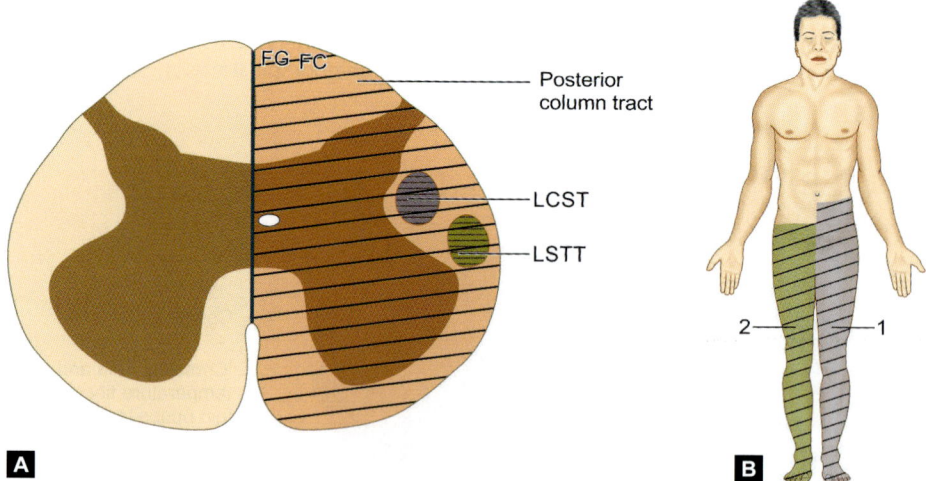

Figs. 16.10A and B: Brown-Séquard syndrome: (A) The obliquely hashed area indicates area/tract affected in Brown-Sequard syndrome; (B) The blue shaded area '1' shows Ipsilateral loss of motor power and posterior column sensation and green shaded area '2' shows contralateral pain and temperature loss slightly below the level of lesion.
(FC: fasciculus cuneatus; FG: fasciculus gracilis; LCST: lateral corticospinal tract; LSTT: lateral spinothalamic tract)

- Pain and temperature loss is from the opposite side, as the lateral spinothalamic tract contains fibers from the opposite side, whereas LCST and PC have ipsilateral side fibers.
- The pain and temperature loss on the opposite side is one or two segments below because the fibers in LSTT cross to the opposite side after ascending a level or two on the same side.
- **Conus medullaris syndrome (CMS)**
  - CMS occurs due to injury or compression of the conus medullaris.
  - The nerves passing via the conus medullaris (S2–S5, coccygeal) innervate the genitals, bladder, bowel, and legs.
  - It may have some UMN signs with increased tone and reflexes.
- **Cauda equina syndrome (CES)**
  - Due to compression of the cauda equina (L2-L5; S1-S5, coccygeal nerve roots)
  - It is an LMN type of lesion.

Table 16.5 outlines the differences between the presentation of CMS and CES.

Table 16.5: Differences between conus medullaris syndrome (CMS) and cauda equina syndrome (CES).

Difference	CMS	CES
Spinal level	Sacral cord and roots	L2-sacral roots
Presentation	Acute	Gradual
Symmetry	Bilateral symmetric	Asymmetric
Radicular pain	Absent/less severe	Frequent, severe
Low back pain	More	Less
Sensory involvement	Bilateral saddle symmetric sensory loss	Asymmetric sensory loss in the saddle area
Motor involvement	Symmetric, less marked, distal paresis of lower limb	Asymmetric, marked, areflexic weakness of lower limb
Reflex	Only ankle jerk affected	Knee, ankle affected
Bladder bowel involvement	Common, sudden, marked	Uncommon, slow involvement
Sexual dysfunction	Frequent	Infrequent

URINARY BLADDER INNERVATION, FUNCTION AND DYSFUNCTION

The urinary bladder (UB) acts as a reservoir for the urine and empties into the urethra with a coordinated autonomic-somatic nervous system reflex.

URINARY BLADDER INNERVATION

The innervation of the urinary bladder is by the sympathetic, parasympathetic, and somatic nervous systems. **Table 16.6** outlines the role of each system in urinary bladder function. **Figure 16.11** illustrates the innervation of the bladder.

Table 16.6: Outline of urinary bladder innervation and function.

Nervous system	Root value	Supplies	Function
Sympathetic (via hypogastric nerve)	D10-L2	Detrusor, IUS	Detrusor—inhibition/relaxation: UB relaxed IUS—stimulation/contraction
Parasympathetic (via pelvic nerve)	S2,3,4	Detrusor, IUS	Detrusor—stimulation/contraction: UB contracts IUS—inhibition/relaxation
Somatic (via pudendal nerve)	S2,3,4	EUS	EUS—contraction/relaxation depending upon cortical response
Sensory (via hypogastric, pelvic and pudendal nerve)			Sensations to the cortex

(IUS: internal urethral sphincter; EUS: external urethral sphincter)

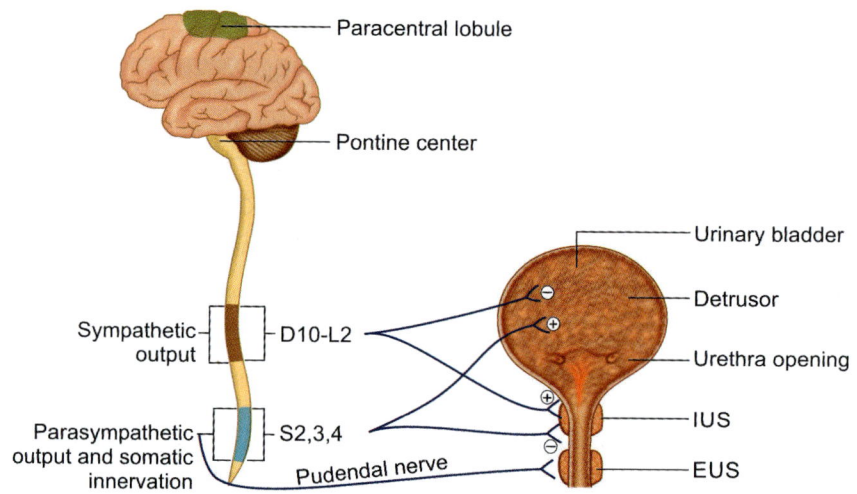

Fig. 16.11: Neurological control of urinary bladder. '+' and '–' indicate stimulation and inhibition, respectively.
(IUS: internal urethral sphincter; EUS: external urethral sphincter)

URINARY BLADDER NEUROLOGICAL CONTROL

UB control is under three centers—cortical, pontine, and sacral spinal center **(Fig. 16.11)**.
- **Cortical micturition centers**
    - The primary center lies in the paracentral lobule on the medial aspect of the frontoparietal cortex. It is "inhibitory" on the pontine center and micturition reflex.
    - Its dysfunction leads to a "loss of social control" of the bladder
- **Pontine center (Barrington's nucleus):** It facilitates and coordinates the micturition reflex.
- **Sacral spinal micturition center (Onuf nucleus)**
    - It is a primitive micturition center and helps in reflex evacuation or micturition
    - However, lone sacral center reflex (without pontine coordination) is ill-sustained and leads to poor detrusor contraction and incomplete bladder evacuation.

URINARY BLADDER FUNCTION
- **The urinary bladder (UB) has two phases of reflex—*filling and emptying*.**
- The state of the reflex (filling/emptying) depends upon the afferent signals going to the higher center, signaling the amount of urine in the bladder, and the conscious signal back to the pontine-sacral centers.
    - The *filling phase is coordinated by the local SYNS,* which relaxes the detrusor muscle and contracts the internal urethral sphincter (IUS). At low urine volume, the afferent firing rate is less; hence, inhibition to micturate from the higher center continues.
    - The *emptying phase or micturition reflex is coordinated by local PSNS and facilitatory signals from the pontine and cortical micturition centre.* Once the bladder starts filling up, the afferent sensory firing increases, and one gets a conscious signal from the brain to void according to social circumstances. Further, the pontine center facilitates the micturition reflex, which signals to local PSNS and pudendal nerve. Local PSNS gets activated, stimulates (contracts) detrusor and relaxes IUS leading to urine outflow from UB. The pudendal nerve gets inhibited and leads to the relaxation of the EUS.

URINARY BLADDER DYSFUNCTION
- **Immediately after acute spinal cord injury**
    - The bladder remains toneless and paralyzed. It accumulates a large amount of urine. It needs to be catheterized for the urine to be evacuated.
    - Later, the behavior of bladder function (UMN/LMN) depends upon the level of SCI.
- **UMN bladder (hyper-reflexic/automatic/spastic bladder):**
    - *Etiology*: The lesion in the spinal cord is above the sacral spinal center (S1) but below the level of the pons. Often seen in complete transection of the spinal cord.
    - *Pathology*: There is a *lack of sensory stimulus from the bladder reaching the higher cortical center, an absence of "supraspinal inhibitory control and a lack of coordination from pons".* However, the entire local reflex arc of the bladder is intact (sensory afferent of UB, center at spinal cord and efferent along with detrusor).
      Often, there is *detrusor-sphincter dyssynergia wherein* there is a simultaneous contraction of the bladder and the sphincter leading to a smaller amount of urine voiding due to the tight sphincter.
      Further, there is *autonomic hyperreflexia if the lesion is above the D6 spinal level.* It is characterized by *sweating, headache, hypertension, and bradycardia.*
    - *Pathofunctioning:* Once the bladder fills up, it causes detrusor stretching, leading to a local reflex arc stimulation, resulting in bladder contraction and the evacuation (complete/partial) of the bladder, often at an inconvenient time. Since the bladder loses control with a higher center, the patient cannot feel the bladder filling up or any inhibitory control. *The bladder empties too quickly and frequently, leading to "urge incontinence."* The lesions above the pons also act like an automatic bladder. However, there is a more coordinated emptying of the bladder resulting in less residual urine leading to a lower chance of infection.
    - *Problems*: The lack of pontine control causes uncoordinated bladder emptying resulting in an incomplete void. However, emptying is more than LMN bladder due to intact reflex arc. Also, the overstretch of the bladder causes vesicoureteral reflex (VUR). Incomplete emptying and VUR predispose the patient to UTI, epididymo-orchitis, vesical calculus and hydronephrosis.

- ♦ ***Treatment:*** Appropriate bladder training, clean intermittent catheterization (CIC) if residual urine volume >100 mL, anticholinergic medications (for detrusor hyperreflexia)
- **LMN bladder (autonomous/areflexic/atonic/flaccid bladder):**
  - ♦ ***Etiology:*** Direct trauma to the spinal center, conus medullaris syndrome, cauda equina syndrome, radical pelvic surgeries damaging the bladder nerves (afferent/efferent)
  - ♦ ***Pathology:*** One or more components of the reflex arc (afferent, spinal center or efferent) are affected in LMN lesion.
  - ♦ ***Pathofunctioning:*** The UB continues to fill with urine. Since the local reflex arc is disrupted, the bladder does not contract due to a lack of neurological stimulus. As rising intravesical pressure (IVP) exceeds the urethral sphincteric pressure, some urine escapes via the urethra. Escaping urine leads to a drop in IVP less than the sphincteric pressure and dribbling stops. It is known as *"overflow incontinence."*
  - ♦ ***Problems:*** In LMN bladder, emptying is less than the automatic bladder, which results in a *large amount of residual urine,* inviting infection, vesical calculus, diverticulosis, epididymo-orchitis, VUR, and hydronephrosis.
  - ♦ ***Treatment:*** Sixth hourly CIC to ensure complete emptying. Patients can also be taught to perform "Crede's maneuver", wherein gentle suprapubic pressure over the bladder is applied to empty the UB.

SPINE/VERTEBRAL INJURIES

MODE OF INJURY

Most spine injuries are a result of **high-velocity injuries** such as:
- RTA, fall from height
- Diving
- Lap seat belt injury
- Whiplash injury.

Occasionally, vertebral fractures can also occur in **low-velocity injury** in a pathological vertebra, such as osteoporosis.

Few facts of spine injury!
- Neurological deficit in 10–15% cases
- ***Most common site of injury is thoracolumbar junction (T10-L2),*** which is uniquely positioned in between the rigid thoracic spine and the mobile lumbar spine. This transition from the less mobile thoracic spine to the more flexible lumbar spine subjects the thoracolumbar region to significant biomechanical stress, resulting in higher incidence of fracture-dislocation.

CLASSIFICATION OF SPINE INJURY

The spine injury can be classified according to the *site of injury, mechanism of injury*, and *stable/unstable injury*.
- According to the **site of injury**
  - ♦ Cervical
  - ♦ Thoracic
  - ♦ Lumbar
  - ♦ Sacral
- **Mechanism of injury (Fig. 16.12)**
  - ♦ Flexion injury
    - Flexion-compression injury
    - Flexion-distraction injury
    - Flexion-rotational injury
  - ♦ Extension type injury
  - ♦ Axial/vertical compression injury

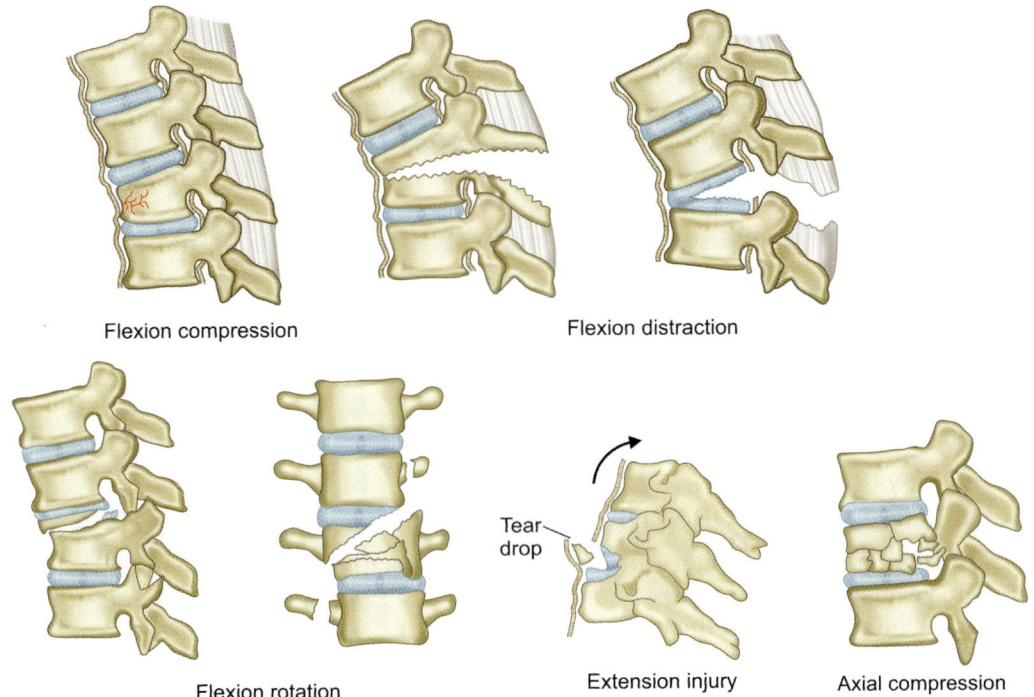

Fig. 16.12: Various common mechanism of injury of the spine.

- Shear or translation
- Direct injury
- Traction injury

Table 16.7 describes various types of injuries with mechanisms and examples.
- **Stable/unstable** spine injury.

Classification		Mechanism	Example
1. **Flexion**	a. *Flexion compression*	Fall on back of head/blow on the back of the head	Wedge compression #
	b. *Flexion distraction*	Seat belt injury	Chance #
	c. *Flexion rotation*	Flexion and rotation of the neck or body	Fracture dislocation
2. **Extension**		Sudden rapid forward acceleration of body	Anterior lip # of the vertebra
3. **Axial/vertical compression**		An object falling on head/head striking the bottom of the pool	Burst #
4. **Shear/translational**			Fracture dislocation, bifacetal dislocation
5. **Direct injury**		Direct penetrating injuries by firearm, sharp objects	
6. **Traction injury**		Muscle and ligament pull the bone resulting in avulsion #	# of transverse/spinous process

Table 16.7: Classification of vertebral fracture based on mechanism of injury (with examples).

What is a stable spine?

Stable spine: White and Panjabi considered spine to be stable if the application of physiological load on the spine does not result into any neurological deficit, pain or deformity.

Clinically, a traumatic spine is considered to be unstable in case of:
- Associated deformity of the spine
- Associated neurological deficit
- Injury to two or more columns of Denis
- Asymmetric gap between the spinous process of the vertebra or rotational malalignment
- If neurological status is not assessed due to polytrauma/unconscious status of patient

CLINICAL FEATURES OF SPINE INJURY

The clinical features of spine injury are due to vertebral fracture and injury to the spinal cord.
- **Due to vertebral column injury**
  - Pain and swelling over the injured part of the spine
  - Pain while attempted sitting/standing
  - Bony tenderness at the injured vertebral level
  - Paraspinal spasm
  - There may be a deformity at the site of injury
  - There may be a step (due to vertebral dislocation) and rotational malalignment felt at the spinous process.
- **Due to associated SCI:** The clinical features (sensory, motor, autonomic and bladder, bowel involvement) depend upon the level of the SCI.
  - ***Sensory assessment:*** *Helps in deciding the level of lesion*
    - Hypoesthesia/anesthesia is per the cervical/dorsal/lumbar injury level.
  - ***Motor assessment (tone, motor power, coordination, reflexes)***
    - *Tone:* Acute SCI causes hypotonia. Later, the patient may develop spasticity or flaccid palsy according to UMN or LMN lesions.
    - *Motor power*: It should be graded it as per the Medical Research Council (MRC) scale.
      - *Cervical spine injury*: Quadriplegia/quadriparesis
      - *Dorsal/lumbar spine injury*: Paraplegia/paraparesis
    - *Coordination*: Assess if power is equal to or more than a grade III. Assess it by performing finger-to-nose test/heel-shin slide test
    - *Reflexes*: Assessment of superficial and deep reflex
      - *Superficial reflex (with root value)*: Abdominal (D7-12), cremasteric (L1-2), and plantar (S1-2)
      - *Deep reflex (with root value):* Biceps (C5-6), supinator (C5-6), triceps (C7), knee (L3-4), ankle (S1-2)
      - *Ankle and patellar clonus*
  - ***Autonomic features:*** More common in cervical spine injuries, and may result in hypotension, bradycardia

- **Involvement of the bladder and bowel**
  - *Acute spinal cord injury*: Flaccid paralysis of the bladder with acute retention of urine is present.
  - Later, the bladder recovers and becomes "automatic" or "atonic", depending upon the level of injury. The bowel remains paralyzed initially but later starts functioning autonomously.
- **Functional assessment with ASIA scoring or Frankel grading**
  - *American spinal injury association (ASIA) scoring*: The functional scoring of a patient to document sensory and motor deficit.
  - *Frankel's grading*
    - *Frankel A*—No motor or sensory function: Complete SCI
    - *Frankel B*—Sensory normal, motor deficit
    - *Frankel C*—Sensory normal, motor power <3/5 (useless)
    - *Frankel D*—Sensory normal, motor power >3/5 (useful)
    - *Frankel E*—Sensory and motor normal: No SCI.

INVESTIGATIONS

- **Plain X-ray of the spine:** AP, lateral view **(Fig. 16.13A)**
  Swimmer's view of cervical spine to visualize lower-level vertebrae (C6–C7). Open mouth view can be taken when there is suspicion of C1–C2 fracture.
- **Computed tomography (CT) scan (Fig. 16.13B)**
  - To understand # configuration, the comminution of fragment
  - Retropulsion of the fragment into the vertebral/spinal canal
  - Associated dislocation/subluxation.
- **Magnetic resonance imaging (MRI):** Due to fracture and/or dislocation of the vertebra, there can be injury to the spinal cord, which can be assessed with MRI. MRI of the spine **(Fig. 16.13C)** may show
  - Contusion
  - Laceration, transection
  - Hematomyelia.

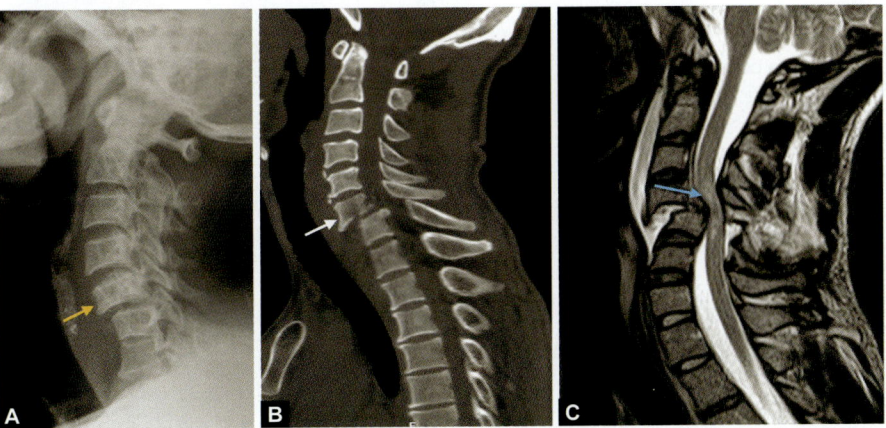

Figs. 16.13A to C: (A) Plain X-ray of cervical spine showing subluxation of C5 vertebra over C6; (B) CT scan of cervical spine showing C6 subluxation over C7 and body fracture; (C) MRI of cervical spine showing compression over the spinal cord due to subluxation of the C6 vertebra (blue arrow).

MANAGEMENT

The principles of management of spine injury are listed in **Box 16.1**.

- **Initial management of the spine injury involves ATLS resuscitation protocol**
- **Protection of the injured part of the spine by immediate immobilization with a brace**
    - *Cervical spine injury*: Hard cervical collar/Philadelphia collar
    - *Dorsal/lumbar spine injury*: Spine board. If there is a dislocation of spine, one must reduce it as early as possible.
- **General management of patient**
    - Proper nutritious, balanced fiber rich diet
    - Adequate hydration
    - Urinary bladder catheterization
- **Definitive management of fracture/dislocation:** While stable vertebral fractures can be managed by braces, unstable ones require operative fixation.
    - *Braces/traction*: It can be used for all stable fractures in all regions of the spine **(Figs. 16.14 and 16.15)**. *Note that Halo immobilization system is the most rigid non-operative method to provide stability in cervical spine injury.*

> **Box 16.1:** Principles of spine injury management.
>
> 1. Initial management with ATLS protocol
> 2. Early protection of spine with immobilization. A dislcoation must be reduced as early as possible
> 3. General management of patient
> 4. Definitive management of fracture
> 5. Care of a paraplegic
> 6. Rehabilitation of patient

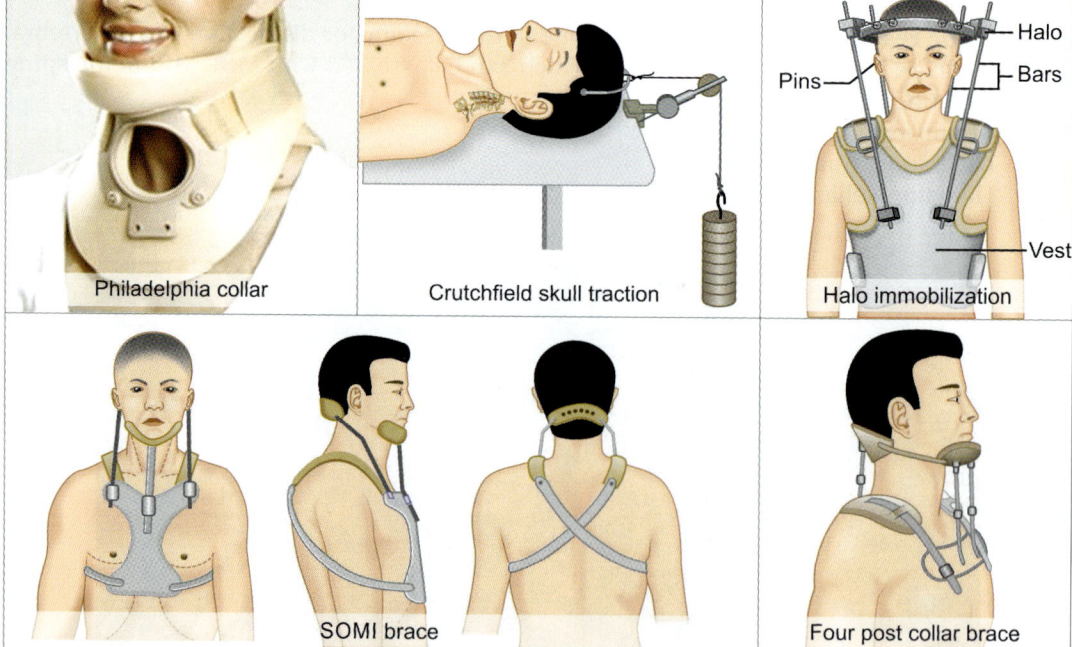

Fig. 16.14: Cervical braces and traction.
(SOMI: sternal occipital mandibular immobilizer)

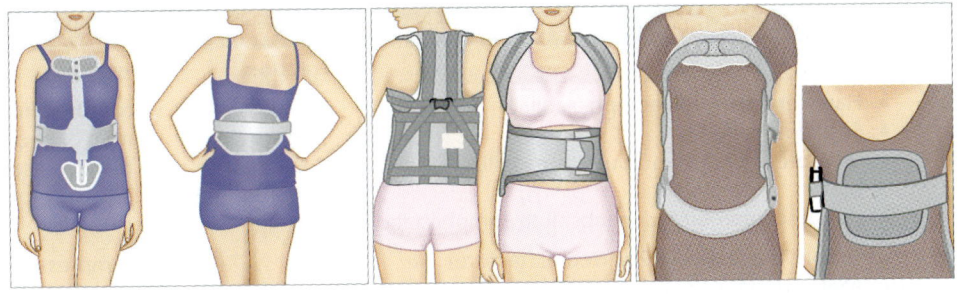

Fig. 16.15: Thoracolumbar braces.
(ASH: anterior spinal hyperextension)

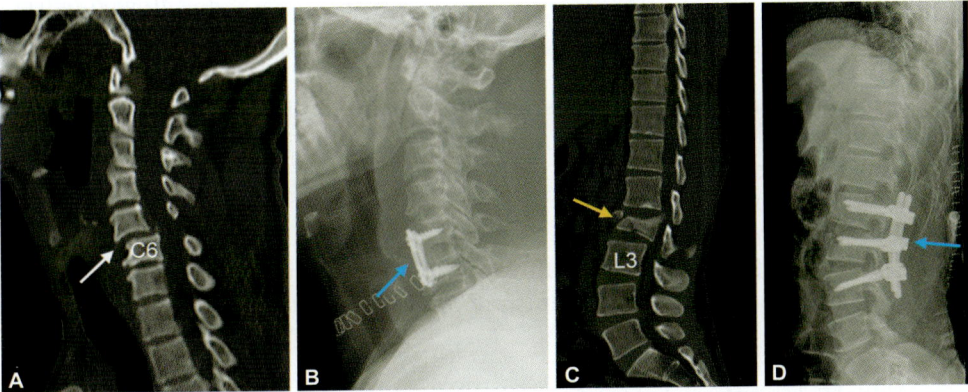

Figs. 16.16A to D: (A) C5 subluxation over C6 (white arrow); (B) Cervical spine fixation with a plate (blue arrow); (C) L2 vertebra fracture (yellow arrow); (D) Lumbar vertebra fixation with pedicle screw system (blue arrow).

- **ORIF of fracture with plates and screws:** The surgical fixation of vertebral fracture is performed for unstable injuries of spine. Typically, the cervical spine fractures (vertebral body) are managed with plates and screws, whereas dorsolumbar fractures (vertebral body) are managed with pedicle screw system **(Figs. 16.16A to D)**.
  The advantage of the surgical fixation of a vertebra in a paralyzed patient is *"early mobilization and faster rehabilitation of the patient and the prevention of complications arising out of recumbent position."* However, the surgical fixation might not hasten or guarantee neurological recovery of the spinal cord.
  Table 16.8 summarizes the treatment (conservative/operative) of the fractures of the spine.
- **Care of a quadriplegic/paraplegic patient:** It involves
  - *Care of the skin of back:* The skin of back is *prone to bedsores,* and that can be prevented by:
    - Two hourly side-side turnings: Use "log roll" method to turn the patient
    - "Six pillow technique" or soft sponges under the bony prominences of the occiput, scapula, elbow, sacrum, greater trochanter, and heel to prevent bedsores.
    - Water bed/alpha or air mattress
    - Keeping the skin of the back dry by the application of talcum powder/spirit
    - Avoiding creases on the bedsheet as creases can act as a pressure point

Table 16.8: Summary of treatment methods for spine injury in different regions.

	Braces	Traction	Operative
Cervical, upper dorsal spine	• Hard cervical or Philadelphia collar • Four post collar • Sterno-occipito-mandibular immobilizer (SOMI) brace • Halo ring immobilization (absolute immobilization)	• Crutchfield tongs • Gardner-Wells tongs	Decompression and fixation of fracture by plate and screws
Dorsal spine	• Taylor's brace (D7-D12 vertebral fracture) • ASH (anterior spinal hyperextension) brace • Modified Jewett brace for dorsolumbar junctions fracture		Decompression and fixation with pedicle screw system
Lumbar spine	Knight spinal brace		Decompression and fixation with pedicle screw system

- **Respiratory care:** These patients are *prone to respiratory infections*, which can be prevented by:
  - Steam inhalation
  - Proper hydration
  - Chest physiotherapy
  - Deep breathing exercises, incentive spirometry exercises
- **Care of the bladder:** These patients are *prone to urinary tract infections* that can be prevented by:
  - Adequate hydration
  - Initial Foley catheterization for a few days followed by sixth hourly clean intermittent catheterization (CIC)
  - Regular change of catheter.
- **Care of the bowel:** Patients are *prone to constipation*, which can be prevented by:
  - Fiber diet, bulk laxatives
  - Plenty of fluid to avoid dehydration
  - Occasional enema.
- **Care of joints and bones:** These patients are *prone to joint stiffness and disuse osteoporosis*
  - Passive mobilization of all affected joints
  - Muscle strengthening exercises
  - Splintage in a functional position (e.g., foot drop splint to prevent equinus)
  - Baclofen to reduce spasticity
  - Mobilization using wheelchair
  - Nutritious diet.
- **Prevention of deep vein thrombosis (DVT)**
  - Compression stockings, gentle passive mobilization of the joints
  - Deep vein thrombosis (DVT) prophylaxis.
- **Psychological support:** Psychological counseling to prevent post-traumatic stress disorder/depression/psychosis.

Complication after SCI involves almost every system of the body!

- **Rehabilitation**
  - Vocational and occupational rehabilitation
  - Wheelchair transfer technique
  - Psychological counseling.

COMPLICATIONS OF SPINE INJURY

- **Complications due to vertebral fracture**
  - Malunion of # leading to deformity and local (neck or back) pain
  - Spinal cord injury leading to paralysis
- **Complications after injury to the spinal cord:** The management of complications could be done on standard lines *(details are out of scope in this chapter).*
  - *Skin: Bedsore*—regular dressing, skin grafting, or flap coverage
  - *Respiratory tract infection (RTI):* Treatment of the RTI
  - *Bladder related*
    - Urinary tract infection
    - Automatic bladder: Urge incontinence
    - *Atonic bladder*: Overflow incontinence—CIC, Crede's maneuver
    - Vesical calculus, diverticulosis and vesicoureteral reflux (VUR).
  - *Bowel related:* Constipation and incontinence
  - *Cardiovascular system*
    - *Heart*: Cardiac arrhythmias, heart block (due to vagal overtone, especially in high cervical spine injuries blocking the sympathetic flow to the heart)
    - *Veins*: DVT
    - *Arterial system*: Hypotension and bradycardia (seen after high cervical acute SCI due to a loss of sympathetic outflow; recovers in a few days)
  - *Central nervous system: Psychosis/post-traumatic stress disorder/depression*
  - *Hepatobiliary system: Cholestasis*
  - *Musculoskeletal system*
    - *Joint stiffness*
    - *Muscle wasting*
    - *Disuse osteopenia*
    - *Myositis ossificans*

PROGNOSIS AFTER SPINAL CORD INJURY

- **Complete SCI:** No sensory or motor sparing or function below the level of the lesion. Poor prognosis for recovery.
- **Incomplete SCI:** Partial sensory or motor sparing below the level of the lesion. Good prognosis for recovery.

SPECIFIC FRACTURES OF THE SPINE

JEFFERSON FRACTURE

- It is the **burst fracture of C1 vertebra** (Atlas) wherein there is *fracture of both anterior and posterior arch* **(Fig. 16.17)**.
- **Etiology:** Due to the impact of the head against the roof of a vehicle or a fall on the vertex, e.g., diving in a shallow pool.

- *Neurological injury is uncommon due to the large space available for spinal cord.*
- Rarely, Jefferson's fracture is associated with vertebral artery blockage resulting in lateral medullary (Wallenberg) syndrome or greater occipital nerve injury.
- **Treatment:** Stable injuries are treated non-operatively with halo traction, and unstable ones are operatively fixed.

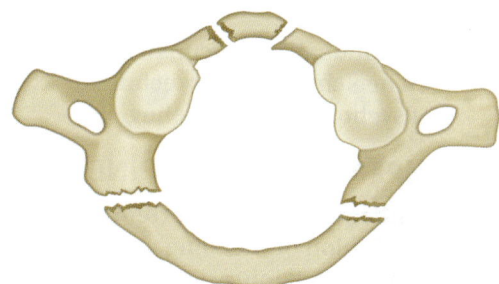

Fig. 16.17: Jefferson fracture showing fracture of both anterior and posterior arch.

HANGMAN'S FRACTURE

- It is *traumatic spondylolisthesis of axis (C2) vertebra*
- Typically described in *judicial hanging with the noose below the chin resulting in traumatic spondylolisthesis of C2 vertebra* (**Figs. 16.18A and B**). Nevertheless, it is commonly seen in RTA with *head-on collision, resulting in hyperextension of the cervical spine* (**Fig. 16.18C**).
- *Neurological deficit is uncommon*
- **Investigations:** X-rays, CT show reveal fracture of both pedicles of C2 vertebra
- **Treatment:** Stable injuries are managed with halo traction, whereas unstable ones are operated.

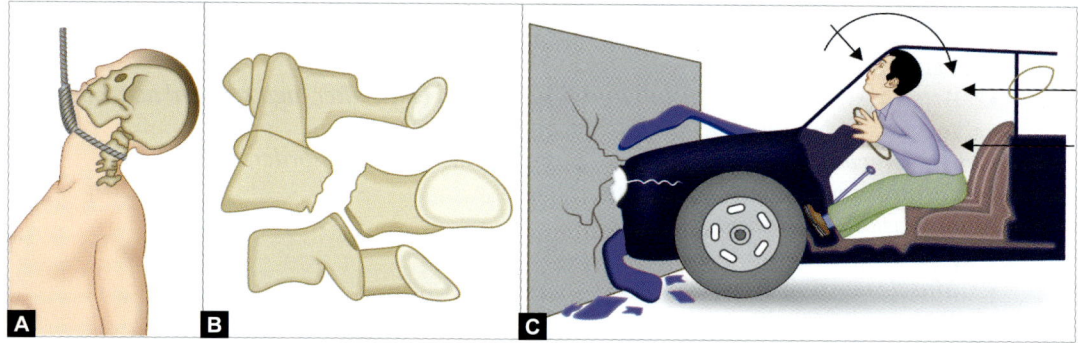

Figs. 16.18A to C: Hangman's fracture: (A) Noose over the neck; (B) Spondylolisthesis of C2 vertebra; (C) Head-on collision causing sudden violent hyperextension of the neck.

HYPEREXTENSION INJURIES OF THE CERVICAL SPINE

- It is *common in old patients with a stiff spondylotic cervical spine*. A stiff spine cannot dissipate the traumatic energy, and it is transmitted to the spinal cord.
- Frequent in spondylotic, ankylosing spondylitis
- *It results in central cord syndrome, which has a relatively good prognosis* (*Refer* **Fig. 16.9**).
- **Treatment:** Conservative with braces or operative fixation depending on displacement of vertebra and cord compression.

WHIPLASH INJURY

- It is common in RTAs with a "rear-end collision" of the vehicle, wherein the head is thrown in *hyperextension followed by hyperflexion* (**Fig. 16.19**).

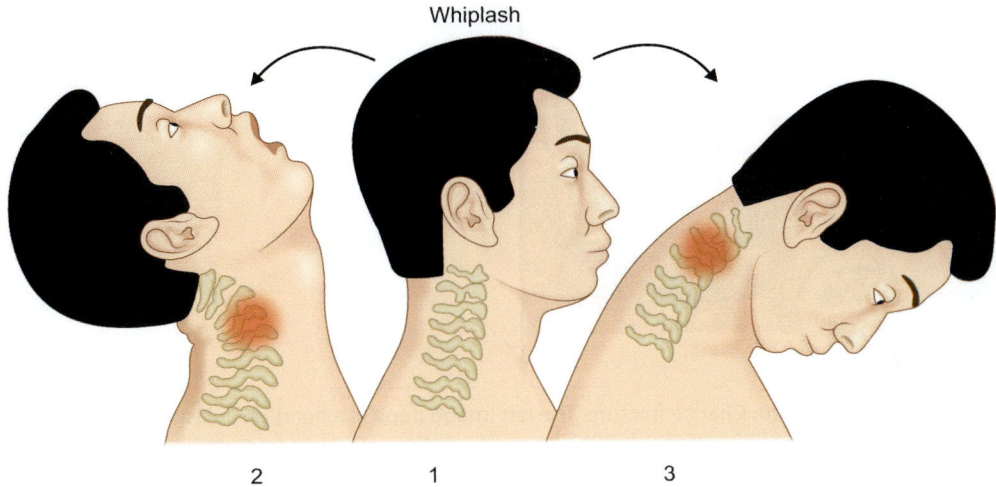

Fig. 16.19: Whiplash injury. Position 1, 2, 3 indicate neutral, hyperextension and flexion, respectively.

- *Usually, no fracture occurs in whiplash injury, but it results in sprain of the capsule and ligaments of the cervical spine.* However, the severe impact may damage the disc, facet joint, ligaments, muscle, and nerve roots. There may be an associated concussion injury to the brain.
- **Clinical features:** Pain and stiffness in the neck is the prime complaint. Sometimes, the pain radiates to both the shoulders and scapula. There may be headache, giddiness, and paresthesia in the limbs. Rarely difficulty in deglutition due to esophageal contusion. There may not be any specific demonstrable neurological sign.
- **Investigations:** Computed tomography and MRI of the spine must be done to rule out any bony/soft tissue injury around the spine or any injury to the spinal cord.
- **Treatment:** Conservative treatment is the mainstay—soft cervical collar, medications, and rehabilitation is the treatment of choice.
- **Complications:** Chronic residual pain and stiffness in the neck are quite common.

CHANCE FRACTURE (SEAT BELT INJURY/JACKKNIFE FRACTURE)

- *Typically seen in the "head-on collision"* of a vehicle with passengers with a seat-belt on. It was more common with "isolated lap seat belt." High chance of associated injury to the duodenum and pancreas. The incidence has reduced with shoulder belt modification.
- **Mechanism:** It is caused by *flexion-distraction injury to the spine resulting in* compression injury to anterior and middle elements (vertebral body) and transverse fracture or distraction through posterior elements (facets, spinous process).
- **Type of Chance fracture:** It is either a **bony Chance fracture** wherein the fracture line runs through the bony components of three columns, or it could be **ligamentous Chance fracture** wherein the injury runs through the intervertebral disc space and posterior ligament complex **(Fig. 16.20)**. The ligamentous chance # is a highly unstable injury which requires surgical fixation.
- **Clinical features:** It is similar to one described for spine injury with sensory, motor, and bladder-bowel affections.

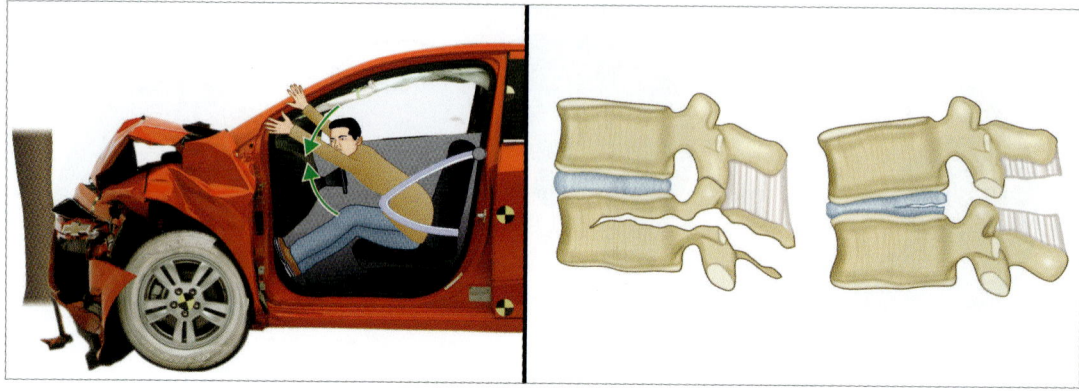

Fig. 16.20: Chance fracture. The left image depicts a head-on collision. The right image shows bony and soft tissue Chance fracture.

- **Investigations:** X-rays, CT and MRI.
- **Treatment:** Most cases require surgical stabilization of the spine.

SPINAL CORD INJURY WITHOUT RADIOLOGICAL ABNORMALITY (SCIWORA)

- It is a specific pattern of spine injury noted in the pediatric population (<8 years).
- There may be associated neurological deficit but no apparent radiological abnormality in the vertebra.
- It occurs due to very elastic ligaments which pull back the vertebra, and hence the radiological abnormality is not seen in the vertebra.
- **Investigations:** X-rays and CT scans are normal. However, they should be done to rule out a bony injury. The MRI of spinal cord can detect the injury to the cord in form of edema, or injury to disc causing compression of the cord.
- **Treatment:** Most cases can be managed with rest, braces and activity modification.

17 CHAPTER

Fracture Acetabulum

INTRODUCTION

Acetabulum fractures are *pelvis fractures that involve the articular surface of the hip joint*. Anatomically, the acetabulum is divided into anterior and posterior columns. The **anterior column** comprises *anterior half of the iliac crest, the iliac spines, the anterior half of the acetabulum, and the pubis*. The **posterior column** comprises *ischium, the ischial spine, the posterior half of the acetabulum, and the dense bone forming the sciatic notch*. The idea of columns is essential while classifying the acetabulum fractures. Since acetabular fractures are intra-articular fractures, an incongruent joint surface due to displaced fracture can result in osteoarthritis of the hip joint. And therefore, they must be managed on the principles of intraarticular fracture *(Refer Chapter 7)*.

MECHANISM OF INJURY

Typically, acetabular fractures are caused by high-energy trauma such as road traffic accident (RTA) or fall from a height.

CLINICAL FEATURES

As acetabular fractures result from high-energy trauma, many patients have injuries to the head, spine, chest, abdomen, and other limb bones. They may present with hemorrhagic shock and therefore, a complete assessment as per advanced trauma life support (ATLS) protocol is a must.

Symptoms
- Pain around the hip joint and pelvis
- Inability to bear weight and move the affected hip.

Signs
- Tenderness is present over the hip joint
- The patient will not be able to perform active straight leg raise
- Movements of the hip are painful and limited
- There may be associated Morel-Lavallée lesion **(Fig. 17.1)**

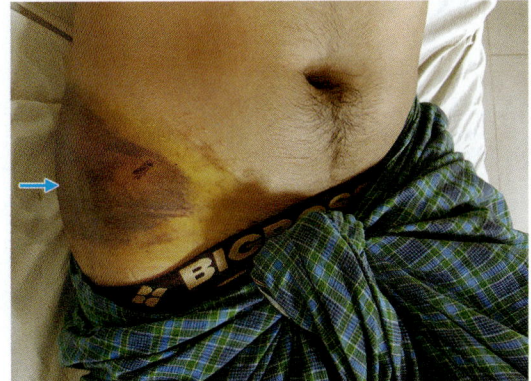

Fig. 17.1: Morel-Lavallée lesion (blue arrow).

- Rule out injury to the sciatic/obturator/femoral nerve—assess the sensation in lower limb, anterior and medial aspects of the thigh. Assess foot movements and knee extension to give an idea about the nerve injuries.

Morel-Lavallée Lesion

It is a closed degloving injury generally occurring over the lateral aspect of the hip and pelvis, characterized by the separation of subcutaneous tissue from underlying fascia, resulting in disruption of vascularity of skin and subcutaneous tissue. In addition, a cavity is created between the deep fascia and subcutaneous tissues. It may result in necrosis, infection, and poor healing (postoperatively) of the overlying skin and subcutaneous tissue.

INVESTIGATIONS

- **Plain X-rays:**
    - AP view of the pelvis (**Figs. 17.2A and B**)
    - *Judet views:* Iliac and obturator oblique views help to visualize the acetabulum in its entirety (**Figs. 17.3 and 17.4**). The iliac view is done in 45° of external rotation of the pelvis, whereas the obturator view is done in 45° of internal rotation.
        - Judet iliac oblique view assesses *posterior column and anterior wall of the acetabulum*
        - Judet obturator oblique view assesses *anterior column and posterior wall of the acetabulum.*
- **CT scan:** It helps to delineate the fracture lines (**Fig. 17.5**). It aids to visualize the entire acetabulum in 3D, which helps in surgical planning.

CLASSIFICATION OF ACETABULAR FRACTURES

Judet and Letournal classification is used to classify acetabular fractures. However, details of the classification are out of the purview of the syllabus.

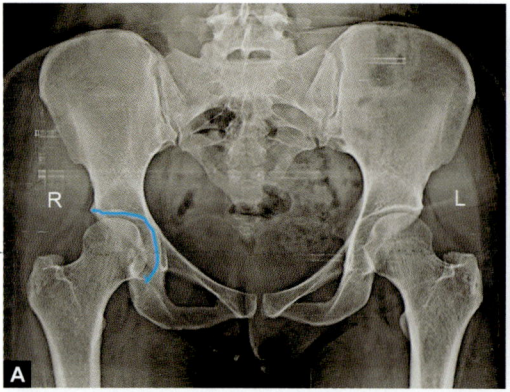 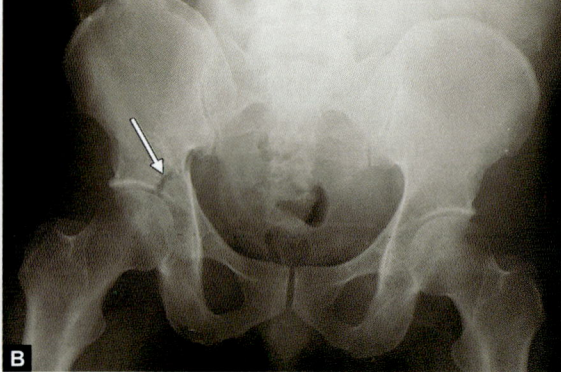

Figs. 17.2A and B: (A) X-ray of a normal pelvis with normal acetabulum (blue line); (B) X-ray pelvis shows right side acetabulum fracture (white arrow).

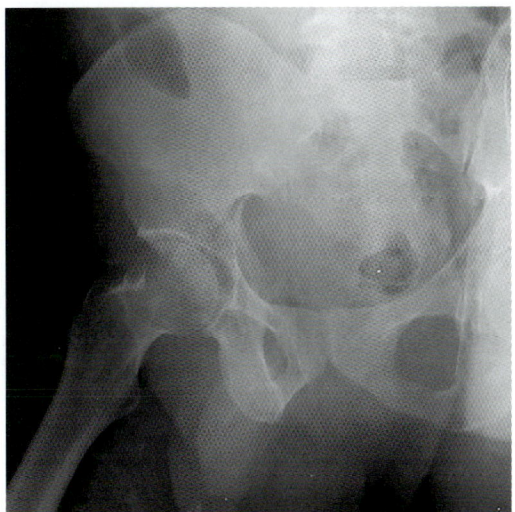

Fig. 17.3: Judet iliac view of the pelvis.

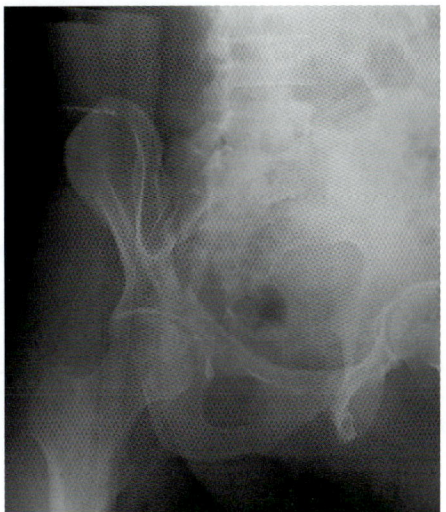

Fig. 17.4: Judet obturator view of the pelvis.

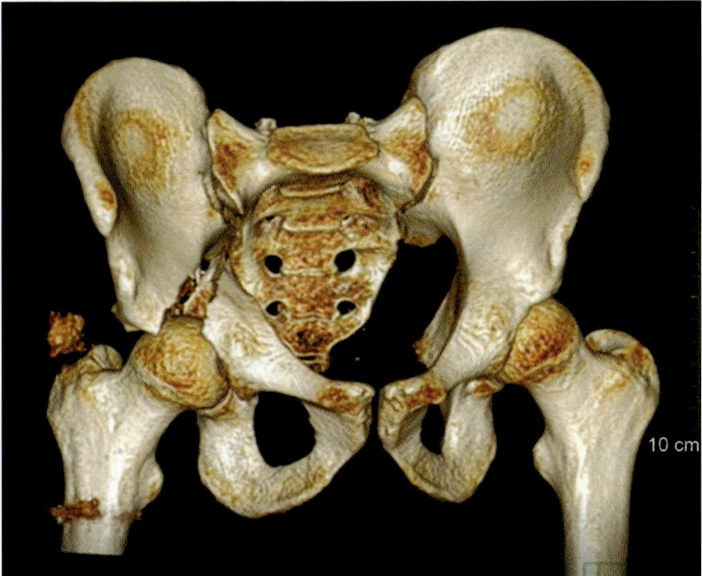

Fig. 17.5: 3D CT scan of the pelvis showing right acetabular fracture.

■ TREATMENT

Acetabular fractures can be managed conservatively or operatively.
- **Nonoperative:** It is indicated in *undisplaced/minimally displaced fractures* and patients with significantly medical comorbidities, which may result in high operative risks or perioperative morbidity/mortality. The patient is on bedrest with or without skeleton traction for 6–8 weeks followed by gradual weight bearing.

- **Operative:** Acetabular fractures are an intra-articular fracture. Therefore, a displaced fractures of acetabulum should be operated to restore the articular surface to provide restore joint congruity. It can be done in two ways:
  1. *Open reduction and internal fixation with plates and screws*
  2. Rarely, *total hip arthroplasty (THR)*, if the surfaces are not reconstructible. THR is also performed in old malunited acetabulum fractures with hip arthritis.

Surgical approaches to the acetabular fracture fixation
Various surgical approaches are described for the acetabulum fractures, such as the **Kocher-Langenbeck approach (posterior approach)** and the **Ilioinguinal approach (anterior approach)**. The selection of approach depends upon the involved column, e.g., *Kocher-Langenbeck and Ilioinguinal approach for posterior wall /column injury and anterior wall/column injury, respectively.*

COMPLICATIONS
- **Acute**
  - Injury to the pelvic organs
  - Hemorrhagic shock
  - Sciatic nerve injury.
- **Subacute:** Morel-Lavallée lesion.
- **Chronic**
  - Post-traumatic degenerative joint arthritis
  - Heterotopic ossification
  - Avascular necrosis of the femoral head.

Notes

CHAPTER 18

Fracture Femur Neck and Intertrochanteric Femur

FRACTURE FEMUR NECK

Fracture neck femur is quite common in older population, especially osteoporotic person. A normal hip X-ray is shown in **Figure 18.1**, while a fracture femur neck is shown in **Figure 18.2**. Before discussing fractures of proximal femur, it is essential to understand certain anatomical facts, such as blood supply of femoral head, bony trabaculae, and calcar femorale, which are relevant in management of the fractures of proximal femur.

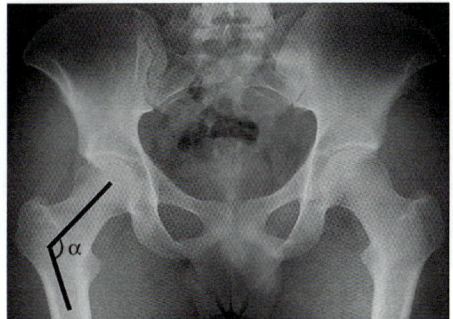

Fig. 18.1: Normal hip radiograph with neck-shaft angle measurement.

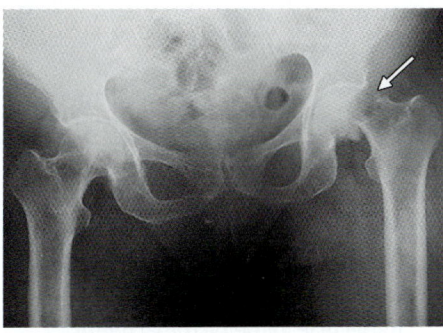

Fig. 18.2: X-ray showing left side fracture neck femur (white arrow).

Normal neck shaft angle (α): 126° (130° ± 7°)
Normal anteversion of femur: 10° ± 7°

SURGICAL ANATOMY REGARDING BLOOD SUPPLY OF HEAD FEMUR AND BONY TRABECULAE

- Blood supply to the femoral head is via three vessels—circumflex femoral, foveal, and metaphyseal (Fig. 18.3).
  1. *Medial and lateral circumflex femoral vessels:* **85%** of the blood supply to the femoral head in an adult is via medial and lateral circumflex vessels, which are branches of the profunda femoris artery. Together, circumflex vessels form an extracapsular circular anastomosis around the greater trochanter. The extracapsular anastomosis gives rise to *subsynovial intracapsular retinacular vessels,* which traverse along the femoral neck to penetrate and vascularize the femoral head.

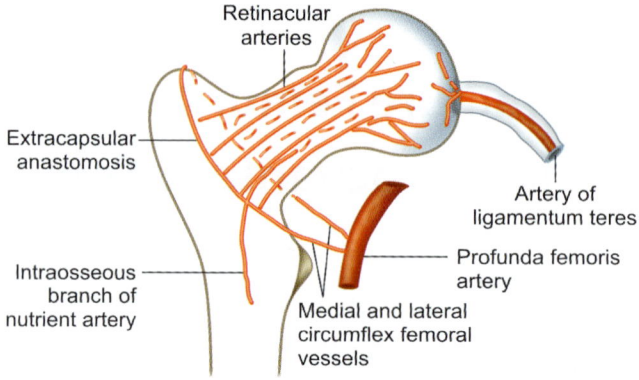

Fig. 18.3: Diagrammatic illustration of vascularity of the femoral head.

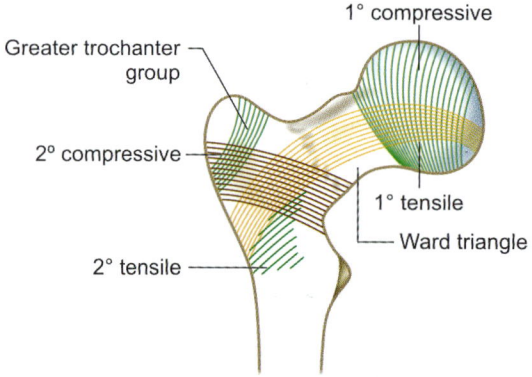

Fig. 18.4: Diagrammatic illustration of bony trabeculae in the proximal femur.

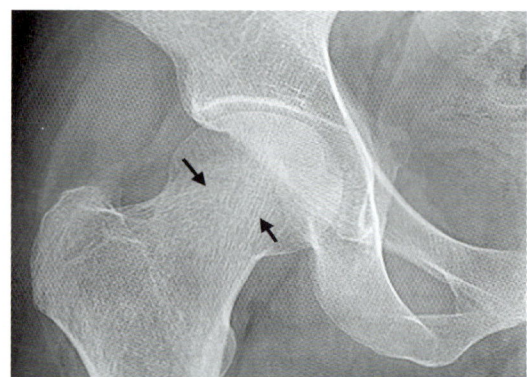

Fig. 18.5: X-ray of the femur showing bony trabeculae (black arrows).

  2. *Foveal vessels:* **10–15%** of the blood supply to the head arises from the foveal vessels (branches of the obturator artery). It penetrates the femoral head via ligamentum teres.
  3. *Intraosseous metaphyseal vessels:* These vessels arise from nutrient arteries.
- **Bony trabeculae of the proximal femur:** There are three groups of bony trabeculae in femoral head and neck area **(Figs. 18.4 and 18.5)**:
  1. *Primary and secondary compression trabeculae*
  2. *Primary and secondary tensile trabeculae*
  3. *Greater trochanter group*
  - These bony trabeculae develop along the lines of maximum stress and provide mechanical support to the proximal femur.
    The grading of trabecular prominence on a plain radiograph is assessed by *Singh's index* (Grades VI to I). Grade VI is normal, and grade I is severe osteoporosis. *Grade III and below is definite osteoporosis.*
  - *Clinical importance of bony trabaculae:* In due course of aging and osteoporosis, progressively, these trabeculae thin out and become less prominent, rendering the neck and trochanteric region weak and susceptible to fracture with minimal trauma.

- **Calcar femorale:**
  - ***Definition***: The calcar femorale is a normal ridge of dense bone that originates from the posteromedial endosteal surface of the proximal femoral shaft near the lesser trochanter. It is vertical in orientation, and the ridge projects laterally toward the greater trochanter. It is thickest medially and thins out as it passes laterally.
  - ***Clinical importance***: Calcar femorale reinforces the femoral neck posteriorly. A weak or resorbed calcar renders the femoral neck prone to fractures. Further, internal fixation of # neck or intertrochanteric femur may not be stable in case of poor/absent calcar. Furthermore, a *prosthesis used during partial hip replacement that sits on the calcar* (Austin Moore) should be avoided in patients with poor calcar femorale. In such a case, Thompson prosthesis is used, which does not require calcar femorale.

Relevant facts about fracture neck femur (NOF) are mentioned in **Box 18.1**.

> **Box 18.1:** Important facts about fracture neck of femur (#NOF)
>
> - Fracture neck femur is an ***intracapsular #***.
> - #NOF occurs in old age due to trivial trauma/fall and is **often associated with osteoporosis**.
> - Typically, it is said that "it is the fracture which causes the fall and not the fall which causes the fracture." Due to osteoporosis, multiple microfractures in the neck area render the neck of femur weak and cause the fall!
> - #NOF in young adults almost always occurs due to high-velocity trauma.
> - In modern orthopaedics, almost all #NOF across the age groups need surgical intervention except undisplaced # in pediatric population and/or a moribund patient who is medically unfit to undergo surgical intervention.

CLASSIFICATION OF FRACTURE NECK FEMUR

There are **three** common classification systems ***based on radiological findings***:
1. **Anatomical:** Based upon the *anatomic location of the fracture line in the femoral neck.*
2. **Pauwels':** Based upon the *angle of the fracture line with respect to the horizontal.*
3. **Garden's:** Based upon *displacement of the fracture.*

Anatomical Classification (Fig. 18.6)

- *Subcapital:* # line just below the femoral head
- *Transcervical:* # line in the middle of the neck
- *Basal:* # line at the base of the neck.

Pauwels' Classification (Fig. 18.7)

- *Type 1*: Less than 30° angle with respect to (wrt) the horizontal
- *Type 2*: 30°–50° angle wrt the horizontal
- *Type 3: 70° or more* angle wrt the horizontal

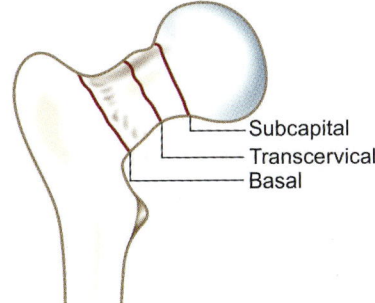

Fig. 18.6: Anatomical classification of fracture neck femur.

> **Practical implication of Pauwels' angle**
>
> *More vertical shear force is applied to the fracture site at higher Pauwels' angles*, making the fracture site more unstable. As a result, *the likelihood of fracture NOF nonunion increases with higher Pauwels' angle*.

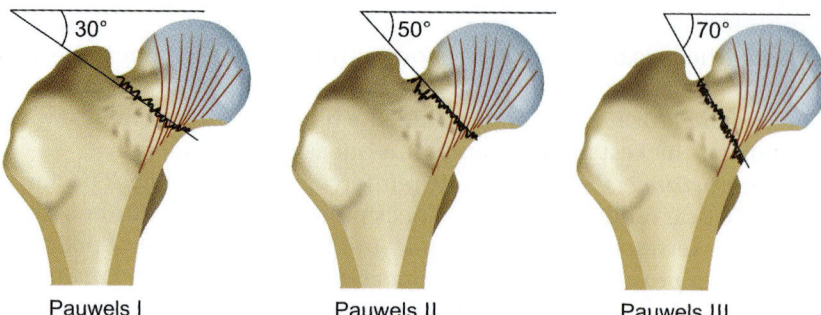

Fig. 18.7: Pauwels' classification (zig-zag black line indicates original fracture line).

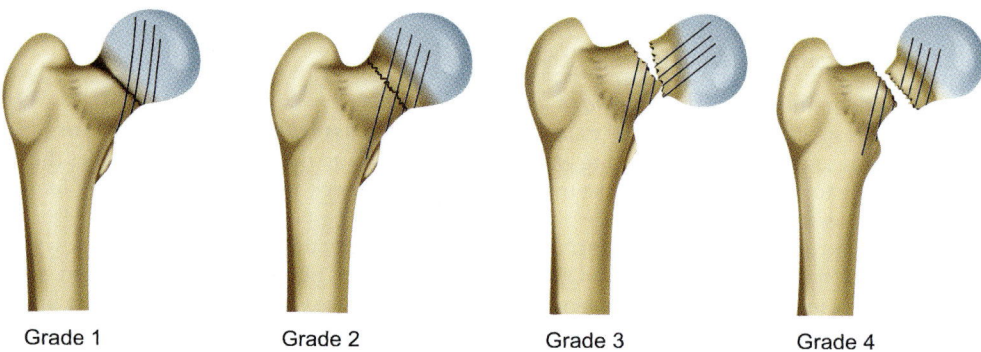

Fig. 18.8: Garden's classification.

Garden's Classification (Fig. 18.8)

- *Type 1*: Incomplete fracture, *trabeculae malaligned with respect to (wrt) acetabular trabeculae*
- *Type 2*: Complete fracture, undisplaced, trabeculae *aligned* wrt the acetabular trabaculae
- *Type 3*: Complete fracture, partially displaced, *trabeculae malaligned wrt* acetabular trabeculae
- *Type 4*: Complete fracture, completely displaced, trabeculae *aligned wrt* acetabular trabeculae.

CLINICAL FEATURES OF FRACTURE NECK OF FEMUR (NOF)

Most cases of fracture NOF occur in **elderly patients with trivial trauma**. Often, there is associated osteoporosis. In contrast, # NOF in a young adult is associated with high-energy trauma such as RTA.

Symptoms
- Pain in the index hip
- Inability to bear weight over the lower limb *(Note—patient can still bear weight in undisplaced or impacted #NOF).*

Signs
- The lower limb is externally rotated and shortened **(Fig. 18.9)**.
- Tenderness is present over Scarpa's triangle

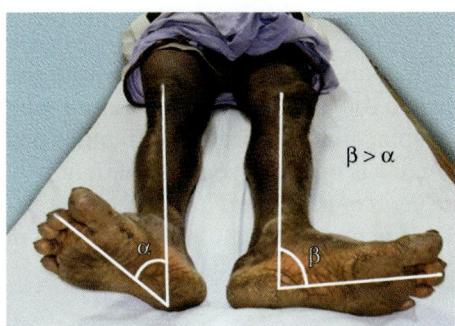

Fig. 18.9: External rotation attitude of the left lower limb in fracture NOF. Alpha and beta denote external rotation angle with vertical. Note that affected side angle is increased.

> **Box 18.2:** Clinical difference between #NOF and # intertrochanteric femur.
>
> "Every clinical feature is extra in intertrochanteric (IT) femur #"
> - Extra age: IT# occurs in more elderly
> - Extra trauma required for IT #
> - Extra pain and swelling over the hip region
> - Extra shortening
> - Extra external rotation.

- Active straight leg raising is not possible
- Attempted hip movements are painful.

The clinical differential diagnosis of fracture NOF is fracture intertrochanteric femur, which also occurs in elderly patient. Box 18.2 reveals the clinical difference between #NOF and # intertrochanteric femur.

INVESTIGATIONS

Plain X-ray of:
- Both hips: AP view **(Fig. 18.10)**.
- Affected hip: Lateral view

The important radiological findings of # NOF are mentioned in **Box 18.3**.

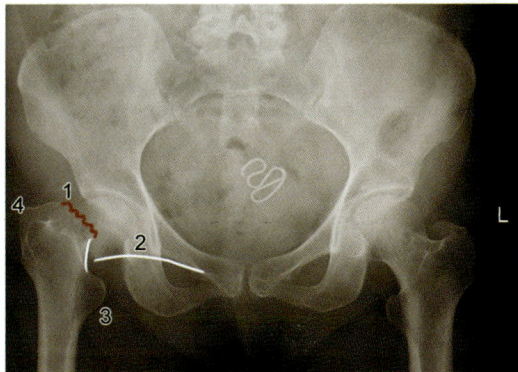

Fig. 18.10: X-ray of #NOF (right side) characterized by (1) Presence of #; (2) Broken Shenton line; (3) Prominent lesser trochanter compared to normal side; (4) Proximal migration of greater trochanter (compared to normal).

> **Box 18.3:** X-ray features of #NOF **(Fig. 18.10)**.
>
> - Presence of fracture line
> - Broken Shenton line
> - Prominent lesser trochanter
> - Proximal migration of greater trochanter (due to externally rotated limb)

TREATMENT

In modern orthopaedics, almost all displaced #NOF in a medically fit patient require surgical treatment. Typically, the essence of the treatment lies in the age of the patient. Since # NOF is associated with non-union and avascular necrosis, replacement is preferred in older patients to avoid risking such complications, whereas fixation of # is opted in younger patients.

- **Age less than 60 years:** The principle is *"save the head of the femur."*
  Plan—closed reduction and internal fixation of the fracture using multiple screws/dynamic hip screw **(Figs. 18.11A and B)**
- **Age over 60 years:** The principle is *"sacrifice the head of the femur."*
  Plan—replacement of femoral head. The replacement could be either hemi/total hip replacement depending upon the arthritic condition of the acetabulum **(Figs. 18.11C and D)**. Note that "undisplaced or minimally displaced" #NOF, even in a patient of more than 60 years, can be internally fixed.

Flowchart 18.1 illustrates the management of the fracture neck of femur.

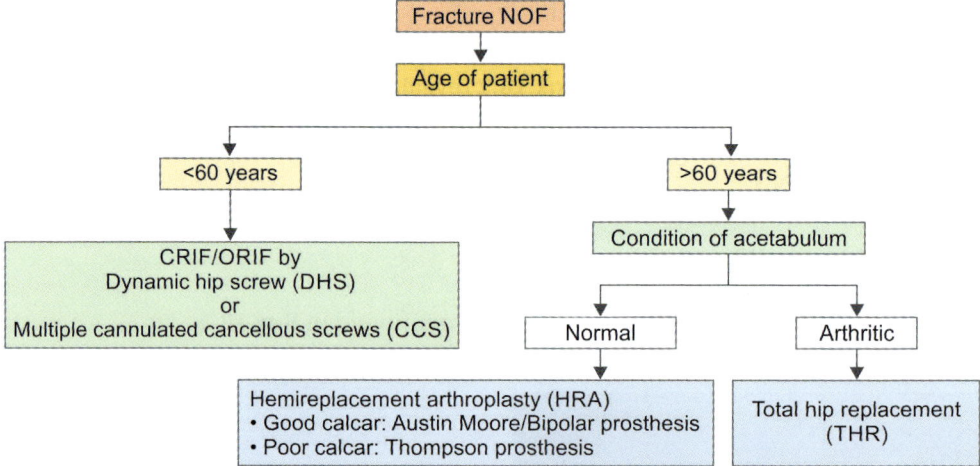

Flowchart 18.1: Treatment algorithm for fracture neck of femur (#NOF).

(CRIF: closed reduction and internal fixation; ORIF: open reduction and internal fixation)

The arbitrary cutoff age of 60 is not absolute, and save/sacrifice options for femoral head can change on either side of age. It is chosen based on various factors, such as longevity of person, co-morbidities, displacement of fracture, expected potential complications, etc. However, to simplify teaching, especially for undergraduates, it is prudent to stick to this cutoff age or follow as per your institutes standard teaching.

Currently, bipolar prosthesis is more frequently used for hemireplacement compared to unipolar Austin Moore or Thompson prosthesis. However, undergraduates can continue using the above algorithm as these prosthesis, especially Austin Moore, are still used in practice and often asked in viva.

Chapter 18: Fracture Femur Neck and Intertrochanteric Femur

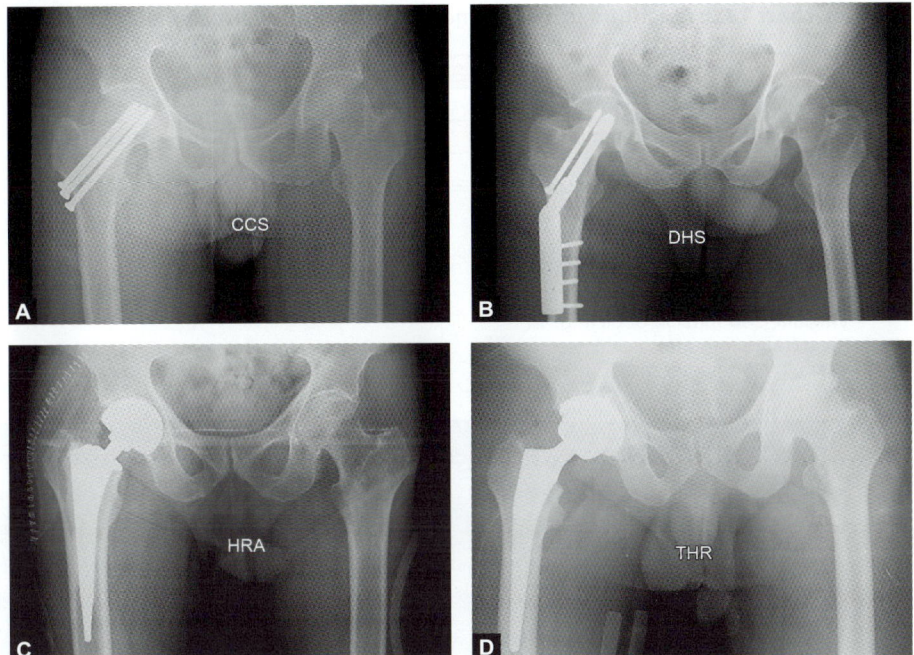

Figs. 18.11A to D: X-rays showing fracture neck of femur (#NOF) treatment.
(CCS: cannulated cancellous screws; DHS: dynamic hip screw; HRA: hemireplacement arthroplasty; THR: total hip replacement)

COMPLICATIONS OF FRACTURE NECK FEMUR

- Nonunion
- Avascular necrosis
- Hip osteoarthritis, which usually follows avascular necrosis of the femoral head.

Nonunion of Fracture Neck Femur

Usually seen after neglected trauma or after failed internal fixation surgery.

- **Clinical features**
    - Mild pain around the hip and difficulty/inability to bear weight
    - Patient limps while walking
    - Shortening and external rotation deformity of the lower limb is present
    - Telescopy and Trendelenburg tests are positive
- **Investigations**
    - *X-ray*: Features of nonunion—gap at # site, resorbed and shortened neck
    - *MRI/bone scan*: To rule out avascular necrosis (AVN).
- **Treatment (Flowchart 18.2)**.

Why nonunion is more common after fracture NOF? It is because of:
- Lysis of fracture hematoma due to synovial fluid
- Absence of cambium layer from periosteum of neck femur
- Disruption of neck vasculature (retinacular vessels) during the trauma leading to poor vascularity.

Section 2: Fractures and Ligament Injuries

Flowchart 18.2: Algorithm to manage nonunion fracture neck of femur (#NOF).

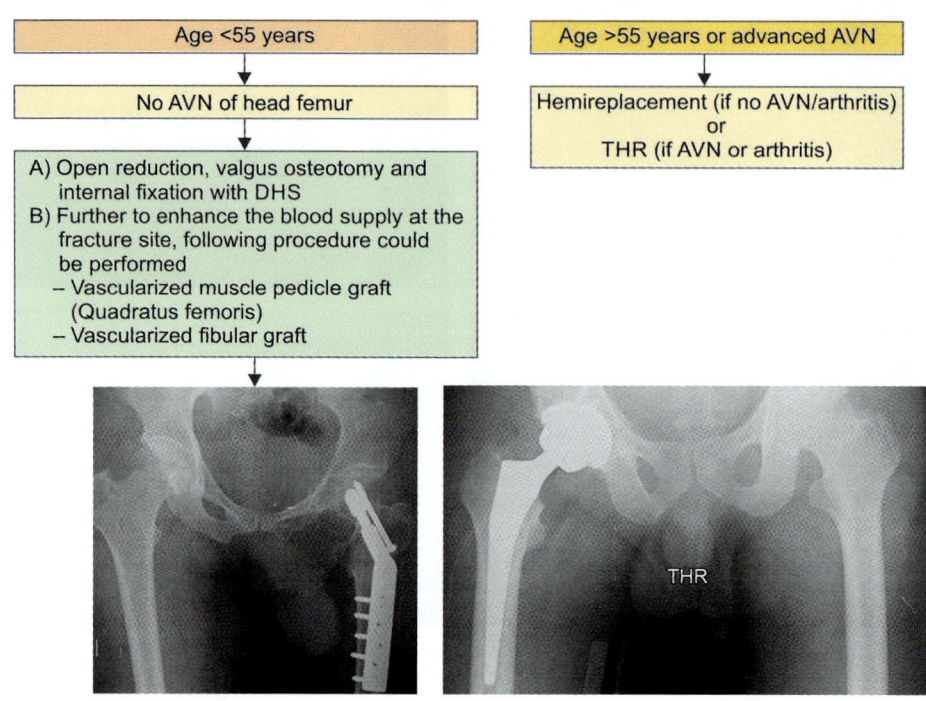

(AVN: avascular necrosis; DHS: dynamic hip screw; THR: total hip replacement)

Rationale of valgus osteotomy

Chronic nonunion of NOF leads to resorption of the neck femur. Hence, the fracture line becomes more vertical (increased Pauwels' angle). The valgus osteotomy (Pauwels') aims to convert this vertical fracture line into a more horizontal line so that the shear stresses at the fracture site are converted into compressive stresses, which helps in the compression and healing of the fracture site.

FRACTURE INTERTROCHANTRIC FEMUR

■ DEFINITION

Intertrochanteric (IT) fracture femur is a type of proximal femur fracture where the fracture line runs between two trochanters (greater and lesser) **(Fig. 18.12)**.

■ CLINICAL FEATURES

The clinical features are similar to # neck femur with some **"extra"** features (*see* **Box 18.2**).
   History of fall, elderly patient. Often, there is associated osteoporosis

Symptoms
- Pain, swelling, and often ecchymosis over the greater trochanter region.
- Inability to stand or bear weight over the affected lower limb.

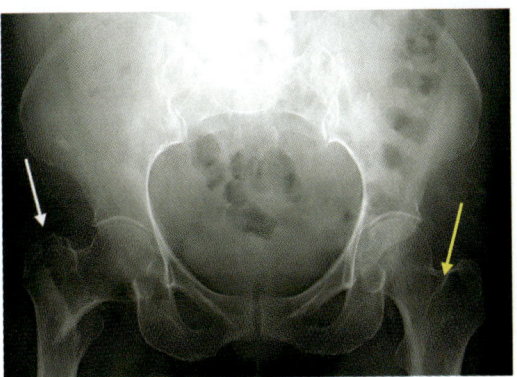

Relevant facts of IT fracture

- Unlike fracture neck femur, IT fracture is an **extracapsular fracture**
- Common in elderly, females, osteoporotic bones
- Unites easily as compared to #NOF due to **rich blood supply and large cancellous area**

Fig. 18.12: X-ray of the pelvis with both hips showing the normal intertrochanteric area of left hip (yellow arrow) and intertrochanteric fracture on the right hip (white arrow).

Signs
- Externally rotated and shortened lower limb
- Bony tenderness over the trochanteric region
- Unable to perform straight leg raise
- Attempted hip movements are painful.

CLASSIFICATION: EVANS' CLASSIFICATION
- **Stable #:** Normal posteromedial cortex
- **Unstable #:** Comminuted with fractured posteromedial cortex.

INVESTIGATIONS
- **Plain X-ray of the pelvis with both hips:** AP and lateral view of the index hip **(Fig. 18.12)**.
- **CT scan of index hip:** It is occasionally required in a comminuted IT fracture, wherein internal fixation is planned.

TREATMENT

Most intertrochanteric fractures can be managed conservatively as the union of # is generally not a concern. However, as IT # occurs in the elderly, they are prone to recumbent position problems arising during conservative treatment for a few weeks, such as DVT, bed sore, hypostatic pneumonia **(Box 18.4)**. These problems could result in increased morbidity and mortality. Further, a malunited IT # results in shortening and external rotation deformity.

Box 18.4: Problems of recumbent position during conservative treatment.
- Deep vein thrombosis (DVT)
- Hypostatic pneumonia
- Bedsores
- Urinary tract infection (UTI)

Therefore, to avoid problems of recumbency and malunion-related issues (shortening and external rotation of the limb), most IT# are operated on in modern orthopaedics. CR/OR and IF with dynamic hip screw (DHS) or proximal femoral nail (PFN) remains the operative choice. After the surgery, the patient can ambulate quickly out of bed, minimizing recumbency complications. *Conservative management is reserved for undisplaced # or medically unfit patients.*

An optimal algorithm for managing IT # is described in **Flowchart 18.3**.

Section 2: Fractures and Ligament Injuries

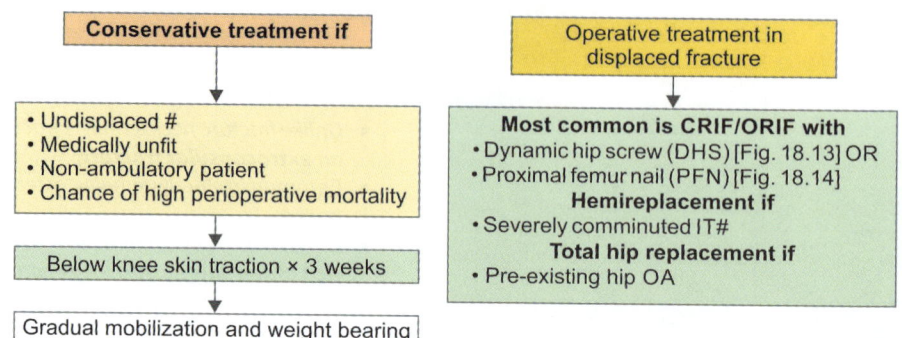

Flowchart 18.3: Treatment algorithm for managing IT fracture (#).

(ORIF: open reduction internal fixation; CRIF: closed reduction internal fixation; IT: intertrochanteric; OA: osteoarthritis)

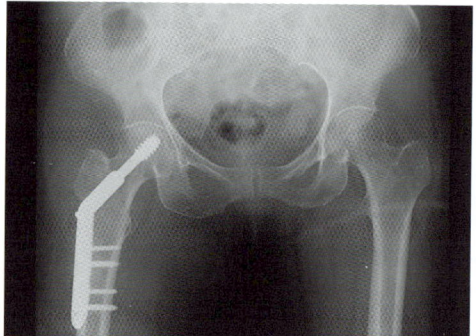

Fig. 18.13: X-ray of the pelvis showing dynamic hip screw fixation.

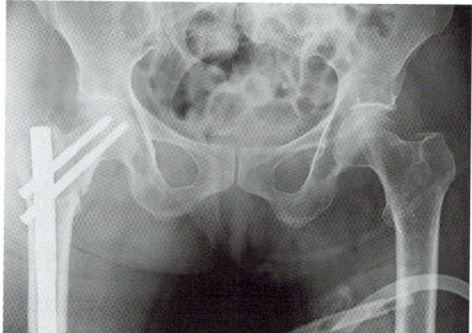

Fig. 18.14: X-ray of the pelvis showing proximal femur nail fixation.

COMPLICATIONS OF INTERTROCHANTERIC

- **Malunion:** The most common complication of IT # is *malunion* resulting in **coxa vara** deformity causing
  - *Shortening*
  - *External rotational deformity of the lower limb*
- **Nonunion:** Quite rare, less than 2%.
- **Complications of recumbent position:** Bedsore, respiratory tract infection (RTI), deep vein thrombosis (DVT) and urinary tract infection (UTI).

Why fracture neck femur and intertrochanteric femur are frequently operated in modern orthopaedics?

In modern orthopaedics, patients with #NOF and IT femur are often offered operative treatment to avoid complications arising out of recumbent position in bed for long (DVT, UTI, bedsore, and hypostatic pneumonia) if managed conservatively. These complications could result in serious morbidity and mortality.

Per se, no patient dies of complication of NOF/IT #, such as nonunion/malunion. However, by fixing/replacing the fracture, patient can be mobilized out of the bed very early, and thereby reducing the complications of recumbent position.

CHAPTER 19

Fracture around Knee—Patella, Distal Femur and Proximal Tibia

FRACTURE PATELLA

SURGICAL ANATOMY OF THE PATELLA

- It is the *largest sesamoid bone* in the body.
- It has two poles—superior and inferior, and there are two surfaces of the patella—articular and non-articular (NA) **(Fig. 19.1)**.
  The articular surface is covered by the thickest hyaline cartilage in the body and has seven articular facets. The NA surface receives attachment of quadriceps tendon (superiorly), patellar tendon (inferiorly), medial patellofemoral ligament (MPFL), and medial retinaculum (medially) and lateral patellar retinaculum (laterally). **Figure 19.2** shows a normal lateral X-ray of the knee showing patella.

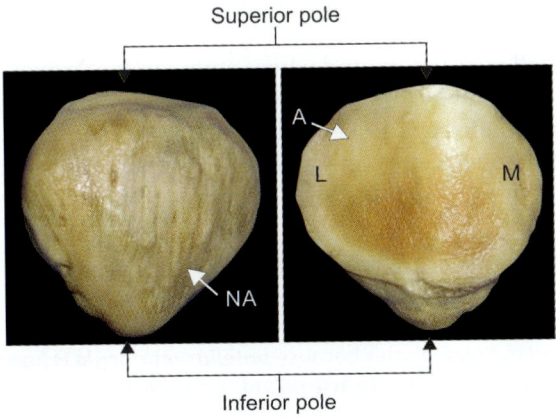

Fig. 19.1: Articular and non-articular surfaces of the patella.
(L: lateral; M: medial; A: articular; NA: nonarticular)

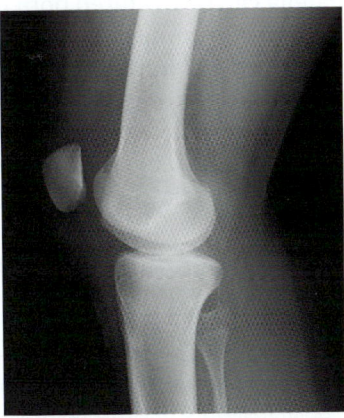

Fig. 19.2: Lateral X-ray of a normal knee showing patella.

FUNCTION OF THE PATELLA

- The most essential function of the patella is to *increase the quadriceps lever arm, facilitating the knee extension'* action by lowering the energy demand of the quadriceps muscle to extend the knee **(Fig. 19.3)**.
  Note: The post-patellectomy knee has decreased lever arm, leading to increased energy requirement in the quadriceps mechanism to extend the knee.

- Other functions of the patella are:
  - It provides shape to the knee.
  - It protects femoral condyles.

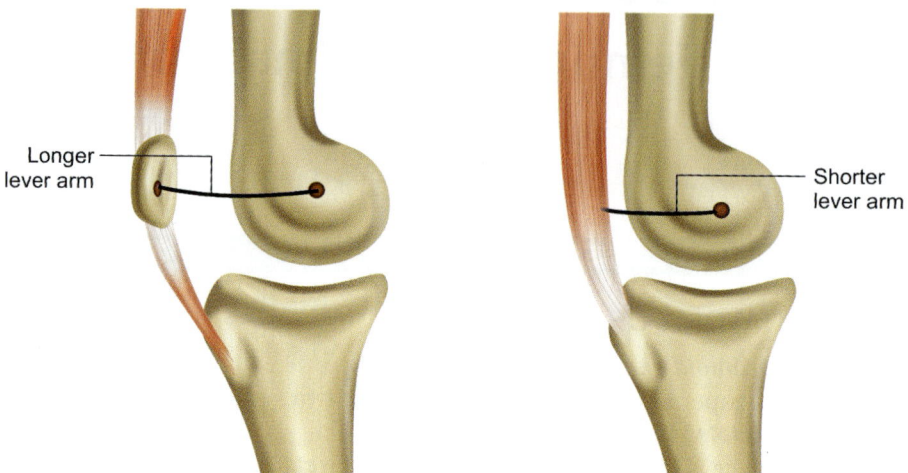

Fig. 19.3: Illustrative image of knee with preserved patella has a longer lever arm (left image), whereas post-patellectomy knee (right image) results in a shorter lever arm.

MECHANISM OF INJURY

Patella can be fractured both in direct and indirect trauma to the knee:
- **Direct trauma** to the knee
- **Indirect trauma:** During a free vertical fall over the ground where a person lands over the foot, the knee can continue to bend due to gravity. The continued bending of the knee is prevented by violent contraction of the quadriceps to keep the knee erect/straight and provide a stable landing, and this forceful quadriceps contraction of the quadriceps could result in a patella fracture.

Surgical implication of direct and indirect injuries causing patella fracture

It is important to differentiate between direct and indirect injuries because ***patellar retinacula is intact in direct injuries*** (stellate/comminuted #s), whereas ***retinacula is torn in all indirect injuries*** (transverse/polar fractures) due to longitudinal force propagating through the retinacula after fracturing the patella. Further:
1. Retinacular tears also contribute to extensor lag
2. Retinacular tears need repair while managing patella #.

CLASSIFICATION

It is based upon the radiological findings of the knee X-ray **(Fig. 19.4)**.
- **Transverse #:** The # line is perpendicular to the long axis of the patella.
- **Polar:** The # line separating the superior/inferior pole of the patella. *The inferior pole # is far more common than superior pole.*

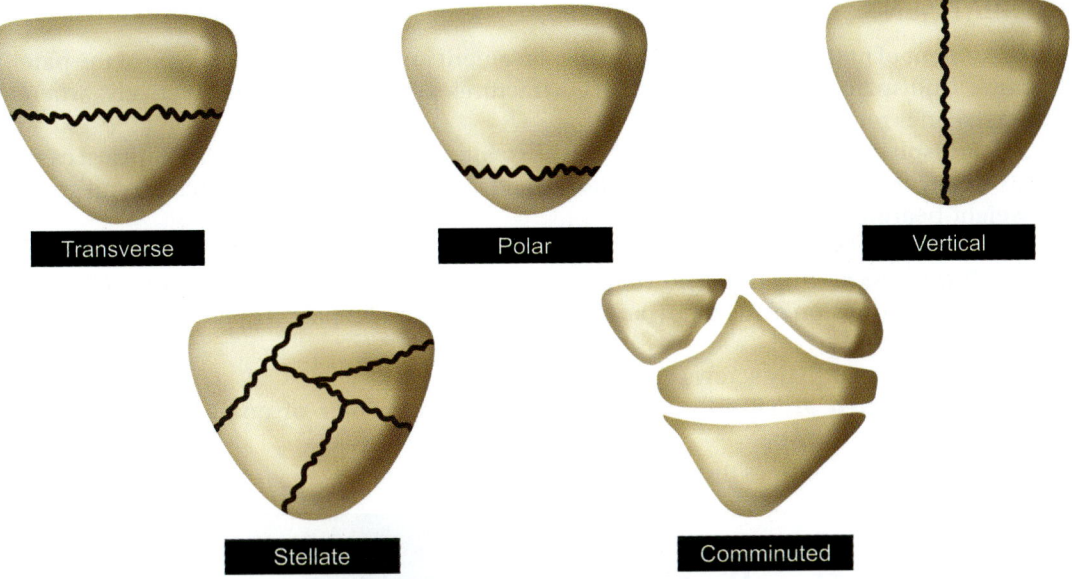

Fig. 19.4: Radiological classification of patella #.

- **Vertical:** The # line is parallel to the long axis of the patella.
- **Stellate:** Undisplaced, comminuted # of the patella.
- **Comminuted:** The multiple fragments are displaced.

Types 1, 2, and 3 can be undisplaced/displaced.

Except inferior pole patella #, all other type of patella # are intra-articular fractures, i.e., the # line breaches the patellar articular surface. Hence, accurate reduction of patella # is must to avoid incongruous articular surface and future patellofemoral arthritis.

CLINICAL FEATURES

Symptoms: Pain and swelling over the knee and inability to bear weight over the injured lower limb.

Signs
- Swelling in the knee (hemarthrosis)
- Bony tenderness present over the patella
- A *palpable gap* is felt over the patella
- Painful and limited movements
- *Extensor lag is present*.

INVESTIGATIONS

Plain X-ray of the knee
- AP and lateral view **(Fig. 19.5)**
- Skyline view is performed to look for vertical #, which may remain obscure on AP and lateral views.

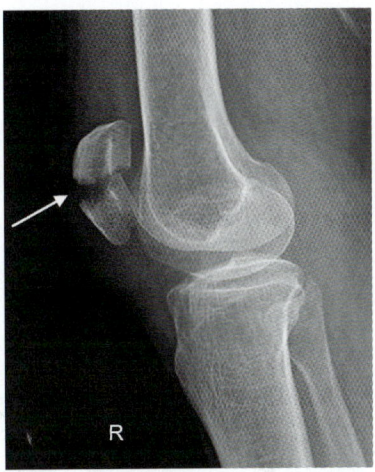

Fig. 19.5: Lateral X-ray of the knee showing # patella.

TREATMENT

The treatment of patella # depends upon displacement and the radiological type of the patella fracture. Undisplaced/minimally displaced fractures are managed conservatively, whereas displaced ones require surgery.

- **All undisplaced fractures/stellate** # can be treated with the above-knee cylindrical cast for six weeks, followed by knee mobilization, quadriceps strengthening exercises, and gradual weight-bearing.
- **Displaced fractures** are treated by the following methods:
  - *Transverse* #: ORIF by tension band wiring (TBW) **[Fig. 19.6]** or screw fixation **(Fig. 19.7)**.
  - *Polar* #: Excision of the pole (partial patellectomy) and repair of quadriceps mechanism **(Fig. 19.8)**.
  - *Vertical* #: ORIF by screws.
  - *Comminuted* #: TBW or total patellectomy and repair of quadriceps mechanism **(Fig. 19.9)**.

Flowchart 19.1 summarizes the treatment of patella fracture.

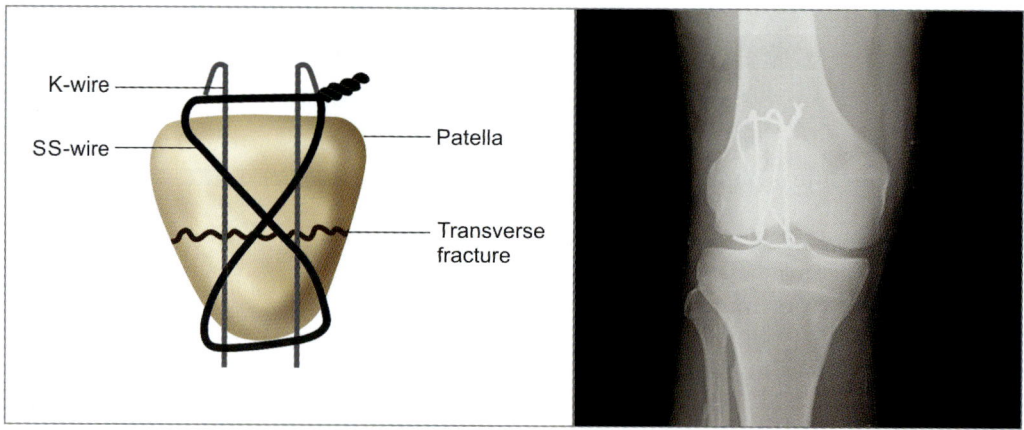

Fig. 19.6: Illustrative image of tension band wiring of transverse # patella (left image), whereas right image shows plain X-ray of the same.
(ORIF: open reduction and internal fixation; TBW: tension band wiring)

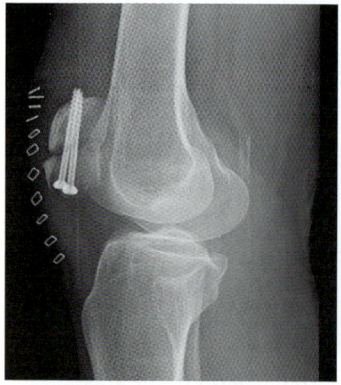

Fig. 19.7: Screw fixation for transverse # patella.

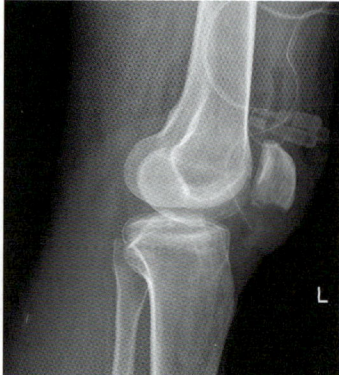

Fig. 19.8: Inferior pole excision for polar # patella.

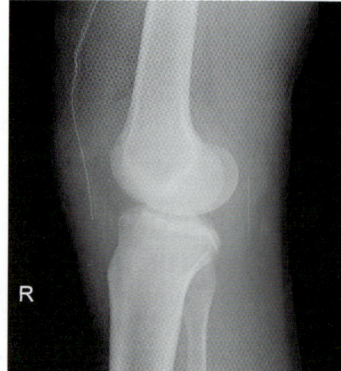

Fig. 19.9: Total patellectomy for comminuted # patella.

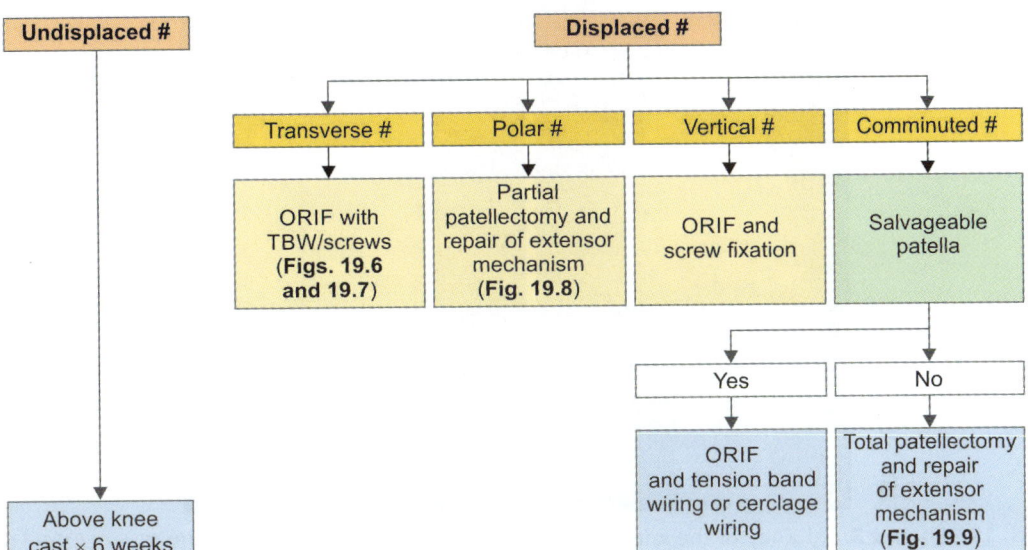

Flowchart 19.1: Treatment algorithm of fracture patella.

COMPLICATIONS OF PATELLA FRACTURE

- **Knee stiffness:** One of the most common complication with varying degree of loss of ROM.
- **Extensor lag:** Extensor lag is a condition that prevents the patient from actively extending the knee *due to weakness in the quadriceps muscle*. However, the patient or physician can passively extend the knee **(Fig. 19.10)**.
- **Patellofemoral osteoarthrosis:** Except inferior pole, all other patella fractures are intra-articular fractures. Any incongruency over the articular surface may result in secondary patellofemoral osteoarthrosis. These patients complain of pain while squatting/sitting cross leg/climbing-descending stairs. Crepitus is felt over the patella.
- **Nonunion**, malunion.
- **Myositis ossificans.**

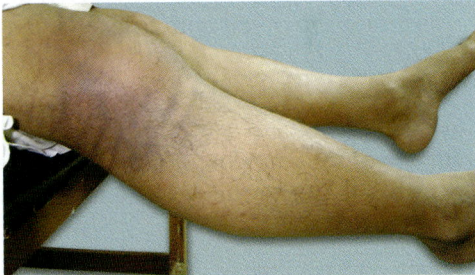

Fig. 19.10: Extensor lag in the right knee after patella #.

DISTAL FEMUR FRACTURE

Distal femur fractures are traumatic injuries involving the region extending from the distal femoral metaphyseal-diaphyseal junction to the articular surface of the femoral condyles. *Distal femur fracture could be supracondylar or intercondylar*. Supracondylar area of the femur is located in the distal 10–15 cm of the femur, whereas intercondylar # of the femur extends into the knee joint and is an intra-articular #.

A fracture in this region would compromise the function of the knee. Therefore, accurate reconstruction of the distal femur anatomy is necessary to restore the function of the knee.

Figure 19.11 shows X-rays of normal distal femur and fracture distal femur.

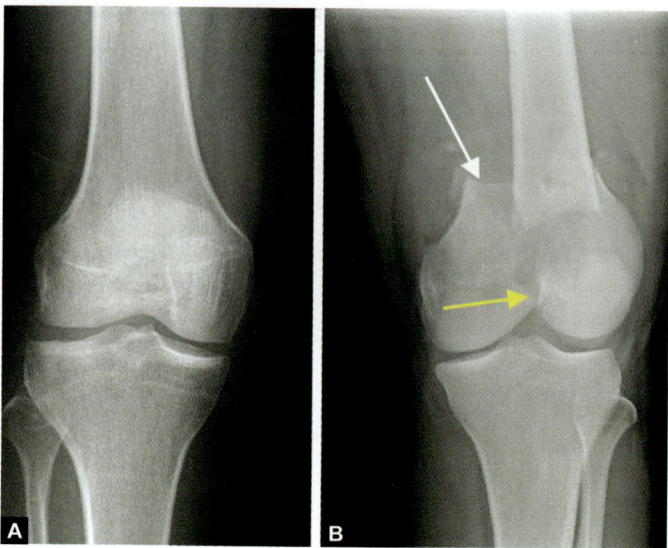

Figs. 19.11A and B: (A) X-ray of the knee (AP view) showing normal distal femur; (B) X-ray of the knee (AP view) showing fracture of supracondylar region of femur (white arrow) with intra-articular extension (yellow arrow).

MECHANISM OF INJURY

- **High-velocity injury:** In young adults, these fracture are usually due to high-energy trauma such as a motor vehicle collision or fall from a height.
- **Low-velocity injury:** In the elderly, the fracture may result from a low-velocity trauma such as minor slip or fall onto a flexed knee due to underlying osteoporosis.

CLINICAL FEATURES

Since most distal fractures result from high-velocity direct trauma, they are often open fractures with comminution and intra-articular extension. The combination of comminuted open fracture with intra-articular extension, makes it very challenging to manage.

Symptoms
- Pain and swelling at the lower end of the femur
- Inability to bear weight.

Signs
- Swelling and deformity present at the lower end of the femur
- Bony tenderness is present at the lower end of the femur
- Any attempt of knee movement is extremely painful
- Assessment of neurovascular status is prudent, as injury to the popliteal artery and adjacent nerves (tibial, common peroneal) is not uncommon.

INVESTIGATIONS

- **Plain X-rays of knee:** AP **(Fig. 19.12)** and lateral views.
- **CT scan** of the distal femur with 3D reconstruction is required for preoperative planning and evaluating intra-articular involvement **(Fig. 19.13)**

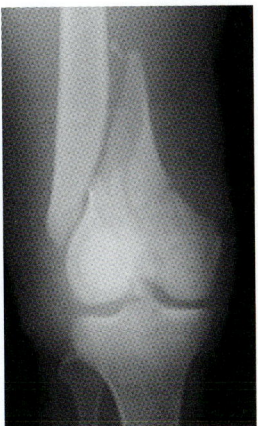

Fig. 19.12: X-ray of the knee (AP view) showing displaced, comminuted supracondylar fracture with intra-articular extension.

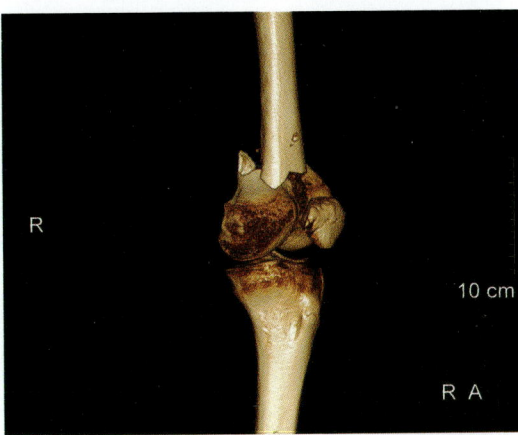

Fig. 19.13: 3D CT scan of supracondylar femur fracture with intercondylar extension.

- **MRI** of the knee aids in evaluating ligamentous injury of the knee. However, it is often not performed in acute stage.

TREATMENT

- **Non-operative:** *Conservative treatment* is indicated for *undisplaced/minimally displaced fractures* with an above knee cast for 6–8 weeks, followed by mobilization.
- **Operative:** *Operative treatment* is indicated in *displaced intra-articular fractures*. The intra-articular fractures must be accurately reduced to restore the articular congruity. The fracture can be treated with ORIF with:
    - Screws alone
    - Plates and screws **(Fig. 19.14)**
    - Distal femoral nail.

COMPLICATIONS

- Knee stiffness
- Post-traumatic osteoarthritis
- Malunion
- Nonunion.

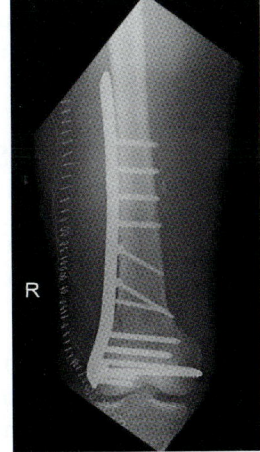

Fig. 19.14: X-ray of the knee showing ORIF of the distal femur fracture with plate and screws.

TIBIAL PLATEAU FRACTURE

Fracture of proximal tibia is also called as tibial plateau fracture. Most proximal tibia fractures are result from high-velocity injury such as RTA or fall from height. It could be closed/open fracture. They are also prone to compartment syndrome. Often, these fractures are intra-articular and comminuted **(Figs. 19.15A and B)**.
- Tibial plateau fractures are intra-articular fractures wherein the fracture enters the tibial articular surface (tibial plateau). The fracture also involves proximal metaphysis and often extends into the shaft. Tibial plateau # is also called as ***bumper fracture***.

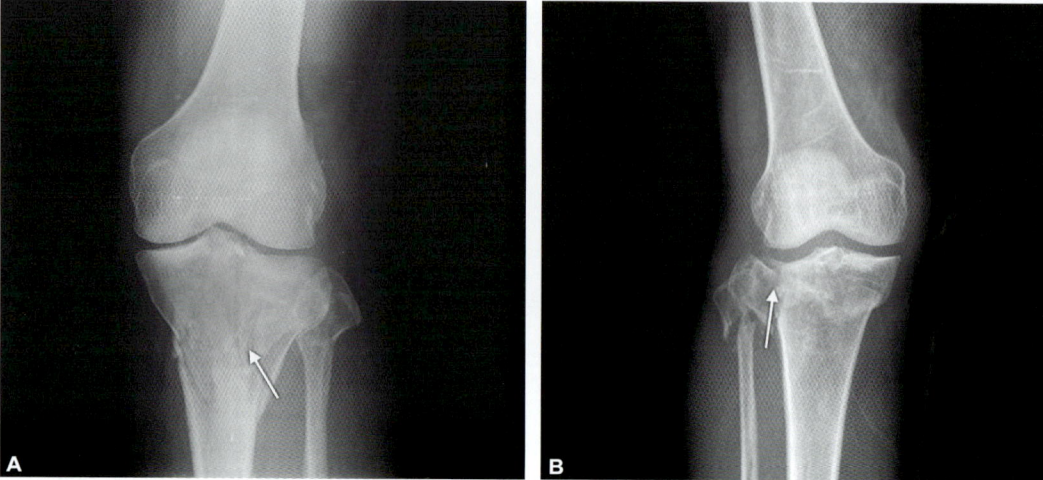

Figs. 19.15A and B: (A) X-ray of the knee showing fracture of proximal tibia; (B) Another X-ray showing intra-articular extension.

- **Mechanism of injury:** High-velocity injuries like RTA, fall from height
- **Classification of tibial plateau fracture:** Schatzker classified tibial plateau fracture into six type—I–VI. Further details of classification are out of scope of this book (for undergrads).

CLINICAL FEATURES

Symptoms
- Pain, swelling, and deformity of the proximal tibia
- Inability to bear weight over the lower limb.

Signs
- Bony tenderness present over the proximal tibia and joint line
- In proximal tibia fractures due to high velocity RTA, *fracture blisters* are often present over the skin indicating compromised blood supply to the skin and underlying soft tissue.
- *High incidence of compartment syndrome*
- *Neurovascular injury* (popliteal vessels, tibial or common peroneal nerve) is not uncommon. Therefore, a thorough neurovascular examination is a must.
- *Associated knee ligament injury* is frequent, and must be ruled out with clinical examination or later with an MRI.

DIAGNOSIS

- **Plain X-ray:** AP and lateral view of the knee and proximal tibia **(Fig. 19.16)**.
- **CT scan of the knee with 3D reconstruction:** To assess comminution and intra-articular extension **(Fig. 19.17)**.
- **MRI of the knee:** To assess ligament injury. In most cases, it is performed after primary management.

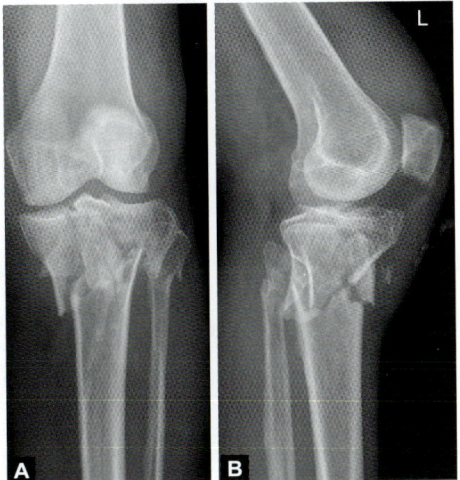

Figs. 19.16A and B: AP and lateral view of X-ray knee showing comminuted tibial plateau fracture.

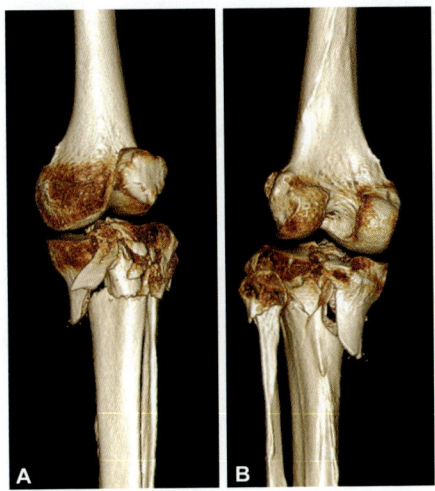

Figs. 19.17A and B: 3D CT scan of proximal tibia showing comminution and intra-articular extension.

TREATMENT (FLOWCHART 19.2)

- **Undisplaced #:** Above knee cast is applied for 6 weeks followed by non-weight bearing knee mobilization for another 6 weeks. Gradual weight bearing is allowed after 3 months.
- **Displaced #**
    - Accurate reduction of intra-articular fracture is essential followed by internal fixation with plate and screws with/without bone grafting **(Fig. 19.18)**.
    - Occasionally external fixator is applied if # is too comminuted or skin condition is poor.
    - Weight bearing is allowed after 12–14 weeks once fracture starts healing.

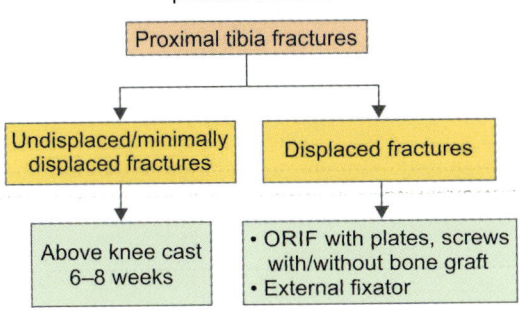

Flowchart 19.2: Treatment algorithm of tibial plateau fractures.

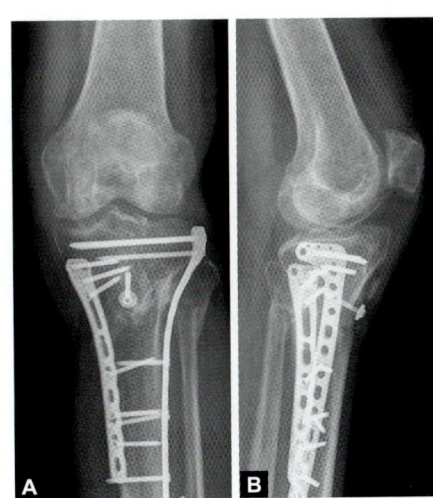

Figs.19.18A and B: AP and lateral view X-rays showing open reduction and internal fixation of fractures by plates and screws.

COMPLICATIONS

Acute
- Compartment syndrome
- Neurovascular injury

Chronic
- Malunion
- Nonunion
- 2° osteoarthritis of knee joint (as it is intra-articular fracture)
- Knee stiffness
- Rarely, knee instability due to 'missed' untreated ligament injury of the knee.

20 CHAPTER

Fracture Shaft Femur and Subtrochanteric Femur

FRACTURE SHAFT FEMUR

INTRODUCTION

- The shaft of the femur lies between the subtrochanteric level to the supracondylar level of the femur.
- Most shaft femur # occurs **due to road traffic accidents (RTA) and other high-velocity injuries.** Since the fracture shaft femur results from high-velocity injury, it is often associated with life-threatening injuries to the head, chest, spine, abdomen, and pelvis. And, therefore, one must examine the patient thoroughly to rule out all other injuries.
- Further, it is important to *note that an isolated fracture femur in an adult could result in blood loss of 1–1.5 liters, whereas it could be as high as 2–2.5 liters if there is an associated fracture of the pelvis*, which could result in *life-threatening hypovolemic shock*.

CLINICAL FEATURES

Symptoms: Pain, swelling, and deformity over the thigh and inability to bear weight.

Signs: In patients with # shaft femur, apart from local signs, one must always assess the features of *hypovolemic shock in patients, if they are brought to the triage within a few hours of the injury*. Further, the features of *fat embolism* should be ruled out for patients who present to triage between 24–72 hours.

The local signs are:
- *External rotation deformity and shortening* of the lower limb.
- Bony tenderness is present over the shaft femur.
- Examine for neurovascular deficit—injury to the femoral artery, femoral or sciatic nerve.

INVESTIGATIONS

Plain X-ray of:
- **Pelvis with both hips anteroposterior (AP):** To rule out pelvic # and ipsilateral # neck of femur (NOF)
- **Index thigh:** AP and lateral **(Fig. 20.1)**.

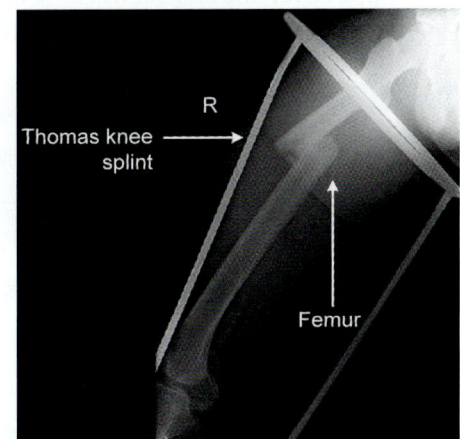

Fig. 20.1: X-ray of the thigh showing fracture shaft femur stabilized with Thomas knee splint.

TREATMENT

It can be divided in two parts:
1. Initial evaluation and treatment
2. Definitive treatment.

Initial Evaluation and Treatment

Initial evaluation and treatment must follow *advanced trauma life support (ATLS) protocol*, as # femur is often associated with multiple injuries. The femur fracture must be stabilized in the *Thomas knee splint*. In patients with hypovolemic shock, the treatment of *hypovolemic shock* must be immediately started on standard principles. Also, watch for *fat embolism* over the next 48–72 hours, wherein patients may develop dyspnea and confusion due to hypoxia.

Definitive Treatment

The definitive treatment of the fracture femur depends upon the patient's age **(Flowchart 20.1)**.
- **Age <6 months**
  - *Pavlik harness*
  - *Thigh to abdomen strapping*: There is a chance of femoral nerve compression
- **Age 6 months–2 years:** Closed reduction of the # and 90-90 hip spica application **(Fig. 20.2)**. 90-90 implies 90-degree flexion at the knee and the hip, respectively.
  Note: In the past, Gallows traction used to be applied in kids <2 years to manage fracture shaft femur **(Fig. 20.3)**. However, it was noted that Gallow's traction was associated with a high incidence of neurovascular deficit, especially sciatic nerve palsy, which led to abandoning the procedure.
- **2–12 years**
  - Closed reduction of femur fracture, above knee skin traction application and stabilization over Thomas knee splint for 2–4 weeks **(Fig. 20.4A)**. After 2–4 weeks, soft callus forms, resulting in a sticky fracture. Then, TK splint is removed and hip spica is applied for another six weeks **(Fig. 20.4B)**. If the reduction is unacceptable or the child does not tolerate Thomas splint, plan for:

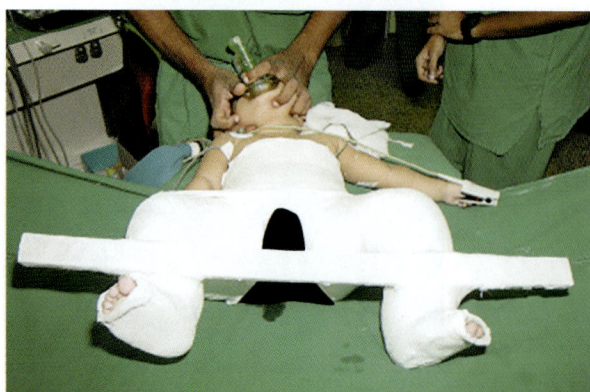

Fig. 20.2: 90–90 hip spica.

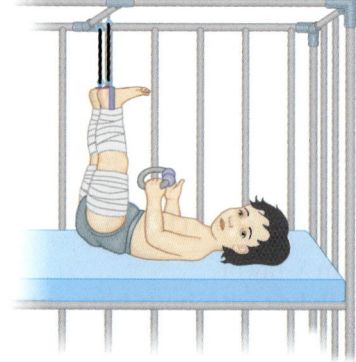

Fig. 20.3: Gallow's traction.

Chapter 20: Fracture Shaft Femur and Subtrochanteric Femur

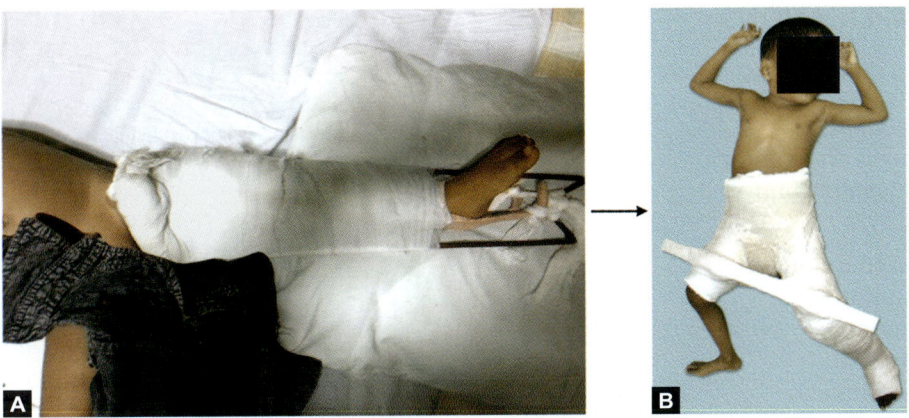

Figs. 20.4A and B: (A) Fracture reduced and maintained in below/above knee skin traction on Thomas knee splint; (B) Fracture further maintained in the one and half hip spica.

- Closed reduction internal fixation (CRIF)/open reduction internal fixation (ORIF) with elastic nails.

  Or
- ORIF with dynamic compression plate (DCP) and screws.
- **Age >12 years**
  - *CRIF/ORIF with intramedullary interlocking femoral nails* is the **current gold standard** (Fig. 20.5)
  - Sometimes, ORIF with DCP and screws.

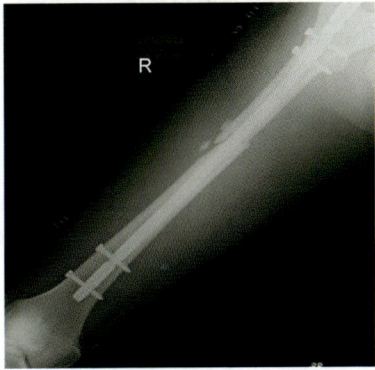

Fig. 20.5: X-ray showing intramedullary interlocking nail in femur #.

Flowchart 20.1: Algorithm to treat fracture shaft femur in various age groups.

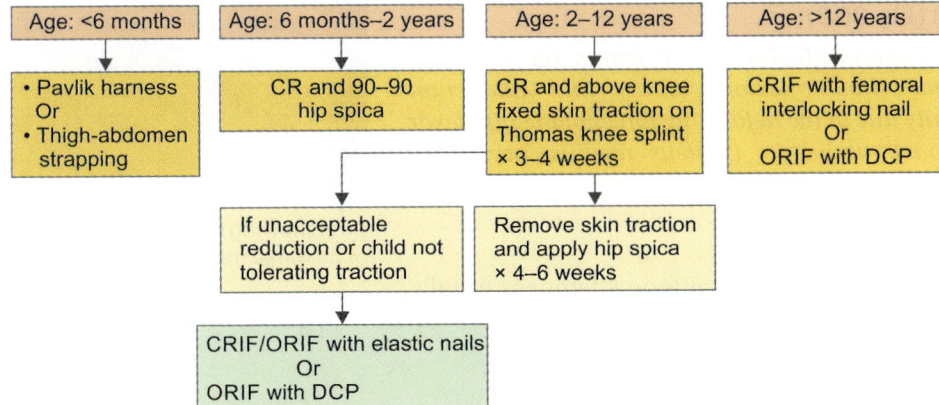

(ORIF: open reduction and internal fixation; CRIF: closed reduction and internal fixation; DHS: dynamic hip screw)

COMPLICATIONS

Acute
- *Hypovolemic shock*
- *Fat embolism*
- Femoral artery injury
- Sciatic nerve injury.

Chronic
- Delayed union
- Nonunion
- Malunion
- Shortening
- Knee stiffness.

FRACTURE SUBTROCHANTERIC FEMUR

INTRODUCTION

The subtrochanteric fracture femur is defined as a fracture 5 cm below the lesser trochanter. It is quite common in young adults.

MECHANISM OF INJURY

- It occurs after **RTA and other high-velocity injuries.**
- Sometimes, it is also observed *after "long-term therapy of bisphosphonates"* (>3–5 years), given for osteoporosis, resulting in brittle quality bone in the proximal femur due to interference in bone remodeling by the bisphosphonates. In such a case, subtrochanteric # can occur after a low-velocity injury, such as a mere fall on the ground.

CLINICAL FEATURES

The clinical features are similar to the # shaft femur.

INVESTIGATIONS

X-ray of the pelvis with both hips AP, index thigh (AP, lateral) **(Fig. 20.6)**.

Note: In the subtrochanteric # femur, the proximal fragment shows flexion, varus, and abduction deformity due to the deforming forces of the hip flexor (iliopsoas), abductors (gluteus medius, minimus), and external rotators.

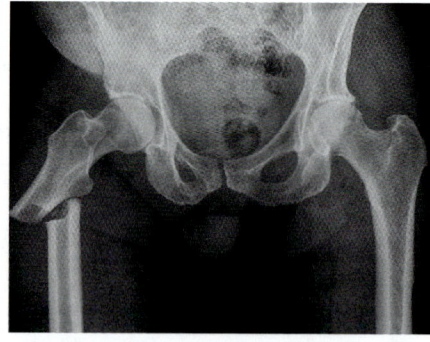

Fig. 20.6: Subtrochanteric femur (right side) showing flexion, varus and abduction of proximal fragment.

TREATMENT

The treatment of subtrochanteric # femur is usually operative with CRIF/ORIF with an intramedullary interlocking nail.

COMPLICATIONS

It is similar to the # shaft femur. However, it is *more prone to nonunion.*

CHAPTER 21

Fractures of Both Bone Leg, Tibial Plafond, Calcaneum and Small Bones of Foot

FRACTURES OF SHAFT TIBIA FIBULA

INTRODUCTION

- Tibia shaft # are quite common # in young patients due to *road traffic accidents (RTA)* or *other high-velocity injuries* (Figs. 21.1 and 21.2). Fibula # is frequently associated with tibial shaft fracture.
- *Many of the shaft tibia # are open fractures,* as the tibia is a subcutaneous bone with minimal soft tissue coverage over the anterior aspect. Direct trauma makes it prone to an open injury.
- *There is a high chance of compartment syndrome in tibia fracture due to three osteofascial compartments* (anterior, lateral and posterior). High-velocity injury may ensue bleeding and edema in the tight osteofascial compartment resulting in compartment syndrome.
- Lower third fractures of the tibia are often associated with nonunion.

MECHANISM OF INJURY

- **High-velocity injury such as in RTA/direct impact**
- **Indirect:** Fall from height, twisting injury to the ankle.

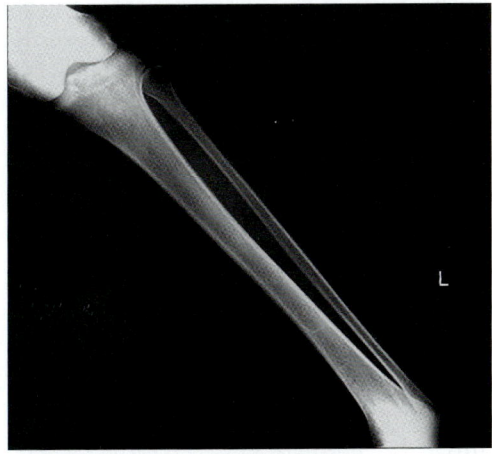

Fig. 21.1: X-ray of the normal leg showing normal tibia and fibula.

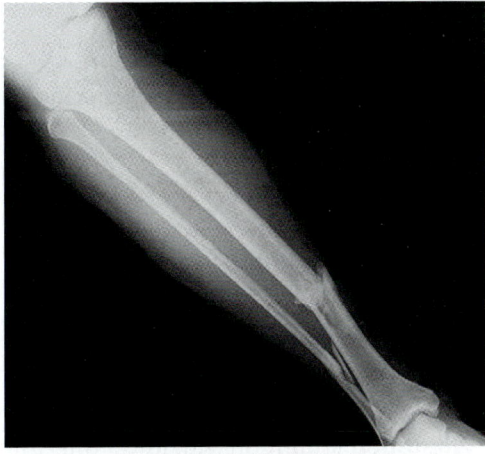

Fig. 21.2: Anteroposterior X-ray of the leg showing fracture shaft tibia fibula.

CLINICAL FEATURES

Symptoms
Pain, swelling, and deformity of the leg and inability to bear weight over the lower limb.

Signs
- Bony tenderness over the shaft of the tibia
- Bony crepitus over the shaft of the tibia (usually not elicited)
- Loss of transmitted movements
- Neurovascular assessment is mandatory
- *Always rule out compartment syndrome* as it is fairly common in fractures of tibia-fibula.

INVESTIGATIONS
Plain X-ray of the leg: AP and lateral view **(Fig. 21.2)**.

TREATMENT
Undisplaced/minimally displaced tibia-fibula fractures are managed with the above-knee cast. After 3–4 weeks, above knee cast is removed and patellar tendon bearing cast is applied. The displaced # are also initially given a trial of closed reduction and above knee cast application. If the reduction is acceptable and stable, the cast is continued. However, if the reduction is not acceptable or the fracture displaces, closed reduction internal fixation (CRIF) with intramedullary interlocking nail is performed. Currently, like femur shaft fractures, **internal fixation with an intramedullary interlocking nail is the gold standard** in the treatment of tibia shaft fractures in adult. Open fractures are managed with debridement and external/internal fixation. The treatment guidelines for tibia # (closed and open) are mentioned in **Flowchart 21.1**.

Patellar tendon bearing cast
PTB cast is a type of functional cast bracing (FCB) based upon principles of **"controlled limited movement at the fracture site is advantageous to the fracture healing"**. Firm compression of soft tissue by the cast stiffens the area and controls alignment. FCBs are applied after few weeks of initial closed reduction and cast application. Further, the joint is free to move which avoids stiffness of the joints. Generally, FCBs are applied in fracture shaft of humerus, radius-ulna, and tibia.

COMPLICATIONS

Acute
- **Compartment syndrome**
- Injury to major vessels and nerves of the leg
- Skin loss

Chronic
- **Infection:** Common in open fractures
- **Nonunion:** Common with lower one-third fractures
- Malunion
- Delayed union.

Lower one-third tibia shaft fractures are prone for nonunion due to:
- Poor vascularity of lower end of tibia
- Periosteal vascular support is poor due to minimal soft tissue coverage of lower third tibia..

Flowchart 21.1: Treatment algorithm of fracture (#) shaft tibia. Types 1, 2, 3 open # is according to Gustilo-Anderson classification.

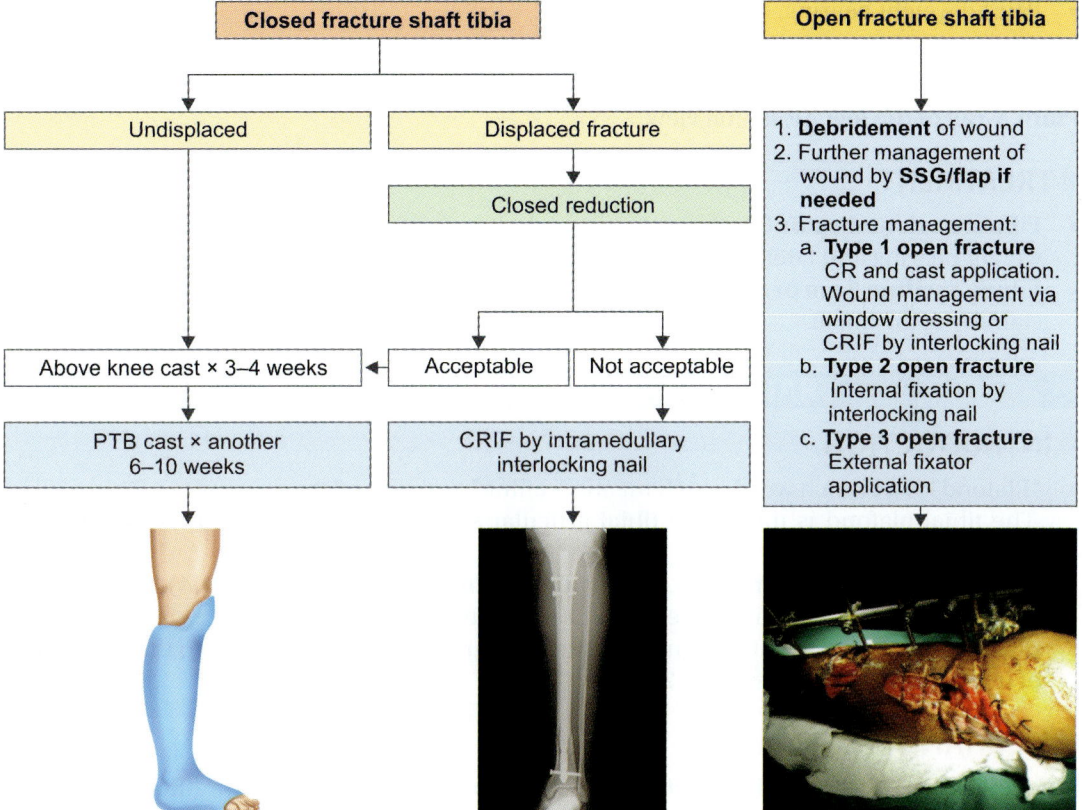

(PTB: patellar tendon bearing; CRIF: closed reduction internal fixation; SSG: split skin graft)

FRACTURE FIBULA

- Isolated # of shaft fibula are rare. They are common with tibial shaft fracture.
- ***Maisonneuve fracture*** is a *spiral fracture of the upper third shaft fibula* that occurs after a twisting injury to the ankle. It is often associated with distal tibia syndesmosis injury, injury of the interosseous membrane and fracture of the medial malleolus.
- As the common peroneal nerve winds around the neck of the fibula, fibular neck fractures may result in injury to the common peroneal nerve, which results in foot drop.
- Quite frequently, fibular shaft fractures occur along with shaft tibia fractures. In combined fractures of shaft tibia-fibula, tibia fracture is managed, whereas fracture shaft fibula is ignored unless fibula fracture is close to the ankle mortise (within 5 cm). Since the latter type of fibula fracture (within 5 cm of ankle mortise) results in unstable ankle mortise, it requires ORIF with plates and screws so as to provide stability to the ankle.

CLINICAL FEATURES OF ISOLATED FIBULA FRACTURE
- Tenderness present over # site
- Painful weight bearing.

INVESTIGATIONS
Plain X-ray of the leg: AP, lateral view.

TREATMENT
- **Fibula neck and shaft fractures:** Non-weight bearing for three weeks followed by partial weight bearing and later full weight bearing.
- **Fibula # within 5 cm of ankle mortise:** It requires ORIF with plate and screws to ensure the stability of the ankle.

FRACTURES OF TIBIAL PLAFOND/PILON

INTRODUCTION
- "Plafond" is a French word which means "ceiling", arched or flat.
  The tibial plafond is the "distal tibial articular surface" **(Fig. 21.3)** and the pilon is the extension above.
- Plafond or pilon fractures are almost **always intra-articular (Fig. 21.4)**. It is usually associated with fibula # and severe soft tissue injury.
- **Fracture blisters** are quite common in such fractures, indicating damage to the vascularity of the skin and soft tissues **(Fig. 21.5)**.

MECHANISM OF INJURY
Most cases result from **high-velocity injury** due to direct impact (road traffic accident) or indirect impact (fall from height).

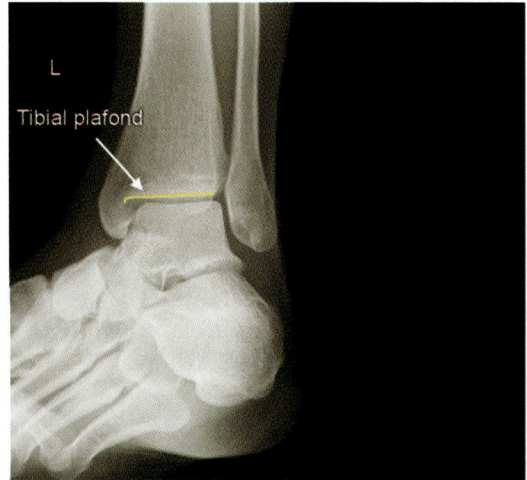

Fig. 21.3: Plain X-ray (AP view) of the ankle showing normal tibial plafond.

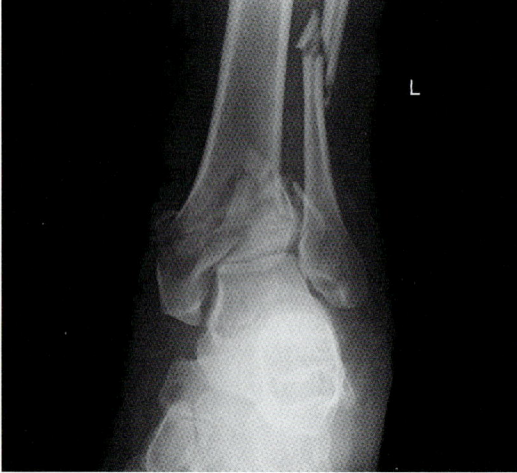

Fig. 21.4: Plain X-ray (AP view) of the ankle showing tibial plafond and fibula #.

CLINICAL FEATURES

Symptoms
Pain, swelling, and deformity of the lower end of the leg and around the ankle. Inability to bear weight over the limb.

Signs
- Deformity is present over lower part of the leg.
- Bony tenderness is present over the lower third tibia.
- ***Fracture blisters are very common* (Fig. 21.5)**.
- The neurovascular examination is a must.

INVESTIGATIONS
- **Plain X-ray of the ankle with leg:** AP and lateral view (*see* **Fig. 21.3**).
- **CT scan with 3D reconstruction (Fig. 21.6)**.

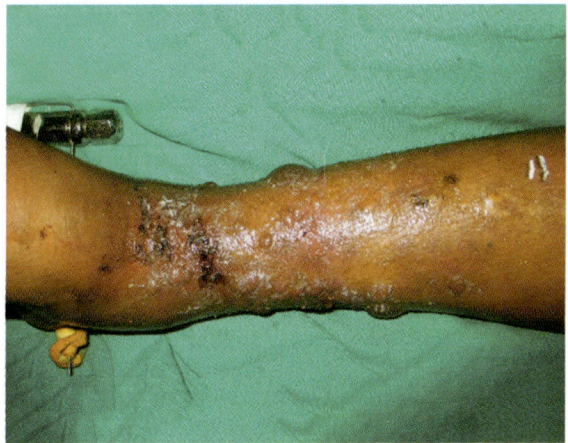

Fig. 21.5: Fracture blisters around lower one-third of leg in pilon #.

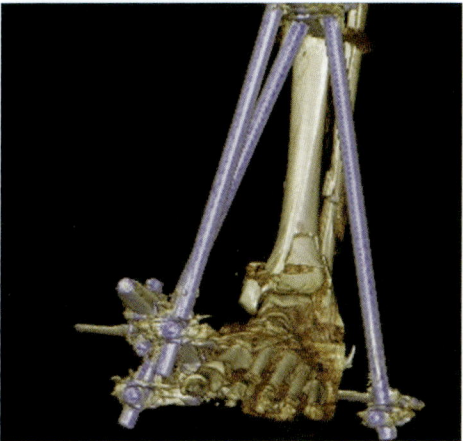

Fig. 21.6: 3D CT scan of pilon fracture with external fixator in situ.

TREATMENT

Tibial plafond # is an intra-articular fracture. The treatment principle involves:
- ***Restoration of the fibula length:*** ORIF with plate and screws.
- ***Accurate restoration of tibial plafond articular surface:*** ORIF with plate and screws.
- Bone grafting, if required.

The **Flowchart 21.2** outlines the treatment of pilon fracture.

COMPLICATIONS

Acute
- Fracture blister formation
- Compartment syndrome
- Skin necrosis and infection, especially after ORIF.

Flowchart 21.2: Treatment of pilon fracture.

```
Undisplaced fracture              Displaced fracture
        │                                  │
        ▼                                  ▼
   Above knee              Initial external fixator
  cast × 6–8 weeks         to let skin condition
                           and edema settle
        │                                  │
        ▼                                  ▼
   Below knee              Continue external
  cast × 6 weeks           fixator for 8 weeks
                                 OR
                           ORIF with
                           plates and screws
```

(ORIF: open reduction internal fixation)

Chronic

- **Nonunion:** Common with lower one-third fractures **(Box 21.1)**
- Malunion leads to deformity, ankle OA
- Delayed union
- Ankle arthritis is quite frequent
- Ankle stiffness

> **Box 21.1:** Causes of nonunion in lower one-third tibia fractures.
>
> - Poor vascularity of lower end of the tibia
> - Periosteal vascular support is poor due to minimal soft tissue coverage of lower third tibia.

FRACTURE OF CALCANEUM

■ INTRODUCTION

Calcaneum is the ***largest of all the tarsals*** and the most caudal heel bone that articulates with the talus superiorly and cuboid anteriorly. The medial side of the calcaneum has sustentaculum tali, which supports the talar neck. Posteriorly, tendo-Achilles is attached to the calcaneal tuberosity. Laterally, peroneal tendons pass between calcaneum and lateral malleolus. Calcaneum forms a joint with talus superiorly (talocalcaneal joint) and cuboid anteriorly (calcaneocuboid joint). And therefore, a fracture line entering either joint results in an intra-articular #.

Calcaneal fracture could be extra-articular or intra-articular. *The calcaneum is the most frequently fractured tarsal bone*. It is also called *'Lover's fracture'* when it occurs due to a fall from height. **Figure 21.7** shows a plain lateral radiograph of the ankle with normal calcaneum, while **Figure 21.8** shows a calcaneal fracture.

■ MECHANISM OF INJURY

Calcaneum is a tough bone, which fractures in **high-velocity injuries**, such as:
- Road traffic accident
- Fall from height and landing on foot.

Box 21.2 lists fractures, which occur due to fall from height.

> **Box 21.2:** Injuries due to fall from height (foot, leg, pelvis, spine, chest, and head).
>
> - Calcaneum #
> - Tibial plafond #
> - Tibial plateau #
> - Pelvis #
> - Spine # (especially atlantoaxial injury)

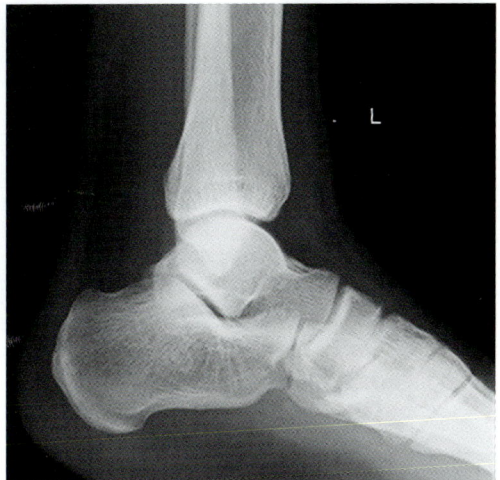
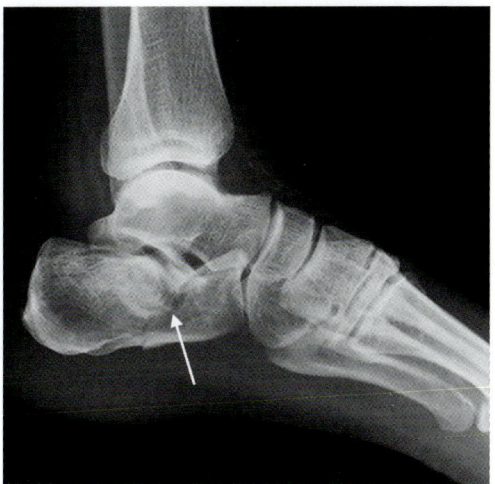

Fig. 21.7: Lateral X-ray of the ankle/heel showing normal calcaneum.

Fig. 21.8: Lateral view of ankle/heel X-ray showing calcaneum fracture (white arrow).

CLINICAL FEATURES

Symptoms

Pain and swelling over the heel and inability to bear weight over the lower limb.

Signs

- Swelling and broadening of the heel is noted
- Bony tenderness is present over the calcaneum
- Painful and restricted movements of the ankle and subtalar joint
- *Fracture blisters* are common in fractures of calcaneum
- *Foot compartment syndrome* is not uncommon

INVESTIGATIONS

- **Plain X-ray of the ankle:** AP, lateral, and axial view **(Figs. 21.9 and 21.10)**. Always look for altered *Bohler's angle* and *angle of Gissane* **(Fig. 21.11)**, which help assess the collapse of the posterior facet of the calcaneum.
- **CT scan with 3D reconstruction:** It is the *gold standard investigation*, and often required to assess the comminution and intra/extra-articular nature of the fracture **(Fig. 21.12)**.

TREATMENT

The undisplaced/minimally displaced calcaneum fractures are managed conservatively in a below-knee cast. Displaced fractures may require ORIF with plate and screws/ K-wires **(Figs. 21.13 and 21.14)**. The management of calcaneum fracture is mentioned in **Flowchart 21.3**.

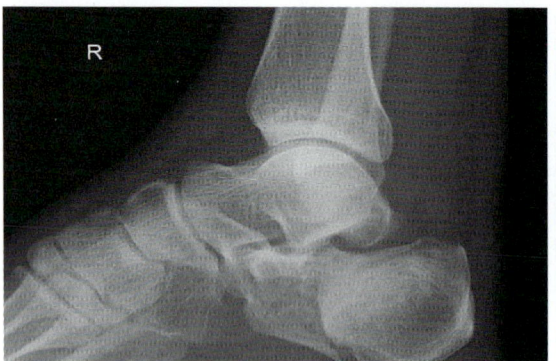
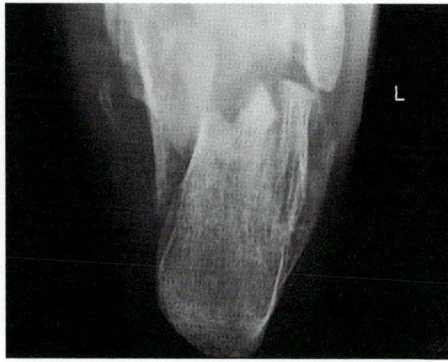

Fig. 21.9: Lateral X-ray of the heel showing # calcaneum with altered Bohler's angle and angle of Gissane.

Fig. 21.10: Axial view of the calcaneum.

Bohler's angle (normal range 20–40°)
This is the angle between the two lines drawn; one from superior calcaneal tuberosity to top of posterior facet (CP) and other one from top of posterior facet to the top of anterior process (PA). A decrease in angle signifies collapse of posterior facet

Angle of Gissane (normal range 100–145°)
This is the angle between the line drawn parallel to the posterior facet to the lowest point on sinus tarsi (PS) and other one from sinus tarsi to the top of sinus tarsi (SA). An increase in the angle signifies collapse of posterior facet.

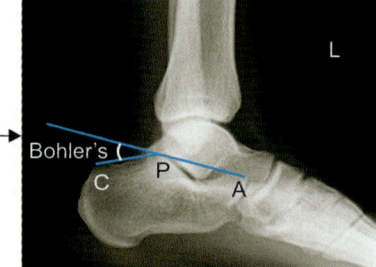
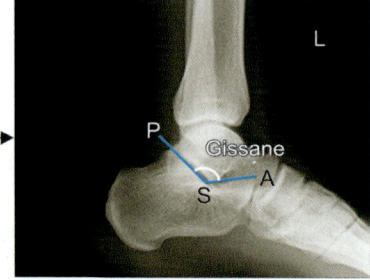

Fig. 21.11: Bohler's and Gissane angle.

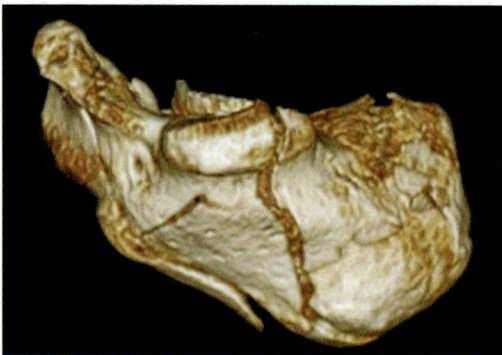

Fig. 21.12: 3D CT reconstruction of calcaneum shows intra-articular comminuted fracture.

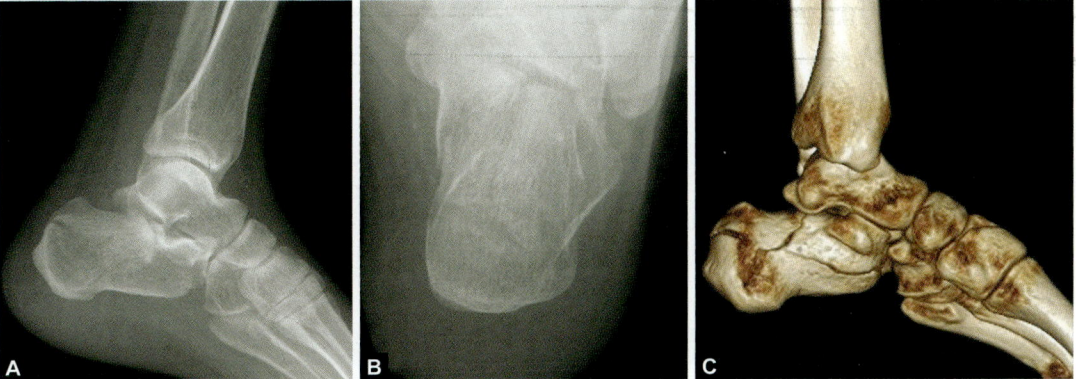

Figs. 21.13A to C: Preoperative lateral X-ray (A), axial X-ray (B), and 3D CT scan (C) of a calcaneum fracture.

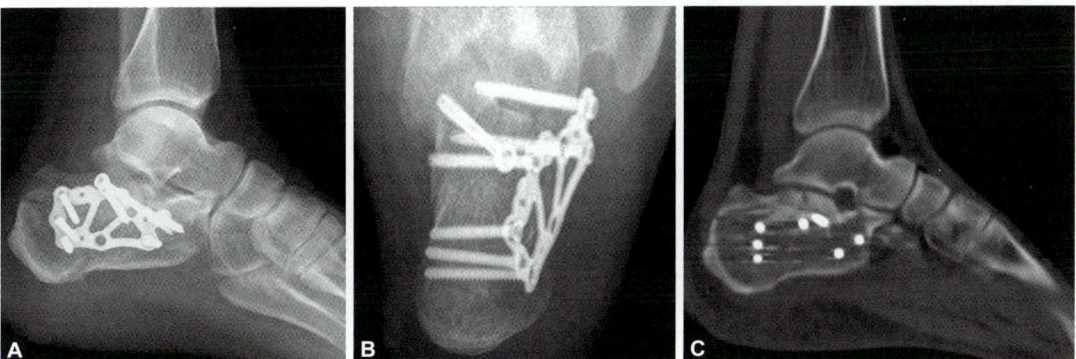

Figs. 21.14A to C: Postoperative lateral X-ray (A), axial X-ray (B), and CT scan (C) of a calcaneum fracture managed with open reduction internal fixation and plate fixation showing restoration of calcaneal articular surface.
(*Courtesy:* Dr Krishna Prasad, KMC, Manipal)

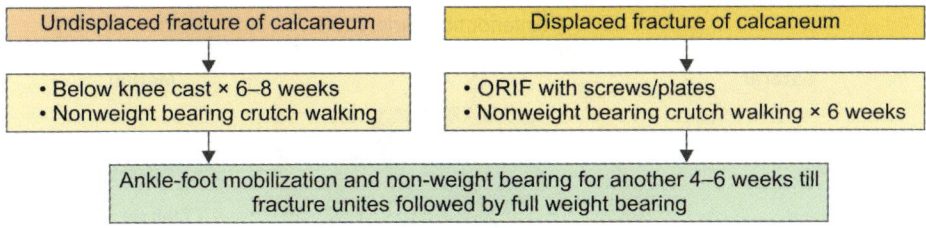

Flowchart 21.3: Treatment algorithm of calcaneum fracture.

(ORIF: open reduction internal fixation)

COMPLICATIONS

Acute

- Fracture blisters
- Ankle–foot compartment syndrome.

Subacute/Chronic

- Complex regional pain syndrome/reflex sympathetic dystrophy
- *Malunion*
- Subtalar joint stiffness
- *Subtalar arthritis* due to malunion of calcaneum fractures: It leads to painful walking, especially on uneven ground. Advanced subtalar arthritis may require calcaneotalar joint arthrodesis to provide pain relief.
- *Peroneal tendon entrapment* due to malunion.

FRACTURE OF TALUS

INTRODUCTION

- Talus has three major parts—head, neck and body. The anterior aspect of talar body is broader than posterior. **Talus is the only tarsal in the foot which has no muscular attachments**.
- The head of the talus articulates with navicular forming talonavicular joint, while undersurface articulates with calcaneum forming talocalcaneal or subtalar joint.
- **Blood supply of the talus:** The blood supply to the talus is **precarious,** derived from the peroneal, anterior tibial and posterior tibial arteries **(Fig. 21.15)**. Injuries such as # *neck talus or talar dislocations often disrupt precarious vascularity resulting in avascular necrosis of the talus.* **Figure 21.16** shows a plain lateral radiograph of the ankle with normal talus, while **Figure 21.17** shows a talus neck fracture.

MECHANISM OF INJURY

- Talar fractures are common in young adults involved in **high-velocity injuries,** such as *RTA or fall from height with forced hyperdorsiflexion of the ankle*. In the latter case, the talus neck gets impinged against the anterior tibial margin resulting in the talar neck fracture.
- Often talus # is associated with dislocation of the subtalar/tibiotalar/talonavicular joint.

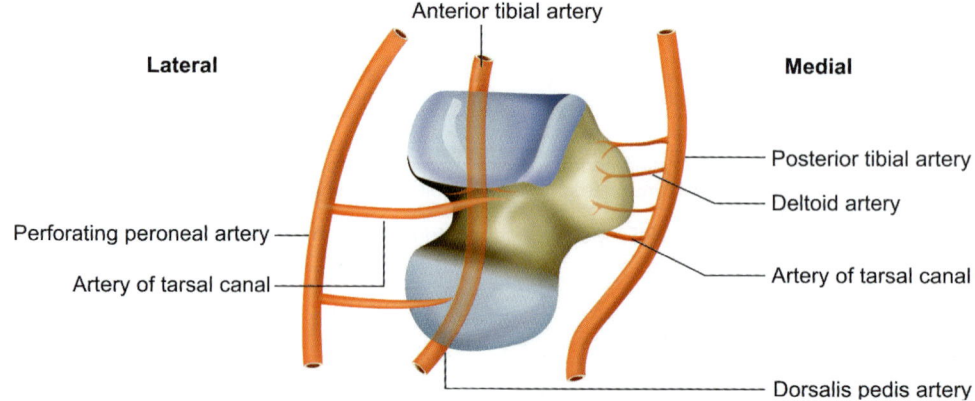

Fig. 21.15: Vascularity of the talus.

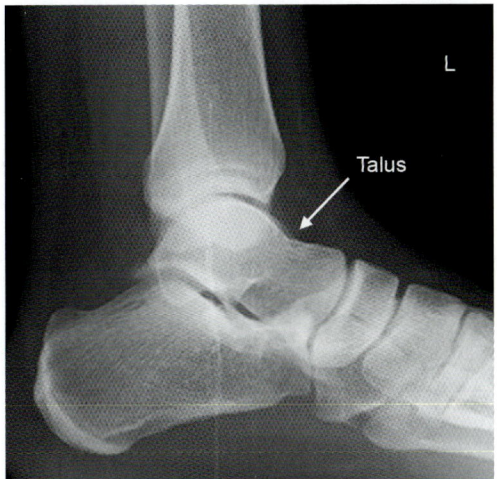

Fig. 21.16: Lateral X-ray of the ankle showing normal talus.

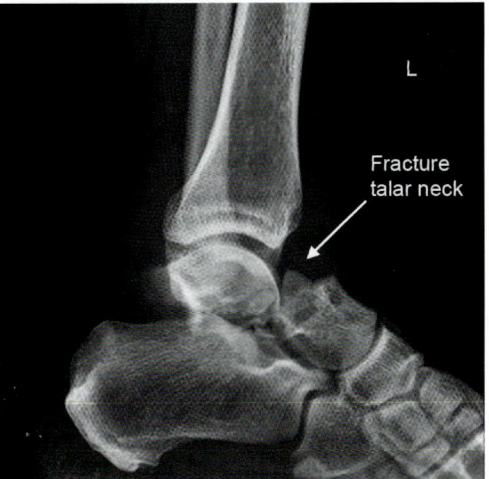

Fig. 21.17: Lateral X-ray of the ankle showing # neck of talus.

Note

The fracture neck of the talus is also known as an ***aviator's fracture (aviator astragalus)***. It is a historical term used to describe talar neck fracture in pilots of crashing fighter planes. During the crash, talar neck # occurred as the rudder bar impacted the plantar aspect of the pilot's feet.

CLINICAL FEATURES

Symptoms
Pain, swelling, and deformity of the ankle and inability to bear weight over the lower limb.

Signs
- Bony tenderness is present over talus
- Painful ankle and subtalar joint movements
- Fracture blisters are common after talus fracture **(Fig. 21.18)**.
- Rule out foot compartment syndrome.

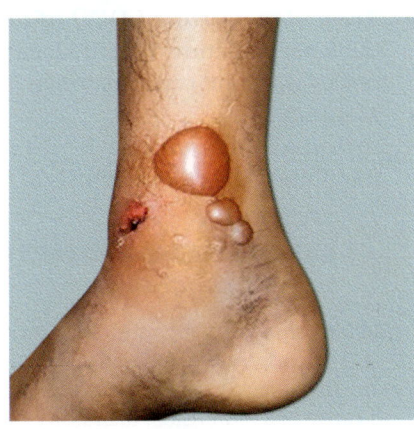

Fig. 21.18: Fracture blisters.

INVESTIGATIONS
- **Plain X-ray of the ankle:** AP and lateral view **(Fig. 21.17)**.
- **CT scan with 3D reconstruction:** To assess other associated fractures and dislocation

TREATMENT
- **Undisplaced fracture:** Conservative—below knee cast for 6–8 weeks.
- **Displaced fracture/fracture-dislocation:** CRIF/ORIF with screw(s).

Flowchart 21.4 outlines the management of a talus fracture.

Flowchart 21.4: Treatment algorithm of the talus fractures.

```
Undisplaced fracture of talus                    Fracture dislocation/displaced fracture of talus
          ↓                                                          ↓
• Below knee cast × 6–8 weeks                    • ORIF with screws
• Nonweight bearing crutch walking               • Nonweight bearing crutch walking × 6 weeks
          ↓                                                          ↓
          Partial weight bearing × 6–8 weeks till fracture unites
```

(ORIF: open reduction internal fixation)

COMPLICATIONS

Acute
- Fracture blisters **(Fig. 21.18)**
- Foot compartment syndrome

Subacute/Chronic
- Complex regional pain syndrome (CRPS)/reflex sympathetic dystrophy/Sudeck's dystrophy
- ***Delayed or nonunion of talus neck fracture***
- ***Avascular necrosis (AVN) of talus body:*** A late complication, especially after displaced talus neck fracture/talar dislocation due to disrupted vascularity. *Hawkins sign* after talus neck # is a good prognostic sign indicating revascularization of the talus.
- Malunion
- *Arthritis of the subtalar joint (50%)* and ankle joint (33%) can occur due to nonunion/malunion/avascular necrosis of talus #.

Hawkins sign is a subchondral lucency noted in the anteroposterior X-ray in the talar body at 8–12 weeks of conservative/operative management. The *presence of Hawkins sign indicates revascularization of the talar body, which suggests that there is a lesser chance of talar AVN. The absence of Hawkins sign is indicative of a high-risk of talar body AVN.*

LISFRANC'S INJURY (TARSOMETATARSAL DISLOCATION)

SURGICAL ANATOMY

The Lisfranc joint is between the tarsals and metatarsals. The first three metatarsals articulate with cuneiform, while fourth and fifth metatarsals articulate with the cuboid **(Fig. 21.19)**.

Note: *Intertarsal joints are also known as 'Chopart joint.'*

DEFINITION

Lisfranc injury is characterized by disruption between the medial cuneiform and the base of the second metatarsal (MT) **(Fig. 21.20)**.

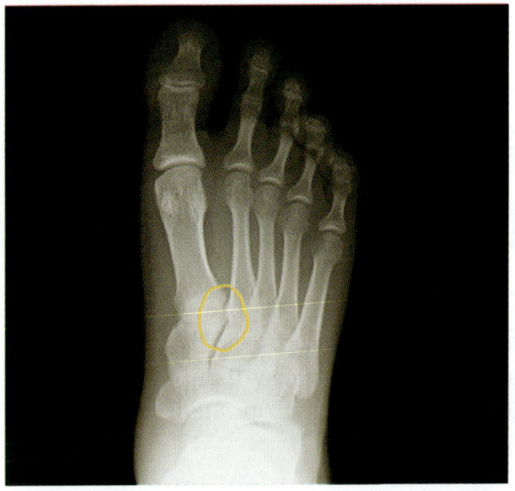

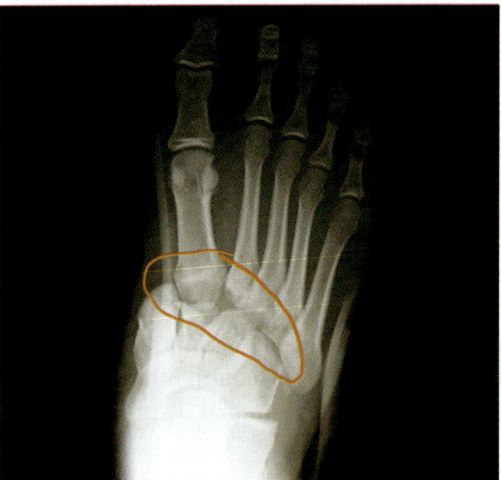

Fig. 21.19: A normal foot X-ray: Normal alignment at medial cuneiform—second MT joint. Yellow circled area shows intact second metatarsal (MT)-cuneiform articulation.

Fig. 21.20: Lisfranc injury: Disrupted medial cuneiform—second metatarsal (MT) joint. Red circled area shows disrupted second MT-medial cuneiform articulation and lateral shift of all MT.

MECHANISM OF INJURY

Lisfranc injury is seen in **high-velocity injuries** such as road traffic accidents.

CLINICAL FEATURES

Symptoms

Pain and swelling of the foot and inability to bear weight.

Signs

- Bony tenderness is present over the base of affected metatarsal and cuneiform
- Foot movements are painful
- There may be a *plantar ecchymoses, which is pathognomonic of Lisfranc injury.*
- *Fracture blisters* may be present
- Rarely, *foot compartment syndrome* can occur.

DIAGNOSIS

- **Plain X-ray of the foot:** AP and oblique views reveal increased space between the medial cuneiform and the second metatarsal base **(Fig. 21.20)**.
- **CT scan of the foot:** It helps assess complex tarsometatarsal injuries.

TREATMENT

- **Undisplaced Lisfranc injury:** Below knee cast for six weeks
- **Displaced Lisfranc injury:** CRIF/ORIF with screws, K-wires.

COMPLICATIONS

- Compartment syndrome
- Fracture blisters
- Chronic arthritis of involved joints

FRACTURE OF METATARSALS

INTRODUCTION

- Metatarsals form an essential part of the longitudinal and transverse arch of the foot
- Any injury to the 1st and 5th metatarsal is more significant as it can disrupt the arch of the foot. Hence, metatarsal displaced injuries should be treated appropriately to restore arch integrity.

MECHANISM OF INJURY

Metatarsal fractures are observed after both high- and low-velocity injuries.
- **High-velocity injury:** Road traffic accident, fall from height
- **Low-velocity injury:** It is observed in twisting injury of the foot.

SPECIFIC FRACTURES OF METATARSALS

The metatarsals can have several specific fractures such as stress fractures involving second or third metatarsal or fractures of the base of fifth metatarsal.

Stress fracture of metatarsals: It is observed in metatarsals in the event of repeated loading in a short period, such as unaccustomed running or walking. *It commonly involves second metatarsal neck, which is also known as the march fracture*, as it is observed in young military recruits after unaccustomed long marches.

Fractures of fifth metatarsal:
- **Avulsion injury of the fifth metatarsal base/tubercle (pseudo-Jones #):** It is a proximal tubercle avulsion fracture of the fifth metatarsal, where the fracture line may enter the cuboid-5th metatarsal joint (intra-articular #). It occurs due to hind-foot inversion injury and pull from peroneus brevis **(Fig. 21.21)**. The nonunion is uncommon in this region.

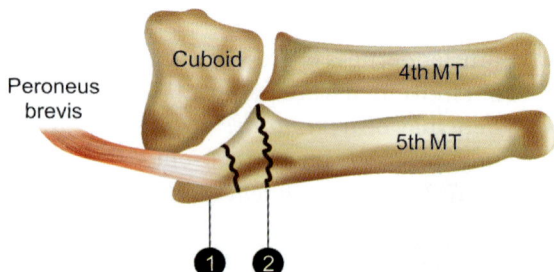

Fig. 21.21: Fifth metatarsal base fractures. 1 indicates pseudo-Jones, while 2 indicates Jones fracture.
(4th: fourth metatarsal, 5th: fifth metatarsal)

- **Jones fracture:** It is an *extra-articular* # of the base of the fifth metatarsal, which occurs at the metaphyseal-diaphyseal junction. It occurs due to forefoot adduction adduction. This area is in watershed zone with precarious blood supply. Therefore, it has higher chance of nonunion (15–25%) compared to pseudo-Jones #.

CLINICAL FEATURES

Symptoms

Pain and swelling in the foot and difficulty bearing weight.

Signs

- Bony tenderness is present over the fractured metatarsal
- Foot movements are painful
- Always rule out foot compartment syndrome.

DIAGNOSIS

X-ray of the foot: AP and oblique views **(Fig. 21.22A)**.

TREATMENT

- **Undisplaced fracture of metatarsals:** Below knee cast for 6 weeks
- **Displaced fracture of base of 5th metatarsal:**
    - *Avulsion fracture*: Suture anchor fixation **(Fig. 21.22B)**
    - *Jones fracture*: Screw fixation **(Figs. 21.23A and B)**.
- **Displaced fracture of other metatarsals:** Below knee cast/K-wire/miniplate fixation.

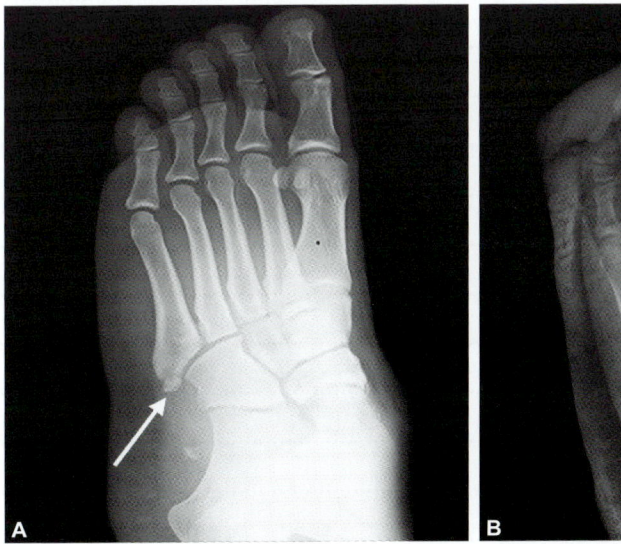
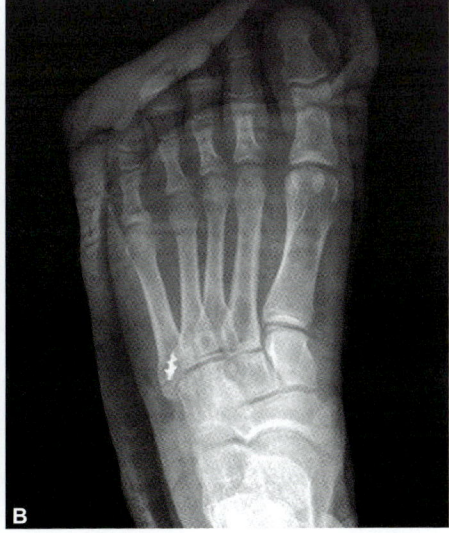

Figs. 21.22A and B: (A) Pseudo-Jones avulsion fracture (white arrow); (B) ORIF with suture anchor.

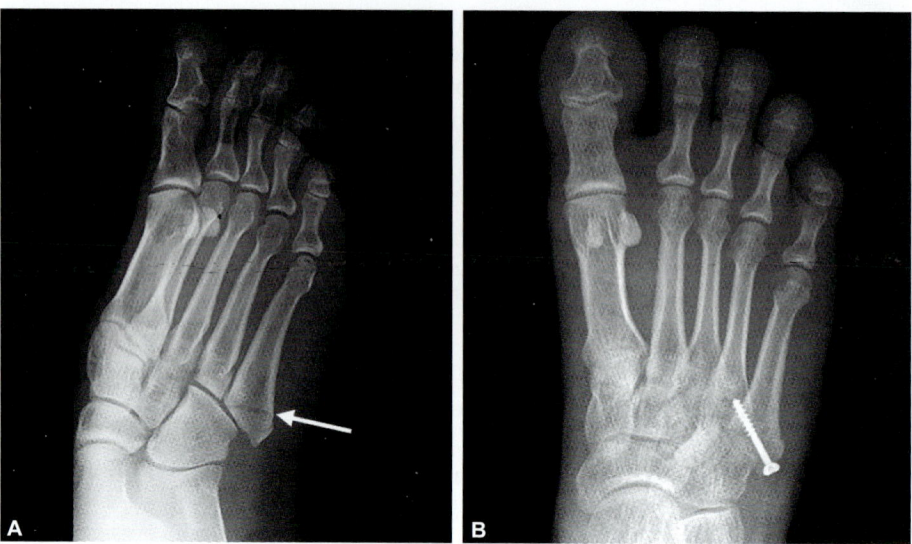

Figs. 21.23A and B: (A) Jones fracture (white arrow); (B) ORIF with screw.

CHAPTER 22

Fracture of the Ankle

POTT'S/BIMALLEOLAR FRACTURE

SURGICAL ANATOMY OF THE ANKLE JOINT

- **Osteology of ankle joint:** The ankle joint is formed by:
  - Lower end of tibia/tibial plafond
  - Three malleoli—medial, lateral and posterior
  - Talus
- **Ankle mortise:** It is the bony arch above the talus, which is formed by:
  - Medial malleolus
  - Tibial plafond
  - Lateral malleolus **(Fig. 22.1)**
- **Major ligaments around the ankle joint:**
  - *Lateral ligament complex:* Anterior and posterior talofibular, calcaneofibular ligament
  - *Medial side of the ankle:* Deltoid and spring ligament
  - *Anterior and posterior syndesmotic ligaments*

Figures **22.1** and **22.2** show a normal ankle, and Pott's fracture, respectively.

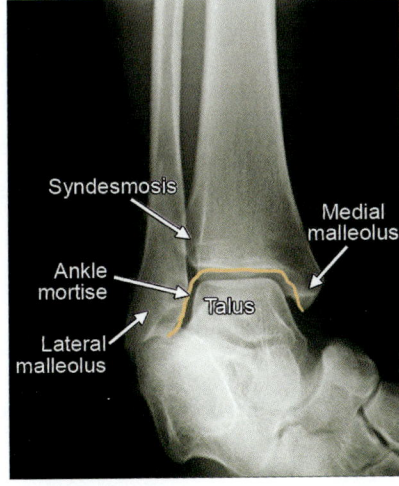

Fig. 22.1: Mortise view (AP in 15 degree internal rotation of ankle) of a normal ankle.

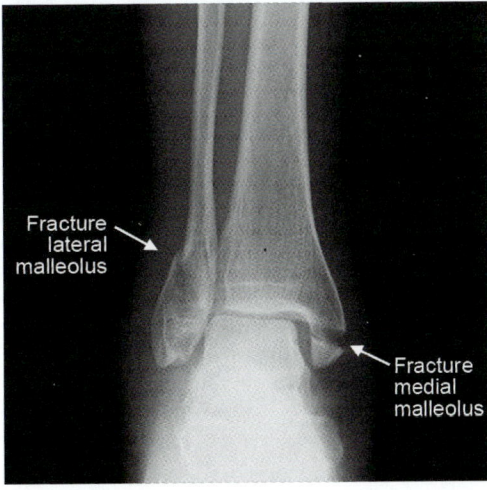

Fig. 22.2: X-ray (AP view) of bimalleolar fracture of the ankle.

Section 2: Fractures and Ligament Injuries

INTRODUCTION

- Ankle fractures typically involve fractures of the malleolus. Malleolar fractures are common in young adults involved in twisting injuries to the ankle/sports/road traffic accidents (RTA). It is also common in elderly patients with osteoporosis.
- Malleolar # could be unimalleolar/bimalleolar/trimalleolar. *Bimalleolar fracture is also known as "Pott's fracture",* whereas trimalleolar # is known as *"cotton's fracture".*

MECHANISM OF INJURY

It involves both low- and high-velocity injury:
- **Low velocity:** Twisting injury to the ankle
- **High velocity:** Road traffic accident

CLINICAL FEATURES

Symptoms

- Pain, swelling, and deformity of the ankle
- Inability to bear weight over the lower limb

Signs

- Bony tenderness over the malleolus
- Painful movements of the ankle
- *Fracture blisters* are quite common in fractures around the ankle **(Fig. 22.3)**.

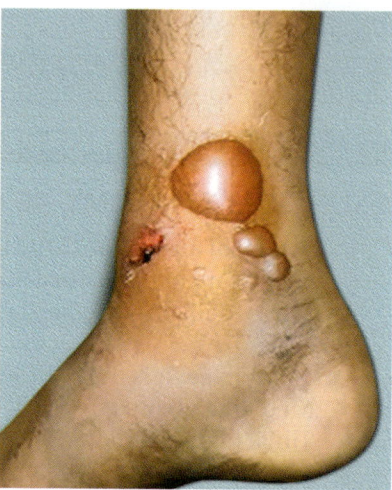

Fig. 22.3: Fracture blister in malleolar fracture.

CLASSIFICATION OF ANKLE FRACTURES: LAUGE-HANSEN CLASSIFICATION (TABLE 22.1)

Table 22.1: Lauge-Hansen classification of ankle fractures (SA-SER-PA-PER).

	Mechanism	Injury sequence and fractures
1.	**Supination adduction (SA)**	- Avulsion # of fibula tip - Vertical # of MM
2.	**Supination-external rotation (SER)**	- Sprain of anterior talofibular (ATF) ligament - Spiral # of LM (# line runs from anteroinferior to posterosuperior) - Sprain of posterior talofibular (PTF) ligament ± # of posterior malleolus - Transverse # of MM/tear of deltoid ligament
3.	**Pronation abduction (PA)**	- Tear of deltoid ligament/transverse # of MM - Injury to syndesmotic ligaments - Transverse # of fibula above the syndesmosis
4.	**Pronation external rotation (PER)**	- Tear of deltoid ligament/transverse # of MM - Tear of ATF - Spiral # of fibula above syndesmosis (# line runs from anterosuperior to posteroinferior) - Tear of PTF or avulsion # of PM

(MM: medial malleolus; LM: lateral malleolus; PM: posterior malleolus)

INVESTIGATIONS (FIG. 22.4)

- Plain X-ray of the ankle; AP, lateral and mortise view.
  Note: Mortise view is an *AP view of the ankle in 15° internal rotation of the leg for assessing the articulation of the tibial plafond and two malleoli with the talar dome*.
- CT scan of the ankle with 3D reconstruction is required if the fracture assessment seems inadequate on a plain X-ray.

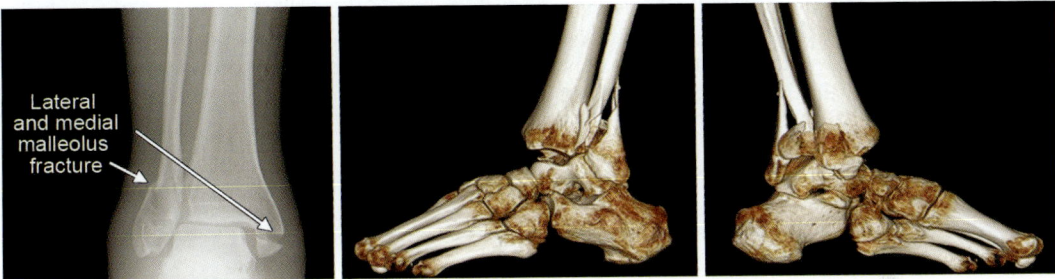

Fig. 22.4: X-ray and 3D CT of Pott's fracture showing fracture of medial and lateral malleolus. CT also shows subluxated ankle.

TREATMENT

The principle of the treatment (conservative/operative) of bimalleolar # is *"restoration of alignment of the ankle mortise and joint"*. Undisplaced fractures can be managed in below knee cast, whereas displaced ones require operative intervention **(Flowchart 22.1)**.

Flowchart 22.1: Management of malleolar fractures.

- Undisplaced fracture of malleolus
  - Below knee cast × 6–8 weeks
  - Nonweight bearing crutch walking
- Displaced fracture of malleolus
  - ORIF with screws and plates
  - Repair of ligaments (if required)
  - Nonweight bearing crutch walking × 6 weeks

Partial weight bearing × 6–8 weeks till fracture unites

(ORIF: open reduction internal fixation)

COMPLICATIONS

Acute
- Fracture blisters
- Foot compartment syndrome

Subacute/Chronic
- *Complex regional pain syndrome (CRPS)*/reflex sympathetic dystrophy/Sudeck's dystrophy
- *Nonunion of malleolus:* Nonunion of the medial malleolus is quite common due to periosteum entrapment in the fracture gap. Hence, during the surgical fixation of medial malleolus, the periosteum is removed from the fracture gap followed by internal fixation.

- Malunion
- Ankle arthritis—due to non/malunion
- Ankle stiffness

The nonunion or malunion of malleolus leads to malalignment of the ankle mortise, which results in uneven distribution of weight over the talus followed by increased stress over the talar cartilage. Uneven distribution of stress over the talar cartilage damages the cartilage, resulting in secondary osteoarthritis of the ankle. Ankle arthritis could be quite disabling, resulting in difficulty in weight bearing.

CHAPTER 23

Complications of Fracture

INTRODUCTION

Many complications happen after the fracture, both **locally and systemic**. *Local complications* are the ones which occur at the local site of trauma involving the skin, nerves, vessels (artery, vein), muscle-tendon, bones, joints, and other local organs. *Systemic complications* can occur in almost all the systems of the body (CNS, CVS, RS, GIT, and genitourinary). The complications could be *immediate* (within a few hours of the injury), *early* (within 2 weeks) or *delayed* (after 2 weeks). **Table 23.1** lists the common local and systemic complications.

Although every complication is essential to understand, this chapter will discuss a few pertinent complications in detail and briefly describe the rest. Several complications are already known to readers as it is discussed in other subjects (tetanus, ARDS, septicemia, delirium tremens, etc.).

Table 23.1: Local and systemic complications of the fracture.

	Local	General/systemic
Immediate	<ul><li>**Skin** injury</li><li>**Nerve** injury</li><li>**Vascular** injury</li><li>**Muscle-tendon** injury</li><li>**Physeal** injury</li><li>**Local visceral injury:** Bladder, urethral injury in pelvis #</li></ul>	<ul><li>Hemorrhagic shock</li><li>Injury to the chest, abdomen, and other organs like the eye, face, ear, etc.</li></ul>
Early	<ul><li>**Skin:** Necrosis</li><li>Fracture blisters</li><li>**Muscle:** Gas gangrene</li><li>**Vascular:** Gangrene of limb, Volkmann ischemia/compartment syndrome, venous thrombosis</li></ul>	<ul><li>Fat embolism</li><li>Pulmonary thromboembolism</li><li>Crush syndrome</li><li>Pneumonia</li><li>Tetanus</li><li>Delirium tremens</li><li>ARDS</li><li>Septicemia (in open #)</li></ul>
Delayed/late	<ul><li>**Skin:** Scarring, contractures</li><li>**Nerve:** Tardy ulnar nerve palsy</li><li>**Muscle:** Contracture, myositis ossificans, Volkmann ischemic contracture</li><li>**Bone/fracture:** Malunion, nonunion, delayed union, growth disturbance, cross union, chronic osteomyelitis, avascular necrosis</li><li>**Joint:** Stiffness, osteoarthritis</li><li>**Others:** Complex regional pain syndrome</li></ul>	<ul><li>Post-traumatic stress disorder</li><li>Renal calculi</li><li>Disuse osteopenia</li><li>Bedsore</li></ul>

Orthopaedic emergencies

Among several complications mentioned above, few are orthopaedic emergencies, such as:
- Hypovolemic shock due to major long bone/pelvis # or major blood vessel injury
- Compartment syndrome
- Acute joint dislocations
- Acute neurovascular transection injuries with/without amputation
- Open fractures
- Septic arthritis
- Crush syndrome
- Cauda equina syndrome

VOLKMANN'S ISCHEMIA (COMPARTMENT SYNDROME)

DEFINITION

A condition wherein *dangerously elevated pressure in the extravascular compartment* results in *microvascular compromise of muscles and nerves of the compartment enclosed in a tight osteofascial space.*
Compartment syndrome is one of the orthopaedic emergencies.

MEAN NORMAL COMPARTMENT PRESSURE IN CHILDREN AND ADULTS
- **Children:** 13–16 mm Hg
- **Adults:** 5–10 mm Hg

COMMON SITES OF COMPARTMENT SYNDROME

Compartment syndrome (CS) can occur in any part of the limb. However, it is common in forearm, leg, hand, foot, elbow joint and knee joint; therefore, it is common after:
- Fractures of both bone forearm, tibia-fibula
- Fractures of hand and feet (metacarpals and metatarsals)
- Injuries around the elbow (elbow dislocation, supracondylar #) and knee (proximal tibia #, knee dislocation)

Compartment syndrome can occur in any space but most commonly observed wherever there are two or more parallel fellow bones like forearm, hand, leg, and foot!

ETIOLOGY

- **Iatrogenic:** *Tight bandage or plaster is the most common cause of compartment syndrome.*
- **Bleeding disorders:** It results in excessive bleeding in the compartment, e.g., hemophilia results in excessive bleeding in the forearm, causing compartment syndrome (CS).
- **Crush injury:** A limb which lies under heavy debris could cause compartment syndrome.
- **Burns eschar around the limb** acts like a tight band around the compartment resulting in compartment syndrome.
- **Postvascular repair (reperfusion injuries):** Reperfusion in the limb after the vascular repair could result in increased pressures in the compartment due to leaky capillaries whose basement membrane was damaged due to prolonged ischemia.

- **Prolonged compression of the limb** while the patient is unconscious.
- **Snake bite:** A cytotoxic effect of snake bite causes vascular endothelial damage, causing increased capillary permeability, which results in extravascular space edema. Further, the systemic effect of snake venom causes coagulopathy, resulting in excessive bleeding in the compartments.
- **Extremely vigorous exercise**: Unaccustomed vigorous exercise can result in CS.
- **Excess intravenous (IV) fluid egress** into the extravascular spaces.

PATHOGENESIS

A 'limb compartment' is a tight non-elastic, enclosed space circumscribed by deep fascia (non-elastic) of a limb, which is often attached to the centrally located bone as intermuscular septums. This tight non-elastic osteofascial space/compartment consists of muscles, nerves, and limb vessels (arteries and veins).

Any condition leading to a rise in pressure inside this tight non-expansile space/compartment could result in excess pressure over the nerves and muscles, and vessels. Compartment syndrome occurs due to a vicious cycle of edema causing hypoxia and acidosis, further increasing capillary permeability and fluid extravasation. This increases volume in the tight closed fascial compartment, which ultimately compromises circulation and causes irreversible muscle and nerve damage. **Flowchart 23.1** describes the pathogenesis of compartment syndrome.

CLINICAL FEATURES

The most important symptom and signs of compartment syndrome are ***pain out of proportion to the injury*** and ***pain on passive stretch*** (of finger/toes), respectively. Other symptoms and signs of compartment syndrome are mentioned in **Boxes 23.1 and 23.2**. The cause of compartment syndrome should always be assessed, whether it is trauma or other causes.

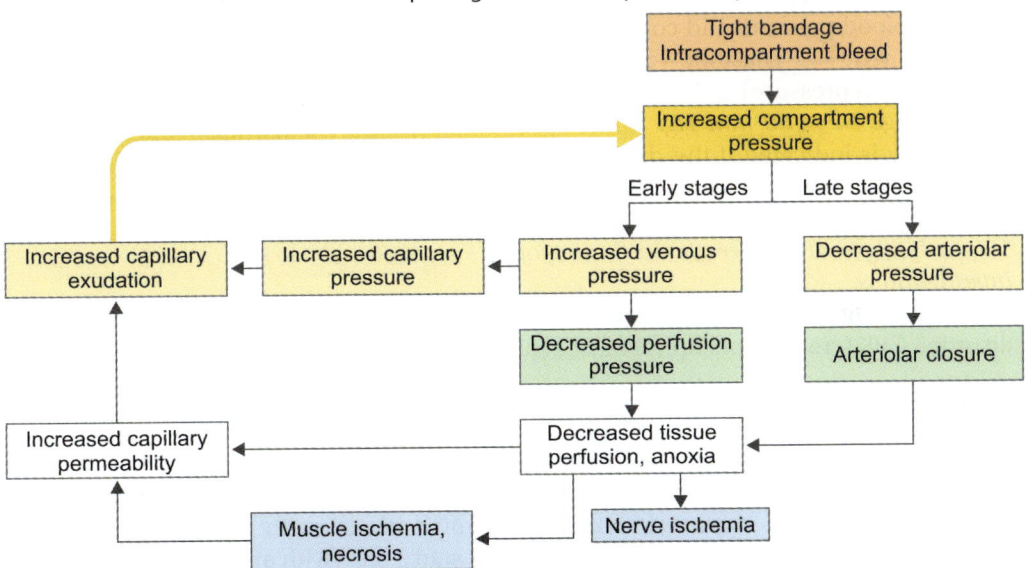

Flowchart 23.1: The pathogenesis of compartment syndrome.

> **Box 23.1:** Symptoms
>
> - **Most important symptom**—severe pain out of proportion of injury
> - Swelling, difficulty in moving limb, and deformity (in case of a fracture)
> - Rest of symptoms depends upon the etiology (fracture, snake bite, etc.).

> **Box 23.2:** Signs (6P's).
>
> - *Pain on passive stretch of digits*—**most important sign!**
> - Pallor
> - Paresthesia
> - Paralysis
> - Pulselessness
> - Other signs depend upon etiology
> - Skin is stretched, shiny, tense with **'woody feel'** (Fig. 23.1). Often skin may show blisters.

INVESTIGATIONS

Compartment syndrome is a clinical diagnosis. However, one must make an attempt to find the etiology.

- **Plain radiograph of limb:** To assess or rule out a fracture or dislocation.
- **Compartment pressure monitoring:** CS is a clinical diagnosis. However, if available, the *Wick catheter method* can measure the compartment pressure. In this method, a catheter is introduced in the compartment to measure the compartment pressure using an arterial transducer. The delta pressure (ΔP) or perfusion pressure is measured, which is the difference between diastolic blood pressure and compartment pressure (ΔP = Diastolic pressure – compartment pressure)

The average ΔP ≥ 80 mm Hg. Immediate fasciotomy is indicated if the difference is less than 30 mm Hg. *However, the decision to perform fasciotomy is primarily a "clinical judgment" rather than a finding of investigations.*

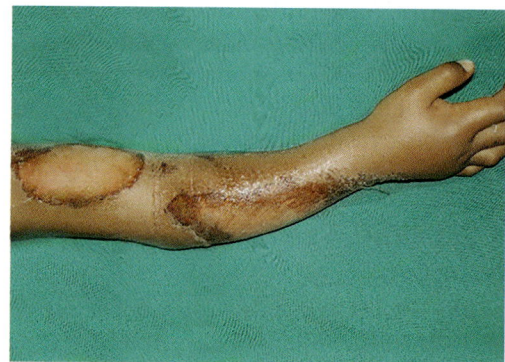

Fig. 23.1: Shiny, tense, and stretched skin in compartment syndrome of the forearm.

Critical compartment pressure over which fasciotomy is required

- Mubarak et al.: 30 mm Hg—more preferred value
- Matsen: 45 mm Hg

- **Other investigations as per etiology.** For example, clotting profile in case of bleeding disorder. CPK (creatine phosphokinase) can be elevated in muscle necrosis.

TREATMENT

- ***Remove any tight bandage*** around the tight compartment. *If not a case of "frank compartment syndrome" or a pre-compartment stage, observe* for any worsening or improvement in symptoms and signs. *Appropriate analgesics* must be given to relieve pain. Treat any underlying etiology such as bleeding disorder or snake bite (with antisnake venom).

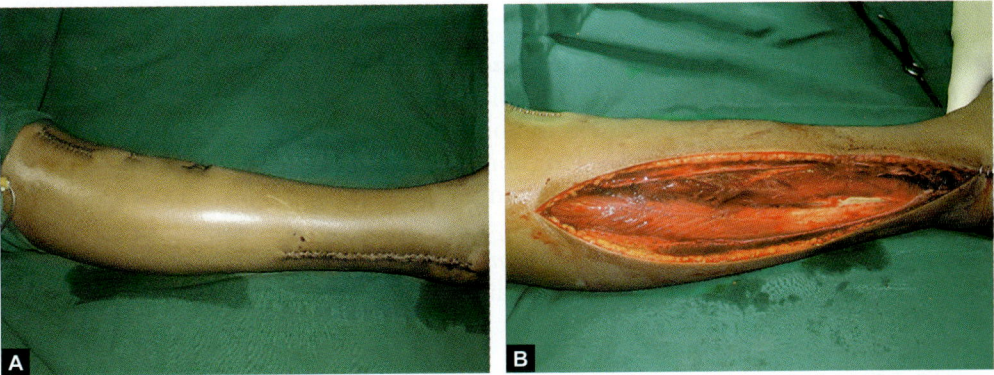

Figs. 23.2A and B: (A) A tense compartment of the right leg; (B) Fasciotomy of the leg.

- **Fasciotomy** should be performed in case of established compartment syndrome (Figs. 23.2A and B). In the case of leg compartment syndrome, *fasciotomy with or without fibulectomy can be done.* Fibulectomy could be required to release all four compartments of the leg. Post-fasciotomy, one must perform the following:
    - **Debridement of the necrotic muscles** of the affected compartment. Do not close the wound to avoid the recurrence of compartment syndrome.
    - **Repeat wound debridement** after 48 hours, followed by 2° closure of the wound (without tension) or split-thickness skin grafting over the fasciotomized area.

COMPLICATIONS

- Volkmann's ischemic contracture *(Refer Chapter 12)*
- Nerve palsy
- Post fasciotomy, there is a risk of crush syndrome, rhabdomyolysis, and renal failure **(Box 23.3)**.
- Infection
- Rarely, amputation.

Box 23.3: After release of compartment syndrome, watch for!!

Crush syndrome: Since the normal circulation is restored after the release of compartment syndrome, the myoglobin and potassium from dead muscle tissue enter circulation causing:
- ***Renal failure*** due to damage of renal tubule by myoglobin-induced mechanical block and direct toxic effect
- ***Cardiac arrest*** due to dangerously elevated levels of potassium

---

FAT EMBOLISM SYNDROME (FES)

DEFINITION

Fat embolism is a syndrome predominantly involving the **"Cerebro-pulmonary"** *system* due to an inflammatory response to the large-scale mobilization of micro fat globules in the circulation, casting mechanical and toxic effects. *Typically, FES appears within 24–72 hours of the trauma.*

ETIOLOGY

Most commonly, FES presents after the *fracture of large long bones of the lower limb* (in isolation or combination) *in young adults*. Most commonly, it is observed after femur shaft fracture. The long bones carry large amounts of yellow marrow, which gets embolized to the systemic circulation causing FES.

Occasionally, *excessive reaming of the medullary canal of a long bone* during intramedullary nailing can result in FES.

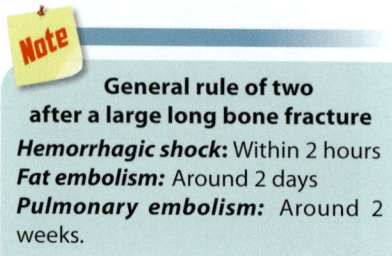

General rule of two after a large long bone fracture
Hemorrhagic shock: Within 2 hours
Fat embolism: Around 2 days
Pulmonary embolism: Around 2 weeks.

PATHOGENESIS

The free fat globules in circulation exert **mechanical and chemical effects** in cerebral and pulmonary capillaries to produce typical *"Cerebro-pulmonary"* features of fat embolism. The mechanical effect of fat globules causes mechanical blockage of the capillaries, whereas the chemical effect is via free fatty acid (FFA) release by breaking down of fat by lipase enzyme. The FFA causes toxic vasculitis to the lung's capillaries, leading to lung injury and ARDS. **Flowchart 23.2** briefly outlines the pathogenesis of FES.

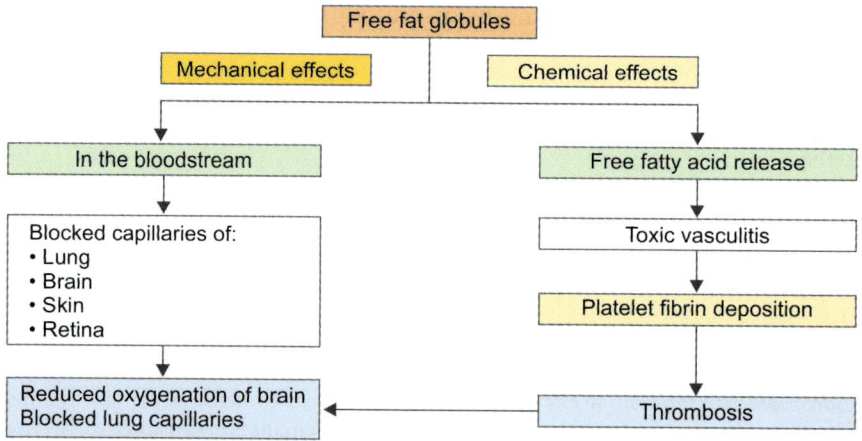

Flowchart 23.2: Pathogenesis of fat embolism syndrome.

CLINICAL FEATURES

The classic picture of FES is described as **'cerebro-pulmonary features along with petechiae'**. Furthermore, these patients have an anxious and agitated look.
- **Cerebral features:** Confusion, restlessness, drowsy, and disorientation
- **Pulmonary features:** Dyspnea, tachypnea
- **Petechiae** are observed in the neck, chest, axilla, and conjuctiva **(Figs. 23.3A and B)**. They are typically observed in the distribution of the superior vena cava area. The petechiae occur due to occlusion of capillaries by fat embolus resulting in erythrocyte extravasation in the tissues.
- **Fever, tachycardia**.

Gurd's criteria of fat embolism syndrome

Gurd's criteria are used to diagnose FES where one major and four minor criteria must be met to confirm the diagnosis of FES **(Table 23.2)**.

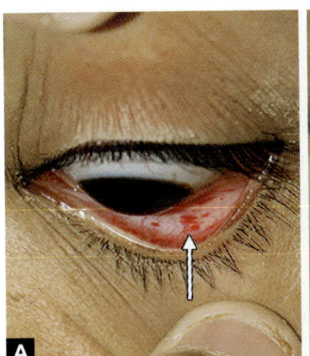
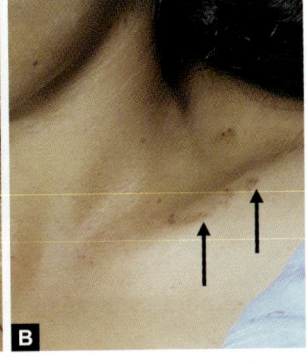

Table 23.2: Gurd criteria for fat embolism.

Major criteria	Minor criteria
Cerebral involvement	Fever, tachycardia, jaundice, retinal change, anemia, thrombocytopenia, renal signs, high ESR, and fat macroglobulinemia
Pulmonary involvement	
Petechial rash	

Figs. 23.3A and B: Petechial hemorrhages over lower conjunctiva (A) and neck (B) in a patient with fat embolism.

INVESTIGATIONS

Four investigations help in establishing the diagnosis of FES; arterial blood gas analysis showing hypoxia, X-ray chest showing pulmonary infiltration, low hemoglobin and platelet counts.

- **Arterial blood gas analysis:** It is the *most important investigation*, which reveals decreased arterial PO_2 (often <60 mm Hg): It is the most significant finding to confirm FES.
- **X-ray chest:** Patchy pulmonary infiltration—snowstorm appearance **(Fig. 23.4)**.
- **Platelet count:** Decreased
- **Hemoglobin:** Low
- **Urine:** Fat globules can be detected using Sudan black dye.
- **Fundoscopy:** Fat globules in retinal vessels, exudates.
- **MRI brain:** It is not performed routinely. However, it may show a typical white matter change outside the vascular territory zone.

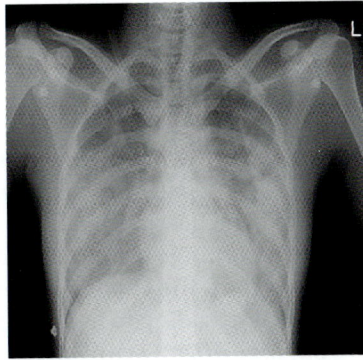

Fig. 23.4: Chest X-ray shows snowstorm appearance of lung.

TREATMENT

The treatment of FES is *essentially conservative* in the form of *"respiratory support"* to ensure adequate arterial oxygenation.
- **Respiratory support in the Intensive care unit:**
    - Early cases may respond to high-flow oxygen alone.
    - Later, the patient may require mechanical ventilation with PEEP (positive end-expiratory pressure).

- **Other supportive measures:** Intravenous fluids to ensure correct intravascular volume, optimal nutrition, and blood transfusion.
- **Fracture fixation:** *Once the patient is hemodynamically stable, the fracture should be fixed as early as possible to reduce further fat embolus showers from unstable fracture ends.*

Currently, there is *no proven beneficial role* of low molecular weight heparin (LMWH), steroid, dextran, or IV alcohol for fat emulsification in treatment of fat embolism!!

CRUSH SYNDROME/TRAUMATIC RHABDOMYOLYSIS/ BYWATERS SYNDROME

DEFINITION

Crush syndrome is characterized by the systemic manifestation of striated muscle damage due to crush injury of local muscle tissue.

CONDITION PREDISPOSING CRUSH SYNDROME

- Crush injury following **limb trapped under the building debris or heavy moving machinery**
- **Ischemia-reperfusion injury of the limb:** Release after prolonged tourniquet
- **Exertional:** Seizures, unaccustomed exertion.

PATHOPHYSIOLOGY

The **principal mechanism causing crush syndrome is the** *"release of myoglobin, potassium, and phosphate from damaged muscle tissue."* These released substances damage the kidney and affect the heart.
- **Renal damage** primarily occurs due to *myoglobin-induced mechanical blockage and toxic damage* to the renal tubules. Further, damaged muscle causes blood stagnation in the muscles, leading to hypovolemia, further reducing renal perfusion.
- **Cardiac effect:** Damaged and crushed muscles release K^+ into the circulation resulting in dangerous hyperkalemia leading to sudden cardiac arrest or arrhythmias.
- **Electrolyte imbalance:** Hyperkalemia, hyperphosphatemia, and hypocalcemia.

CLINICAL FEATURES

- *Renal failure*
- *Cardiovascular instability*: Shock, arrhythmias
- *Metabolic acidosis, DIC*
- *Compartment syndrome, ARDS.*

TREATMENT

It involves the management of limb injury, adequate fluid management, acute renal failure, electrolyte imbalance, and life support.

INJURY TO MAJOR BLOOD VESSELS

It is one of the frequent acute trauma complications.

ETIOLOGY

A major blood vessel can get injured due to direct compression, laceration, or kinked from fracture ends. It can also get compressed from the hematoma.

CONSEQUENCE AFTER INJURY TO A MAJOR BLOOD VESSEL

- **Inconsequential**, especially if there are enough collaterals or another potential blood vessel to the extremity. For example, if the radial artery is damaged, the circulation to the hand remains intact since there is enough blood flow through the ulnar artery.
- **Ischemia and gangrene:** If there is a significant compromise in the circulation.

COMMON SITES OF VASCULAR INJURY

- **Upper limb:**
  - Axillary artery injury during fracture dislocation of the shoulder
  - Brachial artery injury in supracondylar fracture humerus.
- **Lower limb:**
  - Femoral artery injury in femur fractures
  - Popliteal artery injury in knee dislocation or distal femur/proximal tibial fractures.

CLINICAL PRESENTATION

There is usually history of trauma. The most important features of arterial obstruction are **5 Ps**—**p**ain, **p**allor, **p**aresthesia, **p**aralysis, and **p**ulselessness.
- **Cold extremity:** The extremity would be cold and pale. The capillary filling and pinprick is delayed.
- There may be **external bleeding** resulting in **hemorrhagic shock**.
- There can be an **associated fracture/dislocation** in the limb.
- Occasionally, a massive hematoma can form around the bleeding vessel giving rise to massive swelling in the limb.

INVESTIGATIONS

- **Arterial Doppler** scan
- **Computed tomography (CT) angiogram**
- **X-rays** to rule out fractures and dislocation.

TREATMENT

- **Loosen the tight bandage,** if any. Correct the angulation at the fracture site. If pulse returns, then proceed with appropriate management of fracture. If the pulse does not return, then urgent open reduction and fixation of fracture by plate/nail/external fixator followed by exploration of the vessel by a vascular surgeon. The thrombosed and damaged vessel may require:
  - ***Thrombosed vessel:*** Thrombectomy by Fogarty catheter
  - ***Transected/lacerated vessel:*** End-end repair with or without graft.

- Post-vascular repair, patient should be kept on anticoagulants (low-molecular-weight heparin/dabigatran/rivaroxaban) for several weeks to prevent re-thrombosis.

Flowchart 23.3 summarizes the algorithm to manage closed vascular injuries.

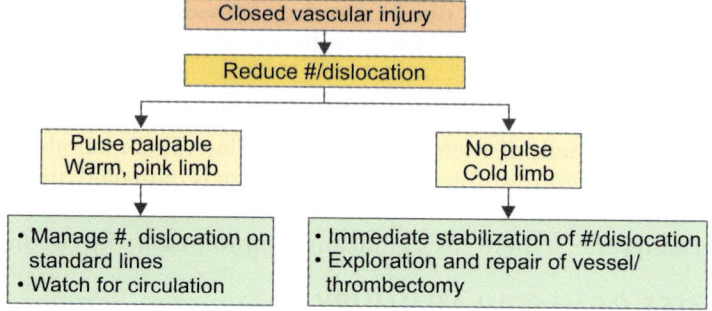

Flowchart 23.3: Treatment algorithm to manage vascular injury of the limb.

COMPLICATIONS

- Gangrene
- Traumatic aneurysm
- Ischemic contracture such as Volkmann ischemic contracture.

DEEP VEIN THROMBOSIS (DVT)

- It is a common complication following trauma, especially when the patient remains bedridden for long periods or in case of pelvic or lower limb surgeries lasting more than 30 minutes.
- Almost 90% of DVT originates from the veins of lower limbs and pelvis.

ETIOPATHOGENESIS

- Any condition which alters the "Virchow's triad" can result in DVT:
    - **Change in blood flow:** Slow/turbulent
    - **Change in the wall:** Injury to vein wall (intima)
    - **Change in blood components (hypercoagulable states):** Polycythemia vera, protein C and S deficiency, and malignancy.

The risk factors for DVT are mentioned in **Box 23.4**.

> **Box 23.4:** DVT risk.
>
> - **Factors stasis:** Trauma, surgery in lower limb and pelvis >30 min, immobility, paralysis
> - **Vessel injury:** Smoking, varicose vein, previous DVT
> - **Hypercoagulable state:** Malignancy, HRT therapy, polycythemia vera
> - **Others:** Smoking, pregnancy, postpartum, obesity

CLINICAL FEATURES

- Often, DVT is asymptomatic except for mild swelling in the limbs. Occasionally, *low-grade fever* may be present.

- There may be **pain, redness and swelling in the calf** with pitting edema. Edema increases after ambulation.
- *Acute massive DVT may result in gross swelling and venous gangrene.* The most severe form of acute lower extremity DVT is called as *Phlegmasia cerulea dolens*, characterized by the triad of massive swelling, cyanosis, and pain due to complete thrombosis of venous outflow.
- In chronic DVT, hyperpigmentation is seen around the lower part of the leg and ankle.
- Moses and Homan's signs may be positive. However, these signs must be elicited carefully in order to avoid dislodgement of the thrombus.
- **Well's clinical probability tool:** A patient with a score <2 is less likely to have DVT. A score ≥2 is likely to have DVT.

- **Well's clinical probability tool for DVT:** It takes ten points in account, such as (1) active malignancy, (2) bedridden patient, (3) paralysis/paresis/immobilization of patient, (4) localized tenderness over deep veins, (5) entire leg swollen, (6) localized swelling, (7) pitting edema, (8) collateral superficial veins, (9) previous DVT, and (10) alternative diagnosis is at least as likely as DVT. All features get one point each, whereas last one gets -2.
- DVT is likely if there are 2 points or more.

INVESTIGATIONS

- **Venous Duplex ultrasound**
- **Quantitative D-dimer assay:** Elevated values of D-dimer are suggestive of DVT.
- **CT abdomen and pelvis** for deep veins of the abdomen and pelvis.

TREATMENT OF DVT

- **Low-molecular-weight heparin** (LMWH; injectable enoxaparin) followed by long-term dabigatran/rivoroxaban/warfarin is the treatment of choice.
- **Limb elevation** and **compression stocking.**
- In patients at risk of a recurrent pulmonary embolism due to chronic lower limb/pelvis DVT, **inferior vena cava filter** placement is required to prevent pulmonary thromboembolism (PTE).
- The risk factors must be corrected.

PREVENTION OF DVT

- Early mobilization of limb and patient, adequate hydration
- Correction of risk factors
- Compression stocking
- Low molecular weight heparin should be prescribed perioperatively in patients with a high risk of DVT.

PULMONARY THROMBOEMBOLISM (PTE)

PTE is almost always is a result of DVT.

There may be risk factors for PTE, such as diagnosis of DVT, old age, obesity, and surgery within last 2 months.

PATHOGENESIS

The clot from DVT breaks away and lodges in the pulmonary artery and lungs, causing poor oxygenation and compromised cardiovascular circulation resulting in hypotension. The symptom and signs of PTE depend upon the size of the clot and the amount of blockade in the lung and pulmonary artery.

CLINICAL FEATURES

The symptoms and signs of PTE are typically sudden in onset and depend upon the embolus size.
- *Smaller embolus:* Mild chest pain, pleuritic rub, and *stable cardiovascular status.*
- *Larger embolus:* Acute chest pain, severe dyspnea, tachycardia, and usually *stable cardiovascular status.*
- *Massive embolus:* Sudden precipitous hypotension, bradycardia, and often cardiac arrest (blue in a bolt), *unstable cardiovascular status.*

Other features are—cough, fever, hemoptysis.

INVESTIGATIONS

- **Chest X-ray:** Oligemia of lung field, enlarged pulmonary artery, wedge shape opacity on the periphery, pleural effusion (bloody)
- **ECG:** Many patterns are observed, such as S1Q3T3, Right bundle branch block, Right ventricular strain pattern, and Right axis deviation.
- **Arterial blood gas analysis:** Hypoxia, hypocapnia.
- **Serum D-dimer levels:** It is elevated. However, it is a highly sensitive but not specific investigation.
- **Multiple detector CT pulmonary angiography of chest** is a *gold-standard investigation.*
- **Ventilation-perfusion scan** would show a mismatch where an area of ventilation is not perfused. It is performed when CT cannot be done.
- **Transthoracic echocardiography:** For right ventricular dysfunction.

TREATMENT

- Oxygen with/without mechanical ventilation.
- Intravenous infusion of LMWH for 7–10 days followed by prolonged oral warfarin.
- Thrombolysis (IV Alteplase) is required, especially in massive PTE. However, massive PTE has a high mortality rate.
- In the case of lower limb/pelvis DVT, IVC filters may be placed to prevent further PTE, especially if anticoagulants are contraindicated.

MYOSITIS OSSIFICANS (MO)

DEFINITION

It is a condition characterized by post-traumatic ossification of the soft tissue around the joint.

COMMON SITES

Although myositis ossificans can occur in any region. However, it is *common around elbow, hip, and knee (in order)* involving brachialis, quadriceps, and gluteal muscles, respectively.

ETIOLOGY

- **Post-traumatic:** It is one of the *most common cause of myositis ossificans*. Often, there is a history of massage/passive vigorous joint mobilization.
- **Post surgical:** It is common after surgery around elbow, hip and knee.
- **Post-head injury:** It is also observed after head injury.

PATHOPHYSIOLOGY

Bleeding into muscles results in hematoma formation and periosteal cell proliferation causing ossification of hematoma **(Flowchart 23.4)**.

CLINICAL FEATURES

Myositis ossificans should be suspected whenever there is a sudden increase in pain and loss of joint movement after the mobilization was initiated during rehabilitation to treat a fracture or a soft tissue injury around the joint. There are two phases in myositis ossificans, and clinical features vary in both phases.
- **Early or warm phase:**
    - A sudden increase in pain following mobilization of joint during rehabilitation.
    - Increased local warmth and tenderness.
    - No myositis mass is palpable.
    - There is a loss of movement, which was initially gained during the mobilization.
- **Late or cold phase:**
    - In this phases, there is reduction in pain and swelling and ROM improves (than warm phase).
    - The typical clinical feature is loss of ROM with a sudden bony block in ROM.
    - The bony mass is often palpable.

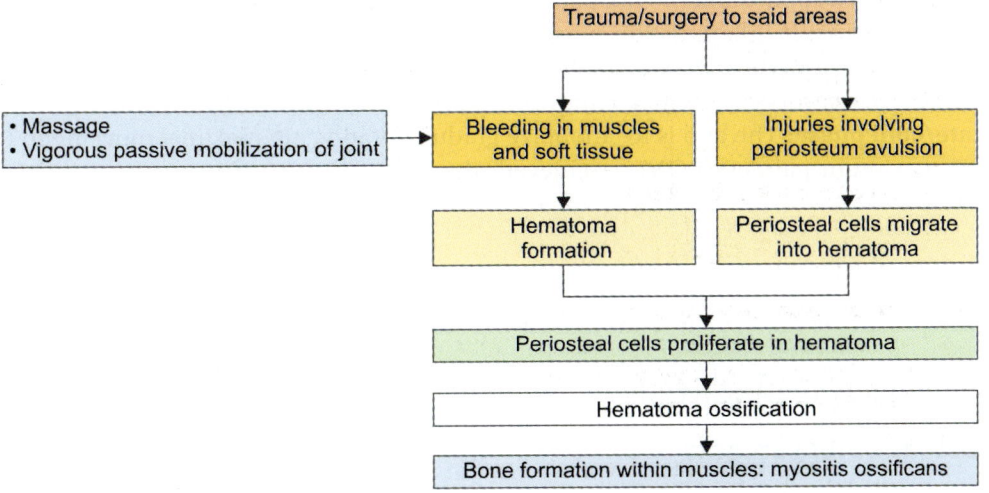

Flowchart 23.4: Pathophysiology of myositis ossificans.

INVESTIGATIONS

- **Plain X-ray:**
    - *Early phase:* Cotton wool appearance (fluffy, irregular edges)
    - *Late phase:* Radiopaque dense mass *away from the bone* (**Fig. 23.5**).
- **Bone scan:** Tc^{99} uptake is increased in the early phase.
- **CT scan:** Eggshell appearance.

PREVENTION OF MYOSITIS OSSIFICANS

- Avoid too many closed reduction attempts of fractures, such as supracondylar #.
- Always avoid massage and heat therapy to local tissues after any acute trauma.
- Avoid vigorous passive mobilization of the joint in acute or subacute phase of injury or surgery. Instead, active mobilization is preferred.
- Drug, such as indomethacin for several weeks postoperatively may help formation of myositis mass.

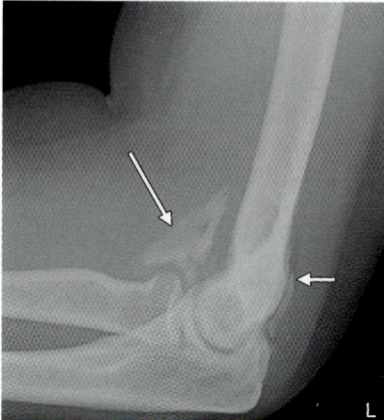

Fig. 23.5: Myositis mass in front and back of the elbow.

Myositis ossificans cannot be stopped once it has begun to develop. It stops enlarging after maturing.

TREATMENT

- **Early/active phase:** The aim is to "let the inflammation subside."
    - *Reimmobilization* for a few days to reduce the inflammation
    - *NSAIDs,* such as *indomethacin,* antiedema measures
    - Cold pack application (*no* hot pack!)
        - Once acute inflammation subsides, start gentle active mobilization
        - Achieve painless maximum ROM in due course of rehabilitation.
    Do not operate for MO excision in the acute phase. Wait for at least six months.
- **Late/cold phase:** The aim is to "mobilize gradually" and gain maximal movement. Once the maximum painless ROM is achieved, the consolidated mature bony mass can be excised.

COMPLICATION

Recurrence after excision of myositis mass is the most common complication.

DIFFERENTIAL DIAGNOSIS

Parosteal Osteosarcoma

It can be differentiated on radiological appearance that parosteal osteosarcoma always arises from the bone, while MO mass is away from the bone.

COMPLEX REGIONAL PAIN SYNDROME/SUDECK'S DYSTROPHY/ REFLEX SYMPATHETIC DYSTROPHY

DEFINITION OF COMPLEX REGIONAL PAIN SYNDROME (CRPS)

Complex regional pain syndrome (CRPS) is a disorder of a body region, usually of the distal limbs, *characterized by pain, swelling, limited range of motion, vasomotor instability, skin changes, and patchy bone demineralization*, which is *out of proportion to injury and time*.

CLASSIFICATION

- **Type 1 CRPS:** Idiopathic
- **Type 2 CRPS:** It is associated with nerve injury. Formerly, it was known as *causalgia*.

ETIOPATHOGENESIS

Although CRPS can affect any site, the most commonly affected areas are *wrist-hand* and *ankle-foot*.

The etiology for the initiation of CRPS is:

1. **Traumatic:** Trauma is the *most frequent event for initiation of CRPS*. CRPS initiates after an **injury to a part** *(fracture or soft tissue injury) or* **surgery**. It also occurs after **nerve injuries**.
2. **Atraumatic** causes, such as stroke, can also result in CRPS.

Several other factors are possibly implicated in CRPS, such as persistent pain and swelling following trauma, poor mobilization of joints or prolonged immobilization, smoking, osteoporosis, and migraine. Possibly, there are genetic, inflammatory and psychological factors too contributing in CRPS.

The **pathophysiology of CRPS** seems *multifactorial* comprising *central and peripheral sensitization, autonomic dysfunction* and *inflammatory changes*.

1. **Central sensitization** occurs due to the release of substance P, bradykinin, and glutamate at the dorsal horn neurons, resulting in *hyperalgesia and allodynia*.
2. **Peripheral sensitization** is triggered by the release of pro-inflammatory markers (TNF-α) after the initial injury leading to *local sensitization and hyperalgesia*.
3. **Autonomic dysfunction** occurs due to the upregulation of sympathetic receptors on nociceptive nerve fibers, resulting in sympathetic hyperactivity causing *local swelling, color, and temperature variations*.
4. **Inflammatory changes:** Elevated levels of *pro-inflammatory cytokines* (TNF-α, interleukins) and *neuropeptides* (bradykinin and substance P) result in vasodilation and tissue extravasation.

The fundamental pathological basis of CRPS is persistent pain and exaggerated sympathetic response following trauma resulting in increased vasospasm induced pain and swelling forming a vicious cycle. CRPS results in sensory, motor, vasomotor and sudomotor features. **(Flowchart 23.5)**.

CLINICAL FEATURES

The onset of CRPS generally occurs within 4–6 weeks of the inciting event. Chief clinical symptoms of CRPS are **pain, sensory changes, motor impairments, autonomic symptoms, and trophic skin changes** in the affected limb. The initial symptoms usually include pain, erythema, and swelling of the affected limb. In most cases, the limb is warm initially, though some are cold at presentation or evolve from warm to cold.

Section 2: Fractures and Ligament Injuries

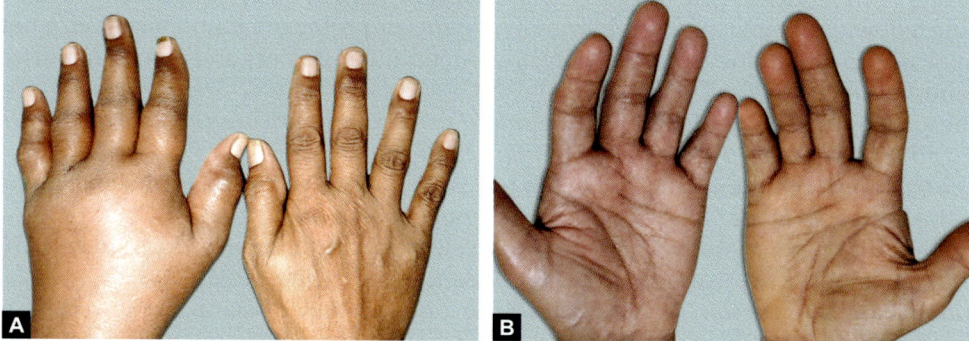

Flowchart 23.5: CRPS pathophysiology.

Figs. 23.6A and B: Complex regional pain syndrome (CRPS) of the left hand showing: (A and B) A swollen hand with mottled reddish colored skin.

Pain is typically the *most prominent and debilitating symptom*. It is described as a *stinging or burning sensation* deep inside the limb. Often, the pain is continuous and undulating but can be paroxysmal. Pain may be worse at night and exacerbated by limb movement, contact, temperature variation, or stress.

Sensory abnormalities, such as *hyperalgesia or allodynia*, are common on examination (hyperesthesia is an abnormal increase in sensitivity, whereas allodynia is pain caused by stimuli which should not trigger a painful response).

Motor impairment is characterized by muscle wasting, reduction of muscle strength, such as handgrip or tiptoe standing, and decreased joint movement.

Autonomic changes are reflected by differences in skin temperature, color (reddish/mottled, shiny skin), hyperhidrosis (increased sweating), or edema (compared to the unaffected side) **(Figs. 23.6A and B)**.

Skin/trophic changes may include increased hair growth, increased or decreased nail growth, loss of pulp fat, brittle nail, and skin atrophy.

INVESTIGATIONS

Primarily, CRPS is a clinical diagnosis, and there are no 'diagnostic investigations' for the same. However, several investigations help corroborate the diagnosis.
- **X-ray:** Patchy osteoporosis in the affected part is characteristic of CRPS **(Fig. 23.7)**
- **Tc^{99} bone scan:** Positive phase III scan.

PREVENTION

- **Early mobilization** of the joints
- **Adequate pain control measures:** NSAIDs or other analgesics, physiotherapy
- **Vitamin C** 500 mg twice a day for 4–6 weeks.

TREATMENT

The essence of the treatment of CRPS is breaking the overactive central, peripheral and autonomic response with **physiotherapy, adequate analgesics, edema control, and other medications.** If medical measures fail, sympathetic overactivity can be controlled by blocking the sympathetic ganglion.
- **Effective control of pain:** NSAIDs/other analgesics, topical analgesics/gels.
- **Physiotherapy:** It aims to mobilize the joints, control edema and pain.
    - *Mobilize the joints:* Whirlpool therapy is quite helpful.
    - *Pain control therapies:* Moist heat, TENS, and local USG massage
    - *Mirror therapy:* Both hands are placed in a box with a mirror separating the two compartments. While moving the normal hand, the reflection is seen in the mirror, which helps move the affected hand.
- **Control edema:** Compression bandage to decrease edema, limb elevation.
- **Other medications:** These medications help reducing pain and allodynia.
    - *Calcium channel blockers* help increase circulation
    - *Tricyclic antidepressants* (Nortriptyline)
    - *Anticonvulsants, GABA agonists*: Carbamazepine, Pregabalin, Gabapentin
    - *Vitamin C* 500 mg bd for 4–6 weeks.
- **Block sympathetic over-activity:** *When physiotherapy and medical measures fail,* blocking the local sympathetic ganglion would temporarily decrease the sympathetic outflow to the limb, thereby reducing vasospasm and improving pain and edema. Chemical/surgical methods can block sympathetic overactivity. To control sympathetic overactivity of upper and lower limbs, *stellate ganglion and L1 sympathetic ganglion* are blocked, respectively.
    - ***Chemical method for sympathetic ganglion block*** using phenol, alcohol
    - ***Rarely, surgical local sympathetic ganglion sympathectomy.***

Budapest criteria for CRPS

Budapest criteria using sensory, motor, autonomic and trophic changes can be used to diagnose CRPS (*details are out of the scope of this book*).

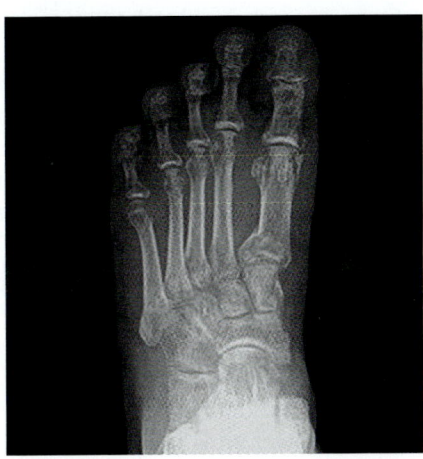

Fig. 23.7: Patchy osteoporosis in CRPS of foot following metatarsal fracture.

Once the hyper-sympathetic activity is controlled, the patient must undergo aggressive physiotherapy to regain movement.
- **Psychotherapy and behavioral therapy** in patients with preexisting or suspected psychologic or psychiatric issues.

NONUNION OF FRACTURE

DEFINITION

A fracture can be said to be in nonunion if it does not unite even after *twice the time it would normally take to unite to a maximum of 9 months* (US FDA).

Another definition of nonunion, which is used in the practical scenario, is a fracture is considered to be in nonunion "when the fracture fails to show any clinical or radiological evidence of union for three consecutive follow-ups (usually at six weeks apart), and the biological process of the union has stopped to such an extent that it will not progress further till the method of treatment is changed."

COMMON SITES OF NONUNION

- Lateral end of the clavicle ⎫
- Lateral condyle of humerus ⎬ Upper limb
- Scaphoid waist ⎭
- Neck of femur ⎫
- Tibia (lower end) ⎬ Lower limb
- Talus neck ⎭

ETIOLOGY

The factors which result in nonunion of a fracture could be local and systemic.

Local Factors (All Start with "I")

- *Infection*: Callus is poorly formed and destroyed amidst infection
- *Inadequate vascularity*: It results in poor callus formation at # site
- *Inadequate immobilization*: Callus cannot bridge due to persistent movement at the # site
- *Improper reduction of fracture or fixation*: Callus cannot bridge due to constant movement or wide gap at the # site
- *Intact fellow bone* (isolated fracture of tibia; fibula intact: Isolated # of radius; ulna intact): Intact fellow bone does not allow the fractured bone site to collapse and approximate for healing
- *Interposition of soft tissue*: Hampers the bridging of callus.

Systemic Factors

- *Use of nicotine in any form*: Smoking, chewing tobacco
- Diabetes mellitus
- Anemia and malnutrition
- Old age
- Hypothyroidism.

CLINICAL FEATURES

Symptoms: Patients report difficulty/inability to use the limb. They may be having difficulty in weight bearing or lifting weights.

Signs:
- *Painless abnormal mobility* at the fracture site is the *most essential sign of non-union*
- *Presence of a gap* at the fracture site
- *Absence of crepitus* at the fracture site (due to smooth # ends). Also, the non-union site is non-tender
- *Deformity and shortening* of the limb may be noticed.

DIAGNOSIS

- **Plain X-ray:** In most cases, plain X-ray is sufficient to establish the diagnosis **(Fig. 23.8)**. The typical findings seen in a case of nonunion are mentioned below:
    - Gap at the fracture site.
    - Smooth, sclerosed fracture ends.
    - Closed medullary cavity.
    - Callus may or may not be present depending upon the type of nonunion—hypertrophic/atrophic (read below).
- **CT scan** of the bone can be done if X-ray fails to establish the diagnosis of non-union.

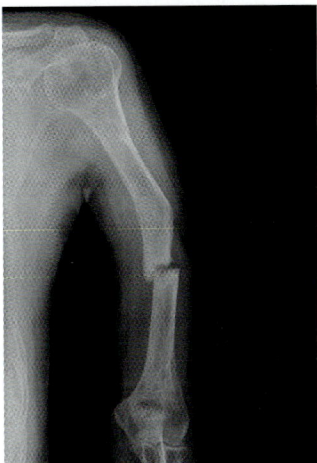

Fig. 23.8: X-ray of nonunion of fracture shaft humerus.

RADIOLOGICAL CLASSIFICATION OF NONUNION—ATROPHIC/HYPERTROPHIC

The radiological classification of a nonunion is based on the amount of callus formation observed at the fracture site. The callus could be none/minimal in atrophic and abundant in hypertrophic type.
- **Hypertrophic type:** Large fracture ends with a gap at the fracture site, while ***callus is abundant***. Hypertrophic nonunion indicates ***adequate vascularity but improper mechanical stability*** at the fracture site. Hence, during treatment, this type of nonunion needs stable fixation to ensure union while bone grafting is not required.
- **Atrophic type:** Small fracture ends with a gap at the fracture site, while ***poor or no callus is observed*** at the # site. It indicates ***poor blood supply at the fracture site***. Hence, during treatment, atrophic type of nonunion needs stable fixation along with cancellous bone grafting to ensure union.

TREATMENT

The treatment of nonunion (conservative/operative) would depend on the patient's functional deficit.

No treatment is required *if there is no or minimal functional deficit*, e.g., clavicle nonunion may not have any functional deficit. And therefore, it can be left alone.

However, most nonunions are symptomatic and require treatment. Furthermore, the nonunion could be aseptic or septic type and their treatment vary **(Flowchart 23.6)**. Aseptic nonunion could have an unstable or stable fixation.

Treatment principles of aseptic nonunion with unstable fixation.
A. **Treatment of the underlying systemic cause:** Stop smoking and chewing tobacco, correct anemia, and control diabetes.
B. **Treatment of nonunion:** The standard surgical principles of treating nonunion with unstable/no fixation are:
   - Open reduction of the nonunion site
   - Freshening of the sclerosed fracture ends till the edges start bleeding
   - Opening of the medullary cavity
   - Internal fixation
   - Bone grafting is required in the case of atrophic nonunion. The hypertrophic type needs only stable fixation and does not require grafting.

Aseptic nonunion with stable fixation: Bone grafting would suffice.

Treatment principles of infected nonunion: It can be managed in two ways, two-stage or single-stage.
1. *Two-stage procedure:* First, treat the infection with radical debridement of the infected site, remove an internal implant (if any), and apply antibiotic-laden bone cement and culture-specific prolonged antibiotics for 6–12 weeks. Once the infection is eradicated, one can proceed with the treatment of aseptic nonunion based on the principles described above.
2. *Single-stage procedure:* Perform the radical debridement of the local infected nonunion site and use the Ilizarov **(Fig. 23.9)** or limb reconstruction system (LRS) to bridge the gap and promote union.

Flowchart 23.6 summarizes the treatment of nonunion.

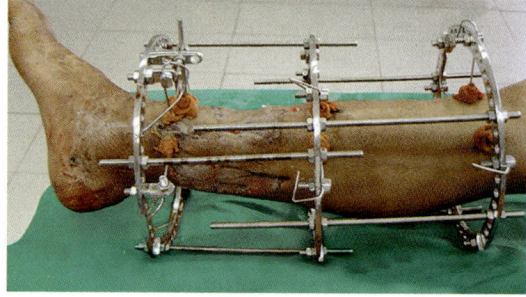

Fig. 23.9: Ilizarov external fixator application on the right leg.

Ilizarov method/LRS system is preferably used when there are more *complex situations, such as nonunion is associated with infection/shortening/deformity* (read about Ilizarov technique at the end of the chapter, page 246).

Why presence of an 'internal implant' (plate/nail) makes it difficult to eradicate infection (osteomyelitis)?
In case of prolonged local bacterial infection, the presence of implant results in a **biofilm formation** over the implant by the bacteria. The biofilm is the **matrix of extracellular polymeric substance** that is secreted by, and encases the bacteria. The key aspect of a biofilm is that it protects bacteria against the antibiotics and immune cells as the **biofilm is impregnable to antibiotics**, resulting in increased resistance to the antibiotics leading to difficult eradication of infection in presence of an implant. In such situation, 'internal' implant has to be removed to eradicate infection and fracture can be stabilized by an external fixator.
Note: *Mycobacterium tuberculosis does not form biofilm easily.*

Chapter 23: Complications of Fracture

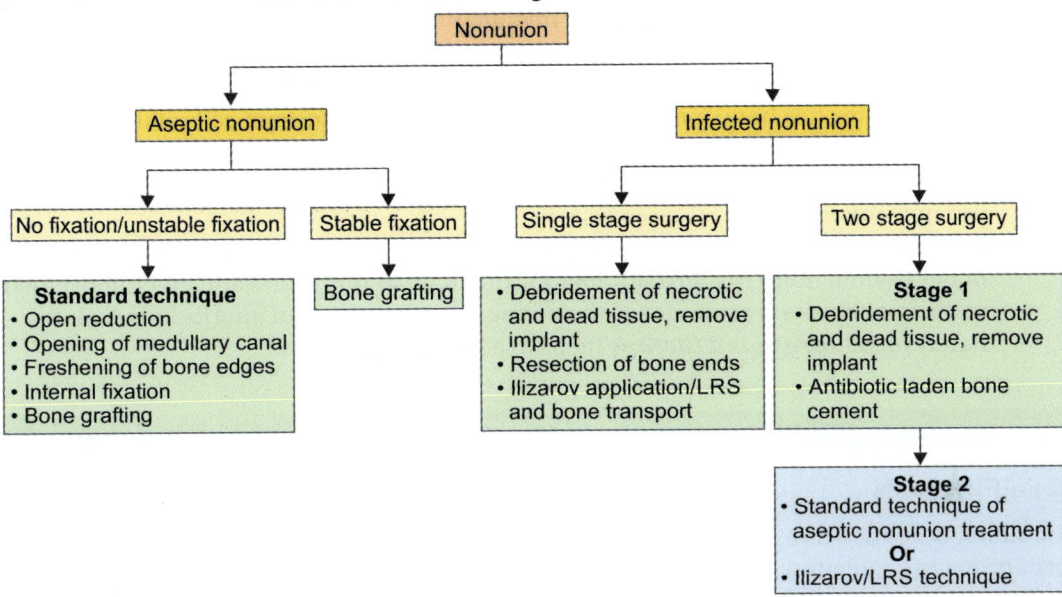

Flowchart 23.6: Treatment algorithm of fracture nonunion.

DELAYED UNION

■ DEFINITION
When the fracture union process is unduly slow, but each clinical follow up at 6–8 weeks does show progressive clinical and radiological union.

■ ETIOLOGY
Most fractures that are prone to nonunion may exhibit the tendency of delayed union. The causes for delayed union are similar to nonunion, such as poor blood supply, inadequate fixation, infection or comminution. Smoking, diabetes, anemia, old age and osteoporosis are some systemic factors that may contribute to delayed union.

■ CLINICAL FEATURES
- Persistent pain at # site
- Inability or difficulty in using the limb
- Occasionally, slight painful abnormal mobility could be present at the # site in the early stages of delayed union.
- Attempted movement at the fracture site would cause pain.

■ INVESTIGATION
The X-ray would reveal a gap at the fracture site at some locations but a union in other areas.

■ TREATMENT
- **Correction of local or systemic factors** such as smoking, local infection, diabetes mellitus, or anemia.

- **Wait and watch:** Unlike nonunion, the same treatment method is continued, and the patient is kept under serial observation until the fracture unites. In case the union fails to progress satisfactorily or if it need to be hastened, the undermentioned methods are adopted.
  - **Bone marrow injection** at the site of the delayed union to stimulate the union process. Bone marrow has bone morphogenic proteins (BMPs) and stem cells which stimulate local cells to convert into osteoblast and enhance the union process.
  - Occasionally **cancellous bone grafting** is performed at the delayed union site to promote union.
  - **Dynamization** of the fracture site. This method is adopted in long weight bearing bones (femur, tibia) treated with interlocking nail. In this procedure, micromovement at the fracture site is promoted by removing one/two screws of interlocking nail.
  - Rarely *local ultrasound therapy* helps in accelerating union.

MALUNION

DEFINITION

Malunion is defined as a condition when the fracture unites in a non-anatomical position. It occurs due to angulation, rotation or overriding.

> **Note**
> **Classic deformity in several # malunion**
> - Supracondylar humerus #: Cubitus varus
> - Colles #: Manus valgus
> - Intertrochanteric #: Coxa vara

> **Note**
> **Possible malalignments between two fragments are:**
> - Angulation
> - Rotation
> - Overriding

COMMON SITES OF MALUNION

- Fracture midshaft clavicle
- Fracture supracondylar humerus
- Colles' fracture
- Intertrochanteric fracture
- Calcaneum fracture.

Fracture in cancellous bones has a higher chance of malunion as cancellous bones have rich vascularity but less strong framework.

CLINICAL FEATURES

- Deformity (due to angulation/rotation) **(Figs. 23.10A and B)**
- Shortening (due to overriding)

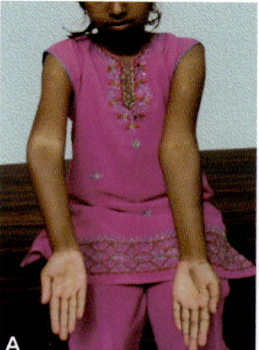
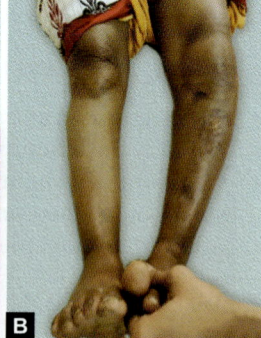

Figs. 23.10A and B: (A) Cubitus varus right elbow due to malunited fracture supracondylar humerus; (B) Varus deformity of the left tibia after malunion of fracture shaft tibia.

- Decreased range of movement
- Pain, stiffness, or other functional limitations/disability
- Poor cosmetic appearance.

INVESTIGATIONS

- **Plain X-ray** of the region
- **CT scan with 3-D reconstruction:** It may help assess complex deformities for further planning.

TREATMENT

The treatment of malunion depends upon the possibility of *future remodelling at the fracture site, functional deficit and/or cosmetic deformity.*
- **No treatment is required in malunion if:**
  - There is no functional disability
  - Younger children with potential remodelling potential with angular deformity in a long bone *(Note: Rotational malunion does not get remodelled).*
- **If there is major functional impairment/poor cosmetic appearance,** malunion can be corrected with the following surgical options:
  - *Corrective osteotomy* to correct deformity with or without internal/external fixation **(Figs. 23.11A and B)**.
  - *Redoing the fracture*: The fracture is recreated in the original plane and fixed with implant.
  - *Osteoclasis*: It is performed in the malunion of greenstick fractures (in children).
  - *Limb lengthening to correct shortening*.

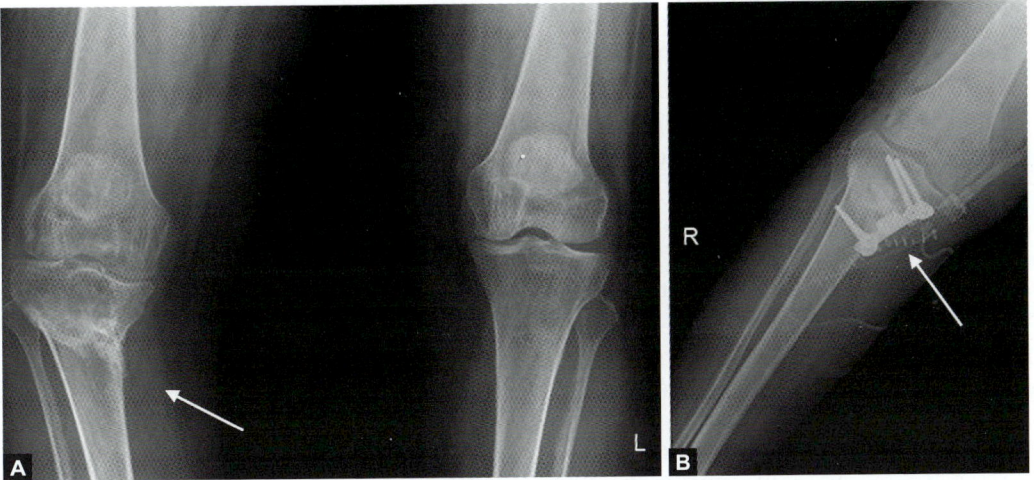

Figs. 23.11A and B: (A) Varus malunion of tibia (white arrow over varus deformity of proximal tibia); (B) Corrective osteotomy and fixation.

JOINT STIFFNESS

INTRODUCTION

- The stiffness of a joint implies that the joint has lost partial or total range of movement, partial or total.
- Complete loss of joint movement or barely perceptible movement at a joint is called "ankylosis."
- Stiffness is a common complication of fracture, especially intra-articular fractures. It is also seen after comminuted fractures close to the joint (meta-diaphyseal).

TYPES OF STIFFNESS

- **Extra-articular:** The cause of stiffness is outside the joint. Common causes of extra-articular stiffness are:
  - Contracture of skin and subcutaneous tissues, fascia, and muscle-tendon
  - Implant adherence (especially plates) to the muscle and adjacent soft tissues results in poor gliding of muscles
  - Myositis ossificans
- **Intra-articular:** The cause of stiffness is inside the joint. Common causes of intra-articular stiffness are:
  - Malunited intra-articular fractures, which alter the shape of the joint surface
  - Capsular and ligaments contractures
  - Intra-articular adhesions
  - Arthritis of the joint
- **Combined:** Combined intra- and extra-articular causes.

PREDISPOSING FACTORS

- **Prolonged immobilization:** Prolonged immobilization results in shortened, contracted muscle—tendon, ligaments, and joint capsules. These structures, especially muscle, get adhered to the # site preventing normal joint movement.
- **Intra-articular fractures** could result in:
  - Intra-articular adhesions
  - Malunited joint surface results in stiffness.
- **Open reduction:** Stripping of various soft tissues (muscle, periosteum, and deep fascia) leads to fibrosis and contractures at the fracture site.
- **Plate fixation:** The overlying muscle gets stuck over the implant and prevents normal muscle slides. Also, dissection of soft tissue leads to fibrosis of soft tissue.
- **Infection:** Extensive fibrosis of soft tissues (skin, subcutaneous tissue, muscle-tendon complex, fascia, etc.).
- **Plastic surgical procedures:** Open fractures with soft tissue defects often require plastic surgical procedures like SSG (split-thickness skin graft) or flaps. This is more likely with ***SSGs as it tends to heal with contracture, whereas full-thickness flaps do not undergo contractures***. Hence, one must avoid SSG over the joint and perform flaps to cover the joint area.

CLINICAL FEATURES
- Reduced range of motion
- Affected joint function.

INVESTIGATIONS
X-ray, CT scan, and MRI.

TREATMENT
- **Early stiffness:** Physiotherapy and active and passive joint mobilization are sufficient to regain an adequate range of motion.
- **Late stiffness:** If the patient presents late, they may require surgical management as the tissues are scarred and not amenable to stretching by physiotherapy.
    - *Skin contractures:* Scar release by Z- or V-Y plasty, scar excision, and flap coverage
    - *Deep fascia contracture:* Releases
    - *Muscle-tendon complex:* Tendon lengthening (V-Y or Z plasty)
    - *Capsule contracture:* Capsulotomy or capsular releases
    - *Myositis mass:* Excision
    - *Ligament:* Limited release of the ligament
    - *Intraarticular adhesion:* Open/arthroscopic release
    - *Bony malunion:* May require corrective osteotomy
    - *Bony ankylosis:* Joint replacement or arthrodesis in the functional position
    - *Severe arthritis:* Joint replacement or arthrodesis in a functional position.

LIMB SHORTENING

A common complication after the fracture, especially with growth plate damage, comminution, bone loss, or infection.

ETIOLOGY
- **Bone loss**
    - After an open fracture leading to bone loss
    - After repeated surgery and bone resection
- **Malunion**
- **Nonunion**
- **Infection:** It leads to bone destruction and surgical excision of bone to eradicate infection
- **Damage to the growth plate**.

TREATMENT OF SHORTENING
- *Address the etiology* such as malunion or infection.
- **If shortening is less than 1 cm:** It can be managed conservatively as shortening gets compensated by pelvic tilt.
- **If shortening 1–4 cm:** Shoe raise can be given up to 4 cm. However, the measures for >4 cm described below too can be applied here if required.

- **Shortening greater than 4 cm**
  - *Limb lengthening*: Using Ilizarov or limb reconstruction system (LRS)
  - *Normal side shortening*: Up to 3" in femur and 2" in the tibia can be performed in kids.
  - *Epiphysiodesis*: In children, the growth of the longer side is slowed by epiphysiodesis.

A NOTE ON ILIZAROV TECHNIQUE FOR LIMB RECONSTRUCTION

Ilizarov technique is based upon the principle of *"Compression-distraction osteogenesis."* It means that when bone ends are compressed or distracted (gradually), it results in new bone formation (osteogenesis). This technique can be used to correct:
- **Shortening**
- **Nonunion**
- **Bone defects**
- **Soft tissue or bony deformities**.

Principle and procedure: The bone is cut transversely mostly at metaphysis keeping the periosteum intact (corticotomy), then two ends are gradually distracted with Ilizarov or limb reconstruction system at the rate of 1 mm/day.

Gradual distraction between two ends leads to new bone formation by intact periosteum by *"distraction osteogenesis"*. In this way, new bone (regenerate) is generated which is required for limb lengthening, correcting bone defects **(Figs. 23.12A to E)**.

In another technique, the two bone ends (of nonunion) can be freshened and further compressed together which result in regeneration of new bone at the compressed site as *"compression osteogenesis"*. This principle is used in nonunion of the fractures.

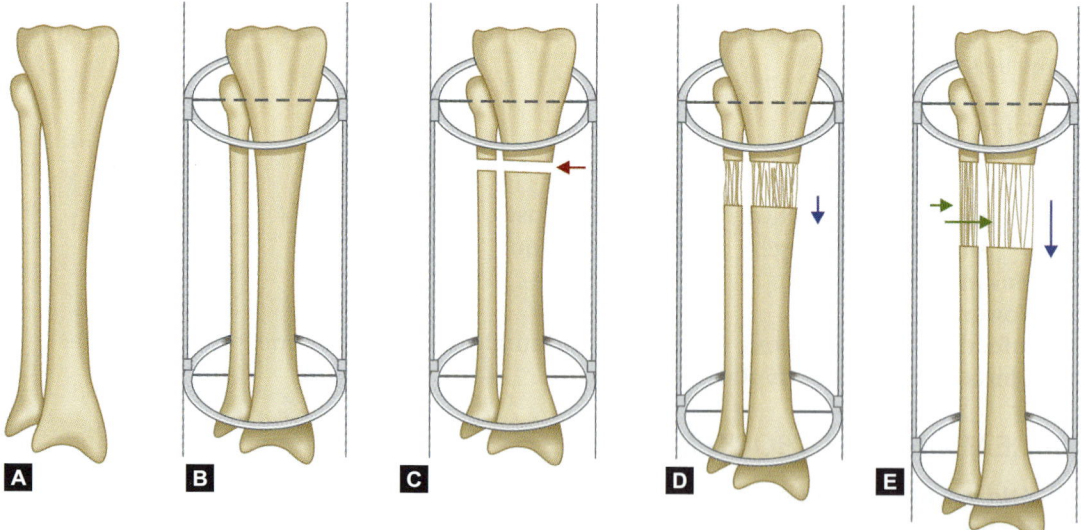

Figs. 23.12A to E: Illustrative images showing distraction osteogenesis using Ilizarov fixator: (A) A short bone; (B) Ilizarov frame application; (C) Corticotomy at metaphysis (brown arrow); (D) Gradual distraction (blue arrow); (E) Further distraction. Green arrow shows regenerate or new bone formation.

One can compress a nonunion site and distract from other end to achieve union and length in same Ilizarov frame **(Figs. 23.13A to D)**.

Also various soft tissue and bony deformity correction can be achieved with Ilizarov's technique.

The *"distraction principle"* is used to correct shortening, bone defect, and gap nonunion, whereas the *"compression principle"* is used in nonunion wherein two freshened ends of the bone are compressed together to achieve union.

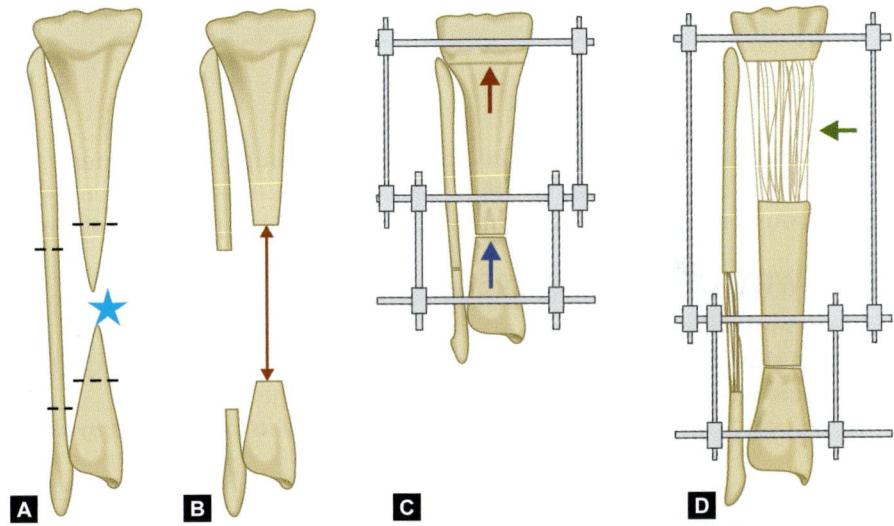

Figs. 23.13A to D: (A) Atrophic nonunion site in bone (blue star); (B) Resection and freshening of the nonunion site (red arrow); (C) Compression at the freshened site (blue arrow) and corticotomy at the other end (red arrow); (D) Distraction at the corticotomy site producing regenerate (green arrow), resulting in regaining the length of bone. New bone also forms at the compression site.

Notes

CHAPTER 24

Open Fracture

DEFINITION

A fracture is said to be open when fracture and/or its hematoma communicates with the external environment through a wound **(Figs. 24.1A and B)**. Previously, open # was also known as a compound fracture, and this term is still being used in many parts of the world.

PROBLEMS WITH OPEN FRACTURE

The primary concerns with open # are:
- **The overlying skin and soft tissue loss** may result in decreased vascularity of the bones involved and increased chance of infection at the fracture site.
- **Infection:** The spectrum may vary from **local soft tissue infection** to **osteomyelitis**.
- **Bone loss**
- **Delayed/nonunion of fracture** are a result of poor vascularity of soft tissue and bone, bone loss and persistent infection.

ETIOLOGY

- Most open fractures are a result of **high-velocity injury, such as RTA**, fall from height, or gunshot injury.

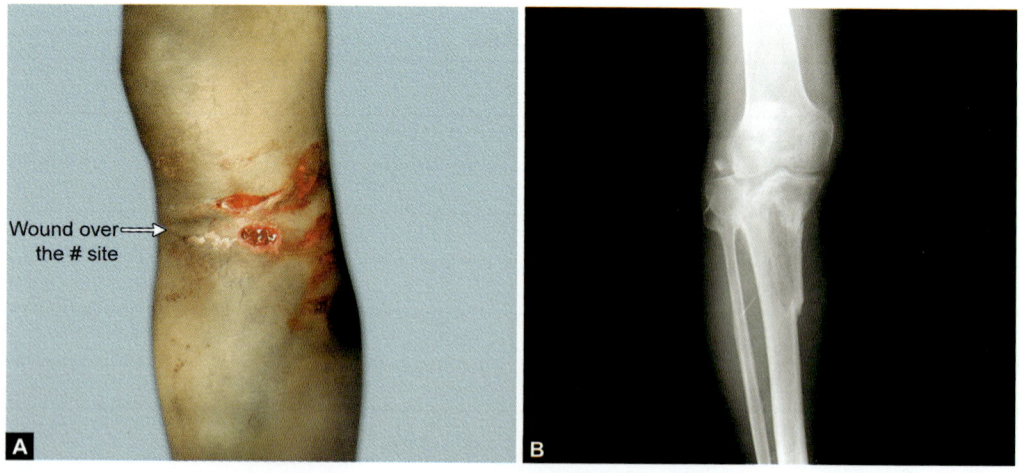

Figs. 24.1A and B: Open fracture with wound: (A) Wound over proximal leg; (B) Concomitant underlying fracture of upper end of the tibia.

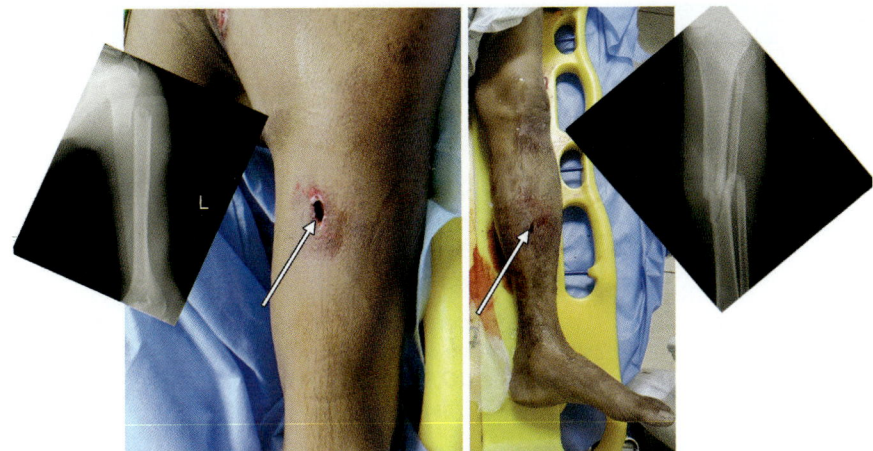

Fig. 24.2: Left image showing an inside out open fracture of humerus and right image shows inside-out open fracture tibia shaft. White arrows are over puncture wounds and inset picture shows corresponding X-rays.

- Sometimes, low-velocity injuries like fall at home or sports injuries could result in open #.

CLASSIFICATION

- **According to the side of open fracture:**
    - *Open from inside*: It implies that the sharp fracture end penetrates the skin from beneath and make a fracture open **(Fig. 24.2)**
    - *Open from outside*: It implies that a high energy injury (a direct blow or a ballistic injury) penetrates the skin, damaging the subtending soft tissues and bone **(Fig. 24.3)**
- **Gustilo–Anderson classification (Table 24.1):** It is the most common classification system used in classifying open fractures. It is further classified into three types (type I-III), considering the following factors.
    - Size of wound
    - Contamination
    - Devitalization of tissues
    - Velocity of injury.

CLINICAL FEATURES

Symptoms: Apart from *pain, swelling, and inability to use the limb*, the most important symptom is the **presence of a bleeding wound** over or around the fracture site. Sometimes, bone is exposed through the wound and is visible to the naked eye.

Inside-out open # are more dangerous because the fractured bone end creates a small puncture wound (small rent) in skin and soft tissue, **gets contaminated** and goes back inside the wound. Hence, it may look innocuous but the contamination at the # site is certain and may get unnoticed due to small size of the wound.

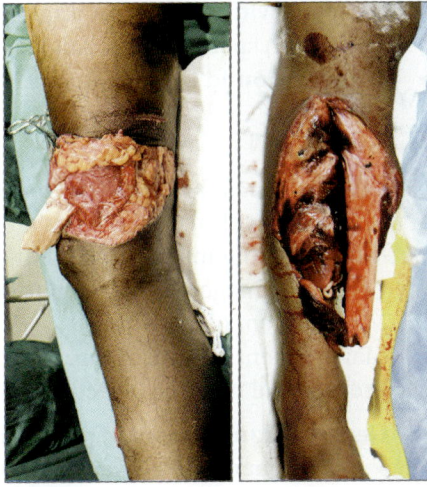

Fig. 24.3: Left and right images shows outside-in open femur fracture and tibia fracture, respectively.

Table 24.1: Gustilo and Anderson classification.

Type	Size	Contamination	Devitalization of tissue	Velocity of injury
I	<1 cm	Minimal	Minimal	Low
II	1–10 cm	Moderate	Moderate	Moderate
IIIA	>10 cm	Severe	Severe with periosteal stripping; the **fracture site can be covered by existing local soft tissues** and **DO NOT require any soft tissue coverage surgery** (SSG/flaps)	Severe
IIIB	>10 cm	Severe	Severe with periosteal stripping; the **fracture site cannot be covered by existing local soft tissues** and **DO REQUIRE soft tissue coverage surgery** (SSG/flaps)	Severe
IIIC	Irrespective of size, any open fracture which *is associated with vascular injury* is considered to type IIIC			

Signs: There is varying skin and underlying soft tissue damage and loss. Further, there may be contamination of the # site by the foreign material through the wound.
- Bleeding through the wound is usually in the form of ooze. Frank arterial bleeds are uncommon.
- Bony tenderness is present over the # site
- Other features: Deformity, shortening of the limb
- Always rule out the neurovascular deficit.

INVESTIGATIONS

- **Plain X-ray:** AP, lateral or other special views
- **Arterial Doppler:** It should be performed in case of feeble or absent distal pulses. Further confirmation of arterial injury can be done with CT angiogram.
- **CT scan (with or without angiography):** CT scan is done for intra-articular fractures or fractures in specific areas. Angiography is added to CT in cases of a vascular injury.
- **Primary wound Gram stain and culture**.

TREATMENT

Note that *'all open fractures' are one of the orthopaedic emergencies*, especially if they arrive at the hospital within 6–8 hours as an early debridement may help prevent infection.
The essential principles of treatment of open fracture are as follows:
A. General management of the **patient**
B. Management of the **wound**
C. Management of the **fracture**
D. Prevent and treat the **infection.**

A. **General management of patient:**
 - Maintenance of airway, breathing, and circulation **(ABC)**. *Assess and manage patient as per ATLS protocol.*
 - **Splint the limb**, and **control bleeding** from the open wound by compression dressing.

- *Appropriate analgesics,* and *tetanus prophylaxis* must be administered. ***Blood transfusion*** if significant blood loss.
- *Systemic antibiotics* should be administered as early as possible (*preferably within 1 hour*), covering gram-positive (1st generation cephalosporin-cephalexin, or amoxicillin-clavulanic acid), and gram-negative (gentamicin/3rd generation cephalosporin-ceftriaxone) microbes. Metronidazole is added presence of fecal or potential clostridial contamination (e.g., farm-related injuries).

    Primary antibiotics are continued for 3–5 days. However, further continuation of antibiotics depends upon secondary infection, which should be according to culture and sensitivity. *Of note: Antibiotics are no alternative for adequate surgical debridement.*

B. **Management of the wound:** *Debridement is the gold standard treatment of an open wound.*

    The first *6–8 hours after the trauma is considered the golden hour to perform debridement to minimize the chance of infection.*
    - ***Debridement*** is defined as the *surgical removal of all dead, devitalized tissue and contamination from an open wound until healthy margins are achieved.* Following tissues must be excised in order to perform an adequate debridement:
        - *Skin:* Extend, and excise 1–2 mm edge or the entire dead margin.
        - *Fascia:* Divide, excise.
        - *Muscle:* Dead muscle is dangerous and should be excised as it can cause gas gangrene, crush syndrome, and tetanus.
        - *Tendon:* Necrotic margins are excised, and the free end is tagged with surrounding tissue for later secondary repair. Primary repair is performed if the wound is clean after debridement.
        - *Nerve:* Necrotic margins are excised, and the free end is tagged with surrounding tissue for later secondary repair. Primary repair is performed if the wound is clean after debridement.
        - *Joint:* Wash with plenty of saline and close the joint.
        - *Wound area and bone:* A bone piece without any periosteum or soft tissue attachment should be sacrificed as it could turn into a future sequestrum (due to lack of blood supply). The wounded area should be given plenty of wash with 6–10 L of normal saline to debulk the contamination and minimize the chance of infection.

    Following debridement, locally antibiotic laden bone cement beads can be placed to prevent infection **(Fig. 24.4)**.

> **Note**
> **Advantages of external fixation**
> - Stabilizes fracture
> - Maintains alignment
> - Allows regular dressing of wound
> - Allows joints mobilization
> - Allows secondary soft tissue coverage procedure such as SSG/flaps

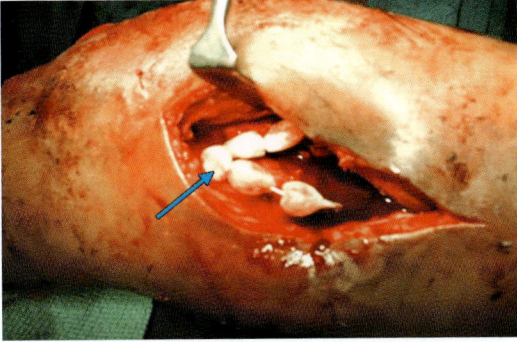

Fig. 24.4: Antibiotic laden bone cement beads (blue arrow) placed in the wound post-debridement.

- *Closure of wound:* Wounds of Gustilo-Anderson type I and II can be closed primarily at the time of debridement. The wound of Gustilo-Anderson type III may be grossly contaminated and require a relook or repeated debridement until the wound is clean. Later, it can be closed with primary suturing (IIIA) or SSG/flaps (IIIB).

C. **Management of fracture:** The fracture should be managed as per Gustilo-Anderson type of fracture (I, II, III). Type I, II can be managed with CR and cast application or internal fixation. External fixators are best suited for Type III **(Table 24.2)**. The type of fixation selected depends upon the type of Gustilo-Anderson wound and fracture personality.
- In case of a closed reduction and POP application of a Type I/II open fracture, the wound/suture dressing is done via a POP window over the wound **(Fig. 24.5)**.

Table 24.2: Outline of management of open # as per Gustilo-Anderson classification.

Gustilo type of fracture	Definitive fracture treatment	Wound coverage
I	***Debridement***, CR, and cast application/internal or external fixation of the fracture	Primary closure of the wound
II	***Debridement***, CR, and cast application/internal or external fixation of the fracture	Primary closure of the wound
III A and B	***Debridement*** and external fixation of fracture **(Figs. 24.6A to C)**	Primary suturing/split skin graft (SSG)/flap
III C	***Debridement***, exploration and vascular repair, external or internal fixation of the fracture	Primary suturing/split skin graft (SSG)/flap

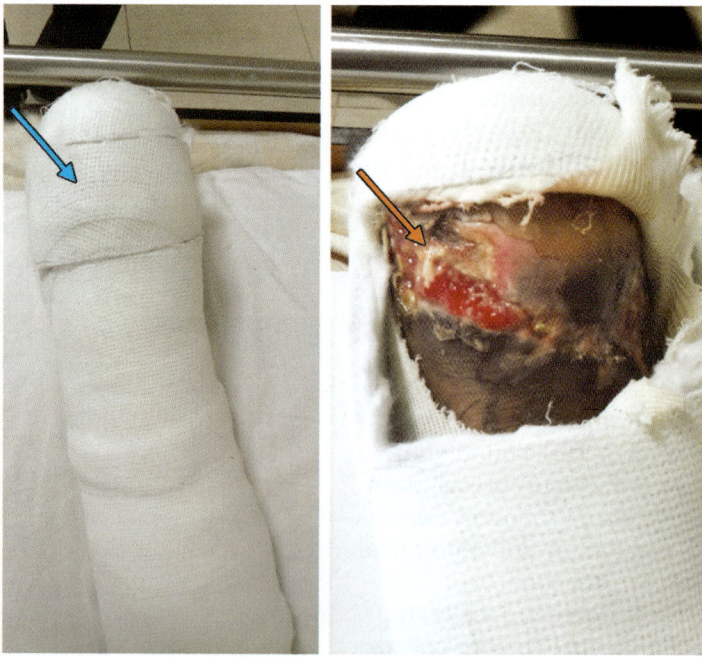

Fig. 24.5: A POP window is created for regular dressing of wound. Blue arrow shows flap of POP while orange arrow shows wound after flap is opened.

Chapter 24: Open Fracture

Antibiotic beads

In cases of localized bone infection, **polymethyl methacrylate (PMMA) bone cement**, which is **non-dissolvable**, is frequently used as an agent to store and gradually release antibiotics locally over a few days to weeks. However, after 6–8 weeks, when the antibiotics have worn off from the beads, the beads must be surgically removed since they can act as a foreign body and cause infection.

Another type of **progressively dissolving antibiotic beads** are available, which are made of **calcium sulphate (stimulan)**. Consequently, a second procedure to remove the bead is avoided.

Note that these agents (PMMA/calcium sulphate) could be preloaded with antibiotic or antibiotic can be mixed just before implantation during surgery. With PMMA, only heat stable antibiotics, such as vancomycin, gentamycin, and tobramycin can be used as PMMA prepration results in exothermic reaction, which can damage a heat labile antibiotic. Although stimulan preparation is not an exothermic process. The United States Food and Drug Administration (FDA or USFDA) has permitted usage of vancomycin, gentamycin, and tobramycin.

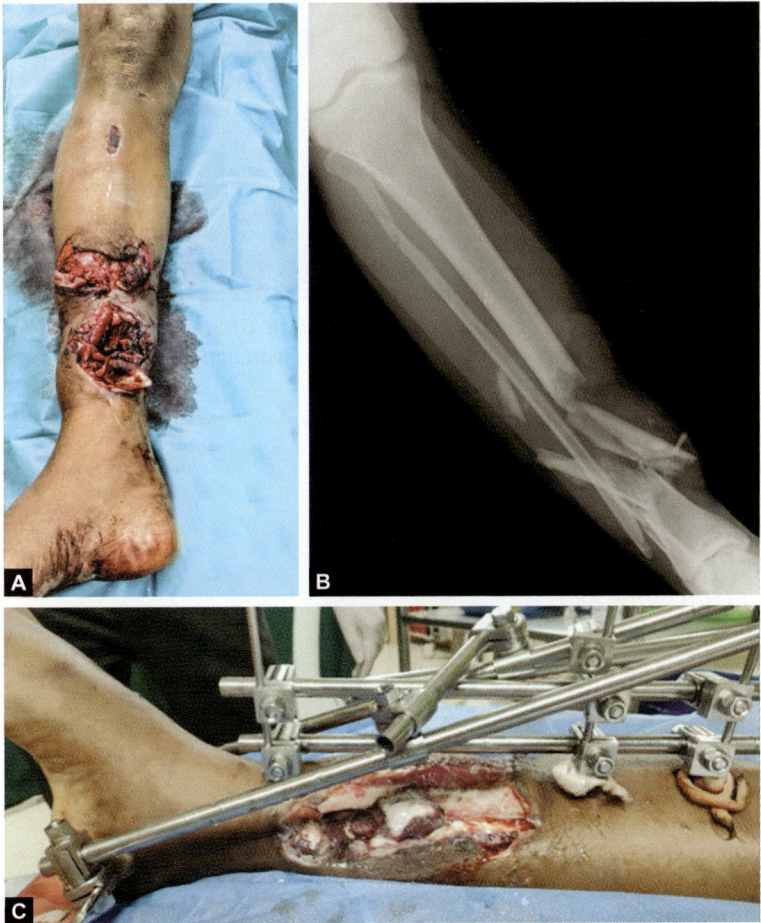

Figs. 24.6A to C: (A) Type III B open fracture of the lower tibia with skin loss; (B) Corresponding X-ray shows comminuted lower third tibia fracture; (C) Debridement and external fixator.

D. **Prevent and treat infection:**
- Repeat debridement, if required. Continue appropriate antibiotic according to culture and for several days-weeks. Antibiotic-laden bone cement can placed during repeat debridement. Note that PMMA beads need to be removed after 6–8 weeks.
- *Once the wound is healthy after debridement, coverage of the open wound should be performed with SSG or flap* **(Figs. 24.7A and B)**. Note that after debridement, wound coverage is the most crucial measure to prevent infection at the fracture site.

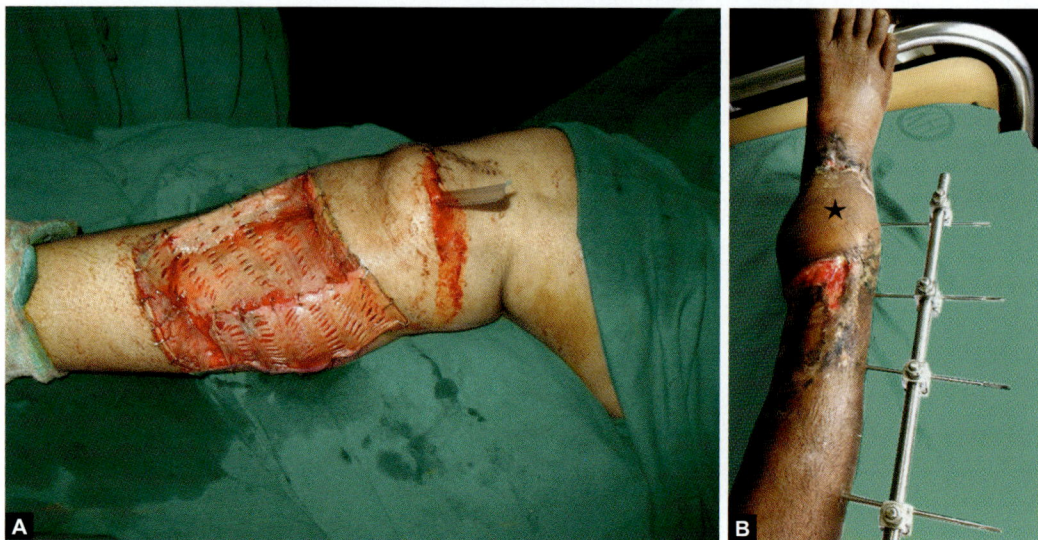

Figs. 24.7A and B: (A) Split thickness skin graft (SSG) over open fracture site; (B) External fixator on fracture shaft tibia with flap (star marked).

COMPLICATIONS OF OPEN FRACTURE

- **Acute**
    - Crush syndrome
    - Gas gangrene
    - Tetanus
    - Bone and soft tissue loss
    - Neurovascular injury
- **Subacute**
    - Septicemia
    - Septic arthritis: If fracture is close to the joint or an intraarticular fracture
    - Local soft tissue and bone infection.
- **Chronic**
    - Chronic osteomyelitis
    - Nonunion
    - Malunion
    - Joint stiffness
    - Shortening
    - Deformity

CHAPTER 25

Ligament Injury of Knee, Ankle and Other Sports Injuries

GENERAL DESCRIPTION OF LIGAMENT INJURY

LIGAMENT

Ligament is a short band of tough, flexible fibrous connective tissue which connects two bones or holds a joint together.

FUNCTION OF LIGAMENT AND CLINICAL APPLICATION

Ligament provides stability to a joint. Therefore, injury, especially complete tear, to the ligament could result in *"instability of the joint"*. It can also result in *pain during activity*. Together, instability and pain result in *joint dysfunction*.

HOW A JOINT REMAINS STABLE DURING MOVEMENT WITHOUT DISLOCATING?

A joint remains stable due to support provided by static and dynamic stabilizers, such as:
- **Static stabilizers**
  - Bony conformation of two articulating surface
  - Ligaments and capsule
  - Negative intra-articular pressure.
- **Dynamic stabilizer:** Muscles and tendons around the joint.

Therefore, any disruption in static/dynamic/both stabilizers may result in an unstable joint.

GENERAL CLINICAL FEATURES OF LIGAMENT INJURY

- **History of injury:** Almost all patients with ligament injury give a history of trauma, which could be a direct trauma to the joint, twisting injury, or a road traffic accident. Rarely, a group of patient may complain of instability without any trauma due to hyperlax tissues or congenital abnormalities in bone (dysplasia) (*Refer Chapter 5, page 29*).
- **Clinical features:** There is *pain and swelling* of the affected part and *difficulty in using the part*. If the patient cannot *stand/bear weight* after injury to the ligaments of lower limb joints, it implies a significant injury to the ligament. *Complaints of instability or giving way* of the joint imply a complete ligament injury.

  In case of *chronic complete ligament injury*, **recurrent instability** *is the key feature*. They may also have mild pain.

Table 25.1: Grade of ligament injury.

Grade of injury	Structural damage	Instability	Functional loss
Grade I	Few fibers sprained	None	None
Grade II	Partial damage	None/rare	Mild
Grade III	Complete tear	Present	Moderate-severe

GRADE OF LIGAMENT INJURY

Most ligament injuries across the body can be classified into 1st, 2nd and 3rd-degree (Table 25.1).

INVESTIGATIONS

- **Plain X-ray:** In a ligament injury, generally the X-rays are normal. However, it is always done to look for:
    - Associated fracture
    - Malalignment of the joint, which could be observed in complete tear of the ligament
    - Soft tissue edema.
- **Stress X-ray:** It is performed to differentiate between *chronic grades 2 and 3 ligament injuries to decide between conservative vs. operative treatment,* as latter would require surgical treatment while former can be managed conservatively. It should be avoided in acute ligament injuries for fear of converting lower grades into higher ones.
- **Magnetic resonance imaging (MRI):** It is the *investigation of choice for musculoskeletal system soft tissue injuries.* It helps in detecting:
    - All grades of ligament injuries
    - Associated cartilage injury, bone bruises, marrow edema, and occult fractures.
- **Computed tomography (CT) scan:** It is usually not required in ligament injuries. However, occasionally, it may be required to assess an associated fracture.

TREATMENT

The treatment of ligament injury depends on various factors, such as duration (acute/chronic), symptoms, age of the patient, and functional requirements.
- **Acute stage of all grades of ligament injury**
    - *RICE* is the mainstay of treatment in the acute stage of all ligament injuries (R: rest to the part; I: ice; C: compression; E: elevation)
    - Nonsteroidal anti-inflammatory drugs (NSAIDs) or other analgesics for pain relief
    - Serratiopeptidase for 3–5 days for edema reduction.
    - Bracing the limb for support and rest.
- **Definitive treatment of ligament injury** depends upon the grade of ligament injury.
    - *Grades 1 and 2:* Most grades 1 and 2 ligament injuries heal with conservative treatment. The conservative treatment offered includes rest, bracing, gradual rehabilitation, followed by resumption of complete activity.
    - *Grade 3:* The option of conservative/surgical treatment depends upon the individual ligament, type of symptoms, patient's age, and activity level. Therefore, various treatment options are:
        - Braces, rehabilitation and activity modification
        - Repair/reconstruction of the ligament.

LIGAMENT AND MENISCAL INJURY OF THE KNEE

The major ligaments and meniscus of the knee are:
- **Cruciates:** Anterior and posterior
- **Collaterals:** Medial and lateral
- **Menisci:** Medial and lateral
- **Medial patellofemoral ligament (MPFL):** It is the major ligament which stabilizes the patella. The details of injury to MPFL, resulting in patella dislocation are discussed in Chapter 5 *(Refer, patella dislocation, page 55)*.

ANTERIOR CRUCIATE LIGAMENT (ACL) TEAR

SURGICAL ANATOMY OF ACL

- The ACL connects the tibia and femur at the knee joint **(Fig. 25.1A)**. Proximally, ACL is attached to the medial wall of the lateral femoral condyle, whereas distally, ACL is attached to the tibia just anterior to the intercondylar eminence. About 90% of ACL consists of type 1 collagen.
- **ACL bundles**—anatomically, there are two bundles of ACL, anteromedial and posterolateral, which are named after their attachment orientation on the tibia. **(Fig. 25.1B)**. Both bundles have different functions:
  - *Anteromedial bundle*: *It is tight in knee flexion,* and it is responsible for the *anteroposterior (AP) stability of the knee.*
  - *Posterolateral bundle*: *It is tight in knee extension,* and it is responsible for the *rotational stability of the knee.*

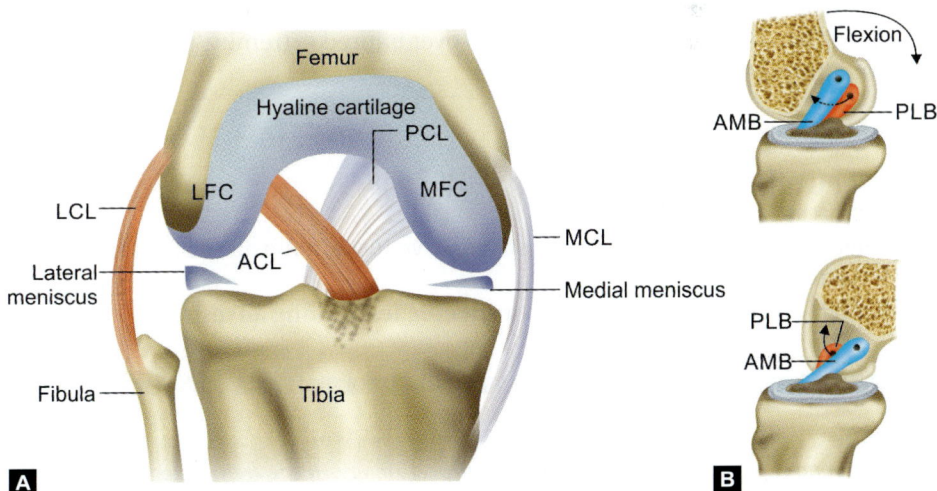

Figs. 25.1A and B: (A) Coronal illustration of the knee in 90° flexion shows knee ligaments; (B) Sagittal illustration shows bundles of ACL in extension (above) and flexion (below).

(ACL: anterior cruciate ligament; LFC: lateral femoral condyle; MFC: medial femoral condyle; LCL: lateral collateral ligament; MCL: medial collateral ligament; PCL: posterior cruciate ligament; AMB: anteromedial bundle; PLB: posterolateral bundle)

- **Blood supply of the ACL:** Middle geniculate artery.
- **Nerve supply of the ACL:** Posterior articular nerve (branch of the tibial nerve).

FUNCTION OF ACL

Typically, the ACL prevents excess anterior translation of the tibia over the fixed femur and provides rotational stability to the knee.

MECHANISM OF INJURY

- **Sports injury:** *It is the most common mechanism of injury to the ACL,* wherein a twisting injury, especially over a semi-flexed knee, tears the ACL. It is often seen in sports requiring pivoting and landing, such as football, basketball, and volleyball. The ACL tear could occur due to contact or non-contact type of mechanism.
- **Road traffic accident (RTA).**

Point to be remembered: Generally, natural spontaneous healing of a complete ACL tear is a rarity. And, therefore, most patient remain symptomatic with knee instability and may require surgical intervention.

CLINICAL FEATURES OF ACUTE ANTERIOR CRUCIATE LIGAMENT TEAR

Symptoms

- History of *injury to the knee* during sports/RTA. During sports, the knee can be injured during a twisting episode/a direct trauma to the knee.
- A ***pop is often heard*** by the patient in case of acute complete ACL tear. It is followed by pain and immediate/early swelling of the knee (hemarthrosis).
- Patient complains of *inability to bear weight* over injured extremity/walk.
- Feeling of *instability/giving way* of the knee.

Signs

- Effusion is present in the knee—positive patellar tap.
- Painful and restricted movement.
- *Lachman test positive,* which is the **most sensitive test** among all the tests for ACL.
- *Anterior drawer test is positive.*
- *Pivot shift test positive,* which is the **most specific test** among all tests.

Facts about tests for ACL tear

Anterior drawer and Pivot shift are difficult to perform in acute injury. Hence, the best test to perform in acute ACL injury is Lachman, which requires only 20–30 degrees of knee flexion. Furthermore, Pivot shift test detects injury to the PL bundle of the ACL, while the anterior drawer and Lachman detect injury to the AM bundle of the ACL.

*Recently, a new test has been described for ACL injury known as **Lelli's test** (students are encouraged to read about the test themselves).*

CLINICAL FEATURES OF CHRONIC ANTERIOR CRUCIATE LIGAMENT TEAR

- *Recurrent instability is the key symptom of chronic ACL injury,* especially while performing pivoting or cutting activities, running, jumping or walking on an uneven surface. However, straight walking on flat ground is usually *not* a problem.
- Quadriceps muscle wasting is almost always present.
- Test for ACL instability (anterior drawer, Lachman, and pivot shift) are positive.

INVESTIGATIONS

- **Plain X-ray of the knee:** AP and lateral view.
    - To look for any bony avulsion of ACL **(Fig. 25.2A)**.
    - *Segond fracture is a hallmark of ACL tear* in which a small bony avulsion is observed adjacent to the lateral tibial plateau **(Fig. 25.2B)**.
- **Magnetic resonance imaging of the knee:** *It is the diagnostic radiological investigation for ACL tear* **(Fig. 25.2C)**. Further, it is also helpful in detecting concomitant injuries of the meniscus, collateral ligament, cartilage injury, bone contusion or occult fractures.
- **Diagnostic arthroscopy:** Occasionally, arthroscopy may be required to confirm the diagnosis if there is a diagnostic dilemma even after clinical examination and MRI **(Figs. 25.3A and B)**.

TREATMENT

The treatment of ACL depends upon the duration of tear (acute/chronic), prevailing symptoms, age, and functional requirements.

- **Acute ACL tear:** Acute injuries are usually managed conservatively.
    - **RICE: R**est, **I**ce application, **C**ompression, and **E**levation
    - Analgesics, bracing
    - **Rehabilitation:** Knee mobilization, hamstring and quadriceps strengthening exercises are started, and gradual weight bearing is encouraged.

> **Important**
> *Spontaneous natural healing of complete ACL tear is rare.* Hence, in most cases of symptomatic ACL tear require ACL reconstruction. Also, the 'repair' of acute ACL tear has largely remained unsuccessful in the past. However, offlate, there has been great progress in ACL repair techniques and results of acute ACL repair.

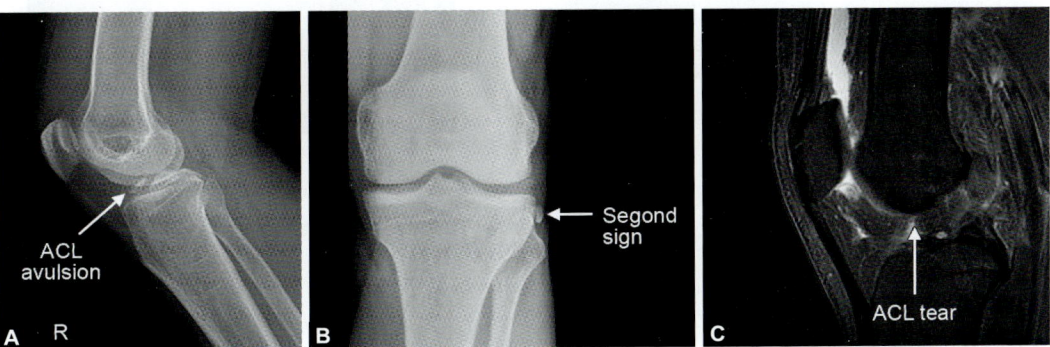

Figs. 25.2A to C: (A) Lateral X-ray of the knee showing ACL bony avulsion; (B) AP X-ray of knee showing Segond sign; (C) MRI of the knee showing ACL tear.
(ACL: anterior cruciate ligament)

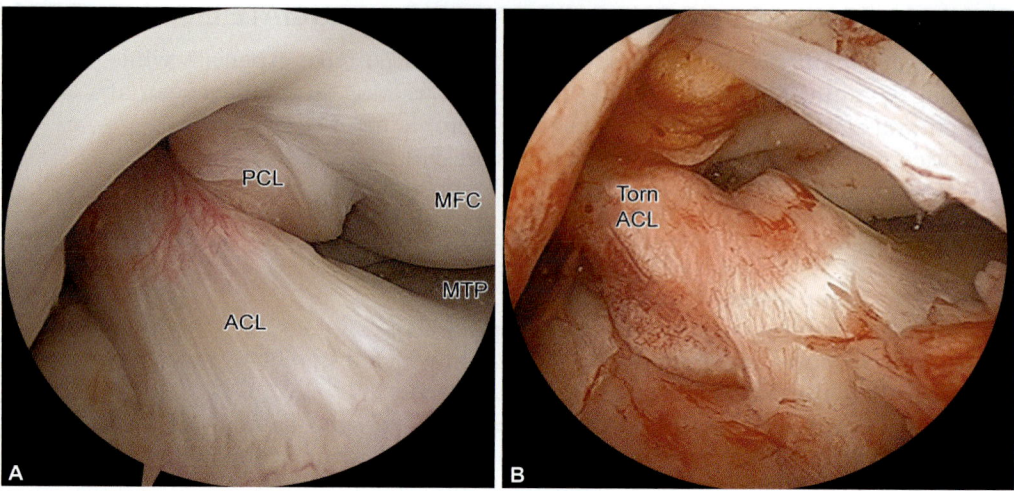

Figs. 25.3A and B: (A) Arthroscopic image of a normal ACL; (B) Arthroscopic image showing acute ACL tear.
(ACL: anterior cruciate ligament; PCL: posterior cruciate ligament; MFC: medial femoral condyle; MTP: medial tibial plateau)

Once acute phase is over and knee is well rehabilitated, **ACL reconstruction** is performed in young patients, especially those with concomitant meniscal and cartilage injury.
- **ACL repair** can be attempted in selected cases.

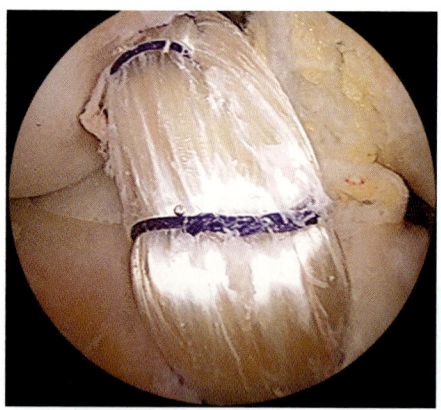

Fig. 25.4: Arthrosocpic image of reconstructed ACL.

Note: The role of hamstring strengthening is vital in the conservative management of ACL tear, as a strong hamstring compensates for ACL tear-induced excess anterior translation of the tibia by pulling the tibia posteriorly, thereby reducing ACL tear-related instability.

- **Chronic ACL tear**
    - *If patient complain of recurrent instability:* Arthroscopic ACL reconstruction is the treatment of choice **(Fig. 25.4)**.
    - *If asymptomatic/occasional instability/old age/low demand patient:* Conservative treatment is advised.
- **Displaced acute ACL bony avulsion:** It should be fixed with pull-out sutures or screws.

Flowchart 25.1 summarizes the treatment of the ACL tear.

Flowchart 25.1: Management of anterior cruciate ligament tear.

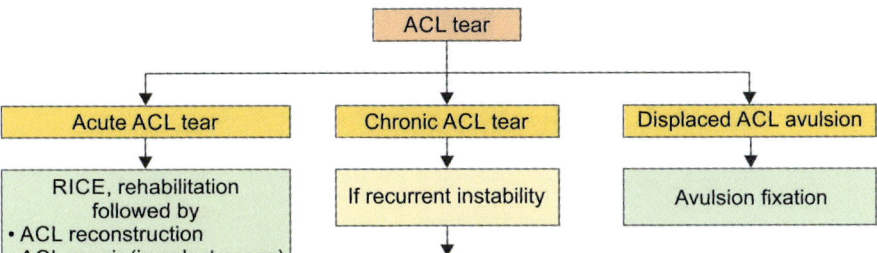

(ACL: anterior cruciate ligament; RICE: Rest, Ice, Compression, and Elevation)

POSTERIOR CRUCIATE LIGAMENT (PCL) TEAR

SURGICAL ANATOMY OF PCL

- PCL connects the tibia and femur at the knee joint. Proximally PCL is attached to the lateral wall of the medial femoral condyle, whereas distally, it is attached to the tibia posteriorly 1-1.5 cm below the tibial plateau in the midline **(Fig. 25.5)**.
- Anatomically, there are two bundles in PCL:
  1. **Anterolateral bundle:** It is *tight in knee flexion*
  2. **Posteromedial bundle:** It is *tight in the extended knee.*

FUNCTIONS OF PCL

- PCL prevents undue posterior translation of the tibia over the femur.
- It is also responsible for the screw home mechanism of the knee during full extension.

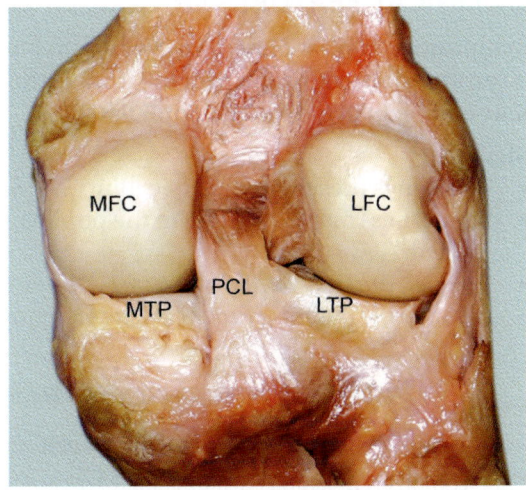

Fig. 25.5: Cadaveric image showing PCL (observed from back of the knee)

(*Courtesy:* Dr Charlie Brown, Abu Dhabi)

(PCL: posterior cruciate ligament; MFC: medial femoral condyle; LFC: lateral femoral condyle; MTP: medial tibial plateau; LTP: Lateral tibial plateau)

MECHANISM OF INJURY

- **Road traffic accident (RTA):** It is one of the most common mechanisms of injury of the PCL. The typical PCL injury is described to occur in '*dashboard injury*' resulting from a posteriorly directed force on the proximal tibia in a flexed knee **(Fig. 25.6)**.
- **Direct blow to the tibia from the front:** It is observed in after a direct fall over the knee in sports/RTA, wherein the patient lands over the front of the knee with knee flexed and foot plantarflexed.

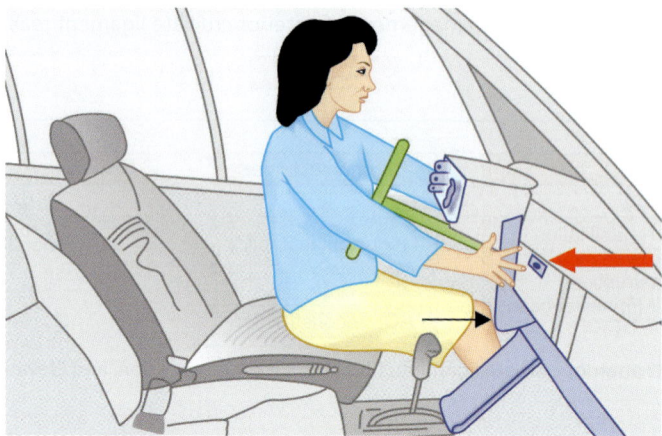

Fig. 25.6: Dashboard injury. Red arrow depicts the force of oncoming vehicle collision while black arrow depicts knee or leg hitting the dashboard.

◼ CLINICAL FEATURES OF ACUTE POSTERIOR CRUCIATE LIGAMENT TEAR

Symptoms: *Pain, swelling, and inability to bear weight* over injured extremity/walk. There may be an abrasion/contusion over the front of the knee in case of direct trauma to the knee. Patient may complain of pain in the popliteal fossa.

Signs
- Effusion is present in the knee joint.
- Tenderness may be present in the popliteal fossa. The range of motion (ROM) is painful and limited.
- *Sag sign and posterior drawer test are positive.*
- Always *rule out injury to the posterolateral corner* of the knee—**dial test**.

What is posterolateral corner (PLC) of the knee?

PLC comprises of lateral collateral ligament, popliteus tendon, popliteofibular ligament, fabellofibular ligament, iliotibial band, biceps femoris and posterior capsule. PLC *provides external rotation and varus stability to the knee.* **Dial test** *is performed to rule out PLC injury.*

◼ CLINICAL FEATURES OF CHRONIC POSTERIOR CRUCIATE LIGAMENT TEAR

Symptoms: A patient with chronic PCL tears *complains of instability, especially while descending stair/ramp.* The patient may also feel unstable while *lifting heavy weights above the head (weight lifter, manual worker)* as the perfect stable knee extension is difficult due to the abnormal screw home mechanism. They may also complain of pain due to degeneration of cartilage of medial knee compartment and patellofemoral joint.

Signs
- Wasting of the quadriceps muscle
- The *posterior drawer test, sag sign,* and *quadriceps active tests* are **positive**.

- The *reverse pivot shift test is positive* **if there is an** *associated posterolateral corner injury*. (*Note:* Reverse pivot shift test is positive only if PLC is injured).

INVESTIGATIONS

- **Plain X-ray of the knee:** AP and lateral view
  - To note avulsion fracture, malalignment
  - Lateral stress X-rays are often required to assess the grade of PCL injury
- **Magnetic resonance imaging of the knee:** *It is the diagnostic radiological investigation*. Further, it is also valuable for assessing concomitant meniscus, collaterals, and cartilage injuries.

TREATMENT

The treatment of PCL depends upon the duration of the tear and prevailing symptoms.
- **Acute PCL tear:** It is often managed *conservatively* with
  - *RICE:* **R**est, **I**ce application, **C**ompression, **E**levation
  - Analgesics, bracing: The knee is immobilized in PCL brace for 3–4 weeks.
  - Static quadriceps strengthening exercises
  - *Rehabilitation:* After 3–4 weeks, knee mobilization and further rehabilitation is initiated.
  - Once acute phase is over, **PCL reconstruction** can be offered in complete PCL tear, especially if patient is young and there are concomitant ligament, meniscal and cartilage lesions.

Does PCL tears heal spontaneously?

Immobilizing the knee in case of a PCL tear for a few weeks may result in spontaneous healing of PCL, unlike ACL, whose spontaneous natural healing after a complete tear is rare.

The quadriceps muscle is strengthened to minimize posterior subluxation of the tibia (c.f. ACL tear where hamstrings are strengthened more than quadriceps).

- **Chronic PCL tear**
  - *If symptomatic with recurrent instability*: Arthroscopic PCL reconstruction
  - *If asymptomatic/low demand patient*: Conservative.
- **Acute displaced PCL avulsion:** PCL avulsion fixation with screw/pull-out sutures.

MENISCAL INJURIES

SURGICAL ANATOMY

- There are two menisci: Medial and lateral. It has anterior and posterior horn, and body **(Fig. 25.7)**. The menisci are semilunar; lateral is more circular than medial. Structurally, they are composed of fibroelastic cartilage.
- *Mobility: Lateral meniscus is more mobile than the medial; hence, the lateral meniscus is less prone to tears.*
- *Vascularity: The periphery of the meniscus is quite vascular. The middle third is partially vascular and the inner third is avascular.* Based on vascularity, meniscus is divided into three zones (red-red, red-white, white-white) **(Fig. 25.8)**.

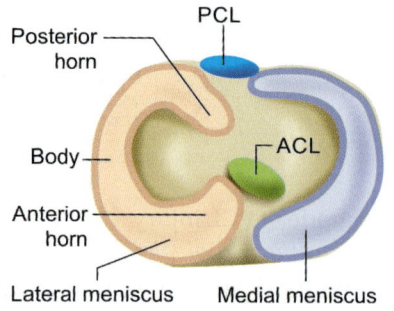

Fig. 25.7: Medial and lateral meniscus.
(ACL: anterior cruciate ligament; PCL: posterior cruciate ligament)

Practical application of meniscal vascular zones

The practical application of knowledge about meniscal zones is that the meniscal tears in vascular zones of meniscus (red-red, red-white) should be considered for repair, whereas meniscal tears in avascular areas (white-white) need excision as repair would not work in the absence of vascularity.

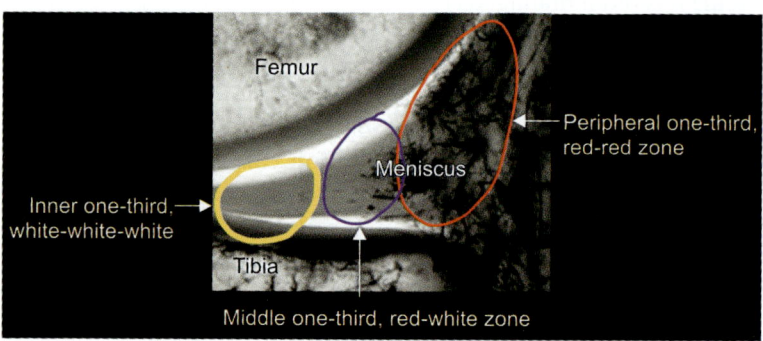

Fig. 25.8: Vascular zones of the meniscus.

FUNCTIONS OF MENISCUS

- Meniscus helps in **load transmission** from the femur to the tibia over a larger surface area avoiding point contact over the cartilage. Therefore, the *meniscus protects the cartilage of the knee joint during vertical loading activities* (walking, running, jumping, squatting). Thus, when the meniscus is completely torn or surgically removed, it renders the knee to premature secondary *osteoarthrosis* due to increased cartilage loading.
- It acts as a **shock absorber**. It also **enhances the knee joint congruity** by increasing the concavity of the tibial plateau, which enhances the joint's stability.
- It also helps in fluid film **lubrication** of the knee joint.

MECHANISM OF INJURY

The most common mechanism of injury is twisting force on a semi-flexed knee. It is common in sports where twisting, landing on a flexed knee, or jumping is involved (football, basketball or volleyball, badminton). It is quite common with ACL tears.
- Degenerative meniscal tears are common in old age where there may not be any history of trauma.

Note: The most common location of meniscal tear is posterior third.

CLINICAL FEATURES

Symptoms
- Constant or *recurrent mechanical pain* is the most common symptom, especially during activities, squatting/sitting cross leg. It may be associated with *recurrent swelling*.
- Occasionally, there can be a *click or locking*. The locking is commonly associated with the bucket handle type of meniscal tear.

Signs
- *Quadriceps wasting* is quite frequent.
- *Joint line tenderness* is often present (sensitive sign)
- *Limited range of motion:* Deep flexion may be limited and painful as the posterior third meniscus is commonly torn, which gets squeezed between femoral and tibial condyles during deep flexion.
- *McMurray's, Apley's grinding*, and *Thessaly test* are positive.

INVESTIGATIONS

- **Plain X-ray of knee:** It is usually normal.
- **Magnetic resonance imaging:** It is a *diagnostic investigation for a meniscal tear*. It helps detect the site and type of tears **(Box 25.1 and Fig. 25.9)**, which helps in planning treatment.
- **Diagnostic arthroscopy:** In case of strong clinical suspicion and inconclusive MRI, diagnostic arthroscopy may be required to confirm the diagnosis.

Box 25.1: Morphological type of tears on MRI and arthroscopy **(Fig. 25.9)**.

1. Longitudinal tear
2. Bucket handle tear
3. Radial tear
4. Horizontal tear: Horizontal split in body
5. Parrot beak
6. Complex tear: Combination of two or more types of tears

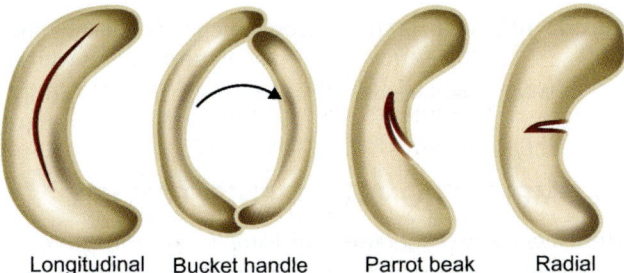

Longitudinal   Bucket handle   Parrot beak   Radial

Fig. 25.9: Morphological types of meniscal tears.

TREATMENT

The treatment of meniscal tear could vary from conservative to operative depending upon size, type and location of tear, symptoms, and failed conservative treatment.
- **Nonoperative:** In small, stable acute tears, or degenerative meniscal tears in older patients, conservative treatment is offered:
  - Analgesics, knee muscle strengthening exercises.
  - Avoid squatting and sitting cross leg as deep flexion is often painful and squats/cross leg sitting may aggravate symptoms of posterior third meniscal tears.
- **Operative:** In large, unstable tears or tears with recurrent locking, or ones with failed conservative treatment, operative treatment is offered. The tears can be managed by meniscal **R**epair/**R**esection (partial—also known as partial meniscectomy).

- *Tear in red-red/red-white zone:* **Arthroscopic repair** of the meniscus is performed **(Fig. 25.10)**.
- *Tear in white-white zone/complex degenerative/irreparable tears:* **Arthroscopic partial meniscectomy** is treatment of choice.
- *In the case of total meniscectomy in a young patient without any significant arthritis:* A **meniscal allograft replacement** (transplant) is a viable option.

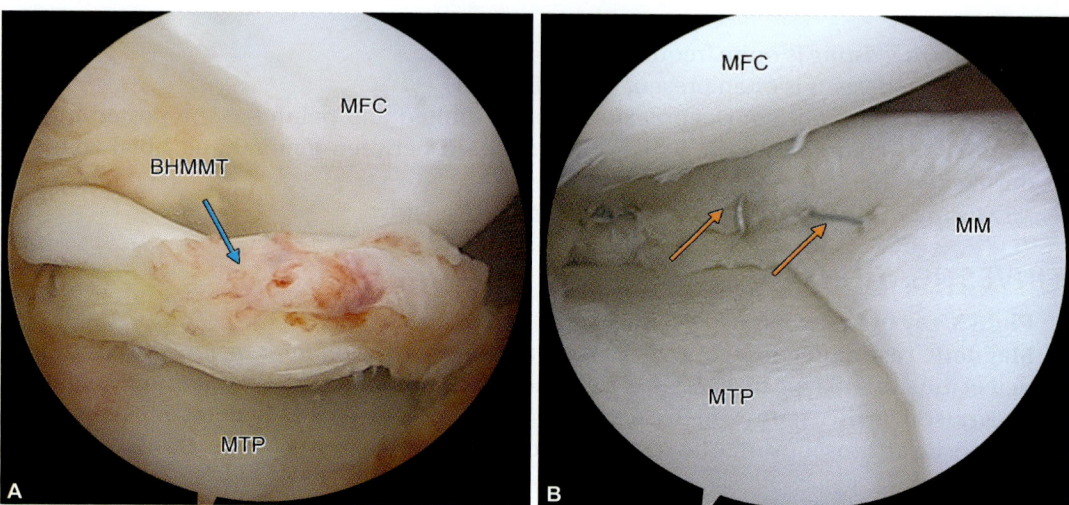

Figs. 25.10A and B: (A) Arthroscopic image of right knee showing bucket handle tear of medial meniscus (blue arrow); (B) Repair of the meniscus with sutures-in-situ (orange arrows).
(BHMMT: bucket handle medial meniscal tear; MFC: medial femoral condyle; MTP: medial tibial plateau; MM: medial meniscus)

COMPLICATIONS OF MENISCECTOMY

Meniscectomy, especially subtotal/total (complete), leads to increased stress concentration over the cartilage resulting in accelerated cartilage damage leading to *secondary osteoarthrosis* of the knee in the long-term.

COLLATERAL LIGAMENTS OF THE KNEE

SURGICAL ANATOMY

There are two collateral ligaments in the knee, medial and lateral. Their proximal and distal attachments are described below.
- **Medial collateral ligament (MCL)**
    - *Proximal attachment:* Medial femoral epicondyle
    - *Distal attachment:* Proximal medial tibia 60 mm below the medial knee joint line **(Fig. 25.11A)**.
- **Lateral collateral ligament (LCL)**
    - *Proximal attachment:* Lateral femoral epicondyle
    - *Distal attachment:* Fibular head **(Fig. 25.11B)**.

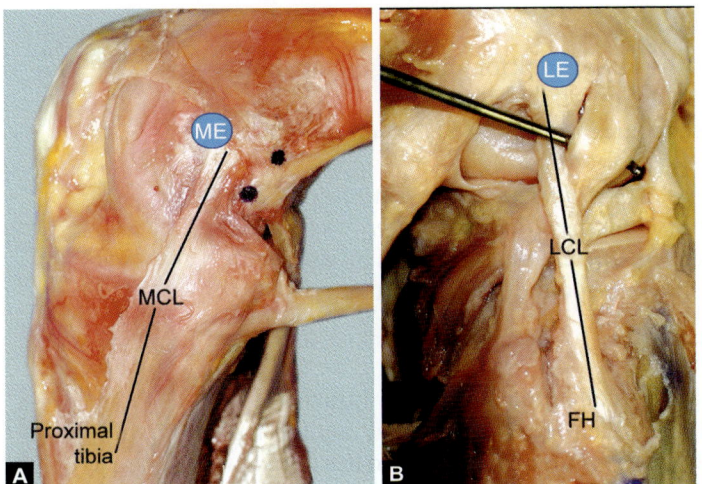

Figs. 25.11A and B: Cadaveric image showing medial collateral ligament (MCL) (A) and lateral collateral ligament (LCL) (B).
(ME: medial epicondyle; LE: lateral epicondyle; FH: fibular head)
(Courtesy: Dr Charlie Brown, Abu Dhabi)

FUNCTIONS

- **Medial collateral ligament:** It provides valgus stability to the knee
- **Lateral collateral ligament:** It provides varus stability to the knee.

MECHANISM OF INJURY

Collateral ligament injury is observed during **sports** or **RTA**. However, collaterals are often injured in combination with cruciate ligament(s) injury. Isolated, lower grade (I, II) injury to collaterals is seen in sports.

CLINICAL FEATURES

Symptoms
- Pain and swelling over the medial or lateral side of the knee *(depending upon MCL/LCL injury)*
- Inability/difficulty to bear weight.

Signs
- Tenderness is present over joint line/substance of collateral ligament or over the proximal/distal bony attachment points of collaterals over femur/tibia/fibula.
- Painful movement of the knee.
- Special tests should be performed to assess the integrity of the collaterals.
    ◆ *Medial collateral ligament:* Valgus stress test in 0° extension and 30° flexion
    ◆ *Lateral collateral ligament:* Varus stress test in 0° extension and 30° flexion.

Varus/valgus test is performed in 30° knee flexion to assess the integrity of the collateral ligament.

Varus/valgus test is performed in 0° knee extension to assess the integrity of knee capsule and cruciate ligaments.

INVESTIGATIONS

- **Plain X-ray of the knee**: Look for joint alignment, bony avulsions of the ligament.
- **Magnetic resonance imaging** *is the diagnostic investigation.*
  Note: *A chronic MCL injury near the femoral end can ossify, giving rise to a radiological sign—Pellegrini-Stieda disease* **(Fig. 25.12)**. *Such patients present with mild medial-side knee pain during activities.*

TREATMENT

All grades of 'acute collateral ligament' injuries are managed on RICE principles, bracing and analgesics. Specifics about the management according to the grade of collateral injury are mentioned below.

- ***Grades 1 and 2 isolated collateral ligament injury***
  - Immobilization in knee extension brace for 2–3 weeks, quadriceps strengthening followed by gradual mobilization in hinged brace **(Fig. 25.13)**.
    Note: *A hinged brace has metallic bars on either side of the knee, preventing excessive side-to-side knee movement while allowing flexion and extension. Untoward side-side movement result in healing of injured collateral ligament in stretched position, which may cause poor functional outcome.*
- ***Grade 3 collateral ligament injury***
  - Isolated grade 3 collateral ligament injury can be managed conservatively. However, femoral bony avulsions or tibial side avulsions may require surgical repair.
  - Repair/reconstruction of grade 3 collateral ligament injury may be required, especially there is an associated cruciate ligament injury.
- ***Chronic collateral ligament tears with instability***
  - Medial collateral ligament/lateral collateral ligament reconstruction with auto/allograft.

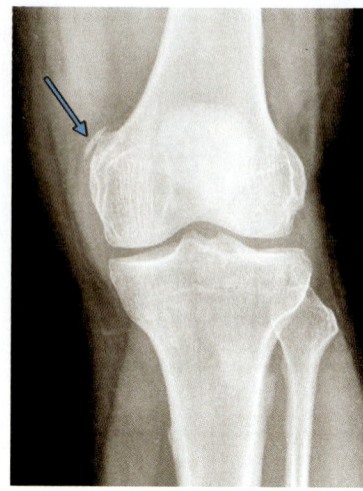

Fig. 25.12: Pellegrini-Stieda disease. Blue arrow shows ossification of MCL at femoral insertion site.

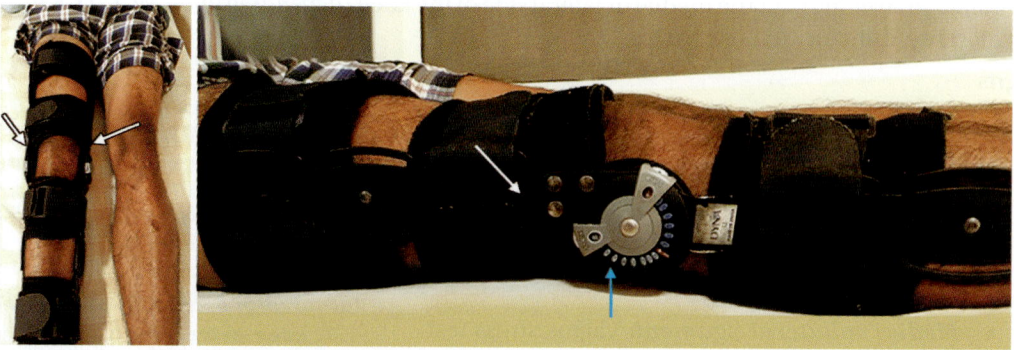

Fig. 25.13: Hinge knee brace. White arrows in right and left image indicate vertical bars on either side to prevent medial-lateral movement. The dial in right image (blue arrow) provides controlled flexion-extension.

ANKLE LIGAMENT INJURY/SPRAIN

SURGICAL ANATOMY OF ANKLE LIGAMENTS

Various ligaments on lateral and medial side of the knee along with syndesmotic ligaments stabilize the ankle.

Lateral Side Ligament

There are several important ligaments of the ankle to provide stability. The lateral ligament complex comprises ATFL, PTFL, and CFL **(Fig. 25.14)**.
- **Anterior talofibular ligament (ATFL)**
  - *It is the weakest among all the lateral ligaments, and is most frequently injured ligament in lateral ankle sprain.*
  - ATF resists "inversion in plantar flexion" and anterolateral translation of ankle.
- **Posterior talofibular ligament (PTFL)**
  - Strongest among lateral ligaments.
  - It resists posterior translation of the ankle.
- **Calcaneofibular ligament (CFL):** Resists inversion in neutral or dorsiflexion.

Medial Side Ligaments

There are two major medial side ligaments:
1. **Deltoid ligament**
2. **Calcaneonavicular ligament (spring ligament).**

Calcaneotalar Ligament

Interosseous talocalcaneal ligament, anterior and lateral talocalcaneal ligament.

Syndesmotic Ligaments (Anterior and Posterior)

Note: Injury to the syndesmotic ligaments is known as a *high ankle sprain*.

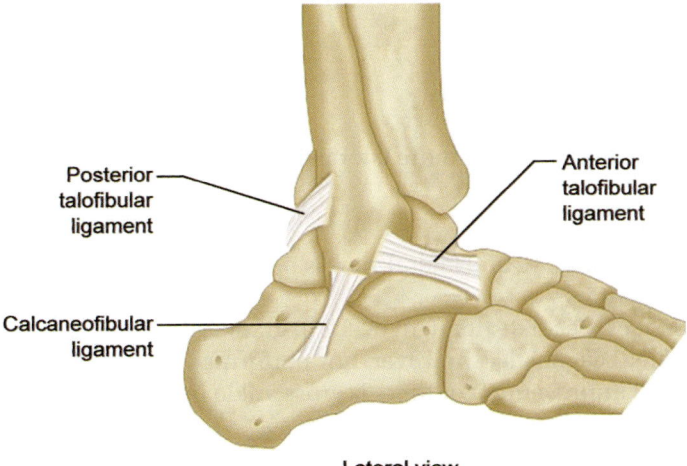

Fig. 25.14: Illustrative image showing lateral ankle ligaments.

MECHANISM OF INJURY

There are two mechanisms of ankle sprain, inversion and eversion.
1. **Inversion injury:** It is the most common type of ankle sprain injury, wherein the lateral ligament complex is injured. The *most commonly injured ligament is ATFL, as it is the weakest among all the lateral ligament complex.*
2. **Eversion injury:** It is a less common type of ankle sprain, wherein the medial ligament complex (deltoid) is injured.

CLINICAL FEATURES

Since lateral ankle sprain is far more clinically common than medial, this section will discuss only lateral ankle sprain.

Clinical Features of Lateral Ankle Sprain (due to Inversion Injury)

Symptoms
- History of *inversion twisting injury* of the ankle. There is *pain and swelling over the lateral aspect of the ankle* (**Fig. 25.15**).
- *Inability to bear weight/weight bearing* increases pain.

Signs
- *Tenderness over the lateral aspect of the ankle* (anterior, inferior, or posterior to the lateral malleolus according to ligament injured).
- *Plantar flexion and inversion are painful as* this maneuver stretches the injured ligaments on the lateral side.
- Bony tenderness may be present if there is an associated fracture of the lateral malleolus/base of the 5th metatarsal, which is occasionally fractured during an inversion injury to the ankle.

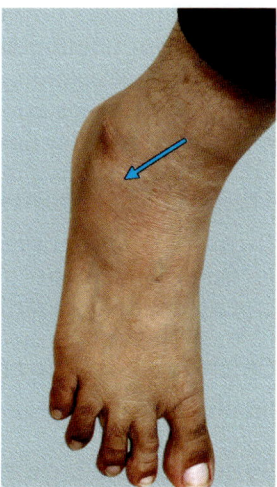

Fig. 25.15: Swelling over the lateral aspect of the ankle (blue arrow).

GRADE OF ANKLE SPRAIN

- **Grade 1:** Stretch of lateral ligaments
- **Grade 2:** Partial tear
- **Grade 3:** Complete tear of one or more lateral ligaments.

INVESTIGATIONS

- **Plain X-ray of the ankle:** AP and lateral view is performed to look for:
  - Associated fractures
  - Malalignment of the ankle: It might occur in grade 3 ligament injuries
- **MRI of the ankle:** Diagnostic—however, not performed routinely in ankle sprain unless there is no clinical improvement or there is gross ankle instability.

TREATMENT

Most ankle ligament injuries are managed conservatively. Acute injuries are managed with RICE, analgesics, and brace or below knee cast (**Figs. 25.16 and 25.17**) followed by rehabilitation.

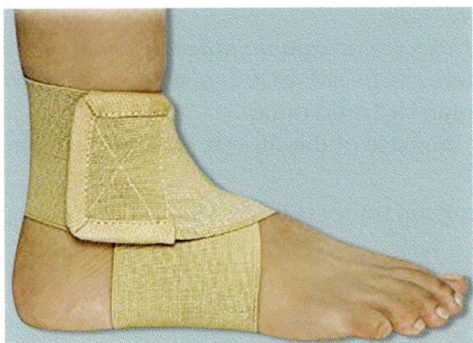

Fig. 25.16: Ankle binder.

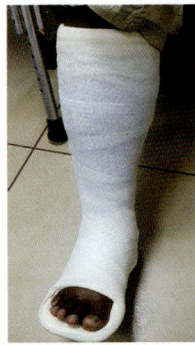

Fig. 25.17: Below knee cast.

Flowchart 25.2: Treatment algorithm of ankle ligament injury.

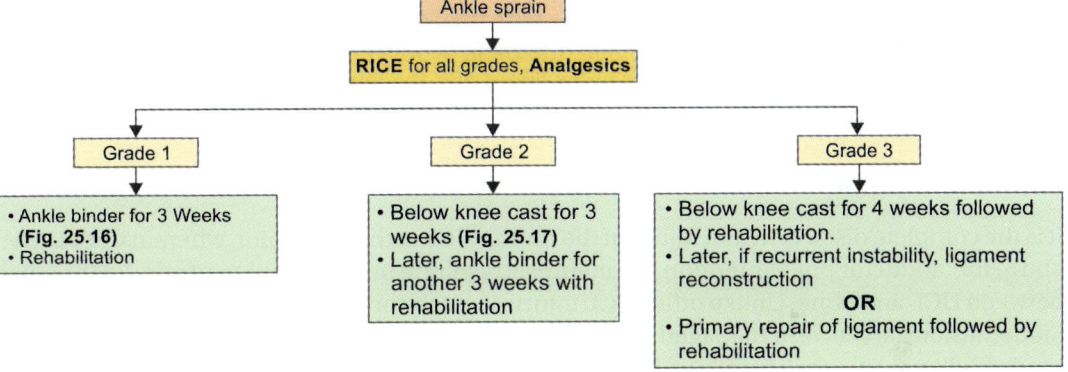

(RICE: Rest, Ice, Compression and Elevation)

However, acute grade 3 in an elite athlete or chronic, recurrent ankle instability may require surgical repair or reconstruction of the ligament (**Flowchart 25.2**).

COMPLICATIONS

- **Recurrent instability:** It may require surgery if rehabilitation fails
- *Persistent ankle edema*
- *Persistent* pain while weight bearing.

MISCELLANEOUS SPORTS INJURIES

GAMEKEEPER'S/SKIER'S THUMB

- Skier's/gamekeeper's thumb refer to injury to the ulnar collateral ligament (UCL) of the MCP joint of the thumb. Although both eponyms imply UCL injury, it is the mechanism of injury that determines the diagnostic terminology.

  Skier's thumb is an acute injury to the UCL while landing on a sking pole (or contact injuries while palying football), whereas gamekeeper's thumb is caused by chronic repetitive injury to the UCL.

- It is *one of the most common sports injury of thumb.*
- **Pathology:** *Injury to the thumb UCL at the metacarpophalangeal (MCP) joint due to hyperabduction or extension of thumb.* There can be Stener lesion, wherein addutor pollicis aponeurosis or tendon is interposed between UCL and bone.
- **Clinical features:** Pain and swelling over the base of the thumb. Patients also have valgus instability of the thumb **(Fig. 25.18)**.
- **Diagnosis:** X-ray help diagnosing bony avulsion injury **(Fig. 25.19)**. USG or MRI can detect ligamentous injury.
- **Treatment**
  - *Partial tear:* Cast immobilization
  - *Complete tear/Stener lesion:* Surgical repair.

Interesting fact about gamekeeper's thumb!

The term "gamekeeper's thumb" was first coined in 1955 by Campbell, who identified ulnar collateral ligament (UCL) injuries as an occupational disease in Scottish gamekeepers. The gamekeepers strangled rabbits using their thumb and index finger, and the repeated valgus stresses resulted in UCL injury and chronic instability of the metacarpophalangeal (MCP) joint.

Stener Lesion of Thumb

It is the complete distal avulsion injury of the thumb UCL at the MCP joint, wherein the UCL lies above the adductor pollicis tendon/aponeurosis resulting in interposition of adductor pollicis between UCL and bone. Unlike other UCL injuries, which can be managed conservatively also, Stener lesions are always managed operatively as interposed adductor pollicis aponeurosis/tendon will not allow spontaneous healing of the UCL to the proximal phalanx.

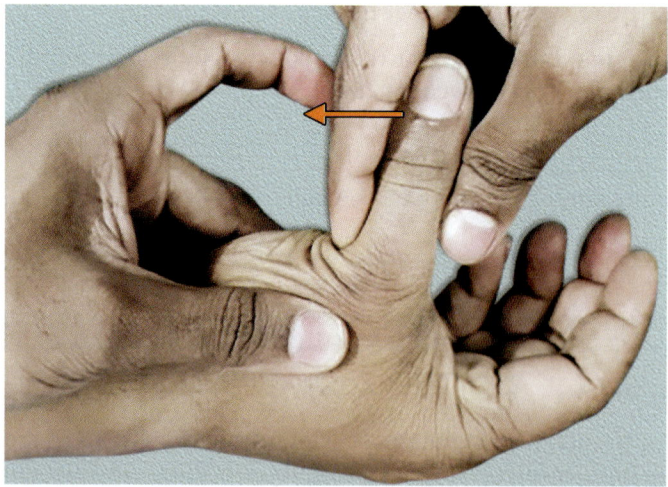

Fig. 25.18: Gamekeeper's thumb with ulnar collateral ligament injury. Orange arrow shows valgus stress resulting in abnormal opening of MCP joint on ulnar side.
(*Courtesy*: Dr Darshan Jain)

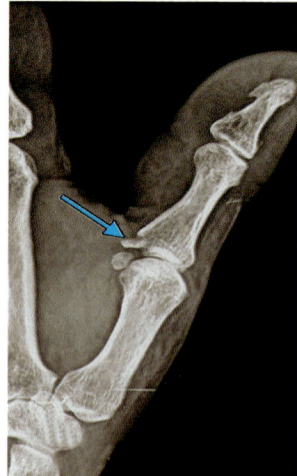

Fig. 25.19: Avulsion injury of ulnar collateral ligament (arrow).
(*Courtesy:* Dr Darshan Jain)

BOWLER'S THUMB

It is a *neuroma of ulnar digital nerve of thumb*. It is observed in spinners who hold the ball between thumb and fingers resulting in perineural fibrosis of ulnar digital nerve **(Fig. 25.20)**.

MALLET FINGER

- **Definition:** It is a *rupture/avulsion injury of the extensor digitorum tendon from the base of the distal phalanx* resulting in flexion deformity of the distal interphalangeal (DIP) joint **(Fig. 25.21)**.
- It is the most common hand tendon injury in sports persons.
- **Mechanism:** Sudden violent flexion of DIP under axial load results in mallet finger.
- **Clinical features:** Pain and swelling at the DIP of the finger. Patient complains of inability to dorsiflex the DIP joint. There is flexion deformity at DIP joint.
- **Diagnosis:** X-ray can reveal bony avulsion **(Fig. 25.22)**. USG/MRI is required for soft tissue avulsion.

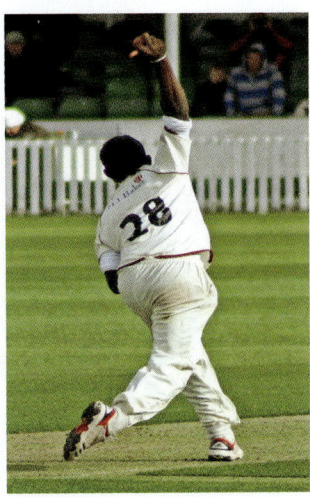

Fig. 25.20: Bowler's thumb-perineural fibrosis in ulnar digital nerve of thumb.
(*Source:* Wikimedia Commons)

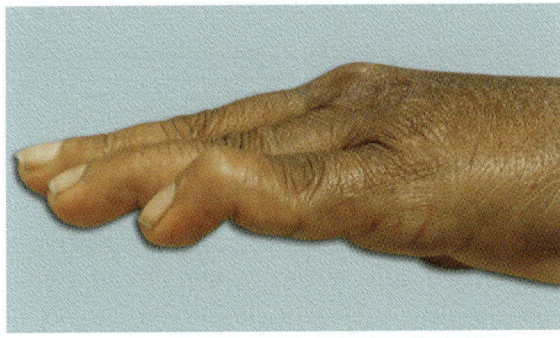

Fig. 25.21: Mallet finger (little finger DIP).

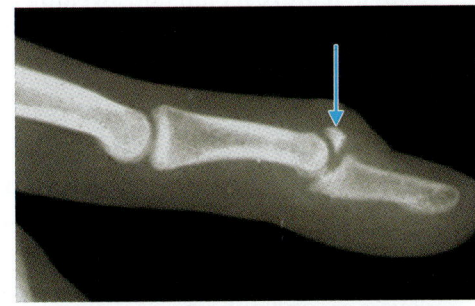

Fig. 25.22: Bony avulsion of extensor digitorum tendon from base of distal phalanx.

- **Treatment**
    - *Undisplaced or minimally displaced bony avulsion:* Mallet finger splint **(Fig. 25. 23)**.
    - *Displaced injury:* Surgical repair.

JERSEY FINGER

- **Definition:** It is a *rupture/avulsion injury of flexor digitorum profundus from the base of the distal phalanx*, resuting in inability to flex the DIP joint **(Fig. 25.24)**.
- Most commonly, ring finger is involved.

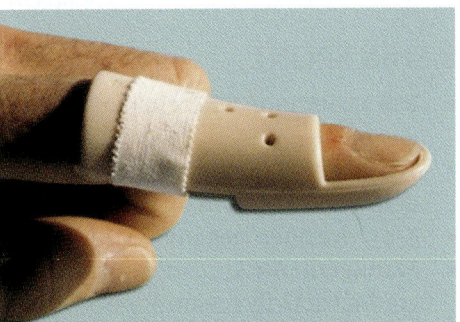

Fig. 25.23: Mallet finger splint.

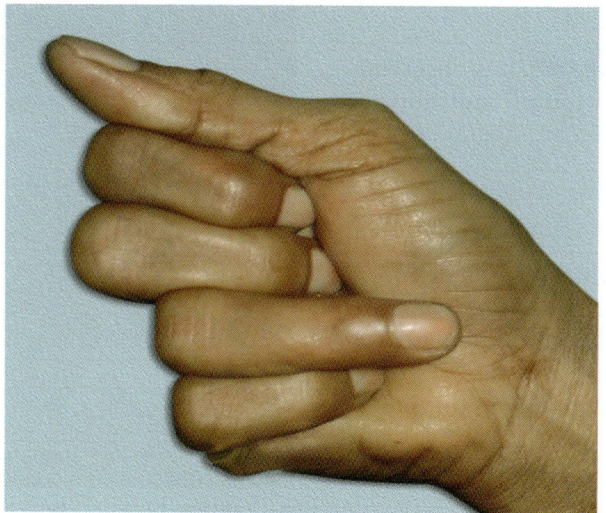

Fig. 25.24: Jersey ring finger.
(Courtesy: Professor Ashwath Acharya, KMC, Manipal)

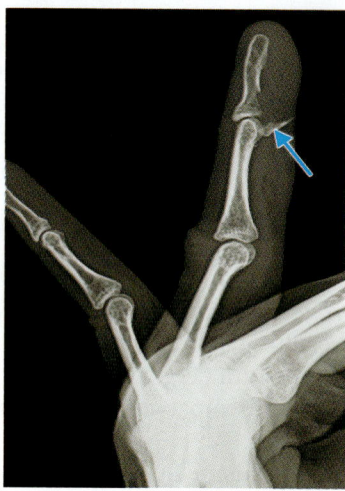

Fig. 25.25: Avulsion of base of distal phalanx in Jersey finger (arrow).
(Courtesy: Dr Darshan Jain, Consultant Hand Surgeon, Bengaluru)

- **Mechanism:** It occurs due to sudden violent hyperextension of DIP under axial load.
- **Clinical features:** Pain and swelling near the DIP and inability to palmarflex the DIP joint.
- **Diagnosis:** X-ray **(Fig. 25.25)**, MRI/USG.
- **Treatment**
    - *Undisplaced:* Splinting
    - *Displaced:* Surgical repair.

LITTLE LEAGUER'S/BASEBALL PITCHER'S ELBOW, LITTLE LEAGUER'S SHOULDER, JAVELIN THROWERS' ELBOW

- **Little Leaguer's/baseball pitcher's elbow:** Medial epicondylar apophysitis in young players around puberty.
- **Little Leaguer's shoulder:** Salter Harris type I injury in children in shoulder.
- **Javelin thrower's elbow:** Painful elbow in javelin thrower either due to ulnar collateral ligament (UCL) tendinitis/triceps insertion tendinitis.

SHIN SPLINT

- It is a condition wherein patient complains of *pain in the legs after unaccustomed running/jogging*.
- Tenderness is felt in posteromedial aspect of lower part of shin due to either **stress fracture of lower third tibia or tendinitis of tibialis posterior/soleus.**
- X-ray are often negative. MRI/bone scan may help in confirming the diagnosis.
- **Management:** Conservative—rest, ice, analgesics. Gradual muscle strengthening and gradual activity resumption.

JUMPER'S KNEE

- Jumper's knee is *patellar tendon tendonitis at the lower pole of the patella.*
- Observed in runners and jumpers
- Diagnosis is established by MRI **(Fig. 25.26)**
- Most cases respond to conservative treatment. Some may require arthroscopic debridement.

IT BAND FRICTION SYNDROME

- IT band friction near lateral epicondyle (LE) of femur due to tight IT band/weak hip abductors.
- Observed in *long distance runners.*
- Pain is felt just above lateral joint line of femur, which increases while patient extends his knee and examiner presses the IT band against LE.

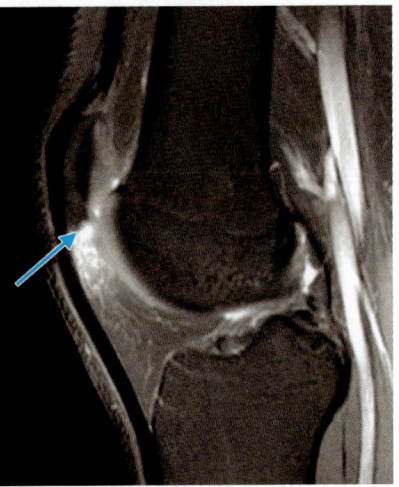

Fig. 25.26: MRI of the knee showing patellar tendinitis (blue arrow).

HAMSTRING STRAIN

- It is the *most common injury in professional footballers.*
- It occurs due to high speed running and muscle overstretch.
- It may occur near distal attachment over fibula head (biceps femoris) or close to ischial tuberosity (semimembranosus).

TENNIS LEG

Tear of medial head of gastrocnemius at the junction of muscle belly and aponeurosis.

DANCER'S TENDINITIS

Tendinitis of flexor hallucis longus in ballet dancer.

TURF TOE

Pain over *1st MTP joint due to hyperextension injury* in American footballers, especially while playing on artificial turf.

HOFFA SYNDROME

Inflammation of infrapatellar fad pad.

CHRONIC EXERTIONAL COMPARTMENT SYNDROME

- Exercise induced compartment syndrome in the leg.
- Pain in leg which increases with exercise and diminishes with rest.

ATHLETIC PUBALGIA/GILMORE GROIN/SPORTS HERNIA

Exertional pain in groin where rectus abdominis inserts over pubic bone.

Notes

# SECTION 3

Musculoskeletal Infection

SECTION OUTLINE

26. Osteomyelitis
27. Septic Arthritis
28. HIV Infections and Orthopaedics
29. Spirochetal Infection of Bones and Joints

Musculoskeletal Infection

CHAPTER 26

Osteomyelitis

OSTEOMYELITIS

■ DEFINITION
Osteomyelitis is defined as an infection of bone and bone marrow.

■ CLASSIFICATION
The osteomyelitis has been classified based on *route of spread, etiology, duration of infection, and Cierny Mader classification* (based on anatomic location of infection and host response).
- **Route of spread**
    - *Direct*: The bone gets infected due to direct inoculation of bacteria due to open injuries/adjacent infective foci, e.g., open fracture resulting in *osteomyelitis, osteomyelitis* of mastoid due to chronic suppurative otitis media, Garre's osteomyelitis due to dental caries.
    - *Indirect/hematogenous:* The infection reaches bone hematogenously with primary foci elsewhere, e.g., primary focus of infection could be in the tonsils/gastrointestinal tract.
- **Etiological type of infection**
    - Pyogenic
    - Tubercular
    - Fungal.
- **Duration of infection**
    - *Acute*: Less than 6 weeks
    - *Primary subacute*: Within 6–12 weeks
        - Brodie's abscess
        - Sclerosing osteomyelitis of Garre's
    - *Chronic*: Greater than 12 weeks.
- **Cierny-Mader classification**: It is based on the anatomic location of infection and host response.

■ PREDISPOSING FACTORS
- ***Infants and children are more prone to bone infection than adults***: Probably due to lesser immunity
- ***Boys are more prone than girls (4:1)*** probably because boys are more prone to trauma
- ***Poor nourishment*** may result in poor immunity
- ***Poor host response*** due to underlying immunosuppresion

- **Sickle cell anemia:** It results in bony infarcts and a microaerophilic environment, which promotes the growth of bacteria. *Salmonella osteomyelitis* is common in Sickle cell anemia.
- Trauma to the metaphysis.

ACUTE BACTERIAL (PYOGENIC) OSTEOMYELITIS

Rutherford–Morrison aphorism (1935)
Atraumatic pain and swelling at the end of a long bone (metaphysis) in a child should be taken as acute osteomyelitis unless proved otherwise!

ETIOLOGY

The common bacteria that cause acute pyogenic osteomyelitis (OM) are:
- ***Staphylococcus aureus:*** *Most common organism* to cause pyogenic OM
- ***Streptococcus pyogenes***
- ***Pneumococci***
- ***Haemophilus:*** Affects children between the age group of 6 months to 6 years
- ***Pseudomonas aeruginosa:*** In IV drug abusers, immunocompromised individuals
- ***Salmonella:*** Multifocal OM, patients with sickle cell anemia
- ***Brucella abortus/suis:*** Due to drinking unpasteurized milk/in direct contact with infected bovine/pig. *Typically, Brucella osteomyelitis causes vertebral osteomyelitis and mimics Pott's spine.*

PATHOGENESIS OF ACUTE HEMATOGENOUS PYOGENIC OSTEOMYELITIS

The most common site for hematogenous osteomyelitis in a long bone is **metaphysis**. Once there is bacterial inoculation in metaphysis, there are *three stages* in the development of pyogenic osteomyelitis.
1. Stage of intramedullary abscess
2. Stage of subperiosteal abscess formation
3. Stage of sequestration and involucrum.

- **Stage of intramedullary intraosseous abscess (Figs. 26.1A to D):** Once bacteremia reaches the bone, the bacteria tend to settle down in the metaphyseal region of the bone due to several reasons:
    - *Hairpin loop structure of the "metaphyseal capillaries":* Hairpin configuration results in blood stagnation and consequent bacterial proliferation.
    - *Rapid growth in metaphysis* leads to discontinuous endothelium at the tip of vessels facilitating the passage of bacteria into the bone during bacteremia.
    - *The metaphysis is metabolically more active* resulting in *high-cell turnover with more cell debris* available for bacterial activity.
    - *Relative lack of phagocytes in the metaphysis* renders easy multiplication of bacteria.

Therefore, local bacterial stagnation, favorable environment, and multiplication results in acute response from the host defense system leading to widespread destruction of bacterial and host cells and a consequent intramedullary abscess formation.

Chapter 26: Osteomyelitis

Note

Fate of intramedullary abscess with respect to growth plate (physis) in various age groups

In infants, there are vascular connections between metaphysis and physis. Therefore, the metaphyseal pus can reach the epiphysis and further into the joint.
In children, the pus cannot reach the epiphysis and joint as the physis is quite thick to be penetrated, and the vascular channels (of infant-hood) between the epiphysis and metaphysis close.
In adults, the pus can enter the epiphysis and joint as the physeal plate thins out after the completion of the growth.

- **Stage of subperiosteal abscess formation (Figs. 26.2A and B):** Once the intramedullary abscess is formed, it usually spreads toward the adjacent metaphyseal cortex resulting in cortical necrosis due to:
    - *Pressure over the cortex* **(Figs. 26.1C and D)**
    - *Thrombosis of the medullary and periosteal vessels* jeopardizes the cortical blood supply.

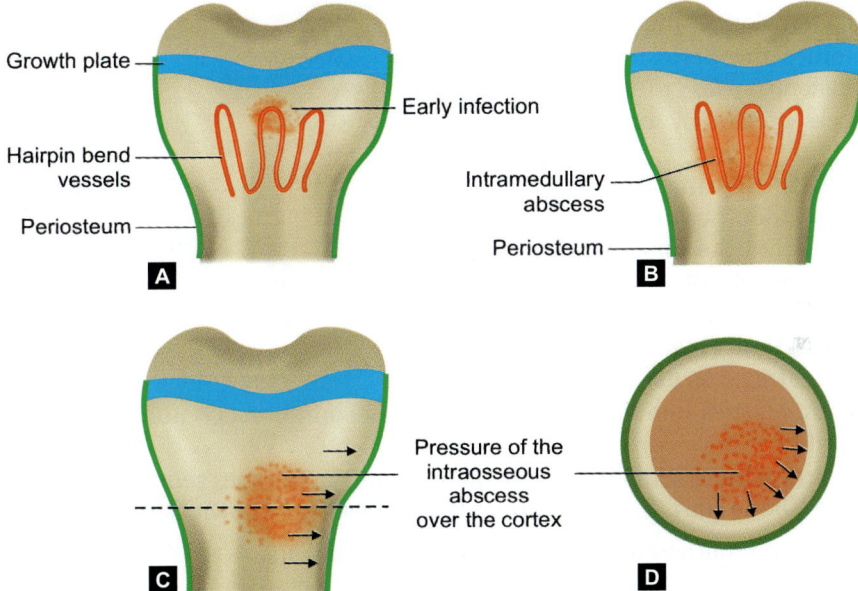

Figs. 26.1A to D: Stage of intraosseous abscess.

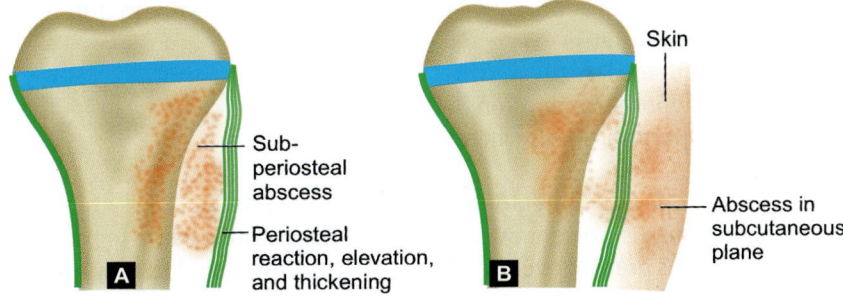

Figs. 26.2A and B: Stage of subperiosteal abscess.

Possible route of metaphyseal intraosseous abscess spread
- Subperiosteal, and then to the soft tissues
- Into the growth plate
- Into the diaphysis
- Into the joint (septic arthritis)

Septic arthritis following metaphyseal osteomyelitis is common in areas where there is 'intracapsular metaphysis'. Once the subperiosteal abscess bursts outside the 'intracapsular metaphysis, the abscess directly opens into the joint.

Location of intra-articular metaphysis:
- Proximal humerus
- Radial head
- Neck femur

Once there is cortical necrosis and erosion, the abscess underlies the periosteum. The periosteum tries to limit the abscess spread by undergoing elevation and thickening **(Fig. 26.2A)**. Further, the abscess erodes the periosteum and escapes into the subcutaneous plane **(Fig. 26.2B)**.

- **Stage of sequestration and sinus formation (Fig. 26.3):** The subperiosteal abscess perforates the periosteum, reaches into the subcutaneous plane, and bursts onto the skin surface via a sinus. Further
  - The cortical bone with inadequate blood supply undergoes sequestration.
  - The new bone starts forming around the sequestrum, known as the involucrum.

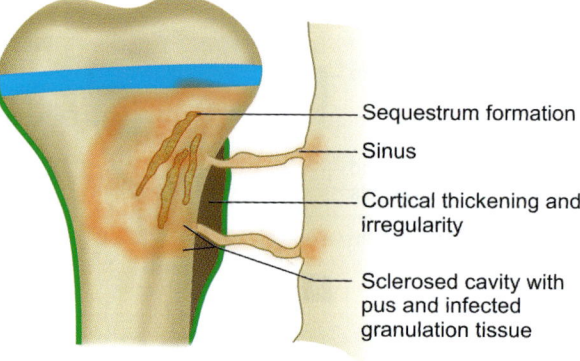

Fig. 26.3: Stage of sequestration and sinus formation.

Flowchart 26.1 summarizes the pathogenesis of osteomyelitis.

CLINICAL FEATURES OF ACUTE OSTEOMYELITIS

The clinical features of acute pyogenic osteomyelitis may vary in different age groups.
- **Neonates and infants**
  - Refusal to feed, restless
  - Fever/hypothermia; often dehydrated
  - Pseudoparalysis of the affected limb.
- **Children**
  - *High-grade fever,* often dehydrated, loss of appetite
  - *Severe pain* is present over the affected part, and unable to move the affected part
  - *Swelling* is present over the affected region, and the skin may have signs of inflammation
  - *Bony tenderness* is present over the metaphyseal area

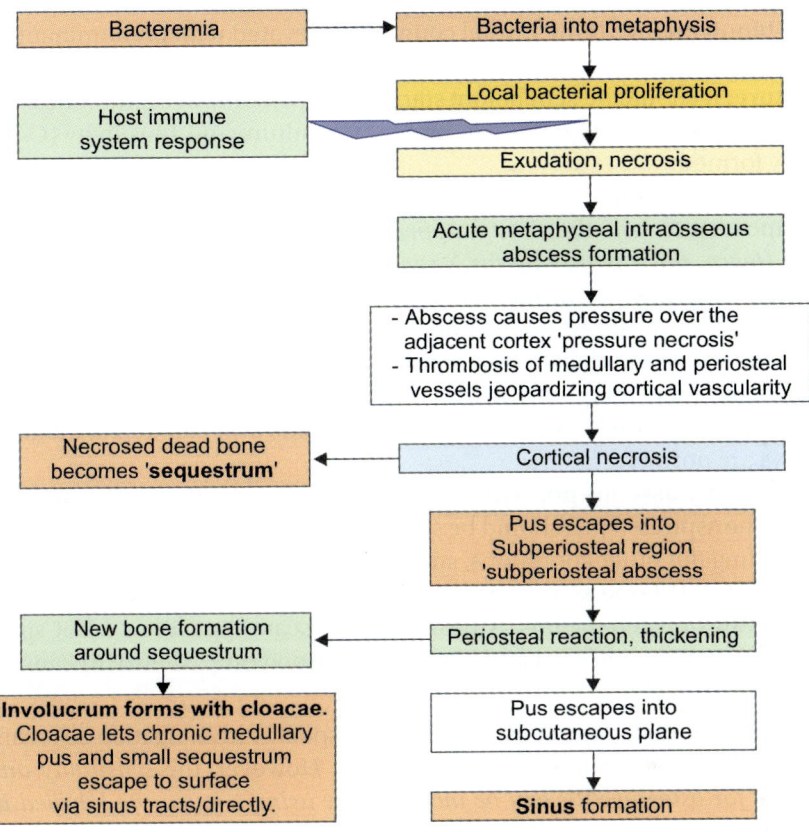

Flowchart 26.1: Pathogenesis of osteomyelitis.

- Due to pain, movements at the joint are severely restricted, which is known as *pseudoparalysis*.
- **Adults**
    - Fever
    - Pain, swelling, and bony tenderness over the metaphyseal area of the bone
    - Painful range of movement.

DIFFERENTIAL DIAGNOSIS

Amidst all differential diagnoses, one must always keep *Ewing sarcoma* in mind, especially in children, as the clinical features are quite similar.
- **Ewing's sarcoma:** Although clinical and radiological features may be similar, Ewing's sarcoma is characterized by diaphyseal involvement of the bone, whereas osteomyelitis is more common in the metaphysis. *The biopsy clinches the diagnosis.*
- **Septic arthritis:** Joint movements are excruciating in septic arthritis, whereas joint movements are painless (albeit less due to adjacent muscle spasm) osteomyelitis. *Presence of pus in joint aspirate clinches the diagnosis.* Note that both osteomyelitis and septic arthritis can co-exist as one can result in either.
- **Scurvy:** It is characterized by multiple areas of swelling and tenderness over many bones due to widespread subperiosteal bleeding.

INVESTIGATIONS

- **Complete blood picture (CBP):** Total counts are elevated with predominant neutrophilia.
- **CRP** is significantly elevated. **ESR** elevated. **Procalcitonin** >0.5 ng%.
- **Blood culture:** It should be sent before starting the presumptive antibiotics.
- **Culture from sinus opening:** Pus can be sent for culture and sensitivity (C/S) if the sinus has already formed.
- **X-ray of the affected bone**
    - It is important to note that *X-rays appear normal till 10–14 days in acute osteomyelitis (OM). Hence, there is no role for X-rays during that period in diagnosing acute OM.* However, it is always performed to rule out any other condition.
    - *After 2–3 weeks,* localized rarefaction, lytic/cavitary lesion in the metaphyseal area, or periosteal reaction in the affected area is often noted **(Figs. 26.4A and B)**.
- **Magnetic resonance imaging (MRI) (Fig. 26.5):** It is the *most sensitive and specific investigation* to diagnose acute pyogenic osteomyelitis as it can detect medullary abscess, while X-rays are normal.
- **Aspiration of intraosseous pus with wide bore needle:** It is the *confirmatory investigation* **(Fig. 26.6)**. The aspirated pus should be sent for Gram stain and culture/sensitivity (C/S). It also helps ruling out other conditions, such as tumor.
- **Technetium (Tc99) bone scan:** It is useful when X-rays appear normal or in the case of multifocal cases of osteomyelitis. A positive bone scan appears as a hot spot. Currently, MRI is preferred over bone scan and latter is performed only when MRI cannot be done or in case of multifocal OM.

Note that the Tc99 bone scan is a sensitive but not a specific investigation as it can be positive (hot spot) in acute trauma, tumors, and infections. However, the *sensitivity and specificity of the bone scan for osteomyelitis can be increased by using a leucocyte-labelled Indium-111/Gallium scan.*

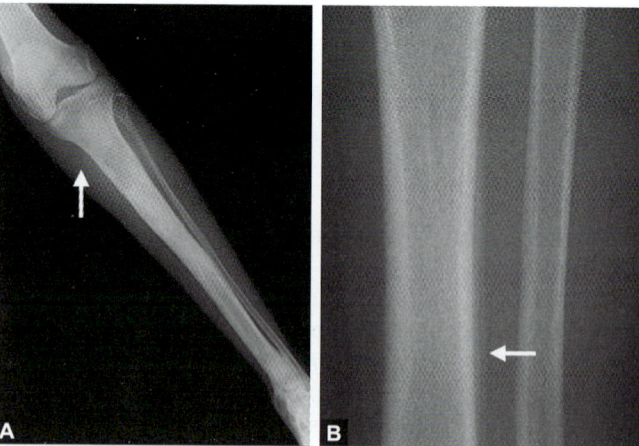
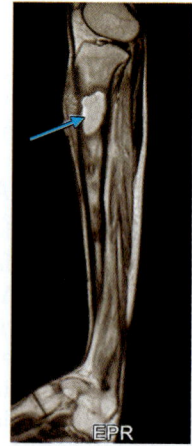

Figs. 26.4A and B: (A) X-ray shows the lytic area in the proximal tibial metaphysis (white arrow); (B) Periosteal reaction (white arrow).

Fig. 26.5: MRI of the tibia shows intramedullary abscess (blue arrow).

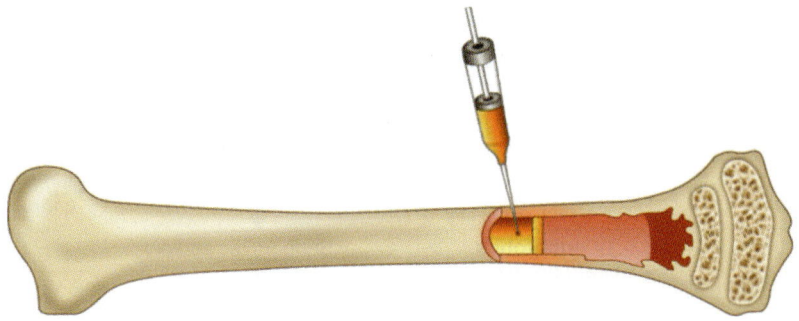

Fig. 26.6: Illustrative image of wide bore needle aspiration of pus from metaphysis.

TREATMENT

The treatment of acute osteomyelitis depends upon the time of clinical presentation (within or after 48–72 hours). An acute OM of *duration lesser than 48–72 hours can be managed conservatively* with antibiotics and other supportive measures, whereas *duration later than 72 hours often requires additional surgical intervention.*

A. **Clinical presentation within 48–72 hours:** Initiate medical treatment and watch for improvement in clinical and serological parameters (decreasing CRP). Surgical treatment is to be added if there is *no* improvement in clinical signs and serological parameters for several days despite the adequate medical treatment.
B. **Clinical presentation after 48–72 hours:** These patients respond best to surgical treatment followed by medical treatment, as a full-fledged abscess in the medullary cavity is hard to treat with mere antibiotics.

Flowchart 26.2 illustrates the treatment of chronic osteomyelitis.

- *General supportive treatment:* Start with all the patients
    - *Analgesics:* For pain relief
    - *Antipyretics and anti-inflammatory medications*
    - *Edema control:* Limb elevation and magnesium sulfate dressings
    - *Intravenous (IV) fluids:* To treat dehydration
    - *Tractions/splint:* To prevent deformity and contractures developing at joints due to pain and spasm.
- *Medical treatment:* The patient is started on broad-spectrum IV antibiotics covering gram-positive and gram-negative microbes, e.g., [flucloxacillin + 3rd gen cephalosporin (ceftriaxone)/aminoglycosides (gentamicin)] or [vancomycin + cefepime] OR [linezolid + cefepime].
  Once the culture sensitivity of the pus is available, specific antibiotics are started.
  Duration of antibiotics: 2–3 weeks of IV antibiotic + 4–6 weeks of oral antibiotic.
  If the patient's clinical features improve, the antibiotic is continued for the above-said duration. However, surgical treatment is opted for if there is no improvement or worsening in clinical features or serological parameters (CRP, blood counts).
- *Surgical treatment:* The typical indications are:
    - No clinical improvement/worsening in symptoms after the IV antibiotics has been administered for 3–4 days.
    - Patient presents after 48–72 hours of the onset of clinical symptoms, as a well-formed intramedullary abscess does not respond to IV antibiotics alone.

Section 3: Musculoskeletal Infection

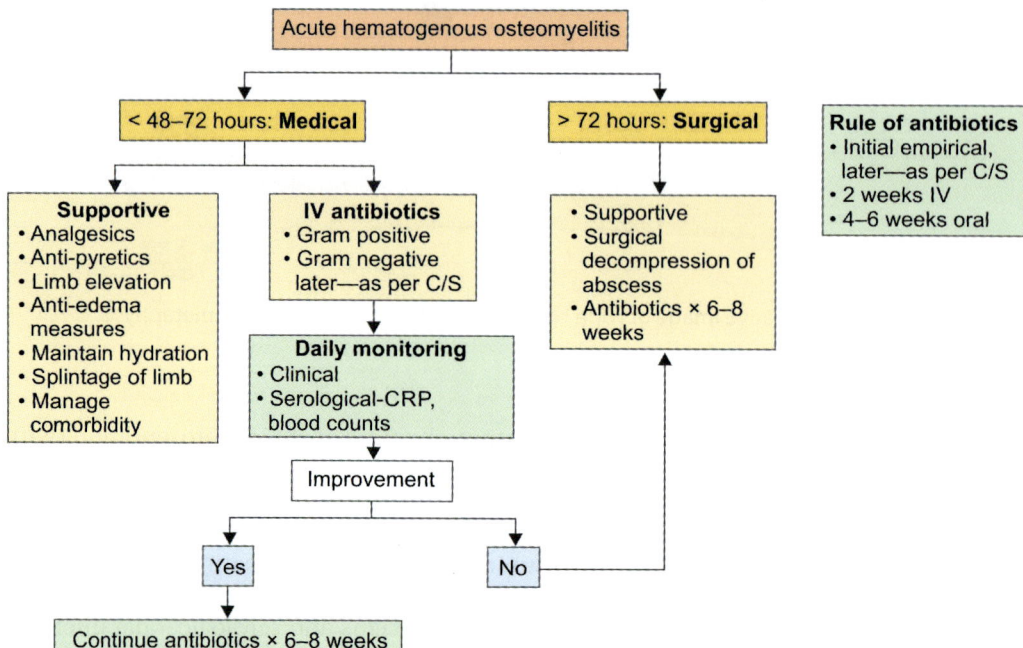

Flowchart 26.2: Treatment algorithm of acute osteomyelitis.

(C/S: culture and sensitivity; IV: intravenous; CRP: C-reactive protein)

The typical surgical steps involve:
- "Opening of the cortical window" in the cortex allows the drainage of the intramedullary pus **(Figs. 26.7A and B)**. The cavity is then curetted and washed with 3–4 liters of normal saline.
- Further, the cavity can be filled with antibiotic-laden bone cement beads for the local release of antibiotics. The preferred antibiotics are vancomycin or gentamicin as they are heat stable. Note that *bone cement preparation is a exothermic reaction, which can damage non-heat stable antibiotics*. The beads are removed after 6–8 weeks *(for types of antibiotic beads, refer page 253)*.
- The IV and oral antibiotic treatment are continued for 6–8 weeks.

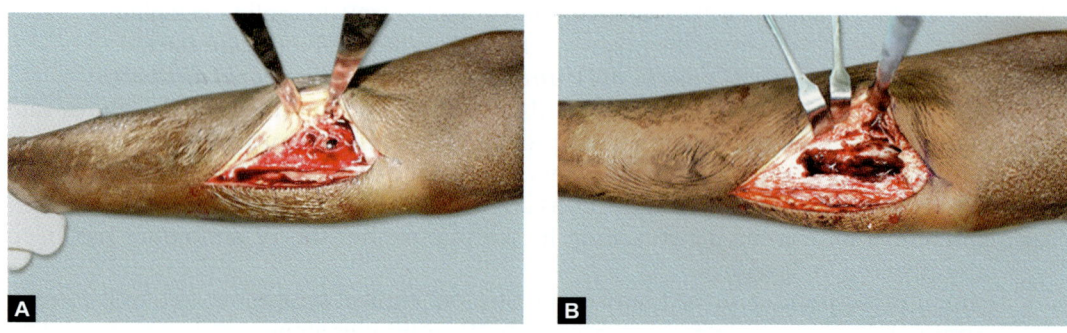

Figs. 26.7A and B: (A) Perforated cortex with pus in the vicinity; (B) Cortical window in the metaphysis.

COMPLICATIONS OF ACUTE PYOGENIC OSTEOMYELITIS

- **Chronic osteomyelitis:** It is the most common complication, which occurs due to inadequate treatment or poor response to the treatment due to various patient-related factors.
- **Growth plate damage** in children (with open physis) results in *limb deformity* and *leg length discrepancy* (shortening, or rarely lengthening).
- **Septicemia** is more common in acute osteomyelitis than chronic as there is no sclerosis around the infected cavity in former, which can limit the spread of the bacteria (and infection) in the blood circulation.
- **Pathological fracture** can occur if the underlying bone is weak due to extensive sequestration and inadequate involucrum formation. It can also occur after surgery due to cortical window resulting in decreased bone strength.
- **Septic arthritis** is more common in infants with osteomyelitis or when osteomyelitis occurs in 'intra-articular metaphyses', such as the proximal humerus, radial head, and neck femur. In latter cases, the ruptured metaphyseal abscess over the bone surface directly opens in the joint.

CHRONIC OSTEOMYELITIS

DEFINITION

Chronic osteomyelitis is a *persistent bone and bone marrow infection* characterized by a sclerosed infected cavity with the sequestrum, involucrum, with or without a discharging sinus.

PREDISPOSING FACTORS

Various causes of chronicity of osteomyelitis are listed below:
- **Untreated/inadequately treated acute osteomyelitis**—results in sclerosed avascular cavity with sequestrum
- **Compromised host defences:** Old age, debilitated patients, diabetes, malnutrition
- **Poor local vascularity:** Periosteal stripping during infection, or open fractures result in loss of soft tissue cover and blood supply of the bone.
- **Bacteria covered in glycocalyx (Biofilm formation):** Typically, it is observed in cases where an implant is in situ (nail/plate) over the bone. The bacteria secrete the glycocalyx layer (biofilm) covering the implant. The biofilm is relatively impermeable to antibiotics and immune cells. Therefore, the bacteria can thrive within the glycocalyx layer, making eradication of infection quite tricky unless the implant is removed.

Why does osteomyelitis become chronic and prevent recurrence after surgical treatment?

- Bacteria survive intracellularly in the osteoblasts
- Bacteria undergo phenotypic alteration in the osteoblast which renders it more resistant to antimicrobials
- Potential protective proteolytic activity is inhibited in the presence of infection
- Bacterial adherence to collagen
- Dead bone (sequestrum) cannot be resorbed
- Rigid bony cavities cannot collapse
- In case of in-situ metal implant, an impregnable biofilm over the implant protects bacteria by resisting antibiotic and immune cell penetration

PATHOPHYSIOLOGY OF CHRONIC HEMATOGENOUS OSTEOMYELITIS

Chronic medullary infection leads to thrombosis of intramedullary blood vessels, while periosteal stripping results in loss of blood supply to the cortex leading to devitalization and destruction of the bone. The devitalised-dead cortical bone separates from normal bones, known as *'sequestrum,'* surrounded by pus and infected granulation tissue. *The sequestrum acts as a substrate for bacterial adhesion and ensures persistent infection.* Due to persistent infection, the purulent material and smaller pieces of sequestrum get discharged to the skin surface via *'sinus tract formation.'* The sinus seals off for a few weeks-months to open later, sometime again. In response to the loss of cortical bone as sequestrum, the bone's healing response results in a *reactive periosteal new bone formation around the sequestrum known as 'involucrum.'* The presence of the involucrum provides strength to the weakened bone as there is a loss of cortical bony support during sequestration of the bone. The involucrum has small fenestrations, known as **cloacae** to let the pus and sequestrum get discharged on the surface directly or via the sinus tract. The infected medullary cavity area in the bone becomes heavily sclerosed to shield the infected cavity from the normal bone. This sclerosis cuts off or diminishes the blood supply to the cavity, resulting in persistent infection.

Flowchart 26.3 summarizes the pathology of chronic osteomyelitis.

Flowchart 26.3: Pathogenesis of chronic osteomyelitis.

```
Intramedullary infection,
thrombosis of blood vessels
            ↓
Loss of cortical blood supply,
chronic infected granulation tissue with pus in the cavity
            ↓
Infected, dead bone known as Sequestrum    →    Formation of sinus tract to the skin to
surrounded by infected granulation tissues and pus    let the pus and sequestrum went out
            ↓
Reactive new bone formation around
sequestrum (Involucrum)
```

CLINICAL FEATURES

Chronic osteomyelitis typically results from inadequately treated acute osteomyelitis or following an open fracture. These patients present with—
- Pain and swelling over the affected bone
- History of *chronic, intermittently discharging sinus* (**Fig. 26.8**)
- History of *discharge of bony spicules* (sequestrum) through the sinus. *If this history is positive, it is the single most important clinical feature in favor of chronic osteomyelitis.*

Examination

Inspection
- Often, multiple scars over the limb are present, which have healed by secondary intention (due to sinus, surgery, old wounds)
- *Single/multiple sinuses* are present. They may be discharging pus/may be quiescent
- Muscle wasting is present.

Note

Types of sequestrum
- **Cortical:** Flat and serrated
- **Ivory:** Syphlitic
- **Sandy/rice grain:** Tubercular osteomyelitis
- **Feathery:** In TB of ribs
- **Black:** Fungal osteomyelitis
- **Ring/annular:** Around amputation stump/pin tracts
- **Diaphyseal:** Seen in children wherein whole diaphysis becomes a sequestrum

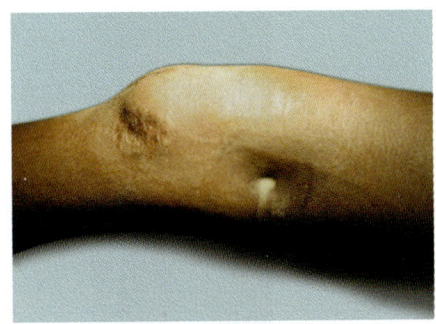

Fig. 26.8: Discharging sinus.

Palpation
- *Bony thickening, irregularity, and tenderness are one of the most notable findings*
- *The sinus (single or multiple) is always fixed to the underlying bone* (not mobile if moved side-side).

Other features
- Joint stiffness, bony deformity
- Limb length discrepancy may be present (due to the growth plate damage/pathological #)
- Regional lymph nodes may be enlarged.

INVESTIGATIONS

Several investigations are performed in case of chronic osteomyelitis, such as plain X-rays, CT, MRI, and sinogram. Among all, X-rays and CT are the most useful.
- **Plain X-ray:** *It is quite diagnostic of chronic osteomyelitis* (**Fig. 26.9**). Key X-ray findings are mentioned below.
    - Cortical thickening and irregularity
    - Periosteal reaction
    - Sequestrum: Dense, irregular, and separate piece from the normal bone
    - Involucrum—usually surrounding the sequestrum.
    - Single/multiple cavities
    - Sometimes, pathological fracture, deformity.
- **CT scan:** If X-rays fail to detect sequestrum, CT is performed (**Fig. 26.10A**).
- **MRI** is routinely not performed in case of chronic osteomyelitis-indicated if there is extensive soft tissue abscess.
- **Sinogram** is performed to delineate the sinus tract pathway. It can be done on a plain X-ray or a CT scan (**Fig. 26.10B**).
- **Culture and sensitivity (C/S):** Purulent material from the sinus opening is sent for C/S. (Note: Pus and tissues from depth of cavity are appropriate material for C/S as secretions from surface can be contaminated).

TREATMENT

The treatment of chronic osteomyelitis is *"essentially surgical" followed by medical treatment.*
There are *two major principles* in treating chronic osteomyelitis:
1. **Treatment of the dead tissues (bone and soft tissues) and chronic infection**
2. **Treatment of the dead space**

The treatment of chronic osteomyelitis is brielfy discussed in **Flowchart 26.4**.

Section 3: Musculoskeletal Infection

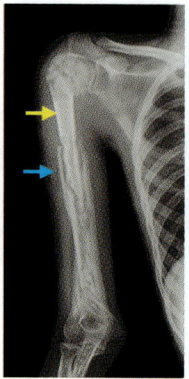

Fig. 26.9: Plain X-ray of the arm showing chronic osteomyelitis of the humerus: Sequestrum (yellow arrow); Involucrum (blue arrow).

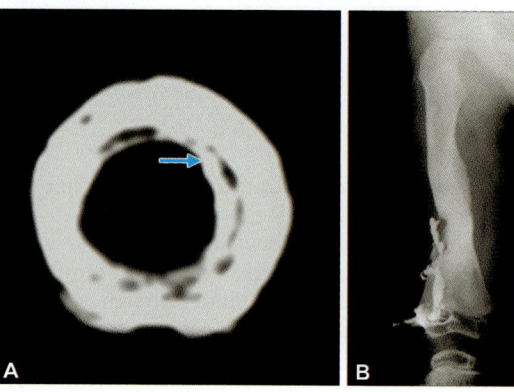

Figs. 26.10A and B: (A) Computed tomography (CT) scan shows sequestrum (blue arrow); (B) Sinogram delineates sinus tract.

Flowchart 26.4: Treatment algorithm of the chronic osteomyelitis.

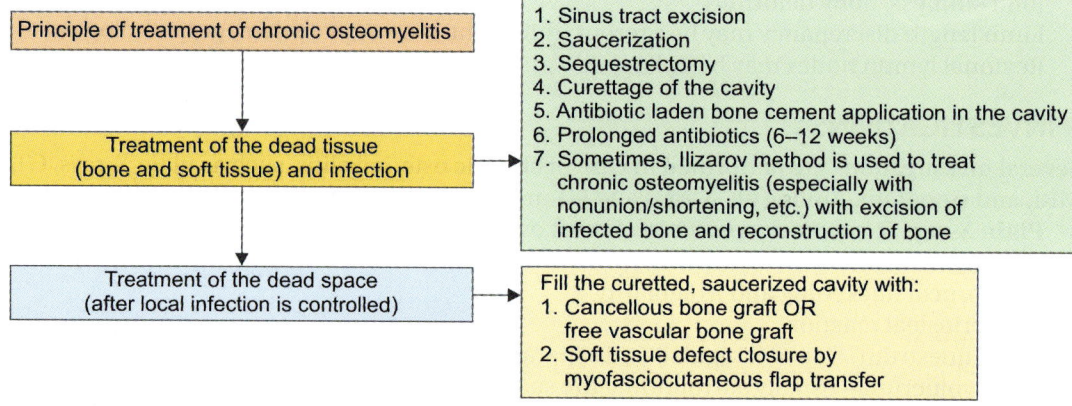

A. Treatment of the dead tissues (bone and soft tissue) and infection involves several steps: *Sinus tract excision, saucerization, sequestrectomy, curettage and/or antibiotic-laden bone cement bead application.*
- **Sinus tract excision:** The infected sinus tract is excised.
- **Saucerization:** *The pitcher-shaped infected cavity is converted into a saucer-shaped cavity by deroofing the cavity* **(Fig. 26.11).** A saucer shape cavity ensures removal of all sequestered bone and proper drainage of the purulent material, which is not possible in an enclosed cavity with narrow opening.
  Note: The saucerization is done only once "adequate involucrum" is formed around the sequestered bone, or else it increases the risk of pathological fracture as saucerization involves the removal of part of a 'normal bone and involucrum' which results in weakening of bone.
- **Sequestrectomy:** The sequestrum is removed once adequate involucrum is formed **(Fig. 26.12).** All the sequestrum must be removed as it is a constant source of infection, and a reason for recurrence of osteomyelitis even after the surgery. The sequestrum should be send for biopsy to confirm the etiology of infection-pyogenic/tubercular/other.

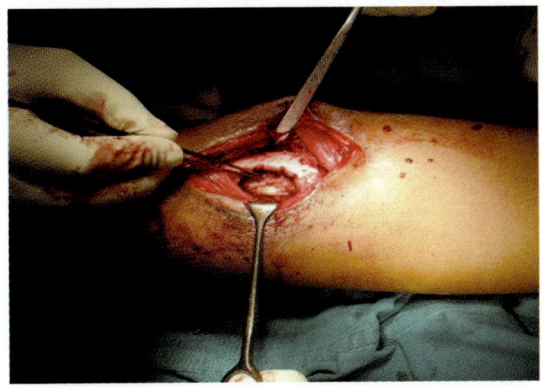

Fig. 26.11: Saucerized cavity of chronic osteomyelitis.

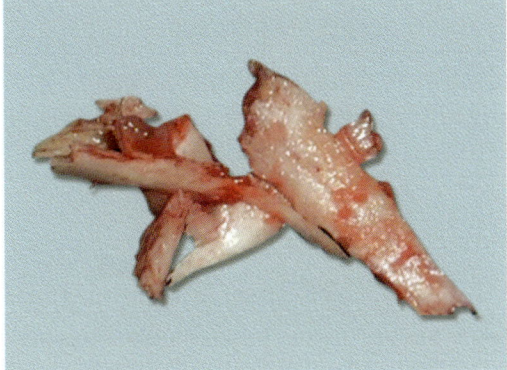

Fig. 26.12: Sequestrum (removed).

- ***Curettage of cavity:*** The entire cavity wall is curetted to remove the sclerosed wall, infected granulation tissue and purulent material. Pus and granulation tissue from the cavity is send for culture and biopsy. Well-curetted cavity walls must reveal fresh bleeding. Furthermore, a well-curetted cavity ensures a robust blood supply to the infected cavity delivering adequate immune cells and systemic antibiotics to the cavity, which helps fight residual infection.
- ***Antibiotic-impregnated bone cement beads:*** After thorough debridement and curettage of the cavity, the beads are in the cavity, ensuring local antibiotic delivery for a prolonged period of 4–6 weeks **(Figs. 26.13A to E)**. 6–8 weeks later, the beads are removed. *Typically, vancomycin/gentamicin are used in bone cement as both are heat resistant.* Absorbable calcium suphate beads with Vancomycin/Gentamicin can also be used, which can be left is place without need of removal.

After the surgical debridement, the culture-specific antibiotics are continued for 2–3 months (2–3 weeks IV followed by another 6–8 weeks oral).

Resistant bone infection with other associated complications such as nonunion, shortening, and deformity are treated best with the Ilizarov method. Here, the dead segment is resected, and the viable segment is transported.

B. Treatment of the dead space: The dead space could result in reinfection and remains a potential risk factor for the pathological factor. Hence, the dead space is managed by:
- ***Delayed, open cancellous bone grafting after 2–3 weeks (Papineau technique)*** once the local infection is controlled. Free vascularized bone graft is also an option.
- ***Myocutaneous flaps/fasciocutaneous flaps***.

COMPLICATIONS OF CHRONIC OSTEOMYELITIS

- **Recurrences after the treatment:** Most common complication.
- **Pathological fractures** occur due to weak bone following infection/saucerization before adequate involucrum is formed.
- **Limb length discrepancy** is observed in children due to damage to the growth plate. Typically, physeal damage results in *limb shortening*. However, there rarely can be *limb lengthening* due to physeal stimulation due to hyperemia in the adjacent infected area. In adults, shortening results from pathological fracture/bone excision during surgeries.

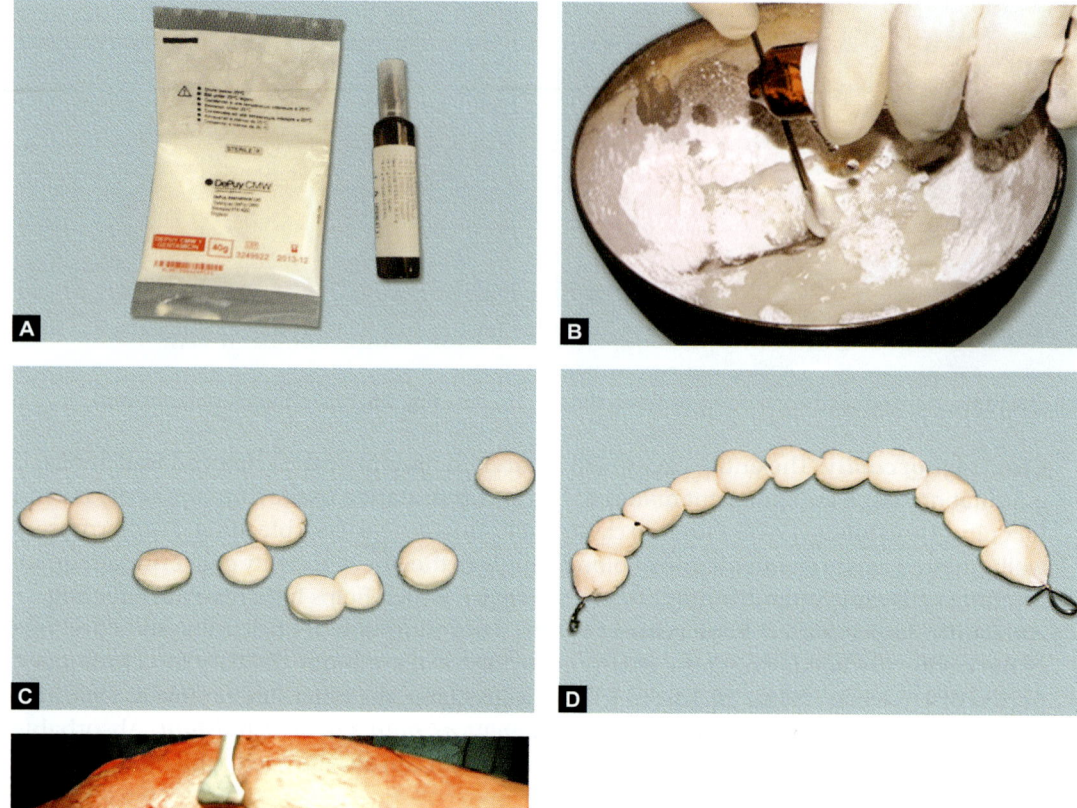

Figs. 26.13A to E: Images showing the preparation of bone cement with gentamicin. (A) Bone cement (PMMA, polymethylmethacrylate) with liquid activator. Antibiotic is mixed in the same stage; (B) Bone cement mixed with activator liquid; (C) Bone cement rolled into semisolid beads; (D) Beads are rolled over the stainless steel wires and let hardened; (E) Beads are placed over the infected area after debridement.

- **Deformity:** Asymmetric physeal destruction results in growth arrest in one part of the physis, whereas the other 'normal' part continues to grow, resulting in a deformity (valgum/varum/flexion/recurvatum).
- **Joint stiffness** occurs due to muscle and other periarticular soft tissue contracture. Sometimes, it could result from concomitant septic arthritis.
- **Rarely, septicemia:** It is uncommon in chronic osteomyelitis due to localized infection in a sclerosed cavity.
- **Sinus tract malignancy:** With sinus persisting for *many years*, it could result in squamous cell carcinoma of the tract.
- **Amyloidosis:** It may result after many years of chronic osteomyelitis.

BRODIE'S ABSCESS AND GARRE'S SCLEROSING OSTEOMYELITIS

BRODIE'S ABSCESS

Definition
It is primary subacute osteomyelitis of hematogenous origin due to low virulence of the offending organism or strong host immune response.

Location
- *The proximal tibial metaphysis is the most common location in a long bone.*
- Sometimes, it can affect distal tibia, fibula, distal radius, carpal, or tarsal bones.

Etiology
Staphylococcus aureus (usually of low virulence or strong host immunity and response).

Clinical Features
Symptoms: Pain and swelling at the upper end of the leg/affected part. Night pain is often present.

Signs
- Bony tenderness at the affected site
- Mild swelling
- Movements at the joint are usually normal. No lymphadenopathy.

Investigations
- Raised ESR
- **X-ray:** Lytic cavitary lesion surrounded by a dense sclerotic rim of bone **(Fig. 26.14)**. No periosteal reaction is observed.
- **MRI:** Lytic lesion with *'penumbra sign'* (a rim of vascularized granulation tissue around a bone abscess cavity with a higher T1 signal intensity than the cavity itself).
- **CT scan:** Lytic lesion with a dense rim around.

Treatment
Surgical drainage and curettage of the cavity followed by culture-specific antibiotics for 6–8 weeks.

GARRE'S SCLEROSING OSTEOMYELITIS

Definition

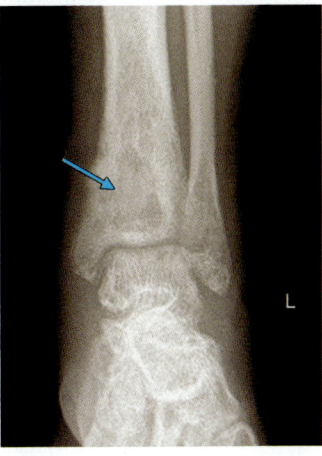

Fig. 26.14: Brodie's abscess in lower end tibia (blue arrow shows lytic area).

It is **primary subacute osteomyelitis in the mandible** due to low-grade infection leading to peripheral periosteal bone deposition (*proliferative periostitis*).

It is common in the mandible of children with dental caries. It may also occur in a long bone.

Clinical Features
- Diffuse, dull aching pain over the involved bone
- Deep tenderness in the involved area
- Associated dental caries in mandibular Garre's.

Investigations
- Raised ESR
- *Orthopantomogram*: Localized periostitis
- MRI and CT scan.

Treatment
The treatment of Garre's osteomyelitis involves removal of the caries tooth, surgical debridement of the lesion, followed by several weeks of antibiotics.

CHAPTER 27

Septic Arthritis

SEPTIC ARTHRITIS

Before we start discussing the various pathological aspects of septic arthritis, it must be noted that all forms of arthritis (septic/inflammatory/tubercular/degenerative/metabolic) ultimately damage *the articular cartilage*.

Damage to subchondral bone (avascular necrosis of bone) or **change in synovial fluid content/type** (inflammatory and infection of joint) affects the nutrition of the cartilage leading to arthritis.

■ DEFINITION

Inflammation and infection of the joint due to *pathogenic inoculation by pus-forming organisms, except tubercular infection,* is known as septic arthritis.

■ ETIOLOGY

- **Risk factors:** Most factors suppress immunity and predispose it to joint infection. Common risk factors include
    - **Age:** Infants/elderly. Infants or young children have not acquired immunity, while older patients lose immunity due to ageing and various comorbidities
    - Diabetes mellitus
    - Rheumatoid arthritis
    - Corticosteroid treatment
    - Septicemia, contiguous skin infection
    - Immunocompromised/immunosuppressed
    - Intravenous (IV) drug abusers.
- **Microbes:** Various microbes have been implicated in the etiology of septic arthritis. ***Staphylococcus aureus* remains the most common cause of septic arthritis in all age groups**. However, there are specific organisms in different age groups/conditions.
    - Neonates: *Escherichia coli* (via maternal genital tract during vaginal delivery)
    - Infants: *Staphylococcus aureus*
    - Adults:
        - *Staphylococcus aureus*: Most common organism
        - *Streptococcus pyogenes*
        - *Gonococcus*: Young sexually active males/females
        - *Salmonella typhi*: In sickle cell anemia
        - *Pseudomonas aeruginosa*: Intravenous drug abusers, elderly
        - *E. coli*: Elderly, IV drug abusers

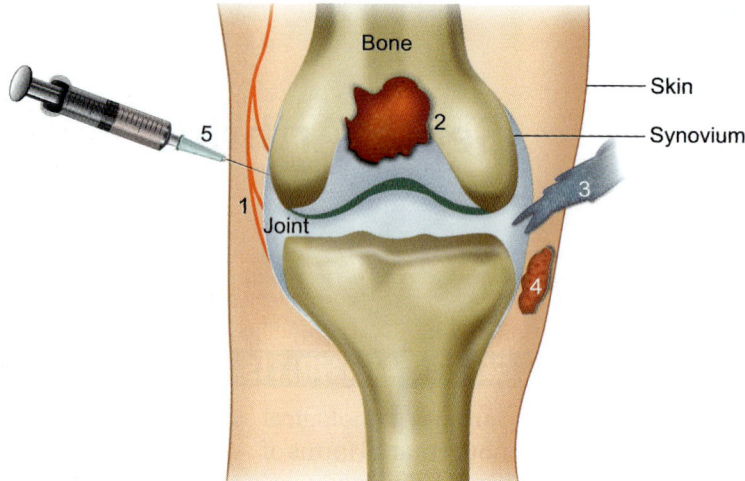

Fig. 27.1: Various routes of spread for septic arthritis. (1) Hematogenous; (2) Osteomyelitis; (3) Direct penetrating injury; (4) Local contiguous infection; (5) Diagnostic or therapeutic intra-articular procedures.

- *Staphylococcus epidermidis:* Prosthetic joints
- *Propionibacterium acnes:* Specially implicated after shoulder joint replacement
- *Brucella:* Spine infections.

Other microbes:
- Anaerobic microbes
- *Fungal:* Histoplasma, coccidioidomycosis
- *Viral:* Hepatitis A, B, C; adenovirus, coxsackie.
- **Route of spread:** The infection in the joint can reach by various routes **(Fig. 27.1)**, such as:
    - *Hematogenously* if there is a focus of infection elsewhere, such as umbilical sepsis, URTI, LRTI, UTI, and GI infection.
    - *Direct* inoculation in the joint due to penetrating injury, injection, open fracture dislocations
    - *Local* spread from osteomyelitis of adjacent bone, bursitis, and pyoderma.

PATHOGENESIS

Once the bacteria reach the joint by local or systemic route, it multiplies, causing infection and damage to the joint. There are three stages of septic arthritis:
1. **Stage of synovitis**
2. **Stage of arthritis**
3. **Stage of deformity or bony ankylosis.**

Stage of Synovitis

The pyogenic organism infects the synovium causing an intense immune response resulting in synovitis. Due to synovitis, there is joint effusion that is initially serous, followed by seropurulent, and further purulent. This stage ends with forming a *"pannus"* over the cartilage **(Fig. 27.2 and Flowchart 27.1)**.

Note: Pannus is a fibrovascular inflammatory tissue that grows over the cartilage.

Chapter 27: Septic Arthritis

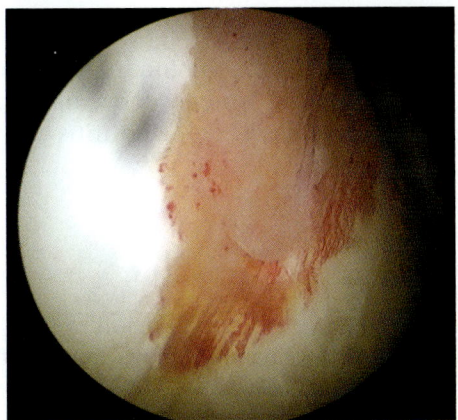

Fig. 27.2: Arthroscopic image of Pannus over the femoral cartilage.

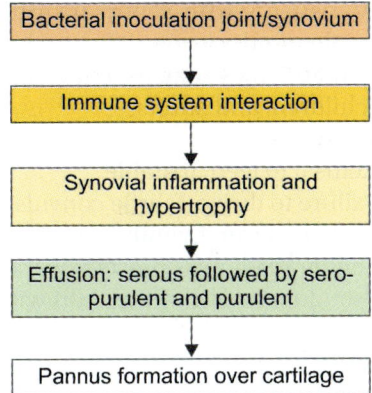

Flowchart 27.1: Pathology of the stage of synovitis.

Stage of Arthritis

Stage of arthritis is characterized by the *destruction of the joint hyaline cartilage* **(Fig. 27.3)** due to several mechanisms **(Flowchart 27.2)**.
- *Pannus* formation over the cartilage results in the choking of cartilage. Therefore, cartilage cannot imbibe nutrition from synovial fluid.
- *Pus* cannot nourish the cartilage
- *Lysosomal enzymes* directly damage the hyaline cartilage.

Stage of Deformity/Bony Ankylosis

Once the hyaline cartilage is destroyed, the subchondral bone of articulating bones is exposed. The bare ends of two articulating bones gradually fuse, leading to bony ankylosis and deformity.

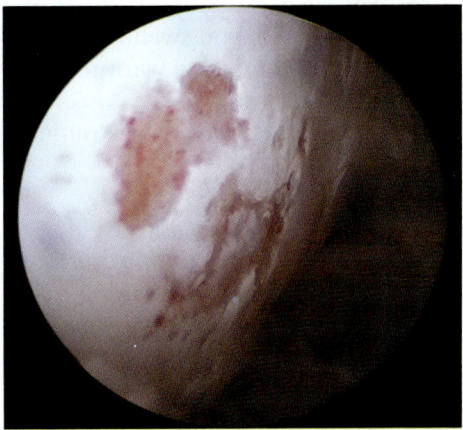

Fig. 27.3: Arthroscopic image of damage to the underlying hyaline cartilage (beneath pannus), which is apparent after pannus removal.

Flowchart 27.2: Pathogenesis of cartilage damage in stage of arthritis.

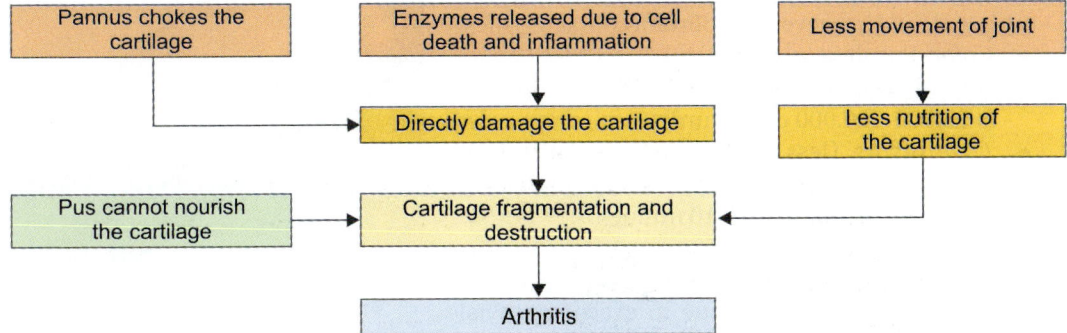

CLINICAL FEATURES

Typically, patients with septic arthritis have pain and swelling over the joint. The joint is warm, tender, and movements are excruciating (cf. osteomyelitis, wherein movements are still preserved). They may have fever. However, the clinical features of septic arthritis vary in infants, children, and adults.

- **Infants**
    - Refusal to feed, irritable
    - Failure to thrive, febrile convulsions
    - High/no fever/hypothermia
    - Tender swelling is present over the joint. There is local warmth and effusion
    - Pseudoparalysis of the limb with severe restriction of passive and active ROM of the joint.
- **Children**
    - Fever, chills, rigors
    - Tachycardia, tachypnea
    - Febrile convulsions
    - Severe pain and swelling of joint, and patient cannot weight bear/walk
    - Effusion and local warmth are present. Features of inflammation may be present over the skin
    - Pseudoparalysis with extremely painful ROM.
- **Adults**
    - Fever
    - Severe joint pain and swelling
    - *Features of inflammation over joint:* Redness, swelling, raised temperature, severe tenderness
    - Very painful ROM (early stage/with serous effusion or patients who are immunocompromised/immunosuppressed may not have very painful ROM).

INVESTIGATIONS

- **Complete blood picture (CBP):** Leukocytosis, neutrophilia
- **CRP, ESR:** Raised
- **Procalcitonin:** >0.5 ng%
- **Blood culture:** It must be sent before initiating presumptive antibiotic therapy.
- **Joint aspiration/arthrocentesis** is the *diagnostic investigation* for septic arthritis **(Fig. 27.4)**. The aspirated fluid has several important characteristics:
    - *Color*: Purulent/turbid
    - *Increased white blood cells (WBCs)* in pus (>50,000–100,000 cells/mm^3)
    - *Low sugars* (less than one-third of serum glucose levels)
    - *Increased lactate levels* >10 mmol/L
- **X-ray of the joint**
    - *Early stage*: Thickened soft tissue shadow, increased joint space (due to excess synovial fluid)

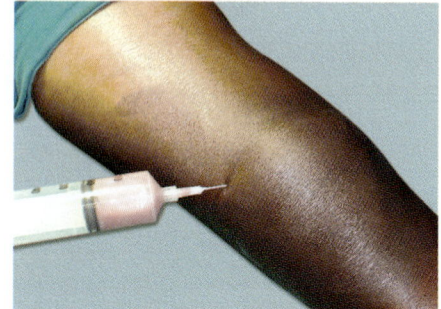

Fig. 27.4: Knee joint aspiration shows pus in the syringe.

- *Late stage*: Decreased joint space (due to destroyed cartilage), periarticular osteopenia, deformity, ankylosis.
- **Ultrasound (USG)** reveals collection in the joint with multiple septations, capsular thickening, synovial hypertrophy
- **Magnetic resonance imaging (MRI)** is performed only to rule out concurrent osteomyelitis.

TREATMENT

The treatment of septic arthritis involves general, medical, and surgical management. Almost all cases require surgical debridement and 6–8 weeks of antibiotics.

- **General management**
    - *Maintain hydration*: Intravenous (IV) fluids
    - Antipyretics, analgesics
    - Splints/traction relieve pain and prevent deformity
    - Correct anemia, if any
    - Treat primary focus, if any.
- **Specific measures involve medical and surgical treatment**
    - *Medical treatment by antibiotics*
        - *Initially:* Start broad-spectrum antibiotics to cover gram-positive (Vancomycin/Clindamycin) and gram-negative microbes (3rd generation cephalosporin). Cloxacillin and gentamycin can also cover gram-positive and gram-negative organisms, respectively.
        - *Later:* Switch over to specific antibiotics according to the culture sensitivity of aspirated pus. The antibiotics should be continued for 6–8 weeks (2 weeks of IV and 4–6 weeks of oral antibiotics).
    - *Surgical debridement of joint* involves drainage of purulent material, removal of florid synovium and pannus and saline wash of the joint. It can be performed by open or arthroscopic technique. Arthroscopic debridement is preferred as it is:
        - Minimally invasive and associated with lesser morbidity
        - Almost every corner of the joint can be reached and debrided with the help of the arthroscope
        - Postoperatively, there is less pain and stiffness due to small incisions
        - Easier rehabilitation due to few stitches and minimal scarring.

COMPLICATIONS

Acute
- Septicemia
- Acute osteomyelitis.

Chronic
- Bony ankylosis **(Fig. 27.5)**
- Secondary degenerative arthritis
- Growth plate damage leading to limb length discrepancy (in growing children), deformity

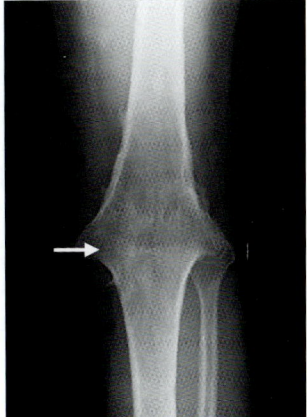

Fig. 27.5: X-ray shows bony ankylosis of the knee, wherein joint space is obliterated and bony trabeculae of femur and tibia are crossing either side.

- Joint stiffness
- Pathological dislocation

Sequalae of untreated/inadequately treated septic arthritis

The sequelae of septic arthritis is bony ankylosis, whereas inflammatory or tubercular arthritis ends as fibrous ankylosis.

TOM SMITH ARTHRITIS
(Syn: Septic arthritis of infancy)

DEFINITION

"Septic arthritis of the hip in infancy" leads to total or partial destruction of the cartilage, causing poor or no development of the head of the femur.

ETIOPATHOGENESIS

The femoral head is cartilaginous in infancy and ossifies at nine months. If septic arthritis happens earlier than nine months, it may result in the total or partial destruction of the femoral head due to the cartilaginous nature of the femoral head.

CLINICAL FEATURES

- The child present with short limb and limp while walking
- Painful hip in early stages, whereas later stages may have painless near full range of motion
- The telescopy test is positive
- Hip joint movements may be exaggerated.

X-RAY

- Absent head of the femur
- Proximally migrated trochanter
- Poorly developed acetabulum.

TREATMENT

- **Early stage:** Arthrotomy and drainage of the pus, antibiotics
- **Late stage:** Salvage procedures like pelvic support osteotomy, limb lengthening
- **Adults:** Total hip replacement.

CHAPTER 28

HIV Infections and Orthopaedics

Various bone and joint manifestations in a patient with HIV are similar to those in a non-HIV patient except for the tumors. However, the course of the disease could be severe.

Various bone and joint disorders in an HIV patient are listed below.
- **Bone disorders**
    - Osteomyelitis
    - Osteoporosis
    - Avascular necrosis
    - Carpal tunnel syndrome
    - Frozen shoulder
- **Joint disorders**
    - Septic arthritis
- **Myopathy**
- **Neoplasms**
    - Kaposi sarcoma
    - Non-Hodgkin's lymphoma
- **HIV and elective orthopaedic surgery**.

BONE DISORDERS

Osteomyelitis
- In HIV patients, both tubercular and non-tubercular infections are common.
- **Tubercular infection:** The spine is the most common site of tubercular infection. The spinal (tuberculosis) TB in an HIV patient is characterized by large paravertebral abscesses and less vertebral body destruction.
- **Non-tubercular osteomyelitis (NTO):** *Staphylococcus aureus* remains the most common offending organism causing NTO.
- Other causes of NTO are syphilis and *Bartonella henselae*.
- **Treatment:** On standard lines.

Osteoporosis
- Osteopenia and osteoporosis are common in HIV patients. The etiology of osteoporosis in HIV patients is multifactorial:
    - Direct inhibitory effect of virus cells on osteoblasts
    - Persistent elevation of TNF-α and IL-1

- **Drug-related:** Many protease inhibitors causes calcium and vitamin D deficiency. Indinavir inhibits bone formation, and ritonavir causes osteoclast differentiation. Further, reverse transcriptase inhibitors cause Fanconi syndrome resulting in hypophosphatemic rickets.
- **Others:** Poor nutrition.
- **Diagnosis:** DEXA scan.
- **Treatment:** Calcium, vitamin D, bisphosphonates. For drug induced Fanconi syndrome osteomalacia, change of drugs and oral phosphate suffice.

Osteonecrosis/Avascular Necrosis

- **Etiology:** Drug-related, dyslipidemia, anticardiolipin antibody, and protein S deficiency
- MRI establishes the diagnosis, and treatment is on standard lines.

JOINT DISORDERS

Septic Arthritis

The most common organism implicated is *Staphylococcus aureus*. Others are *Streptococcus*, *H. influenzae*, and *Salmonella*.

Other Arthropathies

- **Primary HIV arthropathy:** It is a non-erosive oligoarthropathy and is quite common in lower limb joints. However, it is usually transient and subsides within 6 weeks–6 months.
- **Seronegative arthropathy:** Psoriatic and reactive arthropathy are common in HIV patients. The disease is more severe than the usual course. Patients with reactive arthritis may also have enthesopathy.
- **Painful articular syndrome:** It is common in the knee, shoulder, and elbows and lasts 2–24 hours. It presents as acute sharp pain.

MYOPATHIES: INFECTIOUS PYOMYOSITIS, NON-INFECTION MYOSITIS

- **Infectious pyomyositis** is common in the late stages of HIV infection, where the *patient's CD4 count is less than 200/mm³*. The most commonly implicated organism is *Staph aureus*. Pyomyositis undergoes three stages-inflammation, pus formation, and sepsis. The Erythrocyte sedimentation rate (ESR) and C-reactive protein (CRP) are elevated, while creatinine kinase levels are low. MRI is highly sensitive, and pus aspiration may hold the key to the diagnosis. Early diagnosis and aggressive surgical management are the mainstays of treatment.
- **Non-infectious myositis:** It presents as bilateral proximal muscle weakness (shoulder and pelvic girdle), while distal muscle weakness is rare. Dysphagia is observed in 25% of cases. It is characterized by high levels of serum creatinine kinase. ART is one of the common causes of myopathy.

NEOPLASM

- Kaposi sarcoma is the most common associated malignancy in HIV. It involves the skin, mucosa, and lymphatics. However, it rarely involves the musculoskeletal system and can present as bone pain. Osseous lesions are usually lytic in nature.

- **Non-Hodgkin's lymphoma:** The likelihood of NHL is 60 times higher than the average population. These patients are at a higher risk of painful limb swelling and pathological fracture. X-ray shows lytic lesions with soft tissue mass.

HIV AND ORTHOPAEDIC SURGERY

- The risk of renal, pulmonary and infective complications is higher in an HIV patient after routine orthopaedic surgery. Further, the possibility of infection in open fractures is higher than in non-HIV patients.
- **Fracture union:** There is a possibility of delayed union or non-union in patients with HIV, especially if there are high serum TNF-α.

CHAPTER 29

Spirochetal Infections of Bones and Joints

Spirochetes are gram-negative, spiral bacteria with the unique property of endocellular flagella, which are responsible for its motility. The Spirochetales include five genera that are pathogenic for humans. *Treponema* species (syphilis and the endemic treponematoses); *Leptospira* species (leptospirosis or rat fever); *Borrelia* and *Borreliella* species (relapsing fever and Lyme disease, respectively); and *Brachyspira* species (gastrointestinal infections).

■ SYPHILIS

Syphilis is a chronic sexually transmitted infection due to the spirochetal bacterium *Treponema pallidum* (TP) subspecies *Pallidum*. Syphilis includes *primary, secondary, and latent syphilis* less than one year from primary exposure, referred to as "infectious syphilis" and *late syphilis*, which includes tertiary syphilis and latent syphilis of more than one year. Although the disease is rare, it is still an important STD. Musculoskeletal manifestations of syphilis should be kept in mind because of the recrudescence of the disease and because of their frequently misleading expression. In this section, only skeletal manifestation will be discussed.

Musculoskeletal clinical features of syphilis can be grouped into the congenital and adult phase of syphilis.

- **Congenital syphilis:** It can be early and late congenital syphilis.
    - ◆ *Early congenital syphilis:* It appears within two years of life. Skeletal manifestations include periosteal reaction (34%), metaphysitis (24%) and osteitis (0.7%). These changes are typically symmetrical in the involved bone. Femur, tibia, and humerus are commonly involved. X-ray shows enlargement and thickening of the metaphysis with irregularities of the ossification line with alternate dense and lucent bands. Later, the ossification zone disappears and is replaced by deep symmetrical erosions at the inner edge of the involved metaphysis (Wimberger's sign), resulting in epiphyseal displacement. At this stage, there can be severe pain and inability to move limbs, known as Parrot's pseudoparalysis.
    - ◆ *Late congenital syphilis:* It occurs after the age of 2 years, typically between 5–20 years. The most specific sign of late congenital syphilis is *Hutchinson's triad*, consisting of Hutchinson's teeth, eighth cranial nerve deafness, and interstitial keratitis. Syphilitic osteitis may produce periostitis, osteomyelitis, osteitis, and gummatous osteoarthritis. Skeletal manifestations are:
        - *Sabre shin:* Thickened bowed appearance of the tibia due to periosteal thickening (no actual bowing)
        - *Clutton's joint:* Recurrent late arthropathy of the joint characterized by recurrent, large, bilateral effusion of the knee joints without any obvious X-ray findings.

- Hot cross bun appearance of the skull.
- *Parrot's nodes:* Thickened, nodular appearance of the skull.
- *Syphilitic dactylitis:* Painful fusiform swelling of the phalanges.
- **Adult syphilis:** It is characterized by *periosteitis*, which can be observed in long bones as thickening of the bones. In late cases, there can be **tabetic arthropathy** *(neuropathic or Charcot's joint)* characterized by painless destruction of the joints. Progressive absorption of phalanges results in a "pencil sharpening" appearance of the bony ends (decrease in length and width) on an X-ray. Hypertrophic osteophytes are observed in the spine.

Treatment of Syphilis

Congenital Syphilis

- **Early syphilis:** If cerebrospinal fluid (CSF) is normal, procaine penicillin G 50,000 IU/kg/day IM for ten days. If the CSF is abnormal, aqueous penicillin G at the dose of 50,000 units/kg given IM or IV twice daily for ten days.
- **Late syphilis:** Benzathine penicillin G 50,000 IU/kg/week deep IM for three weeks.

Adult Syphilis

Injection of Benzathine penicillin G 2.4 million units deep IM as a single dose.

LYME'S DISEASE

Lyme borreliosis is caused by a spirochete, *Borrelia burgdorferi sensu lato*, transmitted by ticks of the *Ixodes ricinus* complex. The infection has three stages.
- Stage 1 is characterized by characteristic expanding skin lesions, erythema migrans.
- Stage 2 occurs after several days or weeks with the dissemination of infection, characterized by secondary annular skin lesions, meningitis, neuritis, carditis, atrioventricular nodal block, or migratory musculoskeletal pain. Months or years later.
- Stage 3 develops, characterized by intermittent or persistent arthritis, chronic encephalopathy, and polyneuropathy.

Lyme arthritis is characterized by painful intermittent arthritis of one or more joints. The knee joint is most commonly involved. Enzyme-linked immunosorbent assay (ELISA) test reveals high levels of IgG antibody. It can be treated with a month-long course of Amoxicillin or doxycycline. Sometimes, several patients develop inflammatory synovitis and become resistant to antibiotic therapy. They are treated by DMARDs such as hydroxychloroquine and methotrexate.

SECTION 4

Mycobacterial Musculoskelatal Infections

SECTION OUTLINE

30. Skeletal Tuberculosis
    - Overview, Approach and Management of Skeletal Tuberculosis
    - Tuberculosis of Hip, Knee, Spine, Shoulder
    - Tubercular Osteomyelitis
    - Hansen's Disease

2

Mycobacterial Musculoskeletal Infections

30 CHAPTER

Skeletal Tuberculosis

INTRODUCTION

According to a report published by WHO in 2021, the incidence of Tuberculosis (TB) in India is 210 per one lakh population. In 2021, a total of 2.14 million cases were notified in India. 71% of patients were of pulmonary TB. Other important facts are:
- The latent cases outnumber active TB cases.
- Males are more commonly affected than females.
- Among the bone and joint TB, the *spine is the most commonly affected region (50%)*, followed by the hip (15–20%), knee (7%), and SI joint (6%).
- Bone and joint TB is almost always secondary to primary elsewhere, such as lungs, lymph nodes, genitourinary and gastrointestinal tract.
- In contrast to the pulmonary TB where the Mycobacterium load $>10^7$–10^9, most cases of Musculoskeletal TB are paucibacillary wherein the load is $<10^5$.

INCIDENCE OF BONE AND JOINT TUBERCULOSIS

Bone and joint TB has a bimodal presentation, once in childhood and again during older age (Fig. 30.1).

TYPES OF TUBERCULAR INFECTION

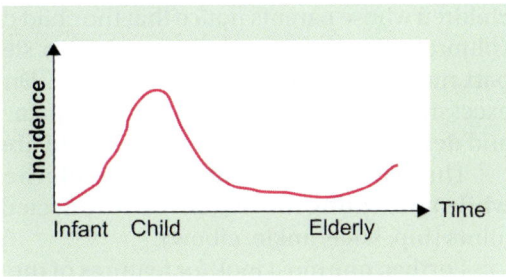

Fig. 30.1: Incidence of TB in various age groups.

1. **Tubercular spondylitis/Caries spine/Pott's spine:** TB of the spine is the most common site (50%) among all areas of affection.
2. **Tubercular arthritis:** Among all the joints, the hip joint is most commonly affected (15–20%), followed by the knee joint (7%), SI joint (6%), and other joints. Typically, tubercular arthritis undergoes three stage changes in the joint—stage of synovitis, arthritis, and advanced arthritis with deformity. The details are mentioned in hip TB (vide infra).
3. **Tubercular osteomyelitis:** It is common in both children and adults. The pathophysiology is similar to that of pyogenic osteomyelitis. However, the sequestrum of TB osteomyelitis is quite typical—*'coarse sand' and 'feathery.'* Coarse sand sequestrum is rarely visible on X-rays, while feathery sequestrum is due to the calcification of caseous material.

ETIOPATHOLOGY OF SKELETAL TB

It is important to note that osteoarticular TB is almost always secondary to primary elsewhere. The main causative organism is *Mycobacterium tuberculosis (MTB)*. Rarely could it be atypical *Mycobacterium*.

The MTB enters the body chiefly via the respiratory route to the lungs or by the gut. Once MTB reaches the target tissue, it causes a granulomatous reaction associated with tissue necrosis and caseation. The infection to the bone reaches via the hematogenous route. The blood supply to the synovial membrane and subchondral bone is similar. Hence, the MTB infection may settle in bone or synovium. Bone TB could be of two types: Caseating and Proliferative.

1. **Caseating/Exudative type:**
    - It is *common in children* and dominated by *caseating necrosis and cold abscess formation*. The tubercular abscesses (cold abscesses) are not red, warm or tender, and contain serum, leucocytes, caseous material, bone debris and tubercle bacilli.
    - It is characterized by *extensive destruction of bone and cartilage*, abscess and sinus formation with constitutional symptoms.
2. **Proliferative/Granular type:**
    - It is *common in adults* and characterized by *cellular proliferation with minimal caseation and tubercular granuloma formation*.
    - Insidious in onset, *less bone destruction*, and *abscess formation is uncommon*.

CLINICAL FEATURES OF SKELETAL TB

The clinical features of musculoskeletal TB comprise **constitutional** and **local**. Constitutionally, patients may complain of *fever, malaise, easy fatiguability, weight loss, and appetite*. Typically, there may be evening rise of temperature. Overall, there may be general debility. The most common local feature is **'bone pain'**, whose intensity may vary from mild to severe. The pain may be continuous and felt more at night (*night cries*). Night cries are typically described in children whose parents notice that the child cries at night. These night cries are due to decreased voluntary muscle tone when the child is sleeping, permitting the movements in the affected part more than when the child is awake. During the day, voluntary muscle guarding prevents excessive joint movement, minimizing pain. As the disease progresses, there may be **swelling** and **deformity** of the affected part. A **cold abscess** may also develop.

The main physical findings are **tenderness** in the affected region, **muscle spasm**, and **pain while attempting movement** of the affected part. **Swelling** and **deformity** are noted over the joints (hip, knee, ankle, elbow).

Further, one must look for features of the primary source [lung/gastrointestinal tract (GIT)/gut/lymph nodes], as musculoskeletal TB is almost always secondary to a primary source of TB elsewhere.

==Note that not all patients with skeletal TB would present with constitutional symptoms, while early local features of pain and difficulty in movements of affected regions are quite nonspecific symptoms. That is why the diagnosis of skeletal TB could be delayed for several weeks/months.==

INVESTIGATION IN SKELETAL TB

The investigations in skeletal TB—general, local and detection of primary source.
1. **General:** General investigations comprise **CBP, ESR,** and **Mantoux** tests. CBP may reveal lymphocytosis while ESR is always elevated. The hemoglobin may be low due to poor

nutrition and anorexia. A negative Mantoux test may help rule out TB, whereas a positive Mantoux test indicates either an active tubercular infection or BCG vaccination.
2. **Local:** The local disease is diagnosed with the help of ***X-rays, CT, MRI, and bone scan***. However, the *diagnosis can be confirmed only with the* **demonstration of Mycobacterium** *(AFB) in ZN stain/culture/Nucleic acid amplification tests/***presence of tubercle granuloma** *in pus or biopsy material* obtained from the affected bone or joint.
    - ***X-rays*** of the affected region may reveal *diffuse osteopenia, bone destruction, joint space reduction, and lytic lesions.* **Phemister triad** is quite typical of TB, consisting of *periarticular osteoporosis, peripherally located bone erosions and diminution of joint space.* Remineralization of bone may indicate healing disease.
    - ***MRI*** may show *bone edema, abscess or local structure compression* (spinal cord in case of spine TB).
    - ***Bone scans*** may be required if *multifocal TB* is suspected in that region, especially in the case of spine TB.
    - ***Pus*** for *AFB staining, MTB culture, and MTB detection via nucleic acid amplification*: One must **aspirate the pus** and send for ZN staining (older method)/auramine-rhodamine dye staining with fluorescent microscopy (newer method) to demonstrate AFB. More than often, one has to perform **biopsy of the affected region** to obtain infected tissues (bone/synovium/pus). The biopsy material must also be sent for **culture** to grow MTB, which remains the *gold standard in diagnosing TB*. The culture can be performed on traditional culture media (Lowenstein-Jensen/Middlebrook 7H10/7H12) or rapid detection culture (MGIT or MODS). Apart from growing MTB on culture media, one must perform *drug sensitivity* as resistance to various antitubercular drugs is high. The material should also be sent for the **Nucleic acid amplification method** (Xpert MTB/RIF assay) for MTB detection and drug resistance assessment. Xpert MTB is also known as GeneXpert. It is a cartridge-based test having high specificity and sensitivity.
    - ***Biopsy:*** Often, the aspirate for pus may be a dry tap. In such cases, a **closed or open biopsy** must be performed, and material should be sent for *Xpert MTB/RIF assay* (popularly known as GeneXpert), *culture*, and *histopathology*. The histopathology can demonstrate classic tubercle granuloma.
3. **Detection of the primary focus of TB infection:** As musculoskeletal TB is almost always secondary to a primary elsewhere, the clinicians must attempt to investigate the primary source of infection, which may be present in the lungs, gastrointestinal tract, genitourinary tract, or lymph nodes. *Chest X-rays or CT scans, abdomen-pelvis USG or CT scans, and urine examinations* may help diagnose the primary source.

TREATMENT OF SKELETAL TB

The treatment of musculoskeletal TB comprises general, medical and/or surgical treatment.
- **General treatment** involves managing pain, spasm, deformity, anemia with analgesics, traction, braces and treatment of anemia, respectively.
- **Medical treatment:** The *most important aspect of skeletal TB management is antitubercular treatment (ATT) for 12–18 months* depending on the response. There are two phases of ATT—intensive and continuation. In case of no resistance, 1st line drugs are used for ATT
    - ***Intensive phase:*** All four standard 1st line drugs are used in this phase for two months—Isoniazid, Rifampicin, Ethambutol, and Pyrazinamide (HREZ—Isoniazid, Rifampicin, Ethambutol, Pyrazinamide). Along with ATT, 10 mg/day of Pyridoxine is added to

Table 30.1: 1st line antitubercular drugs, action, dose, and common side effects.

Drug	Action	Dose (in mg/kg/day)	Common side effects
Isoniazid	▪ BC against IC and EC bacilli ▪ BS against resting bacilli	5–10	Peripheral neuropathy
Rifampicin	BC against IC and EC bacilli	10	Hepatitis
Ethambutol	Bacteriostatic	15–20	Optic neuritis
Pyrazinamide	Bactericidal	20–30	Hyperuricemia
Streptomycin	Bactericidal against rapidly dividing EC bacteria	15	Ototoxic, nephrotoxic

(BC: bactericidal; BS: bacteriostatic; EC: extracellular; IC: intracellular)

Table 30.2: Commonly used 2nd line antitubercular drugs, action, dose and common side effects.

Drug	Action	Dose (in mg/kg/day)	Common side effects
Amikacin	Bactericidal	12–18	Ototoxic, nephrotoxic
Kanamycin	Bactericidal	12–18	Ototoxic, nephrotoxic
Thioacetazone	Bacteriostatic	2.5	Gastrointestinal disturbance
Para-aminosalicyclic acid	Bacteriostatic	10–12	Gastrointestinal disturbance
Ethionamide	Bacteriostatic	15–20	Gastrointestinal disturbance
Cycloserine	Bacteriostatic	0.5–1 g	Psychosis

counter the peripheral neuropathy side effect of INH. Currently, Streptomycin is not routinely used.
- **Continuation phase:** Three drugs (HRE) is used for remaining duration, i.e., 10-16 months.

The dose and side effects of 1st line drugs are mentioned in the **Table 30.1**.

The 2nd line drugs are used in case of resistance against MTB. Common 2nd line antitubercular (ATT) drugs, their doses and side effects are mentioned in **Table 30.2**. Fluoroquinolones, such as ofloxacin, levofloxacin, moxifloxacin are also used as second line drugs.

- **Surgical treatment:** It varies from debridement, decompression of abscess, sequestrectomy and stabilization of the affected part. The details of procedure are discussed in the specific regional TB of hip, knee and spine.

TUBERCULOSIS OF THE HIP JOINT

INTRODUCTION

- TB of the hip is the second most common (15–20%) site of infection after TB of the spine (50%).
- It commonly affects **(Fig. 30.2):**
    - The roof of the acetabulum
    - Head of the femur
    - Neck of the femur (Babcock's triangle)
    - Greater trochanter
    - Trochanteric bursa.

PATHOLOGY OF HIP TB

The MTB reach the bone or synovium via the hematogenous route. The primary lesion could be in the bone or synovium. The initial lesion is tubercular granuloma with caseation and necrosis.

Primary lesion in the bone: If the lesion is in the femoral head, neck and trochanter, it rapidly enlarges and involves the bone forming abscesses and necrotic bone fragments.

Soon, lesions destroy the cortex, involve the joint, and further affect the synovium. The destruction of the acetabular roof is slow and joint involvement is late. However, once the roof is destroyed, it results in superior migration of the head femur.

Primary lesion in synovium: Sometimes, the lesion may directly start in the synovium, resulting in hyperemia and hypertrophy of synovium, leading to significant effusion. A pannus of granulation tissue extends from synovial reflection over the cartilage resulting in gradual articular cartilage destruction. The pannus also grows beneath the cartilage and separates it from the subchondral bone. The bone at the joint edge may show bony erosion.

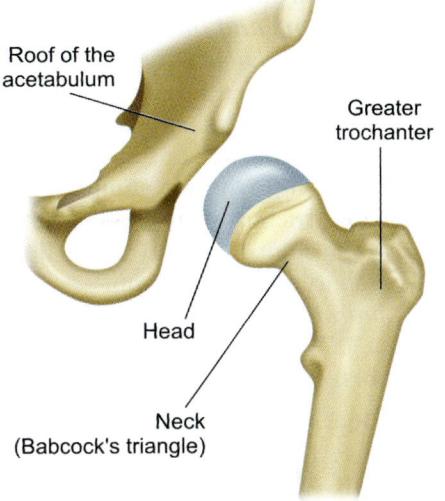

Fig. 30.2: Site(s) of tuberculosis around the hip.

Sequalae of hip tuberculosis:
- Damaged cartilage may promote *fibrous ankylosis of the hip joint.* Occasionally, bony ankylosis may occur if there is a secondary pyogenic infection. Extensive bony and soft tissue destruction results in subluxation/dislocation of the hip.
- The tubercular infection of the hip forms a *cold abscess,* which further damages the cartilage and breaks open out of the capsule. Usually, a cold abscess follows neurovascular bundles or fascial planes. The cold abscess from the hip may track toward the femoral triangle, posterior, inferior or medial to hip joint or in the ischiorectal fossa.

PATHOLOGICO-CLINICAL STAGES OF HIP TB

There are three pathological stages in the development of hip tuberculosis—stage of synovitis, arthritis and fibrous ankylosis. Each one has a different clinical presentation.
A. **Stage of synovitis** (stage of apparent lengthening)
B. **Stage of arthritis** (stage of apparent shortening)
C. **Stage of fibrous ankylosis/dislocation** (stage of true shortening)

A. **Stage of synovitis:** This stage is characterized by an *infection in the joint affecting the synovium and* ending with effusion and pannus formation. Due to effusion, the joint attains a position of ease or maximum capacity.
   Clinically, the hip assumes a position of *flexion, abduction, and external rotation* with the anterior superior iliac spine (ASIS) of the affected side at a lower level. This stage is also known as the *"stage of apparent lengthening."*
B. **Stage of arthritis:** This stage is characterized by the *destruction of articular cartilage* due to pannus, pus and destructive lysosomal enzymes in the joint.

Due to arthritis and adductor spasm, *clinically, the hip assumes a position of **flexion, adduction, and internal rotation*** with the ASIS of the affected side at a higher level. This stage is also known as the *"stage of apparent shortening."*

C. **Stage of dislocation or fibrous ankylosis:** This stage is characterized by *chronic infection and arthritis* damaging the hip joint and soft tissue due to:
- Ligament and capsular destruction
- Lesions in the acetabulum cause the widening and destruction of the acetabulum
- Destruction of the head of the femur and discrepant size of the head and the acetabulum
  The joint may end up in fibrous ankylosis, subluxation, or dislocation with a true shortening of the limb.

*Clinically the hip assumes a position of **flexion, adduction, and internal rotation*** with the ASIS of the affected side at a higher level. This stage is also known as the **"stage of true shortening."**

Table 30.3 summarizes the clinicopathological staging of hip TB.

CLINICAL FEATURES

In patients with hip TB, the clinical features comprise constitutional and local.
A. **Constitutional features:**
- Low-grade fever, which may typically show evening rise and night sweats. Patients may also complain of weight loss, loss of appetite, and malaise.
- *Features of TB in the primary area may be present*: Present or past history of TB in other areas of the body, e.g., pulmonary, genitourinary tract (GUT), and cervical lymph nodes.
- There may be history of contact with a person with TB.

B. **Local clinical features:**
Symptoms:
- *Localized hip pain* is the most common complaint, which is more at rest. Children may also have *night cries*.
- Patient may complain of *difficulty in standing, walking, or squatting*.

Signs:
- *Gait*: Stiff hip/antalgic gait
- *Muscle wasting* of the thigh and gluteal region may be noted.
- Scars from previous surgery (biopsy/debridement) may be present over the hip
- Discharging sinuses ±
- *Deformity:* The hip may show deformity as per the pathological stage **(Table 30.3)**.

Table 30.3: Clinicopathological staging of hip tuberculosis.			
Pathological stages	**Clinical appearance (deformity, limb length)**		**Cause**
Stage of synovitis	Abduction, flexion, ER	Apparent lengthening	Effusion causes joint to assume position of ease
Stage of arthritis	Adduction, flexion, IR	Apparent shortening	Spasm of flexor and adductors
Stage of deformity	Adduction, flexion, IR	True shortening	Arthritis, dislocation, subluxation

(ER: external rotation; IR: internal rotation)

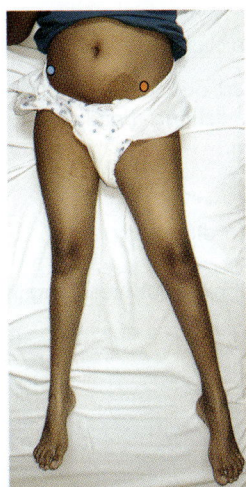

Fig. 30.3A: Stage of apparent lengthening of left hip—flexion, abduction and external rotation of left hip. Left ASIS (orange circle) is lower than right ASIS (blue circle).

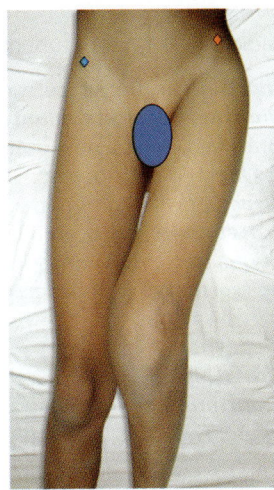

Fig. 30.3B: Stage of apparent shortening of left hip. Flexion, adduction and internal rotation deformity at the left hip. Left ASIS (orange star) is higher than right ASIS (blue star) (ASIS: anterior superior iliac spine).

- *Stage of apparent lengthening:* Flexion, abduction, and external rotation. anterior superior iliac spine (ASIS) would be at a lower level **(Fig. 30.3A)**.
- *Stage of apparent shortening:* Flexion, adduction, and internal rotation. ASIS would be at a higher level **(Fig. 30.3B)**.
- *Stage of true shortening:* Flexion, adduction, and internal rotation. ASIS would be at a higher level.
- *Hip joint line tenderness* is present.
- The *ROM of the hip is painful and restricted.*
- Often, there is a *shortening of the limb.*
- *Trendelenburg test* may be positive.
- *Telescopy test* may be positive if the hip is dislocated or resorbed.
- *Cold abscess* may be present in the femoral triangle/gluteal region/greater trochanter.

INVESTIGATIONS

The investigation of any musculoskeletal tuberculosis is three-pronged. Assess and stage the local pathology and detect the primary foci in the lung/GUT/urinary tract.
A. **General investigations for local pathology:**
   - ***Complete blood picture (CBP):*** Low hemoglobin, raised lymphocyte count
   - ***ESR:*** Raised
   - ***Mantoux test***
B. **Investigations for local pathology:**
   - ***X-ray of the hip:*** Anteroposterior (AP) and lateral view. It may reveal:
     - *Phemister triad*: Periarticular osteopenia, osteolytic lesions in bones (acetabulum roof, femur head and neck, greater trochanter) and decreased joint space **(Fig. 30.4)**.
     - Various types of radiological presentation of hip TB may be noted on hip X-ray **(Box 30.1)**.

> **Box 30.1:** Radiological types of tubercular hip (Shanmugasundaram classification).
>
> 1. **Normal hip:** Normal joint space, no major destruction; cyst in head, neck or acetabulum.
> 2. **Wandering/traveling acetabulum type:** Acetabular roof is affected; hence head migrates upwards and femoral head forms a new pseudo-joint proximally with ilium.
> 3. **Dislocated hip:** Hip is dislocated.
> 4. **Perthes' type:** X-ray features mimic Perthes disease.
> 5. **Protrusio acetabuli type:** Acetabulum cavity is eroded deep protruding into pelvis.
> 6. **Atrophic type:** Decreased joint space due to subchondral erosions.
> 7. **Pestle and mortar type:** Destruction of femoral head or acetabulum or both resulting in articular surface 'size' mismatch.
> 8. **Unclassified type:**
>   – **Ankylosed hip**
>   – **Pseudoarthrosis coxae:** Head and neck is destroyed
>   – **Triradiate:** The focus of TB infection is in floor.

- **MRI of the hip:** It can detect synovitis, effusion, bony lesions in the femoral head, neck, and acetabulum and periarticular abscess.
- **Pus aspiration:** Send for
  - For acid-fast bacillus (AFB) staining and MTB culture
  - *GeneXpert:* It is a type of real-time polymerase chain reaction (PCR) technique which can rapidly detect MTB in a sample within 2–3 hours. It is very sensitive in patients with HIV or immunocompromised status. It also provides information regarding "resistance against Rifampicin, if any".
- **Biopsy from bone and synovium:** The biopsy from the affected area is diagnostic. The material is sent for biopsy and GeneXpert.

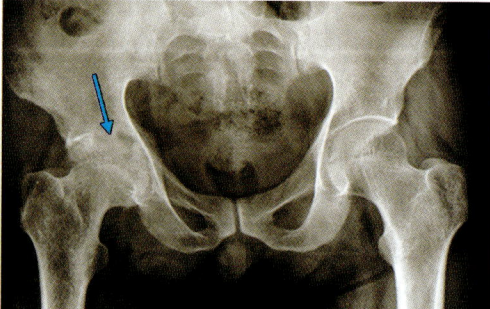

Fig. 30.4: X-ray of the pelvis showing osteolytic lesion in femoral head and joint space reduction in right hip, whereas left hip joint is normal.

C. **Investigations for primary foci:**
   - For pulmonary TB: Chest X-ray and sputum for AFB, culture
   - For GI and genitourinary TB: USG and CT abdomen and pelvis
   - Urine examination is performed to assess the genitourinary TB. It may show sterile pyuria.

TREATMENT

The principles of treatment of hip TB are:
- General support and treat active TB infection
- Control disease progression and manage complications
- Manage the sequelae of TB hip

A. **General management:**
   - Nutritional support: Balanced diet
   - Correct anemia

- *Antipyretics and analgesics:* To control fever and pain
- *Traction to correct and prevent deformity:* Especially in synovitis or early arthritis stage where the contractures are not established **(Fig. 30.5)**.

B. **Medical management:** *Daily* antitubercular treatment for 12–18 months
   - *Isoniazid (INH):* 5 mg/kg/day
   - *Rifampicin (RIF):* 10 mg/kg/day
   - *Ethambutol (ETM):* 15 mg/kg/day
   - *Pyrazinamide (PYZ):* 20 mg/kg/day
   - *Vitamin B_6:* Pyridoxine (10 mg) to counter the peripheral neuropathy effect of INH.

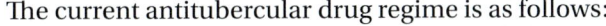

Fig. 30.5: Above knee skin traction in a patient with left hip TB.

The current antitubercular drug regime is as follows:
- *The intensive phase of 2 months:* HRZE (INH + RIF + PYZ + ETM)
- *Continuation phase of 10–18 months:* HRE. The continuation phase is longer in musculoskeletal TB and can go on from 10–18 months as per physician's discretion and response of TB to ATT.

C. **Surgical:** There are different options in various stages of the disease:
   Early stages of the disease: Stage of synovitis, early lytic lesion with normal hip joint
   - *Synovectomy and debridement of the joint:* Open/arthroscopic
   - Curettage of the lesion and drainage of cold abscess

   Late stages of the disease: Advanced arthritis/fibrous ankylosis/dislocated or subluxated hip. There are various options, such as:
   - *Total hip replacement:* It provides a painless, stable, and mobile hip **(Fig. 30.6A)**
   - *Arthrodesis* implies surgical fusion of the joint surfaces, which provides a painless, stable hip but no movement **(Fig. 30.6B)**. However, post-arthrodesis, the patient cannot squat/sit cross-leg.
   - *Excision arthroplasty:* It is also known as *Girdlestone arthroplasty*, which provides a painless, but unstable hip with shortening of the limb **(Fig. 30.6C)**. Therefore, patient can walk (short-limb gait), squat and sit cross-leg.

> **Note:** Girdlestone arthroplasty is an excision arthroplasty performed in advanced stages of TB hip wherein the damaged head and neck of the femur are excised.

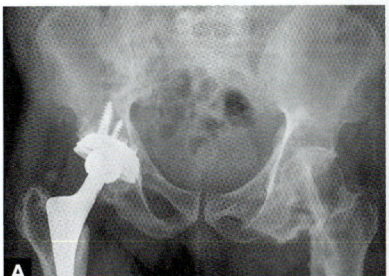
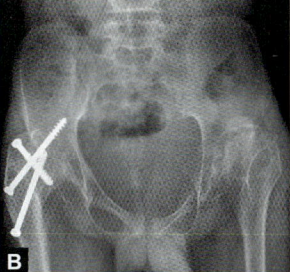
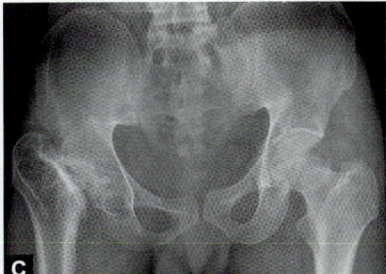

Figs. 30.6A to C: (A) Total hip replacement of right hip; (B) Arthrodesis of right hip; (C) Girdlestone excision arthroplasty of right hip (the femoral head and neck has been excised).

TUBERCULOSIS OF THE KNEE JOINT

Tubercular lesions in the knee could be present in:
- *Femur*: Lower end
- *Tibia*: Upper end
- *Synovium* of the joint.

PATHOLOGICAL STAGES OF KNEE TB

Similar to the hip joint, there are three pathological stages:
1. **Stage of synovitis/bony lesion**
2. **Stage of arthritis**
3. **Stage of triple deformity/triple dislocation:** Triple dislocation is a misnomer, as there is no dislocation. A combination of three deformities characterizes this stage—
    i. Flexion deformity of the knee joint
    ii. Posterior subluxation of the knee joint
    iii. External rotation of the leg

   The combination of three deformities is known as triple dislocation/triple deformity **(Figs. 30.7A and B)**. It is due to:
   - Joint destruction, capsule and ligament damage
   - Spasm of the lateral hamstring (biceps femoris tendon) typically results in external rotation deformity.

Later, patient will have *fixed deformities* with *fibrous ankylosis*.

CLINICAL FEATURES

A. **Constitutional features:** Similar to hip TB
B. **Local clinical features**

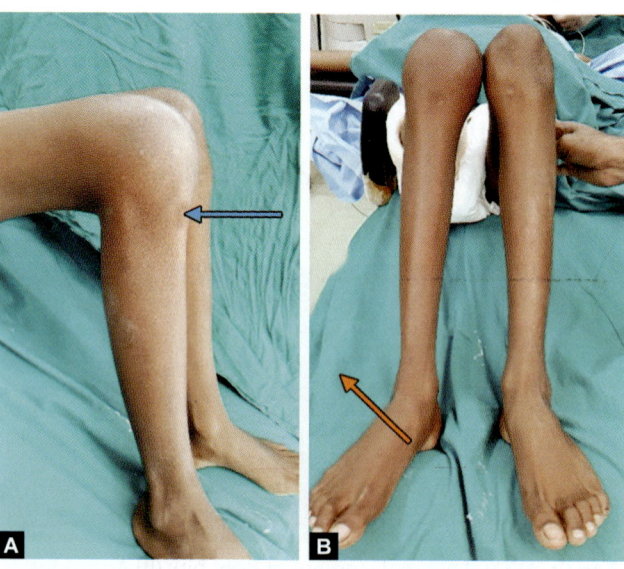

Figs. 30.7A and B: Triple deformity of TB knee: (A) Flexion deformity and posterior subluxation of right knee (blue arrow); (B) External rotation deformity of right leg (orange arrow).

Symptoms:
- Pain and swelling over the knee joint. Pain is felt more at night
- Difficulty in walking, sitting cross leg/squatting.

Signs:
- Flexion deformity is common. Later, there may be triple deformity
- Wasting of the quadriceps muscle
- Synovial hypertrophy and effusion **(Fig. 30.8)**.
- The joint line is tender.
- The movements are painful and decreased.
- Cold abscess, or sinuses may be present around the knee with puckered skin.

INVESTIGATIONS

Almost all investigations are similar to one discussed in general description, except few such as:
A. **X-ray of the knee:**
   - Periarticular osteopenia, erosion of articular surface with lytic lesions in the bones (femur/tibia), and reduction of joint space (*Phemister triad*) **(Fig. 30.9)**
   - Deformity.
B. **MRI of the knee:**
   - Synovial hypertrophy
   - Cold abscess
   - Damage of articular cartilage.
C. **Pus aspiration, synovial and bone biopsy:** The samples must be sent for AFB staining, cultures, GeneXpert, and biopsy.
D. **Evaluate the primary foci** in lung/GIT/gut.

TREATMENT

A. **Conservative:**
   - General and medical treatment (as described in introduction section/Hip TB-vide supra)
   - Splinting or below-knee traction (skin/skeletal) prevents spasm or flexion deformity, especially in the early stages of synovitis or early arthritis. *If there is triple deformity*, it requires biaxial traction to correct the deformity **(Fig. 30.10)**.
   - Once the deformity is corrected, start gentle mobilization of the knee and muscle strengthening.
B. **Surgical treatment**
   - Abscess drainage, synovectomy and curettage of the bony lesion
   - *Later stages of arthritis or painful fibrous ankylosis*: Arthrodesis or total knee replacement **(Figs. 30.11A and B)**.

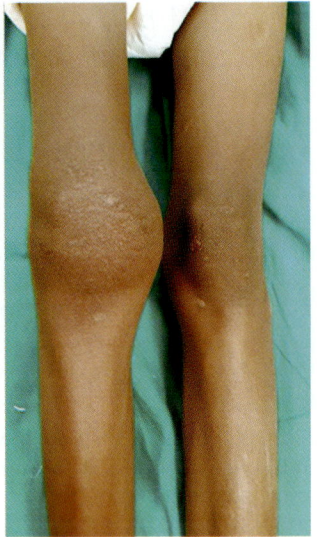

Fig. 30.8: Swelling present over the right knee.

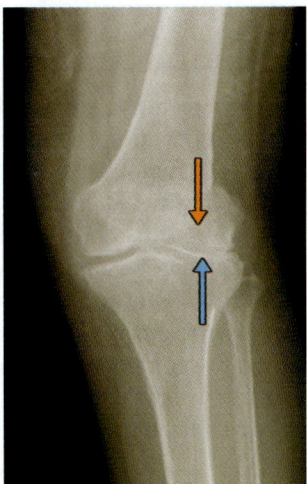

Fig. 30.9: X-ray of the left knee showing reduction in lateral joint space (blue arrow) and osteolytic lesions in lateral femoral condyle (orange arrow). Note-medial joint space is normal.

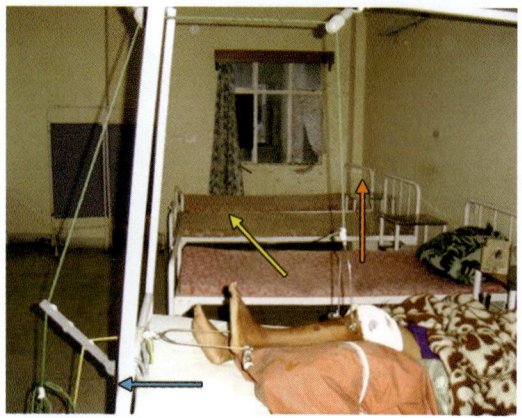

Fig. 30.10: Biaxial traction (lower and upper tibia) in TB knee. Orange and blue arrow indicate vertical and horizontal component of the traction. Yellow arrow shows resultant vector.

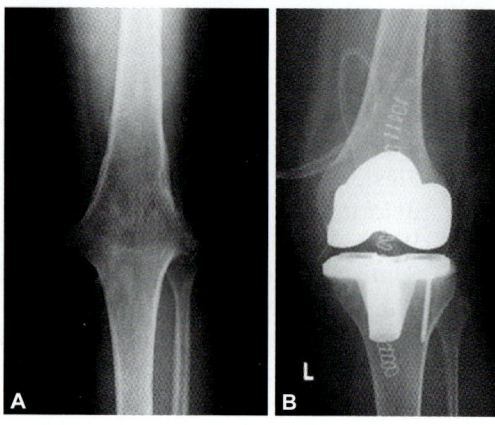

Figs. 30.11A and B: (A) Arthrodesis of left knee (note no joint space and crossing trabeculae); (B) Total replacement of left knee.

TUBERCULOSIS OF THE SPINE

(Syn: Pott's spine/Caries spine)

INTRODUCTION

- ***Commonest*** among all bone tuberculosis (TB) (50% of all cases)
- The most common region to get affected is the ***dorsal spine (42%),*** followed by the Lumbar (26%), dorsolumbar (12%), cervical (12%), cervicodorsal (5%) and lumbosacral (3%).
- ***It is always secondary to a primary elsewhere***: The primary may remain overt/covert in lymph node, chest, gastrointestinal or genitourinary system. The hematogenous tubercle bacilli spreads into the vertebra via 'Paravertebral Batson's venous plexus'.
- **Surgical anatomy:** *Blood supply of vertebra follows an embryological pattern wherein branches of segmental intercostal or lumbar artery supply adjacent halves of 2 vertebra, i.e., the lower half of the upper vertebra and upper half of the lower vertebra and the intervening intervertebral disc* **(Fig. 30.12)**. This occurs as this vertebral complex (halves of upper and lower vertebra) and intervening disc develops from the same somite.

Due to this peculiar blood supply, the MTB infection is more common in the 'paradiscal region' of two adjacent vertebrae.

Further, ***Batson's paravertebral venous plexus*** in the vertebra is a valve-less system that allows free flow of blood in both directions depending upon the pressure generated by the intra-abdominal and intrathoracic cavities following strenuous activities like coughing. The spread of the TB infection via the intraosseous venous system may be responsible for central vertebral body tubercular lesions.

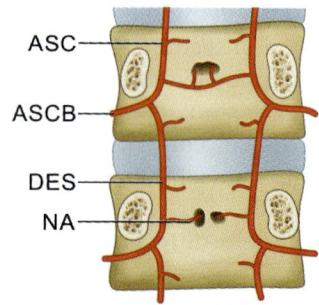

Fig. 30.12: Blood supply of adjacent vertebra via a common ASCB.

(ASCB: anterior spinal canal branch; ASC: ascending branch; DES: descending branch; NA: nutrient artery)

COMMON SITE FOR SPINE TUBERCULOSIS (FIG. 30.13)

- **Paradiscal (90%):** It is the commonest site of vertebral TB, adjacent to disc spaces.
- **Anterior:** Over the anterior surface of the vertebral body.
- **Central:** Center of the vertebral body.
- **Posterior:** In neural arches—pedicle, lamina, transverse, and spinous process.

ETIOPATHOGENESIS

The primary source of Mycobacterium Tubercle bacilli (MTB) in the bone is usually from the lymph nodes, lungs, genitourinary or gastrointestinal tract. The MTB reaches the vertebra via a hematogenous route, arterial or venous.

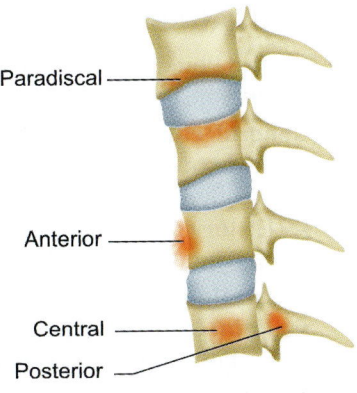

Fig. 30.13: Site(s) of tuberculosis (TB) in the spine.

An arterial arcade forms a rich vascular plexus in each vertebra's subchondral region, which facilitates the hematogenous spread of the infection in the paradiscal regions. From visceral organs, it reaches the vertebra via prevertebral Batson's venous plexus.

Most commonly, MTB affects the paradiscal area (90%). Sometimes, it can also affect multiple vertebrae or can have skip lesions. The pathogenesis of Spinal TB is discussed in **Flowchart 30.1**.

Post-treatment, the spinal TB heals with the formation of new bone at the site of lysis, resulting in **bony ankylosis** of the vertebrae (*Note: In peripheral joints, the sequelae of TB is 'fibrous ankylosis'*).

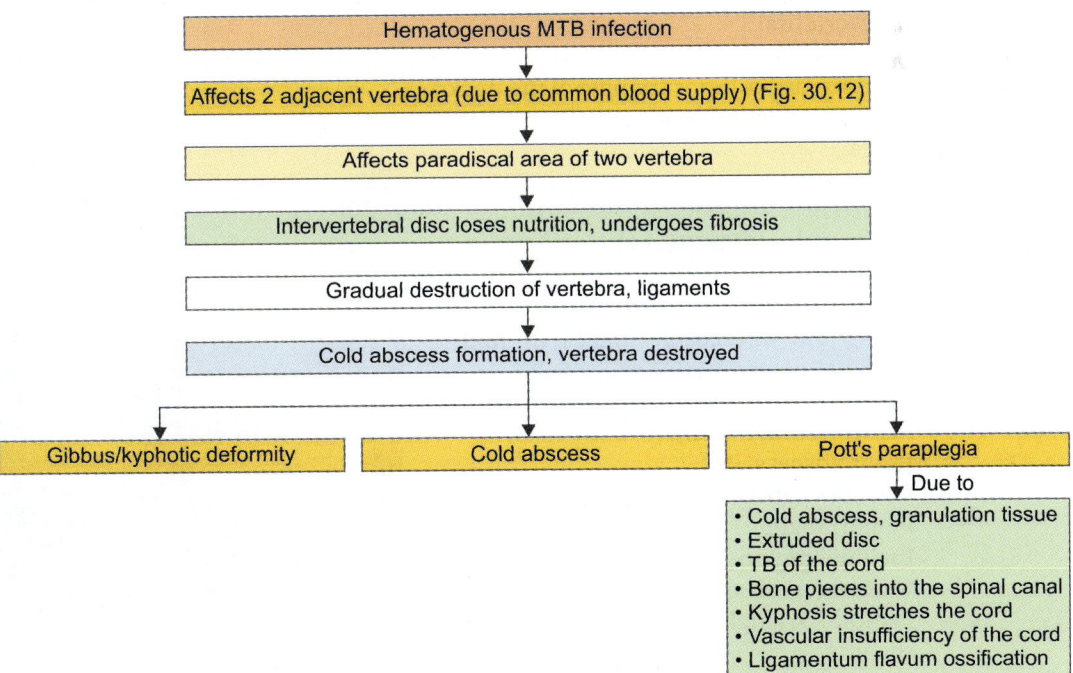

Flowchart 30.1: Pathogenesis of tubercular spine.

CLINICAL FEATURES

Sir Percival Pott described the classic symptoms of TB of the spine as *constitutional symptoms, back pain, spasm, deformity, cold abscess, and 'Pott's paraplegia.'*

A. **General/constitutional features:**
   - Fever (evening rise of low-grade temperature), night sweats
   - Weight loss, loss of appetite, and malaise
   - History of contacts with patients of TB, history of TB in other parts of the body (lung, GIT, gut, lymph node).

B. **Local clinical features:**
   - ***Pain:*** It is one of the most common features of the TB spine.
     - Local moderate-severe pain over neck/back (depending upon region). The pain is often present at night as *night cries*.
     - There is an associated paraspinal spasm.
     - Pain could be referred to the limbs if there is root compression.
   - ***Stiffness in the back***: It is felt due to paraspinal spasm.
   - ***The kyphotic deformity (Gibbus)*** is observed due to vertebral destruction. There are three types of deformity—knuckle, angular and round back.
     - *Knuckle*: Single vertebra destroyed
     - *Angular*: Two to three vertebra destroyed
     - *Round back deformity*: Four or more vertebra destroyed.
   - ***Cold abscess formation:*** It is almost invariable in spine TB and usually tracks along the lines of nerve plexus or musculofascial planes. Hence, usually, it is detected far from the site of the original infection. The location of cold abscesses in TB of various spine regions is mentioned below:
     - *Cervical TB:*
       - Paravertebral
       - Retropharyngeal
       - Anterior or posterior triangle of the neck
       - Infraclavicular region
       - Axilla
       - Mediastinum.
     - *Thoracic TB:*
       - Paravertebral **(Fig. 30.14)**
       - Mediastinal
       - Parasternal
       - Along the intercostal spaces in mid-axillary line or anterior chest wall.
     - *Lumbar TB:*
       - Paravertebral
       - Psoas abscess
       - Iliac fossa abscess
       - Petit triangle
       - Inguinal region
       - Gluteal region along the sciatic nerve
       - Femoral triangle along femoral nerve sheath.

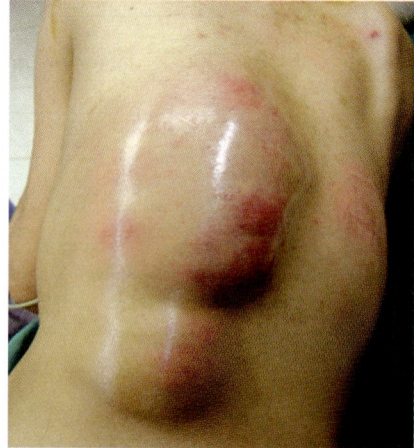

Fig. 30.14: Large paravertebral cold abscess in the thoracolumbar region.

- **Bony tenderness** is present over the affected vertebra. **Paraspinal muscle spasm** is also present.
- **Movements:** The movements of the affected region of the spine are decreased and painful.
- **Neurological assessment:** A detailed neurological evaluation of upper and lower limbs, including bladder and bowel status, is necessary as cold abscesses and other debris often compress the spinal cord or nerve roots.

C. **Pott's paraplegia/Tubercular paraplegia:**
Definition: The paralysis of lower limbs (paraplegia) due to compression of the spinal cord and/or nerve roots due to tuberculosis of the spine is known as Pott's paraplegia.

The reasons for paraplegia are compression/involvement of the spinal cord are due to:
Extrinsic/Mechanical causes (outside the spinal cord)
- Caseous material, granulation tissue
- Sequestrated and extruded disc, vertebral bony fragments
- Vertebral canal stenosis, and kyphotic deformity

Intrinsic causes (in the spinal cord)
- Prolonged cord stretching
- Cord edema, infarction and myelomalacia
- Spinal artery thrombosis
- Tubercular meningomyelitis
- Syringomyelia changes: Dilation of the central spinal canal.

Classification of Pott's paraplegia: It is based on the *time of onset* and *type of motor weakness*.

1. **Time of onset of paraplegia:** Early (within two years of disease) and late-onset (after two years)
2. **Based on motor weakness:**

1. **Based on the time of onset:** *Griffith's classification*
    - Early-onset paraplegia: Within two years of disease onset:
        - During the active phase of TB.
        - It occurs due to pressure on the cord due to granulation tissues, abscess, mechanical debris, and arterial thrombosis.
    - Late-onset paraplegia: After two years of disease onset
        - During the healed phase of TB.
        - It occurs due to mechanical pressure on the cord due to a transverse ridge in the spinal canal with severe kyphosis, ligament ossification, and dural fibrosis.
2. **Based on motor weakness:**
    - Stage I: Patient unaware of deficit; clinician detects Babinski/ankle clonus
    - Stage II: Patient aware of the deficit but walks with support
    - Stage III: Nonambulatory, *paralysis in extension*, sensory deficit less than 50%
    - Stage IV: Nonambulatory, *paralysis in flexion*, sensory deficit greater than 50%; sphincters involved.

INVESTIGATIONS

The investigations performed are general, for local disease, and to detect the primary foci of infection.

- **General investigations:**
  - CBP: Elevated lymphocytes, low Hb (if anemia)
  - ESR: Elevated
  - Mantoux test
- **Investigations for local disease:** The local disease is assessed with the help of a *plain X-ray, MRI, and bone scan*. However, the confirmation of the disease is established by *biopsy*.
  - *Plain X-ray* (**Fig. 30.15**): Various findings noted are:
    - Narrowed Disc space ⎫ These are the earliest changes
    - Localized osteopenia ⎭
    - Osteolytic lesions in the vertebra
    - Kyphosis
    - *Pre-/para-vertebral abscess:* In thoracic spine TB, paravertebral abscess gives a typical fusiform or *"bird nest"* appearance (**Fig. 30.16**).
    - Disuse osteoporosis

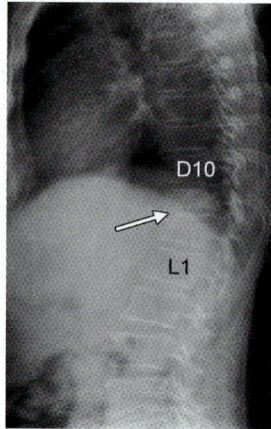

Fig. 30.15: Narrowed disc space between D11 and D12 vertebra.

Concertina collapse: Central body TB could result in collapse of vertebral body
Aneurysmal sign: Erosion of anterior part of body due to anterior surface TB

- *MRI scan of the affected part of the spine:* Various findings noted are:
  - Vertebral edema and destruction, cold abscess (**Fig. 30.17**)
  - Spinal cord—edema, compression, and myelomalacia
- *Bone scan:* It is performed to detect skip lesions, which may be seen in 15% of cases.

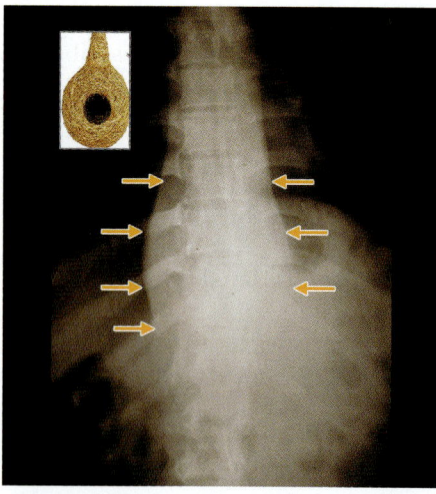

Fig. 30.16: Bird nest appearance in thoracic spine TB. Inset picture shows bird nest.

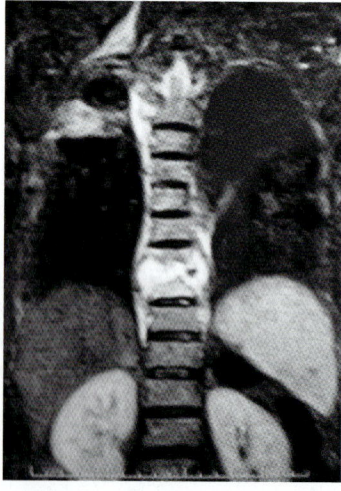

Fig. 30.17: Magnetic resonance imaging of dorsal spine shows vertebral destruction and paravertebral abscess.

- **Vertebral biopsy:** Image/CT-guided biopsy of the affected vertebra is a *'diagnostic investigation'* of spinal TB. The aspirated material is sent for:
  - Acid-fast bacillus (AFB) staining
  - Culture and susceptibility (C/S) along with drug resistance testing
  - GeneXpert test
  - Biopsy
- **Investigations to detect primary foci of TB, if any**
  - Sputum for AFB, C/S, PCR for MTB and *Chest X-ray* to rule out pulmonary TB
  - USG/CT scan of abdomen and pelvis to rule out abdominopelvic TB
  - Mantoux test: A negative Mantoux is more helpful as it may rule out TB
  - Sterile pyuria may indicate TB of the urinary system.

TREATMENT

Most cases of spinal TB respond to conservative treatment involving general measures, ATT and braces. Few selected cases may require surgical management.

Tuli's middle path regime: Conservative treatment is for all the patients, while few require surgery.

A. **General:**
   - *Rest:* It is essential for pain relief to prevent further collapse of the vertebra and any possible neurological deficit.
   - *Nutritional support* must be provided as these patients are malnourished. Correct underlying anemia.
   - *Analgesics* for pain relief and *muscle relaxants* (tizanidine, thiocolchicoside) to reduce muscle spasm.
   - If the patient has paraplegia, adequate care must be provided to prevent the complications of recumbency *(for the care of people with paraplegia—read Chapter 16 on spine injury).*

B. **Medical treatment and brace support:** ATT with spinal orthosis is the mainstay of spinal TB in most cases.
   - *Standard ATT* for 12–18 months must be instituted. *2 months of Intensive phase (HREZ)* followed by *10–16 months of maintenance phase (HRE).*
   - *Orthotic support* to the affected part of the spine
     - Cervical spine TB: Hard cervical collar/four post brace
     - Dorsal spine TB: Taylors brace or custom-made jackets **(Fig. 30.18)**
     Braces are usually continued for 8–12 months, depending upon the extent of the lesion.
   - Gradual mobilization with braces once pain at the local site decrease.

C. **Surgical treatment:** It is indicated if there is—
   - Paraparesis develops during treatment, increasing neurological deficit
   - No improvement in paraparesis with treatment
   - Large prevertebral abscess causing dyspnea/difficulty in deglutition (in cervical spine TB)

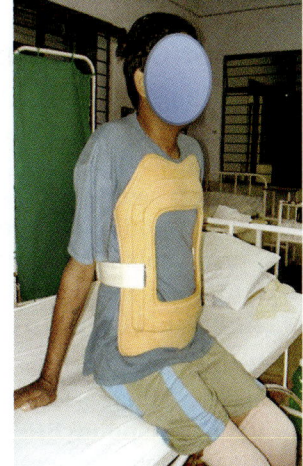

Fig. 30.18: Custom made brace for dorsal spine TB.

- Progressive deformity, Kyphosis greater than 40°
- Pott's stage IV paraplegia.

The principles of surgical treatment of spinal tuberculosis are:
- *Debridement* of infected bone and *drainage of the paravertebral abscess*
- *Decompression* of the spinal canal
- *Correction of the spinal deformity using structural grafting ± cage*
- *Instrumentation* (usually posterior) to support the vertebral column after debridement and grafting **(Fig. 30.19)**.

Various surgical procedures performed are:
- ***Anterolateral decompression:*** Resection of part of rib + transverse process + pedicles + part of vertebral body
- ***Hong-kong procedure:*** Anterior decompression via thoracotomy + abscess drainage + debridement + canal decompression + bone grafting and instrumentation.
- ***Costotransversectomy:*** Resection of part of rib + transverse process
- ***Laminectomy:*** It is performed only in case of posterior element disease or spinal tumor syndrome.

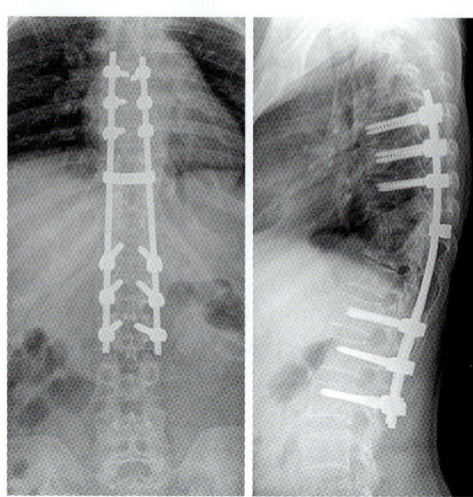

Fig. 30.19: AP and lateral view of dorsolumbar spine showing spinal instrumentation after debridement and decompression.

COMPLICATIONS OF SPINAL TUBERCULOSIS
- Early- or late-onset quadriplegia/paraplegia (depending upon the level of infection)
- Bladder and bowel involvement
- Cold abscess
- Deformity.

PROGNOSTIC SIGNS
The prognosis of spinal TB is better, if:
- Short duration of disease
- Early onset paraplegia
- Younger patients with slow progression of the disease
- <60° kyphotic deformity
- Normal spinal cord on MRI.

DIFFERENTIAL DIAGNOSIS
- **Brucella spondylitis:** It is common in the lumbar region. The disc involvement is late, the vertebral body is less involved, and the paraspinal abscess is well localized and small.
- **Pyogenic spondylitis:** It is common in the lumbar region. Disc involvement is early, while the paraspinal abscess is less well-defined.
- **Secondaries:** The disc space is normal, the pedicle is involved, and there is no abscess formation.

TUBERCULOSIS OF SHOULDER

- Tuberculosis of shoulder is uncommon, and affects adults.
- There are three clinical types of TB shoulder:
    a. **Caries sicca (dry variety):** It is the classic dry form of TB shoulder. There is marked wasting of muscles around shoulder and painful restriction of ROM.
    b. **Caries exudata:** It is characterized by swelling, sinus and cold abscess formation.
    c. **Caries mobile:** The patient has restriction of active movements while passive is preserved.
- **Diagnosis:** X-ray shows osteopenia of involved bones, joint space reduction, lytic lesions and destruction of joint surface.
- **Management:** Biopsy would confirm the diagnosis. ATT must be continued on standard lines. Arthroscopic debridement may be required to excise synovium, granulation tissue and pannus.

TUBERCULAR OSTEOMYELITIS

SALIENT FEATURES

- Tuberculosis of bones (TB osteomyelitis) is uncommon than tuberculosis of joints (TB arthritis).
- The periosteal reaction and sequestrum formation in TB osteomyelitis is less common than pyogenic osteomyelitis.
- **TB dactylitis (Spina ventosa):** TB of small bones of hand and feet is called as TB dactylitis. It presents as swelling around the affected bone. The X-rays of spina ventosa show a cystic cavity with wind-blown widening of the cavity and central lucency.

OTHER MUSCULOSKELETAL TB

Poncet tubercular rheumatism: It is a polyarthritis which resembles RA in patients with TB. Such patients should be treated with ATT and polyarthritis resolves.

HANSEN'S DISEASE

DEFINITION

It is a chronic infectious disease caused by *Mycobacterium leprae* characterized by one or more of the following features:
- Hypopigmented or erythematous skin patches with sensory loss
- Peripheral nerve involvement characterized by:
    - Sensory loss
    - Motor weakness in hand, feet, or face.

ETIOLOGY

Mycobacterium leprae is the cause of Hansen's disease. It has several characteristics:
- It is an acid-fast bacillus (AFB)
- It grows very slowly in *macrophages and Schwann cells*
- It *prefers low temperatures (27–32°C) to proliferate, therefore, its affection involves the skin and superficial peripheral nerves.* It is also found in respiratory tract.

CLASSIFICATION

- Lepromatous leprosy
- Borderline leprosy
- Tuberculoid leprosy
- Indeterminate leprosy.

PATHOGENESIS

Leprosy infection possibly happens via:
- Respiratory tract: Main route
- Broken skin.

After infection, a variable response happens:
- **Indeterminate leprosy:** With the adequate immune response, vague hypopigmented patches on the skin. Mostly resolves spontaneously
- **Tuberculoid leprosy:**
  - Due to delayed hypersensitivity to *M. leprae*
  - Focal, well-circumscribed granuloma.
- **Lepromatous leprosy:**
  - In patients who are unable to mount effective cell-mediated immunity against *M. leprae*
  - Diffuse granuloma, the entire body's skin may be affected
- **Borderline leprosy:** Indeterminate leprosy with some features of Tuberculoid and Lepromatous.

Peripheral nerves are always affected in leprosy especially cutaneous nerves and some other major nerve trunks. Affected nerves undergo:
- Thickening of epi- and peri-neurium and endoneurial fibrosis
- Demyelination and axonal degeneration
- In chronic Hansen's, the nerves could be damaged due to immune complexes or so-called 'reactions.'

CLINICAL FEATURES

Skin Involvement

- The Hansen's disease results in affecting skin and nerves
- Hypopigmented skin patches with impaired sensibility
- *Skin lesion in Tuberculoid leprosy*: Sparse, well demarcated, anesthetic
- *Skin lesion in Lepromatous leprosy:* Diffuse, extensive, some sensory impairment, leonine facies, nasal septum destruction.

Peripheral Nerve Involvement
- Thickened and tender nerves. Following nerves are commonly affected:
  - Ulnar nerve
  - Median nerve
  - Radial cutaneous nerve
  - Greater auricular
  - Common peroneal nerve
  - Posterior tibial nerve
- **Sensory loss:** Trophic ulcers, especially in hand and feet
- **Muscle palsy:** Claw hand, foot drop, contractures
- Charcot's joint occurs in very late stages.

INVESTIGATIONS
- Skin smear
- Nerve biopsy.

TREATMENT
The Hansen's diseases is typically managed medically with antileprosy drugs—Rifampicin, Dapsone and Clofazimine. The orthopaedic management depends upon the early, late palsy or chronic residual sensorimotor deficit.
- **Early palsy: "Stage of active neuritis"**
  - *Oral steroids*: Reversal of neuritis
  - Splintage to prevent deformity
  - Physiotherapy to mobilize the joint and prevent stiffness
- **Late stage of nerve involvement: "Stage of perineural abscess"**
  - Drainage of abscess
  - Neurolysis of nerves
- **Chronic nerve palsy: Sensorimotor deficit**
  - *Motor palsy:*
    - Reconstructive surgery—
      - *Correct deformity*: Contracture release
      - *Tendon transfer* to restore power in paralysed joints
    - Orthotic support to the limb: AFO for foot drop
  - *Sensory loss:* It leads to neuropathic ulcers, especially in the foot.
    - Rule out osteomyelitis of underlying bone and treat it
    - Debridement of ulcer
    - Total contact cast with Bohler's walking frame
    - Prevent further ulcerations: Soft MCR footwear
    - Correct deformity to prevent further ulcer formation
    - Care of foot.

Notes

SECTION 5

Arthritis

SECTION OUTLINE

31. Overview of Arthritis, Osteoarthrosis Knee
    - Arthritis—General Descriptions and Classification
    - Primary Degenerative Osteoarthrosis of the Knee
32. Rheumatoid Arthritis
33. Seronegative Arthritis and Other Arthritis
    - Seronegative Arthritis—Ankylosing Spondylitis, Psoriatic Arthritis, Reactive Arthritis, and Enteropathic Arthritis
    - Crystal Arthritis—Gout, Pseudogout
    - Neuropathic Arthritis/Charcot's Arthropathy
    - Miscellaneous Arthritis—SLE Related Arthritis, Hemophilic Arthritis, Alkaptonuric Arthritis, and Juvenile Rheumatoid Arthritis, Mseleni Joint Disease, and Kashin Beck Disease

Arthritis

CHAPTER 31

Overview of Arthritis, Osteoarthrosis Knee

DEFINITION OF ARTHRITIS

Arthritis is a condition wherein the *joint cartilage is damaged*, resulting in pain and stiffness in the joint.

Figures 31.1A and B show arthroscopic image of the joints with a normal cartilage and damaged cartilage of an arthritic joint.

Note: Arthralgia refers to joint pain without any damage to the cartilage.

CLASSIFICATION OF ARTHRITIS

Arthritis can be classified in several ways, such as etiology, seropositivity (or seronegative), and number of joints involved.

Etiological

- ***Infective***
  - Septic
  - Tubercular
  - Others—viral, fungal.

Note

Clinical manifestation of an arthritic joint
- Joint line tenderness
- Crepitus
- Painfully restricted range of motion

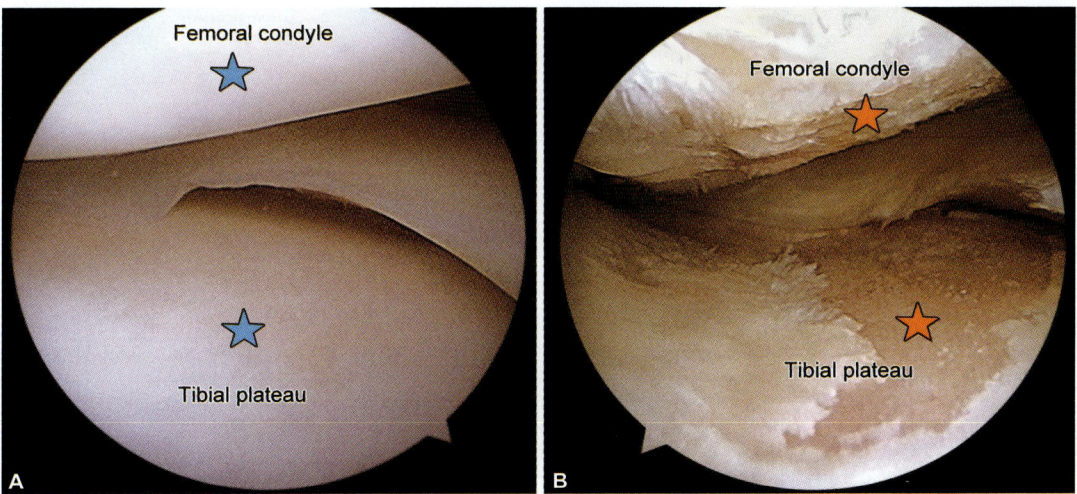

Figs. 31.1A and B: (A) Arthroscopic image of cartilage of a normal joint (blue stars); (B) Damaged cartilage of arthritic joint with exposed subchondral bone (orange stars).

- **Inflammatory**
  - *Seropositive (RA factor positive)*: Rheumatoid arthritis
  - *Seronegative*: A class of arthritis with RA factor negative
    - Ankylosing spondylitis
    - Reiter's disease
    - Psoriatic
    - Enteropathic.
- **Degenerative:** Typically known as primary degenerative osteoarthritis/osteoarthrosis
- **Metabolic:** Gout, pseudogout
- **Traumatic**
- **Neuropathic (Charcot's):** It is *only arthritis that results in painless joint destruction*, whereas all other etiologies result in a painful joint. The common causes of Charcot's arthropathy are:
  - Diabetes mellitus: Most common cause of neuropathic arthropathy
  - Leprosy (Hansen's)
  - Syringomyelia
  - Syphilis.
- **Associated with the bleeding disorder:** Hemophilia.

Seropositive and Seronegative

Another method of classifying arthritis is seropositive or seronegative arthritis, which is based upon the presence or absence of the rheumatoid arthritis (RA) factor. The presence of the RA factor in serum is known as seropositive arthritis. In contrast, arthritis without RA factor in serum is known as seronegative arthritis. Seronegative arthritis could be inflammatory or non-inflammatory **(Flowchart 31.1)**.

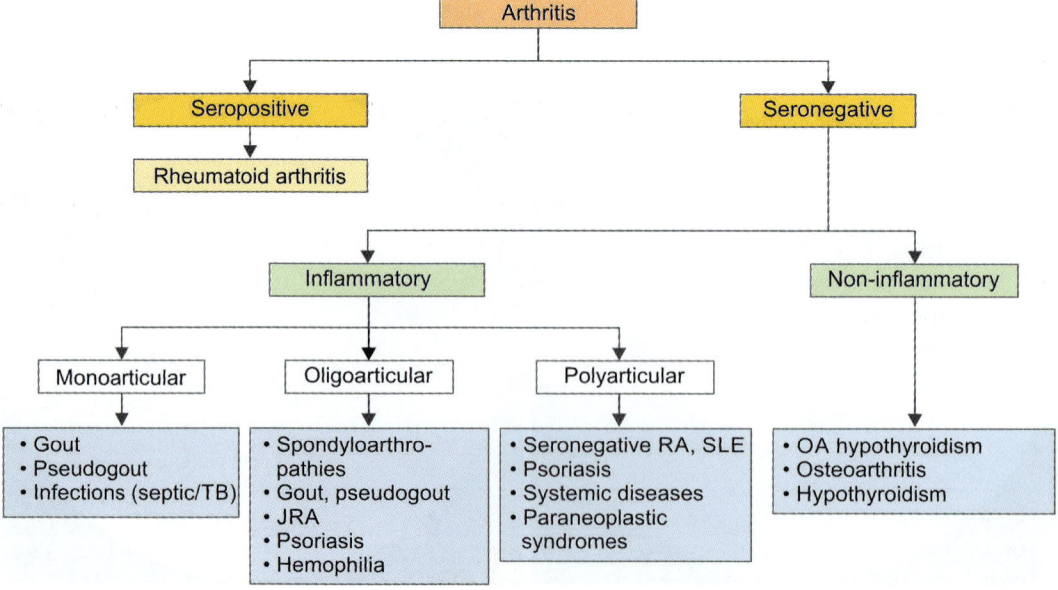

Flowchart 31.1: Seropositive (RA factor +) and seronegative arthropathy.

(RA: rheumatoid arthritis; SLE: systemic lupus erythematosus; OA: osteoarthritis; JRA: juvenile rheumatoid arthritis)

Number of Joints Involved

- **Monoarthritis** is when commonly a single joint is involved at a time, e.g., gout, infective, or post-traumatic.
- **Oligoarthritis** is when two-four joints are involved, e.g., juvenile idiopathic arthritis, spondyloarthropathy.
- **Polyarthritis** is when five or more joints are involved, e.g., rheumatoid arthritis, SLE.

OSTEOARTHRITIS/OSTEOARTHROSIS

▌INTRODUCTION AND DEFINITION

The term "osteoarthritis" is a misnomer as it is not primarily an inflammatory disorder. Hence, the appropriate term is *osteoarthrosis (OA)*.

Osteoarthrosis is defined as wear and tear-related progressive damage of the articular cartilage followed by new bone formation as osteophytes.

Before the understanding of various arthritis, one must understand the basic structural anatomy of a synovial joint.

▌SURGICAL ANATOMY OF A SYNOVIAL JOINT (FIG. 31.2)

A synovial joint is formed between two bones. The ends of the bone are covered by hyaline cartilage and synovium covers the joint from inside. The subchondral bone supports the cartilage **(Fig. 31.2)**.

- **Synovium:** It has two types of cells—type A and type B.
  - **Type A cells** have *macrophage-like action*, which helps clear the joint debris and acts as the first line of defense against microbes.
  - **Type B cells** *release hyaluron*. The presence of hyaluron in synovial fluid help *lubricate the joint and nourish the cartilage*. The synovial fluid has several characteristics, such as:
    - It is an **ultradialysate of blood mixed with Hyaluronic acid (HA).** It is 96% water and its pH is 7.3–7.6. Synovial fluid does not clot.
    - It has **thixotropic properties,** i.e., viscosity decreases with increased rates of shear and allows non-Newtonian kinetics
    - **Function of synovial fluid**—lubricates, nourishes and protects the joint.
- **Hyaline cartilage** covers the end of the articulating bones. *Hyaline cartilage is avascular, alymphatic, and aneural.* Nutrition of hyaline

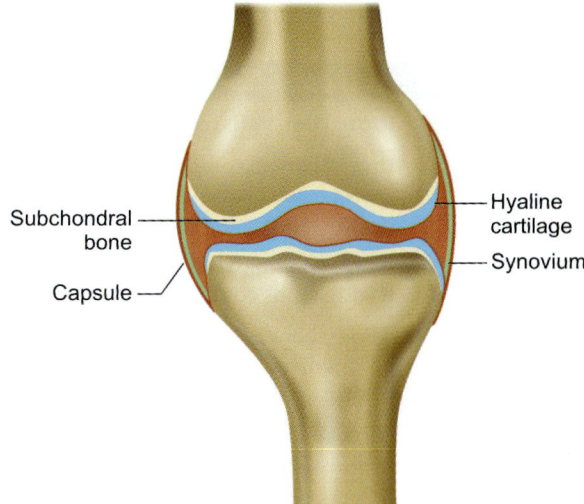

Fig. 31.2: Surgical anatomy of a synovial joint.

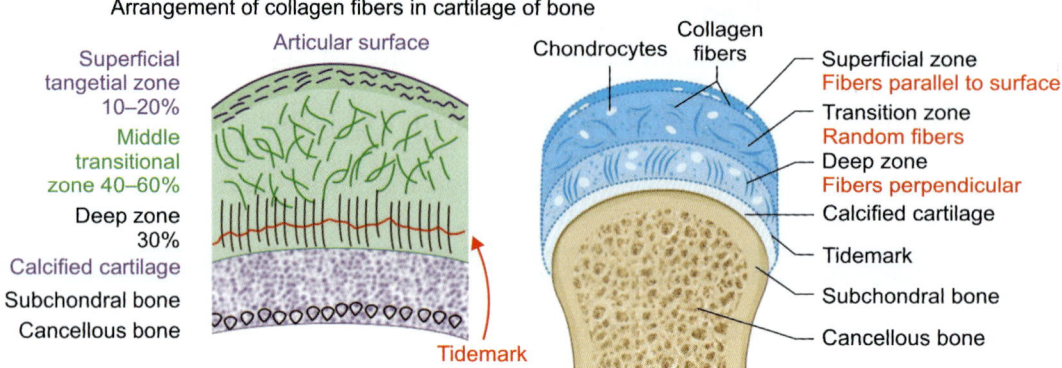

Fig. 31.3: Layers of cartilages.

cartilage is derived from *synovial fluid diffusion and subchondral marrow*. Since the hyaline cartilage is almost avascular, it results in poor regeneration capacity 'as hyaline cartilage' following the injury. And therefore, *it heals as fibrocartilage, which carries inferior mechanical properties to withstand stress and strain compared to hyaline cartilage*.

- Hyaline cartilage is 80% water and electrolytes, whereas 20% constitutes cells and collagen
- *Predominant type of collagen in hyaline cartilage is type II*. Others are IV, V, VI, X, and XI.

Histologically, the hyaline cartilage has five layers—superficial, deep, middle, tidemark and calcified layer **(Fig. 31.3)**. **Table 31.1** briefly describes the layer and function of each layer.

- **Subchondral bone** is beneath the cartilage. It has following functions:
    - It provides mechanical and nutritional support to the cartilage.
    - It is highly vascular and rich in nerve supply. Therefore, rubbing of exposed subchondral bone due to loss of articular cartilage (in arthritis) results in pain.

Table 31.1: Characteristics and function of different layers/zones of cartilages.

Layer/zone	Properties, cells, collagen, proteoglycan	Water
Superficial/1	Upper (lamina splendens)—no cells, thinnest Lower—flat, ellipsoid chondrocyte It withstands shear force over the cartilage	More
Middle/2	Active spheroidal chondrocytes, more proteoglycans, thick collagen It withstands compressive force over the cartilage	Less
Deep/3	Largest zone, most active chondrocytes, highest proteoglycans, thickest collagen, metabolically most active It withstands compressive force over the cartilage	Least
Tidemark	Separates uncalcified cartilage with calcified 'undulation barrier' It withstands shear force over the cartilage	
Calcified layer/4	It has *metabolically least active chondrocytes* and *hydroxyapatite crystals* This layer anchors the cartilage to the subchondral bone	

Note: Once hyaline cartilage is damaged, naturally it does not regenerate by forming hyaline cartilage but forms "fibrocartilage", which carries inferior biomechanical properties.

CLASSIFICATION OF OSTEOARTHROSIS

Osteoarthrosis (OA) is classified as primary and secondary.
- *Primary OA:* Without any antecedent cause.
- *Secondary OA:* With the previous insult to the joint, either traumatic/pathological.

Table 31.2 lists the various causes of secondary OA.

RACIAL INFLUENCE IN PRIMARY OSTEOARTHROSIS

- **Asians:** Knee joint more involved > hip joint > ankle
- **Caucasians:** Hip > knee > ankle.

ETIOLOGY OF PRIMARY DEGENERATIVE OSTEOARTHROSIS

- **Age:** Usually, after 50–55 years of age
- **Gender:** Females are more prone to OA than males
- **BMI:** Obese persons are more prone to OA
- **Weight-bearing joint:** Lower limb joints are more prone compared to upper limb
- **Other risk factors:** Trauma to the joint, smoking, positive family history.

Table 31.2: Classification of osteoarthritis.

Primary: Without any antecedent cause	
Secondary: With the previous insult to the joint, either traumatic/pathological	
Developmental Epiphyseal dysplasia DDH SCFE in hip	*Endocrinal* Acromegaly
Traumatic Intra-articular fractures Meniscectomy	*Aseptic/avascular necrosis* Sickle cell anemia Corticosteroid usage Caisson's disease
Infection Pyogenic arthritis Tubercular arthritis	*Neuropathic* Diabetes mellitus Syringomyelia Hansen's disease
Metabolic Gout Pseudogout Alkaptonuria Wilson's disease	

(SCFE: slipped capital femoral epiphysis; DDH: developmental dysplasia of the hip)

Joints commonly involved in primary osteoarthritis: Most common joint affected in primary OA is knee followed by 1st carpometacarpal joint (of thumb), proximal interphalangeal (PIP), distal interphalangeal (DIP), hip, cervical and lumbar spine.

PATHOPHYSIOLOGY OF PRIMARY OSTEOARTHROSIS

The mainstay in the pathology of primary osteoarthritis (OA) is an *imbalance between cartilage matrix synthesis and degradation, resulting in the reduced formation of the cartilage* (Flowchart 31.2). There are two theories to explain OA.
1. **Gradual aging and wear- and tear-related damage to the cartilage** lead to osteoarthritis followed by bone changes.
2. **Repeated loading causes subchondral bone changes** leading to cartilage damage causing OA.

In primary OA, the *cartilage loss is more in the area of stress or loading* (cf inflammatory arthritis, where the cartilage loss is uniform across the joint). Once the cartilage is damaged, the denuded subchondral bone of either side rubs against each other. The *subchondral cysts* form under the exposed subchondral bone. The osteoblastic activity increases in the subchondral bone resulting in *subchondral sclerosis and osteophyte formation*.

Flowchart 31.2: Pathophysiology of osteoarthrosis of synovial joints.

```
Aging ─┐                                              ┌─ Obesity
        │                                              │
Metabolic diseases ─┤ Abnormal cartilage │  │ Abnormal stresses on joint │ ├─ Anatomic abnormality (malaligned joint)
        │                                              │
Inflammation ─┘                                        └─ Instability
                          │              │
                          ▼              ▼
              ┌──────────────────────────────────┐
              │ Biophysical changes              │
              │ • Collagen framework breaks      │
              │ • Cartilage cell degenerate      │
              │ Biochemical changes              │
              │ • Increased metalloproteases MMPs│
              │   (proteolytic enzymes)          │
              │ • Inhibitor reduction            │
              └──────────────────────────────────┘
                            │
                            ▼
                  ┌───────────────────┐
                  │ Cartilage damage  │
                  └───────────────────┘
                            │
                            ▼
                  ┌───────────────────────┐
                  │ Subchondral sclerosis │
                  │ Osteophyte formation  │
                  │ Subchondral cyst      │
                  └───────────────────────┘
```

(MMP: matrix metalloproteinases)

PRIMARY DEGENERATIVE OSTEOARTHROSIS OF THE KNEE

Risk factors: Aging, obesity, smoking, and genetic factors.
Etiopathology: Usually, OA knee affects patients older than 55–60 years, who are often obese. In a human knee joint, there are three compartments—medial and lateral tibiofemoral and patellofemoral. The latter is between patella and femoral trochlea. The tibiofemoral compartment is more loaded during activities while person is standing due to vertical load. In contrast, patellofemoral (PF) compartment is more loaded during the activities while the knee is flexed (squatting, cross leg sitting) or quadriceps is under intense load (stair climbing/descending). Since the significant weight transfer of the body occurs via the medial compartment of the knee,

the medial tibiofemoral is commonly involved in primary knee OA, while the lateral tibiofemoral compartment is involved in later stages. Patellofemoral joint is also involved in primary OA of the knee, especially in people who tends to do more squatting, sitting cross leg and ascending or descending stairs as these activities load PF compartment. The tibiofemoral compartment OA, especially medial, results in pain while weight-bearing (walking) as this compartment is loaded more during standing. Excess wear out of medial compartment cartilage results in genu varum deformity. In contrast, the patellofemoral compartment OA results in more pain on squatting, cross-leg sitting and stair climbing/descending as the PF compartment experiences high pressures during these activities.

CLINICAL FEATURES

Symptoms

These patients present with mechanical pain, intermittent swelling, and knee joint deformity.
- **Pain:** The pain is predominantly mechanical, which is felt during weight bearing, walking, standing for long, squatting, sitting cross-leg, and stair climbing.
  Patients with patellofemoral OA present with pain while squatting, sitting cross-leg, or climbing stairs, wherein the patella is in deep contact with the femoral trochlea.
- **Swelling** may be present due to effusion, synovial hypertrophy, or both.
  Sometimes, the patient may report a swelling at the back of the knee, which is most likely a Baker's cyst.

Signs

Often, patients moderate to advanced OA knee present with genu varus deformity **(Fig. 31.4A)**.
- **Deformity:** Most common—genu varum; uncommon—genu valgum
- **Joint line tenderness**
- **Crepitus on movement**   } *Three classic signs of OA*
- **Painful restriction of movement**

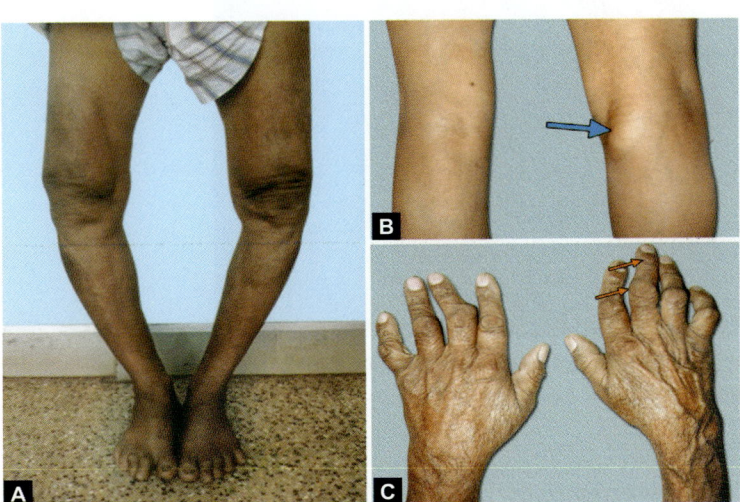

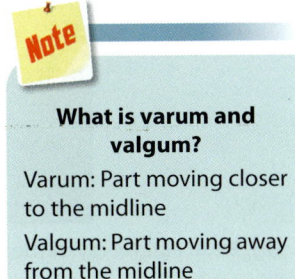

Note

What is varum and valgum?
Varum: Part moving closer to the midline
Valgum: Part moving away from the midline

Figs. 31.4A to C: (A) Bilateral genu varum deformity; (B) Bakers cyst in right popliteal fossa (blue arrow); (C) Bouchard and Heberdon nodes at PIP and DIP joint, respectively (orange arrow).

One must examine the popliteal fossa to look for **Baker's cyst** (**Fig. 31.4B**). Further, these patients may also have *1st carpometacarpal joint arthritis*, *Bouchard and Heberden nodes* (**Fig. 31.4C**). Bouchard and Heberdon nodes indicate arthritis of PIP and DIP joints, respectively.

INVESTIGATIONS

- **Plain X-ray of the knee** *is diagnostic of OA knee.* Anteroposterior (AP) in standing (**Fig. 31.5**), lateral and skyline view are performed to assess OA in all three areas (medial and lateral tibiofemoral compartment as well as patellofemoral joint). The classical findings are:
    - Decreased joint space (due to loss of cartilage)
    - Osteophyte formation
    - Subchondral cysts
    - Subchondral sclerosis
    - Prominence of the tibial spines
    - Deformity (genu varum/valgum)
    - Loose body (if any).
- **Magnetic resonance imaging (MRI) of the knee joint:** It is not performed routinely. However, it is performed in case of poor response to conservative treatment to look for any meniscal tears or cartilage flaps, especially if there is a history of trauma.

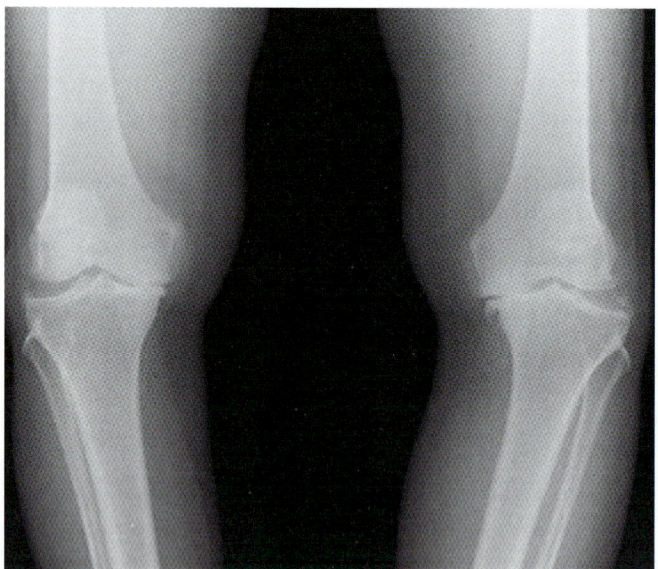

Fig. 31.5: Plain X-ray of the knee (AP view) showing decreased medial joint space, medial osteophytes, prominent tibial spine, and genu varum.

TREATMENT

Conservative treatment is the mainstay of treatment in mild to moderate OA of the knee, whereas advanced OA may require surgical intervention. The conservative treatment involves general measures, physiotherapy, orthotics and medical measures.

General Measures
- Weight reduction, especially in obese patients, is one of the important measures to unload the joint
- Avoiding activities that exacerbate pain (squatting and cross-leg sitting)
- Using a western toilet (to avoid deep squats in the Asian type).

Physiotherapy, Orthotics
While physiotherapy aims to reduce pain, strengthen muscles, and improve ROM, orthotics help change the mechanical axis to relieve pain.
- *Moist heat/shortwave diathermy/TENS* to the knee to relieve pain
- *Quadriceps strengthening exercises:* It is one of the mainstays of conservative treatment
- *Walking stick* to unload the affected joint
- Cycling and swimming
- *Unloader braces* marginally shift the lower limb's mechanical axis from the medial to the lateral compartment of the knee joint, and that helps relieve pain as weight is shifted to lesser affected lateral compartment (Fig. 31.6).
- *Footwear modification:* Lateral border shoe raise (shifts mechanical axis laterally slightly unloading the damaged medial area and helps relieve pain).

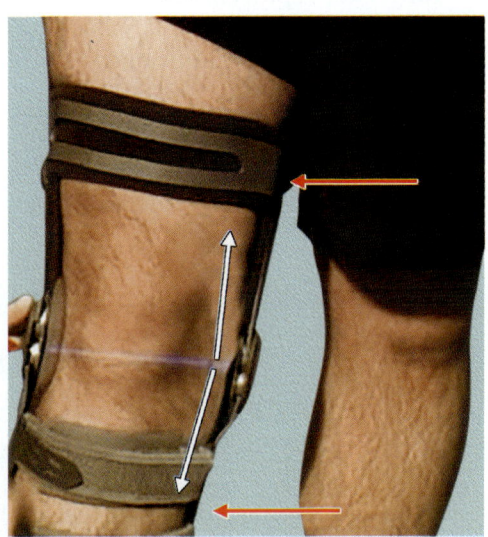

Fig. 31.6: Unloader brace for OA knee.

Medical Management
It includes medications to relieve pain and inflammation. Further, newer measures such as stem cells or platelet-rich plasma aim at cartilage regeneration.
- *Analgesics:* Nonsteroidal anti-inflammatory drugs (NSAIDs), cyclooxygenase-2 (COX-2) inhibitors, paracetamol, or other analgesics to relieve pain.
- *Proteoglycan synthesis stimulator*: *Glucosamine and chondroitin sulphate* are two drugs that have been used to treat OA. However, recent literature has not supported the beneficial effect of these drugs in OA knee.
- *Intra-articular steroid injection* is given if there is an acute exacerbation of pain due to inflammation.
- *Intra-articular hyaluronic acid injection:* Improves viscosity and relieves pain.
- *Intra-articular injection of platelet-rich plasma or stem cell (autologous/allogenic):* These two measures have recently gained much traction as they seem to help cartilage regeneration. However, long term results are awaited.

Surgery
- *Arthroscopic debridement* can be performed in early cases of OA knee, if there is a loose body, cartilage flaps, and meniscal tears.

- ***High tibial osteotomy*** is indicated in OA in *young patients* with genu varum deformity or isolated medial compartment OA knee. It helps shifting the load into the lesser affected lateral compartment **(Fig. 31.7A)**.
- ***Distal femur osteotomy:*** It is performed in the case of OA knee of a young patient with lateral compartment OA with genu valgum deformity
- ***Unicompartmental knee replacement:*** It is an option for single (usually medial) compartment OA knee, especially in a younger patient (45–55 years) **(Fig. 31.7B)**.
- ***Total knee replacement*:** It is the procedure of choice, especially in advanced OA of older patients **(Fig. 31.7C)**.
- ***Arthrodesis*:** Rarely indicated.

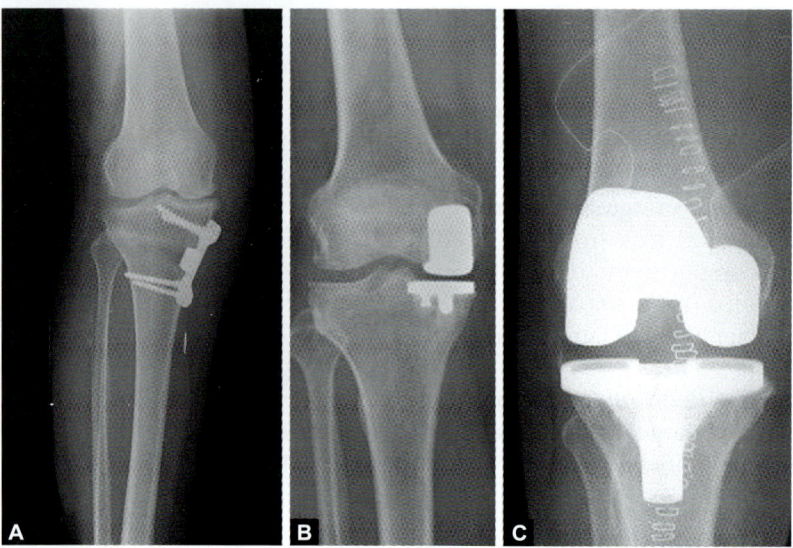

Figs. 31.7A to C: Surgical treatment of OA knee: (A) High tibial osteotomy; (B) Unicondylar replacement; (C) Total knee replacement.

Notes

CHAPTER 32

Rheumatoid Arthritis

DEFINITION

Rheumatoid arthritis (RA) is a chronic inflammatory disease of the connective tissue, chiefly affecting the synovium.
  Note that synovium is present in synovial joints and surrounds the tendons as tenosynovium. Therefore, RA affects synovial joints and tendons.
- **Age group affected:** Typically, it affects younger patients who are in the age group of 20–50 years.
- **Gender:** Females are more affected than males (4:1).

ETIOLOGY AND PATHOGENESIS

The exact etiology of RA is unknown and seems to be multifactorial, such as:
- **Hereditary/genetics:** HLA-DR4, DR1, and DW5. The risk of RA is three times higher chance of RA if a 1st-degree relative is affected
- **Unknown virus, degraded B-cell products**
- **Autoimmune:** Cell-mediated immunity, antigen-antibody complex
- Environmental factors.
  The essence of the pathogenesis of RA is the deposition of immune complexes over synovium resulting in synovitis. The brief pathogenesis of rheumatoid arthritis is depicted in **Figure 32.1**.

PATHOLOGY

RA affects both ***articular and extra-articular structures.*** Typically, RA affects the synovium of the joints and tendon sheath, resulting in synovitis, which is the key to the pathogenesis of RA.
- **Articular pathology:** The joint pathology or involvement undergoes three stages—synovitis, arthritis and deformity.
  1. **Stage of synovitis:** Initial immune-mediated antigen-antibody-complement reaction causes immune complex deposition in the synovium, resulting in *synovial inflammation, hypertrophy* **(Fig. 32.2A)**, and *effusion*. The *stage of synovitis ends up with pannus formation*, which is an abnormal fibrovascular tissue growth over the cartilage from the synovial junction (**Fig. 32.2B and Flowchart 32.1**).
  2. **Stage of arthritis:** The stage of arthritis is characterized by the destruction of cartilage due to the following:
     - The *pannus chokes the articular cartilage;* therefore, cartilage cannot get nourishment from synovial fluid, leading to cartilage destruction.
     - The *proteolytic enzymes* released by the lysosomes (from cells of inflammatory fluid) destroy the cartilage.

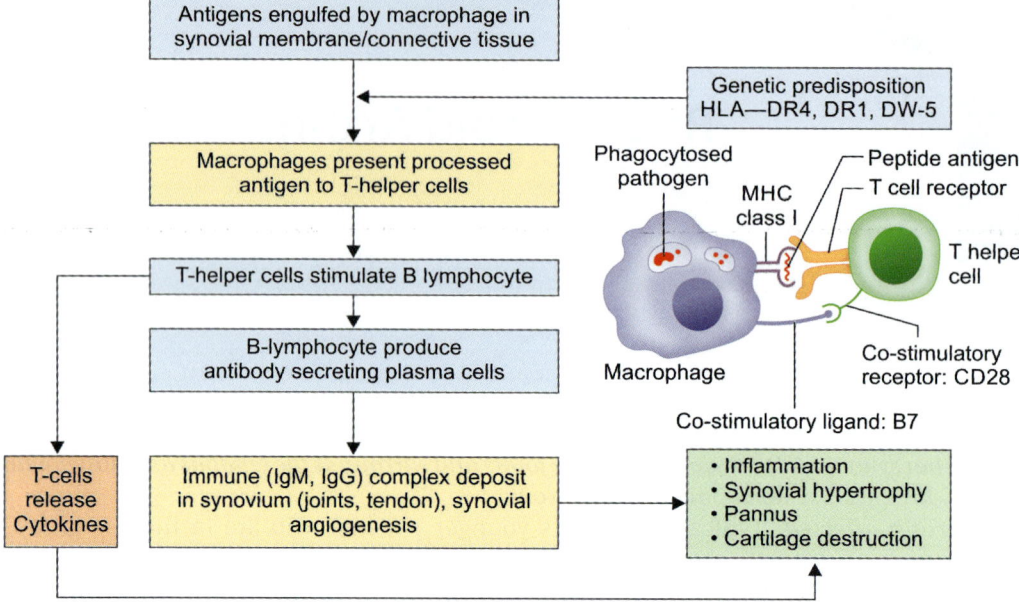

Fig. 32.1: Pathogenesis of rheumatoid arthritis (in brief).

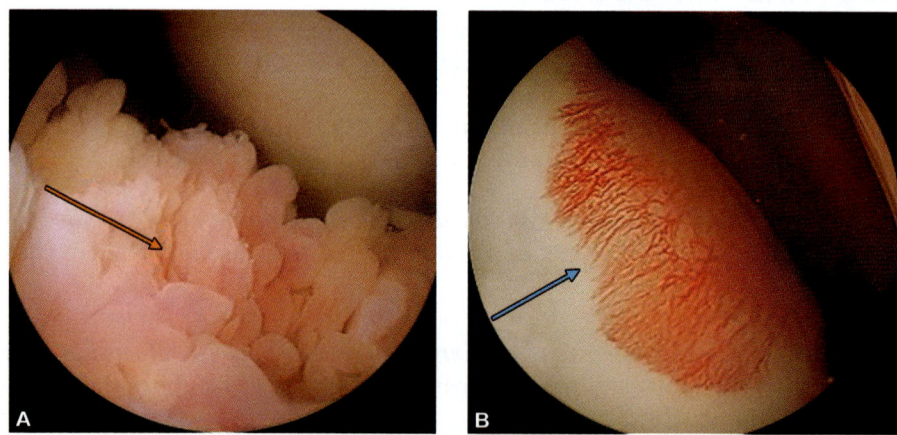

Figs. 32.2A and B: Arthroscopic image of a rheumatoid knee undergoing synovectomy: (A) Synovial hypertrophy (orange arrow); (B) Pannus over femoral condyle (blue arrow).

Flowchart 32.1: Pathogenesis of rheumatoid arthritis in stage of synovitis.

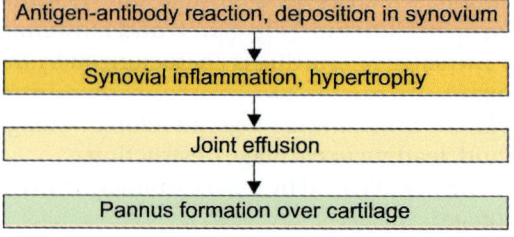

Once articular cartilage is damaged, it results in exposure of the subchondral bone and arthritis **(Fig. 32.3)**. **Flowchart 32.2** explains the destruction of the cartilage.

3. **Stage of deformity, fibrous ankylosis:** The inflammatory process subsides, but the arthritic joint gradually becomes stiff and deformed due to cartilage destruction and adhesion formation between joint surfaces.
    - Muscle spasm
    - Capsular contracture or stretching
    - Tendon rupture
    - Ligament stretching.
    - Finally, fibrous adhesions form between joint surfaces leading to **fibrous ankylosis**. Sometimes, the supporting ligaments and capsule stretch out significantly, leading to joint subluxation. Rarely, there could be *bony ankylosis*.

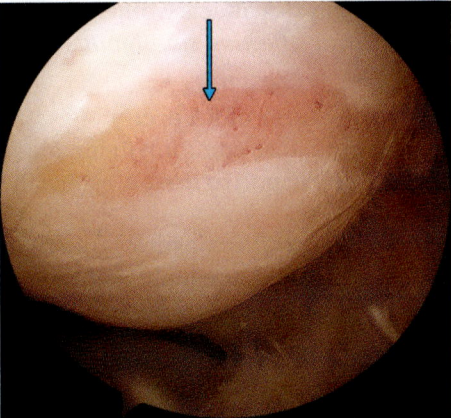

Fig. 32.3: Arthroscopic image of loss of cartilage and exposure of subchondral bone over medial femoral condyle (blue arrow) surface after pannus removal.

The inflammatory damage of RA is not only limited to joints; it also involves synovial tendon sheaths resulting in thickened and inflamed tendons, especially in the hand and foot. These inflamed tendons may rupture, causing deformity and dysfunction.

- **Extra-articular involvement**
  - Vasculitis
  - Lymphadenopathy and splenomegaly
  - **Muscle weakness:** Due to myopathy or neuropathy
  - **Perineural fibrosis:** Leading to neuropathy
  - **Visceral changes:** Heart, lung, kidney, GIT, and brain.

Flowchart 32.2: Pathogenesis of rheumatoid arthritis in stage of arthritis.

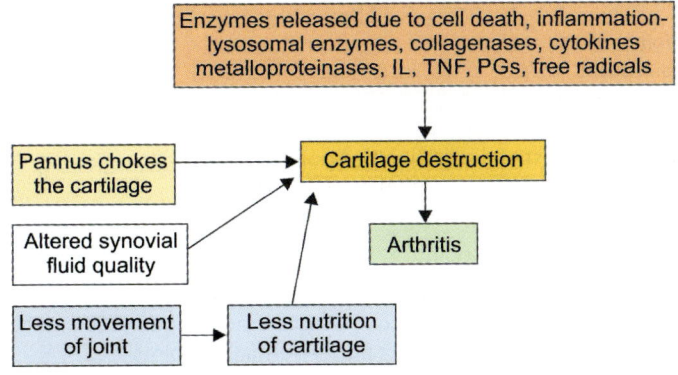

■ CLINICAL FEATURES

Classically, RA is a disease of the appendicular skeleton affecting synovial joints. *Except the "upper cervical spine (C1-C2)",* RA does not involve rest of the spine and the sacroiliac joints.

Typically, RA affects women in their 20s–40s. The onset of RA is insidious, with *symmetrical polyarthritis affecting small joints of hands and feet, with morning stiffness lasting more than an hour.*

The key features of RA are:
- *Gender:* More common in females than males (4:1)
- *Symmetric polyarthritis*, especially of small joints of the hand and foot, lasting more than six weeks
- *Morning stiffness* lasting more than one hour
- *Deformities* in the hand and wrist.

ARA and EULAR criteria are used to diagnose RA, as mentioned in **Boxes 32.1** and **32.2**.

Box 32.1: American Rheumatism Association (ARA) 1987 revised criteria to diagnose rheumatoid arthritis.

Patient is said to have RA if patients have four out of seven criteria and points 1–4 are present.

1. **Morning stiffness** in joints last more than 1 hour
2. **Arthritis of three or more joints:** Simultaneously have soft tissue swelling
3. **Arthritis of wrist or hand:** At least one swollen area in wrist, metacarpophalangeal (MCP) or proximal interphalangeal (PIP) joint
4. **Symmetric arthritis**
5. **Rheumatoid nodules:** Observed on extensor surface of forearm/bony prominences
6. **Serum rheumatoid factor**
7. **Typical changes in the X-ray** of the wrist and hand

Box 32.2: American College of Rheumatism (ACR)/European League Against Rheumatism (EULAR) criteria 2010.

Any patient having six or more point is said to have RA. Patient need to have at least one joint involvement and at least one joint to have typical RA changes.

Joint distribution
- 1 large joint: 0 point
- 2–10 large joints: 1 point
- 1–3 small joints: 2 points
- 4–10 small joints: 3 points
- Greater than 10 joints (at least one small joint): 4 points

Symptom duration
- Less than 6 weeks: 0 point
- Greater than or equal to 6 weeks: 1 point

Serology
- Negative rheumatoid factor (RF) and anticitrate citrullinated peptide (CCP) antibody: 0 point
- Low positive RF and anti-CCP antibody (<3 × upper normal): 2 points
- High positive RF and anti-CCP antibody (>3 × upper normal): 3 points

Acute phase reactant
- Normal erythrocyte sedimentation rate (ESR) and C-reactive protein (CRP): 0 point
- Raised ESR and CRP: 1 point

Articular Features

Deformities in hand (Figs. 32.4A to E)
- *Swan neck deformity*: PIP hyperextension and DIP flexion **(Fig. 32.4A)**. It is due to rupture of volar plate of PIP joint.
- *Boutonniere's deformity*: Distal interphalangeal (DIP) hyperextension and PIP flexion **(Fig. 32.4B)**. It is due to rupture of central slip of extensor expansion of finger.
- *Metacarpophalangeal joint subluxation* leading to prominent knuckles **(Fig. 32.4C)**.
- *Ulnar deviation at the MCP joint* **(Fig. 32.4D** yellow arrow shows ulnar deviation**)**.
- *Z deformity of the thumb* **(Fig. 32.4D** Blue lines over thumb**)**.
- *Radial deviation of the wrist* **(Fig. 32.4D,** gray arrow indicates radial deviation of wrist**)**.
- *Dorsal subluxation of the ulna.*
- Tenosynovitis of hand tendons, trigger fingers and thumb.

Extensive tenosynovitis of wrist and hand tendons and joint could result in typical syndromes, which are mentioned in **Box 32.3**.

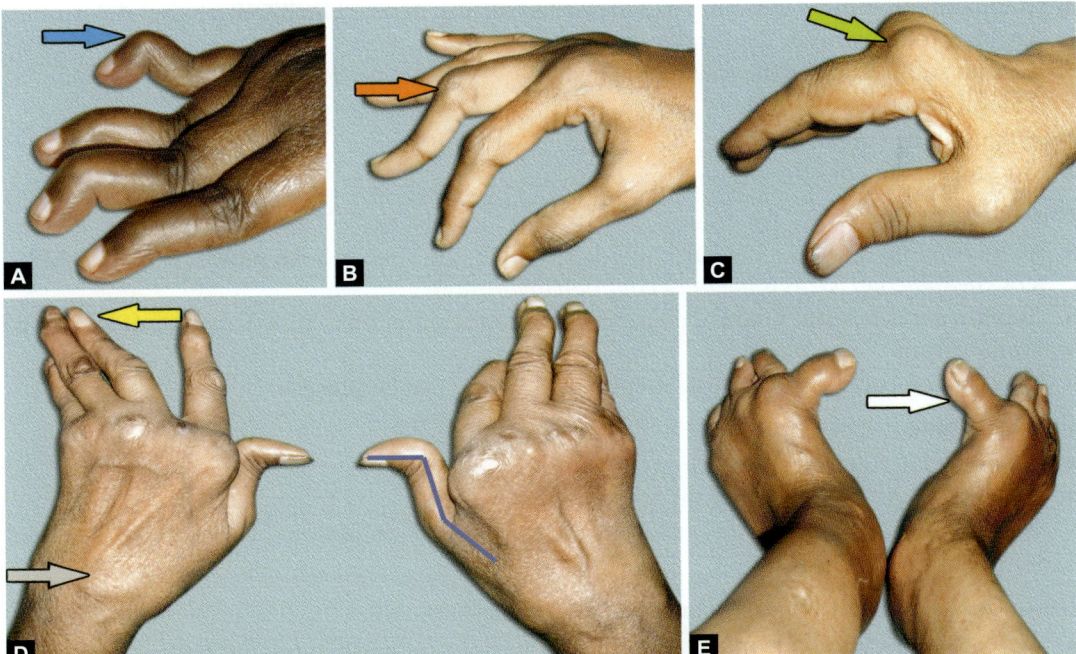

Figs. 32.4A to E: Various deformities of RA in hand and feet. (A) Swan neck deformity (blue arrow); (B) Boutonniere's deformity (Orange arrow); (C) Subluxation at MCP joint (green arrow); (D) Radial deviation of wrist (grey arrow) and ulnar deviation of fingers at MCP joint (yellow arrow), Z deformity of thumb; (E) Hallux varus (white arrow).

Box 32.3: Hand syndromes in RA.

- **Mannerfelt syndrome:** Rupture of flexor pollicis longus in the carpal tunnel due to scaphoid osteophytes.
- **Vaughan–Jackson syndrome:** Rupture of hand digital extensor tendons starting from the ulnar to the radial side.
- **Arthritis mutilans:** Gross destruction and deformity of the hand. Radiologically, pencil in cup changes in phalanx are present. It is also present in psoriatic arthritis.

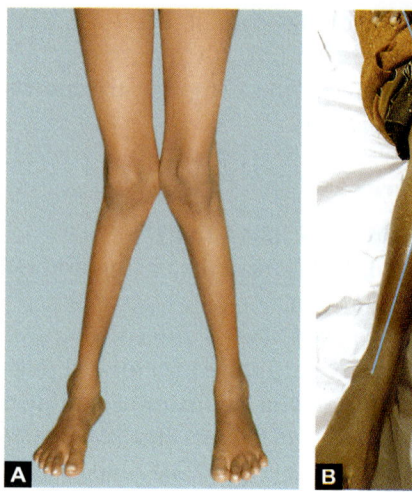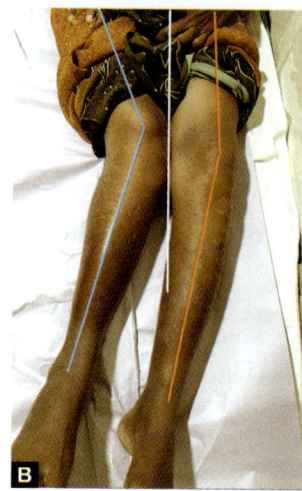

Figs. 32.5A and B: (A) Genu valgum deformity in RA; (B) Wind swept deformity. Note genu valgum in right knee (blue lines) and genu varum in left knee (orange lines). White line indicates midline.

Foot deformities
- Hallux valgus is quite common. Hallus varus can also occur **(Fig. 32.4E)**. Other deformities are claw toes, hammer toes and bunion.
- Plantar subluxation of the metatarsal head
- Lateral deviation of the toes
- Valgus at the subtalar joint
- Equinus at the ankle.

Knee deformities
- *Genu valgum:* It is the most common deformity in the knee of a RA patient **(Fig. 32.5A)** (*cf.* OA knee wherein varus is the most common deformity)
- *Windswept deformity:* One knee has valgus, and the other has varus deformity **(Fig. 32.5B)**
- Genu varum
- Flexion deformity. Rarely, triple deformity (like TB) can be present.

Cervical spine
- Atlantoaxial, subaxial subluxation
- Basilar invagination of odontoid process.

Note that above findings are radiological changes in cervical spine. Patient may complain of neck pain and stiffness.

Other musculoskeletal manifestations
- Tenosynovitis, tendon rupture result in various deformities of hand and foot.
- *Carpal tunnel syndrome:* It happens due to extensive tenosynovitis of the flexor tendons in the carpal tunnel.
- *Tarsal tunnel syndrome (in foot):* It happens due to tenosynovitis of the flexor tendons lying under the foot flexor retinaculum.

Extra-articular Manifestations

- **Constitutional features:** Generalized fatigue, low-grade fever, weight loss, and loss of appetite
- **Hematological:** Anemia of chronic disease, leukopenia, thrombocytosis, generalized lymphadenopathy
- **Rheumatoid nodules** are non-tender subcutaneous nodules on extensor surfaces, especially on forearm near the olecranon **(Fig. 32.6)**. Rarely, they could be present on pleura and meninges. *The presence of subcutaneous nodules indicates the severity of the disease.*

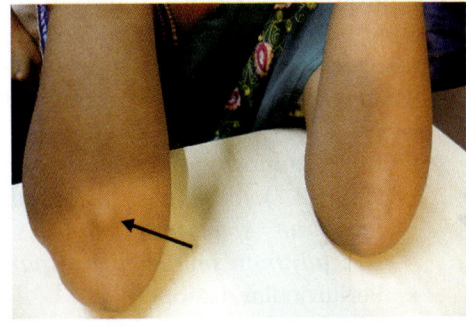

Fig. 32.6: Rheumatoid nodule over extensor surface of right forearm (black arrow).

- **Vasculitis:** It can involve any organ. Vasculitis of vasa nervosa (vessel supplying arteries) could result in mononeuritis multiplex, which is an asymmetric sensorimotor peripheral neuropathy involving different nerves.
- **Abdomen:** *Felty's syndrome*—hepatosplenomegaly with RA
- **Lungs:** *Caplan's syndrome* characterized by nodules, effusion, and bronchiolitis
- **Heart:** Pericarditis, myocarditis, endocarditis, pericardial effusion
- **Eyes:** Episcleritis, scleritis, and scleromalacia.

> **Important**
>
> **Dictums in acute monoarticular exacerbation in rheumatoid arthritis**
>
> An acute exacerbation of a single joint inflammation and synovitis in a patient with RA indicates septic arthritis unless proved otherwise. And therefore, intra-articular steroid should not be administered until joint infection is ruled out.

INVESTIGATIONS

- **Complete blood picture (CBP):** It may be normal or may show several specific findings, such as:
  - *Low hemoglobin*: The possible causes are anemia of chronic disease, poor appetite, etc.
  - *Total white blood cell (WBC) count:* It could be elevated in acute exacerbation of RA.
- **ESR and CRP** are raised, especially if the disease is uncontrolled or there is acute exacerbation.
- **Rheumatoid (RA) factor:** RA factor is a sensitive test; *positive in 60–70% of cases only.* RF titers >1:40 by latex method are considered positive. A titer value correlates with severity of the disease. It can be false positive in 5% of healthy individuals and other inflammatory conditions such as Sjögren's syndrome, SLE, and mixed connective tissue disorder. It is also positive in 25% of elderly population above 65 years of age. In such cases, one must rely upon other clinical features and titer value >1:640.

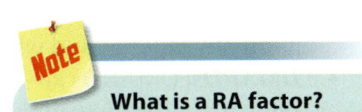

Note

What is a RA factor?
RA factor is IgM antibody against Fc fragment of IgG antibody.

Note: Several patients have clinical features of RA, but their RA factor is negative. They generally have better prognoses.

- **Anti-CCP antibody (anti-citrate citrullinated peptide):** It is positive in 98% of cases. It carries superior specificity compared to the RA factor. It is positive even when RA factor is negative.
  Note that ANA may also be raised in RA.
- **X-ray**
  - In RA, uniform joint space reduction is noted (**Fig. 32.7**). *(cf. primary osteoarthritis, wherein the joint space reduction is asymmetric, typically more on medial compartment).*
  - Periarticular osteopenia
  - Subchondral erosions and cysts
  - Soft tissue swelling.
- **Synovial fluid analysis** shows typical features of inflammatory arthritis. However, it is not performed routinely, except in the case of suspected septic arthritis.
- **Synovial biopsy**: It can be performed in cases where serological investigations are non-specific.

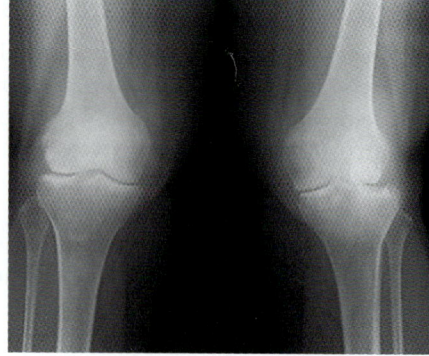

Fig. 32.7: X-ray of the rheumatoid knee showing a uniform reduction in joint space and periarticular osteopenia.

TREATMENT

The treatment of RA is comprehensive, involving a multidisciplinary approach. The therapy involves general, medical, physiotherapy and occupational therapy, and/or surgical measures. Generally, most RA patients need lifelong/long-term medical treatment in form of DMARDs.
- **General measures**
  - Nutritional support, correct anemia
  - Counseling about the disease process and the importance of continuing the medical treatment.
- **Medical measures:** The *mainstay of RA treatment is pharmacologic*, which comprises **NSAIDs** to relieve pain and inflammation, disease-modifying anti-rheumatoid drugs **(DMARDs)** to control the disease in the long-term, and/or **steroids** to control inflammation. Severe cases of RA, which cannot be controlled with DMARDs, require **biological agents**.
  - ***NSAIDs:*** Naproxen and Diclofenac are commonly used NSAIDs. They are required to control pain and inflammation, while DMARDs are yet to act and reduce inflammation.
  - ***Steroids:*** It can be given in systemically or locally (intra-articular). They are quite valuable for controlling the severe form of the disease and inflammation in the acute phase along with NSAIDs, while DMARDs are yet to provide relief. Oral steroids can be gradually tapered and withdrawn after a few weeks-months.
  - ***DMARDs:*** DMARDs are the drug of choice in RA. DMARDs are *beneficial in the stage of synovitis, wherein they can prevent/slow down the further progression of the disease into the stage of arthritis.* And therefore, the early introduction of DMARDs helps control RA and its consequences.
    DMARDs may take 12–16 weeks to provide substantial relief. It also helps maintain remission. Following are the commonly used DMARDs in RA.
    - Methotrexate
    - Hydroxychloroquine (HCQ)

- Sulfasalazine
- Leflunomide

Commonly, DMARDs are used in combination of two or three. *Methotrexate and HCQ are the most commonly used DMARDs.* If there is no clinical response to DMARDs to 3–4 months, other DMARDs/biological agents are added.

- **Biological agents:** Typically, biological agents are added if DMARDs fail to control the disease for 3–4 months. There are two categories of biological agents; TNF and IL-1 antagonists.
    - TNF (tumor necrosis factor) antagonist
        - Etanercept
        - Infliximab
        - Adalimumab, golimumab, certolizumab.
    - IL-1 antagonist
        - Anakinra.
- **Physiotherapy and occupational therapy:** Along with medical management, physiotherapy is essential for optimal outcomes.
    - *Splinting* to prevent or correct deformities of various joints
    - *Muscle strengthening* exercises
    - *Joint mobilization* to prevent stiffness
    - *Heat therapy*: Moist heat, short-wave diathermy, and wax bath
    - *Cold therapy*: Useful in acute exacerbation.
- **Surgical treatment:** The choice of surgical treatment depends upon the structure involved (tendon/synovium/joint) and the specific pathological stage (synovitis/arthritis). Various surgical procedures, which are performed on RA patients are:
    - *Synovectomy:* It is helpful in the stage of synovitis to excise inflamed synovium and pannus, which can prevent damage to the cartilage.
    - *Joint replacement*: In the late stages of arthritis, deformity
    - *Arthrodesis*: Badly arthritic and deformed joints can be surgically fused when joint replacement is not an option. It is quite common for small joints of the hand and foot.
    - *Resection arthroplasty*: Occasionally performed in the upper limb when joint replacement is not an option
    - *Osteotomy*: For correction of bony deformities
    - *Tendon repair, tendon transfer, or tenodesis* in cases of tendon rupture
    - *Capsular surgery*: For capsular contractures or laxity.

DIFFERENTIAL DIAGNOSIS

The differentials to exclude are SLE, viral arthropathies (post-chikungunya), and Reiter's syndrome.

CHAPTER 33

Seronegative Arthritis and Other Arthritis

DEFINITION

"Seronegative arthritis" comprises a group of inflammatory arthritis without positive rheumatoid factor (RF). Various common seronegative arthritis are mentioned in **Box 33.1**.

SERONEGATIVE SPONDYLOARTHROPATHY

Seronegative spondyloarthropathies are a group of inflammatory arthropathy, which is RF negative, commonly affects **young men** (more than women), characterized by **inflammation of sacroiliac joints and axial skeleton**, and often **HLAB27 positive**.

The fundamental pathology in seronegative spondyloarthropathy is *'enthesitis.'*

Note: The enthesis is the connective tissue between the tendon, ligament, and bone.

The key features of seronegative spondyloarthropathy are mentioned in **Box 33.2**.

> **Box 33.1:** Various seronegative arthritis.
>
> - Seronegative spondyloarthropathies
> - Crystalline arthritis
> - Inflammatory arthritis
> - Systemic diseases
> - Infective arthritis
> - Neoplastic or paraneoplastic arthritis

> **Box 33.2:** Key features of seronegative spondyloarthropathy (SpA).
>
> - Gender: Male preponderance
> - Age of onset: Usual onset in less than 40 years of age
> - Seronegative, i.e., RA factor negative
> - Most cases are HLA B27 positive
> - **Pathological hallmark SpA is "enthesitis."** It presents with pain at the site of insertion of tendon or fascia (plantar fasciitis, tendo-Achilles tendinitis, etc.).
>
> **Cardinal clinical presentations are:**
> - Inflammatory back pain with morning stiffness
> - Essential feature is "sacroiliac joint involvement"
> - Peripheral joint involvement usually oligoarticular and asymmetric
> - Extra-articular manifestations like uveitis, cardiac involvement are not uncommon

The common seronegative spondyloarthropathies are:
- Ankylosing spondylitis
- Psoriatic arthritis
- Reactive arthritis/Reiter's syndrome.

- Enteropathic arthritis: Due to inflammatory bowel disease
- Synovitis, acne, pustulosis, hyperostosis, and osteitis (SAPHO) syndrome
- Undifferentiated.

==A typical patient of seronegative arthropathy is a young male who presents with back pain and stiffness, which increases after a period of rest, and improves with activity. The sacroiliac joints are almost always involved in seronegative spondyloarthropathy, and HLAB-27 is often positive.==

ANKYLOSING SPONDYLITIS/MARIE-STRÜMPELL DISEASE/ BECHTEREW'S DISEASE

DEFINITION

Ankylosing spondylitis (AS) is a systemic seronegative spondyloarthropathy characterized by:
- HLA-B27+ (in 90% of cases), RA factor negative
- Typically, AS is characterized by the *involvement of the axial skeleton comprising the SI joint and spine*. Rarely, large appendicular joints (hips, knee, shoulder) are involved.

> **Note:** HLA-B27 is located on B locus of the sixth chromosome.

PATHOPHYSIOLOGY

- **Genetic:** More than 90% of patients are *HLA-B27 positive*. HLA B-27 is said to aggregate with joint peptides and damage the joint.
- **Enthesitis** commonly occurs at the sacroiliac (SI) joint, spine ligaments, spinal facet and apophyseal joint. Inflammation of enthesis leads to bony erosion, ossification, and eventual bony ankylosis.
- **Intervertebral disc space involvement** leads to syndesmophyte formation.

CLINICAL FEATURES

AS is more common at a *young age (20–50)*, and *males are more affected (male:female = 4:1)*. Clinically, typically, AS involves the sacroiliac joint, lumbar-dorsal-cervical spine (usually in ascending order), and costovertebral joints. SI joint and spine involvement results in stiff spine, whereas costovertebral joint involvement results in reduced chest expansion. Other *peripheral joints* like the hip, shoulder, knee, and hand, especially hip joints are involved. *Extra-articular structures* like the eye and heart are often involved.

Symptoms: Almost all patients complain of *low back pain and stiffness around the SI joint*, which may gradually progress towards lumbar spine. Typically, pain is felt after a period of rest and is relieved after activity. *Morning stiffness or stiffness after a period of rest is common.* In advanced cases, the patients complain of pain in the thoracic and cervical spine regions. Furthermore, involvement of costovertebral joint might results in stiffness in the chest (affected rib expansion).

Signs
- *Tests for SI joint involvement:* Tenderness is present over the *SI joint. Figure of four* and the *Gaenslen test* for SI joint arthritis are positive.
- *Tests for lumbar spine involvement:* Schober's test is positive, which indicates the stiffness of the lumbar spine.
- *Tests for chest involvement:* Chest expansion is decreased (<2–3 cm)

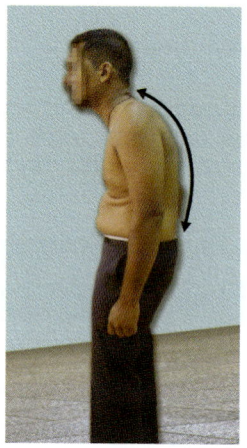

Fig. 33.1: The round back kyphotic deformity in dorsal spine (black curve) in ankylosing spondylitis.

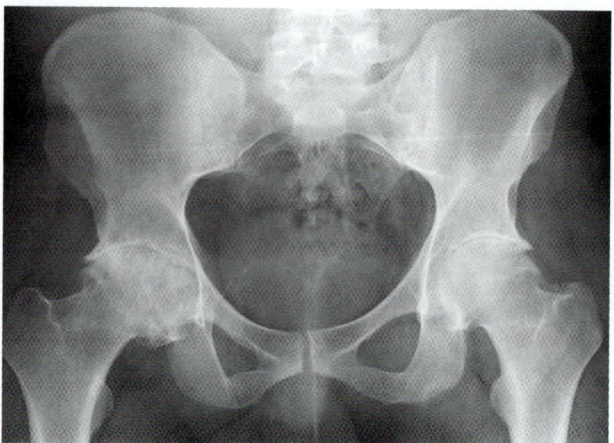

Fig. 33.2: X-ray pelvis anteroposterior (AP) showing bilaterally diminished sacroiliac (SI) joint space, sclerosis, and bilateral hip arthritis.

- Advanced cases of AS involving the dorsal spine result in *roundback deformity* **(Fig. 33.1)**. *Occiput-to-wall distance* is increased if the dorsal and cervical spine is stiff. Later, the patient may assume a 'question mark' posture.
- Rarely, bony ankylosis of the hip (more frequent) and knee result in stiff hip and knee.
- Costosternal joint, plantar fasciitis and tendo-Achilles tendinitis indicate peripheral enthesitis.
- ***Extra-articular manifestations***
    - *Eyes:* Uveitis and iritis
    - *Heart:* Cardiac conduction abnormality, aortic stenosis and regurgitation
    - *Lungs:* Apical pulmonary fibrosis
    - *Klebsiella pneumoniae* synovitis.

INVESTIGATIONS

The investigations of AS are radiological and serological.
- **X-ray of the SI joint—AP view:** The involvement of the *bilateral SI joint is a classic finding* of AS showing SI joint erosion, sclerosis, and diminished SI joint space **(Fig. 33.2)**. *The iliac side of the SI joint is first involved.* Late stages show SI joint fusion.
- **X-ray lumbodorsal spine**
    On lateral view
    - ***Squaring of the vertebra:*** Anterior vertebral border is straight rather than concave **(Fig. 33.3A)**.
    - ***Syndesmophyte:*** Thin vertical dense spicules bridging the vertebral bodies **(Fig. 33.3B)**.
    On AP view
    - ***Bamboo spine:*** It is a pathognomonic X-ray finding in spine that occurs as a result of vertebral body fusion by marginal syndesmophytes and annulus fibrosis ossification. Therefore, the resulting radiographic appearance, is that of thin, curved, radiopaque spicules that completely bridge adjoining vertebral bodies **(Fig. 33.3C)**.
    - ***Trolley track sign:*** Central dense line due to ossification of supra- and interspinous ligament along with two lateral lines due to ossification of apophyseal joints gives rise to Trolley track sign. **(Fig. 33.4)**

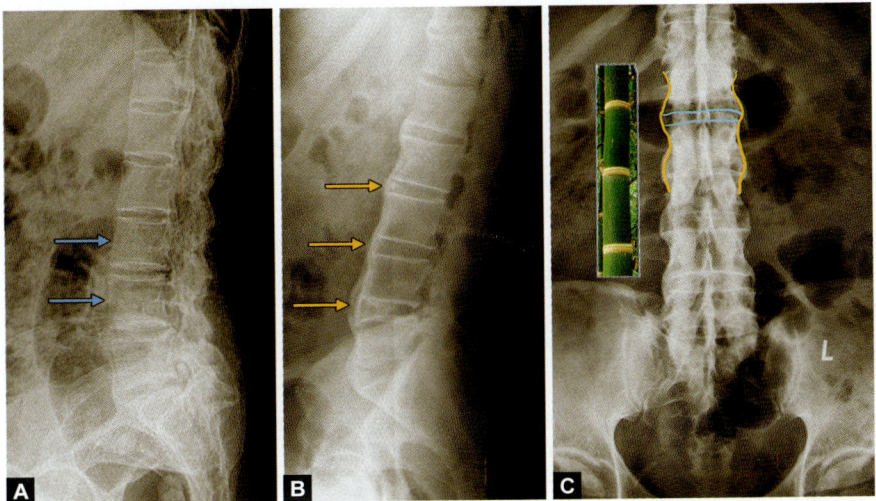

Figs. 33.3A to C: X-rays lumbar spine in ankylosing spondylitis: (A) Lateral view of lumbar spine showing squaring of the vertebra (blue arrow); (B) Lateral view showing anterior syndesmophytes (yellow arrow); (C) Bamboo spine.

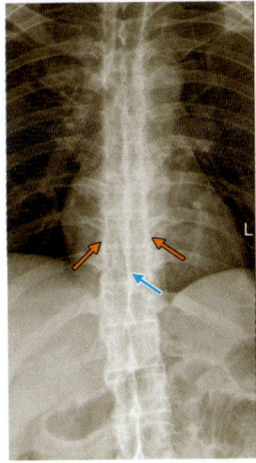

Fig. 33.4: AP X-ray of dorsolumbar spine showing dagger spine (blue arrow) and trolley track sign (orange arrows).

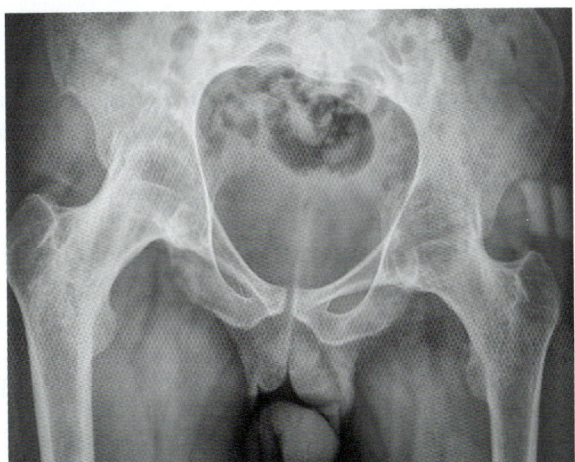

Fig. 33.5: Bony ankylosis of both hip joints. There is no hip joint space and bony trabaculae of femur and acetabulum are crossing the obliterated joint space.

- *Dagger spine*: Single central dense line on AP X-ray due to supra- and interspinous ligament ossification **(Fig. 33.4)**

In advance cases, the entire spine including cervical spine is ankylosed.
- **Apophyseal and costovertebral ankylosis**
- **X-ray hip:** Arthritis, protrusio acetabuli followed by bony ankylosis **(Fig. 33.5)**.
- **X-ray shoulder—AP view:** *Hatchet lesion* (bony defect on anterolateral part of the head)
- **MRI of the SI joint** is performed if X-rays appear normal. It can detect SI inflammation in early stage.

- *Romanus sign:* Small erosion on anterosuperior and anteroinferior corners of the vertebra.
- *Andersson sign:* Spondylodiscitis in AS.
- **Serology**
    - HLA-B27: It is positive in 90% of cases.
    - Erythrocyte sedimentation rate (ESR) is often elevated.
- **Pulmonary function test** is performed in cases where the chest expansion is limited, it may result in restrictive lung disease.

The diagnosis of AS can be established with the help of **Modified New York criteria** (1984), which comprises clinical and radiological criteria **(Box 33.3)**.

Box 33.3: Modified New York criteria for ankylosing spondylitis.

1. Clinical criteria
- Low back pain >3 months which improves with activity, and not with rest
- Limited lumbar spine mobility in sagittal (forward) and frontal (lateral bending) plane
- Limited chest expansion

2. Radiological criteria
- Bilateral sacroiliitis of grade ≥2
- Unilateral sacroiliitis of grade 3 or 4

The diagnosis of AS is made if the patient fulfills atleast one clinical and radiological criteria.

TREATMENT

Conservative treatment is the mainstay using medications and physiotherapy. Treatment aims to maintain the mobility and flexibility of involved structures and prevent or minimize the disease progression. Surgical treatment is offered to the joints that are entirely fused causing serious functional impairment.

- **Physiotherapy**
    - Physical therapy to *maintain flexibility* in the spine and other joints
    - Deep breathing exercises for chest.
- **Medical treatment:**
    - *Analgesics:* NSAIDs (indomethacin, diclofenac) and cyclooxygenase-2 (COX-2) inhibitors (etoricoxib) are used to relieve pain. Among all, Indomethacin is the most commonly used NSAID.
    - *Disease-modifying agents:* Sulfasalazine, methotrexate
    - *Biological agents:* TNF-alpha blocking agents—infliximab, etanercept. They are used if analgesics and disease-modifying agents fail to control symptoms.
- **Surgical treatment**
    - Total joint replacement for bony ankylosis of hip, shoulder, and knee joints.
    - *Spinal osteotomy* can be performed to correct severe thoracic kyphosis.

COMPLICATIONS

- Bony ankylosis of the involved joints **(Fig. 33.5)**
- Restrictive lung disease due to involvement of costovertebral joints
- The AS is very stiff, and fracture of a stiff cervical spine could result in central cord syndrome
- Recurrent uveitis and iritis affecting vision
- Progressive severe kyphosis can lead to limited visual distance.

PSORIATIC ARTHRITIS

DEFINITION

It is a seronegative arthropathy characterized by ***sacroiliitis*** (causing low back pain), ***psoriatic skin lesions***, ***arthritis of small joints of the hand*** (typically distal interphalangeal joint), and ***nail changes***.

About 30-40% of cases with psoriasis develop psoriatic arthritis.

GENETICS

50% of cases are associated with HLA-B27.

CLINICAL FEATURES

The clinical features of psoriatic arthritis comprise back pain along with skin lesions and nail changes. They may also have features of enthesitis, eye symptoms and gout.

- **Age group:** 30–50 years; **gender:** Equal male/female ratio
- **Low back pain and stiffness** due to sacroiliitis. Usually, sacroiliitis is unilateral.
- **Skin:** Psoriatic lesions over the body **(Fig. 33.6A)**. Usually, skin lesions precede arthritis.
- **Arthritis of hand joints**
  - Arthritis of the DIP joint is typical **(Fig. 33.6B)**. Rarely, PIP and MCP may be involved.
  - *Sausage digits/dactylitis*—swelling of a complete finger/toe
  - *Arthritis mutilans*

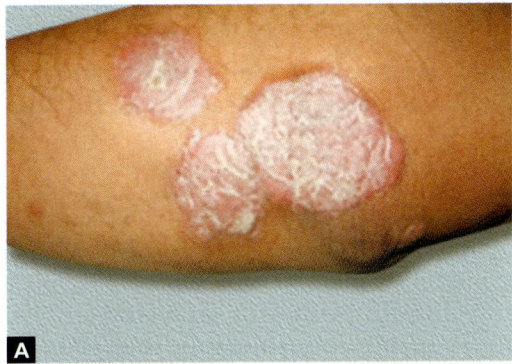
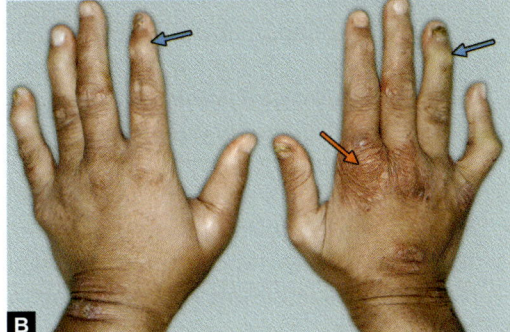
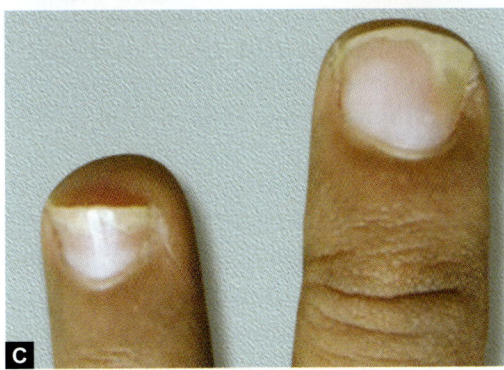

Figs. 33.6A to C: (A) Psoriasis over the elbow; (B) DIP arthritis in hands (blue arrows) with psoriatic lesions (orange arrow); (C) Nail features of psoriasis.
(*Source:* Professor Pratik Gahlaut, SKIMS, Bareilly)

Arthritis mutilans

It is observed in psoriatic and rheumatoid arthritis characterized by severe inflammation damaging the IP and MCP joints of hand and feet resulting in severe deformity. The digits are shortened and subluxed that can be telescoped producing classical 'opera glass deformity', which gives rise to 'pencil in cup' appearance on X-ray.

- **Nail involvement (Fig. 33.6C)**
    - *Onychodystrophy*: Nail pitting
    - *Onycholysis*: Nail bed lifts distally
    - *Ridging and yellowish discoloration of the margin*
- **Enthesitis:** Patients may have heel pain due to plantar fasciitis or tendon Achilles tendinitis.
- **Eye symptoms:** 30-40% of patients may have symptoms of uveitis, blepharitis, or keratoconjunctivitis sicca.
- **Gouty arthritis:** Sometimes, intermittent swelling of synovial joints is observed due to hyperuricemia associated with psoriasis.

Note: **Wright and Moll's diagnostic criteria** are used to diagnose psoriatic arthritis [Inflammatory arthritis (sacroiliitis, DIP arthritis) with clinical features of psoriasis].

INVESTIGATIONS

- **X-ray hand:** AP and oblique views
    - Distal interphalangeal *arthritis* **(Fig. 33.7)** with distal phalanx *acrolysis*
    - *Fluffy periosteitis (whiskering)*: Proliferative bone changes along the shaft of the metacarpal and metatarsal
    - Pencil-in-cup deformity in case of arthritis mutilans
- **X-ray of SI joint and spine**
    - Sacroiliitis: Usually unilateral
    - Syndesmophytes in the spine with skip areas (unlike AS, where it is in the continuum)
- **MRI of the SI joint**: In case of strong clinical suspicion of psoriatic arthropathy where X-ray fails to show sacroiliitis, MRI can detect sacroiliitis.
- **Serology**
    - **HLA-B27+** (in 50% of cases)
    - **Serum uric acid:** Often, serum uric acid is elevated in psoriasis as latter is a high cell turnover condition.
    - **Others:** Elevated ESR, CRP in acute exacerbation.

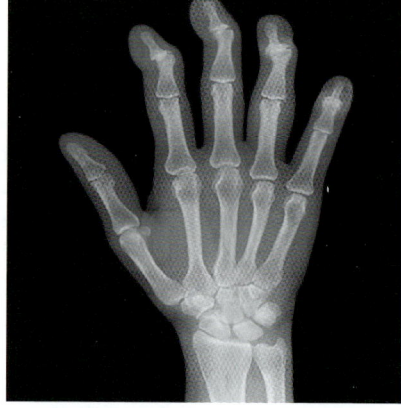

Fig. 33.7: Distal interphalangeal arthritis in Psoriasis sparing MCP and PIP joint.

TREATMENT

The *mainstay of treatment is to control psoriasis*, which is managed by retinoids, psoralens, and PUVA therapy. Psoriatic arthropathy is managed conservatively by NSAIDs for pain relief and DMARDs to prevent joint damage.

- **Medical treatment**
    - Pain relief: NSAIDs
    - Disease-modifying agents: Sulfasalazine, methotrexate
    - Biological agents: *Anti*-TNF drugs
- **Surgery:** Interphalangeal (IP) joint fusion (arthrodesis) for pain relief and improving hand function.

REACTIVE ARTHRITIS/REITER'S SYNDROME

DEFINITION

Reactive arthritis is an inflammatory seronegative spondyloarthropathy that results from a nonpurulent infection elsewhere (typically gastrointestinal or genitourinary).

Classic triad of reactive arthritis
Postinfection nonerosive arthritis, nongonococcal urethritis, and conjunctivitis, which generally occurs 3–4 weeks after the primary infection **(Fig. 33.8)**.

ETIOLOGY

Commonly, reactive arthritis occurs after an episode of gastrointestinal infection or genitourinary infection due to certain bacteria, which are mentioned below.
- **Gastrointestinal:** *Shigella, Salmonella,* and *Campylobacter jejuni*
- **Genitourinary:** *Chlamydia trachomatis, Mycoplasma genalium, Yersinia*

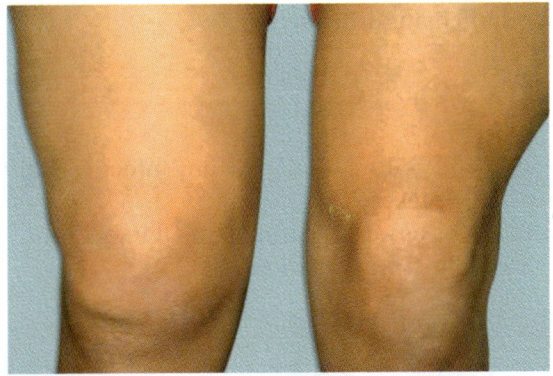
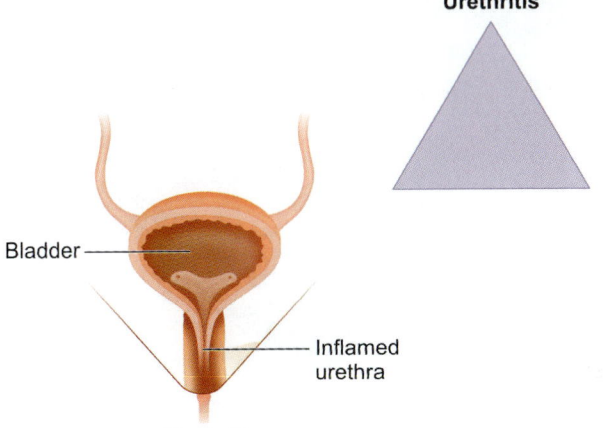
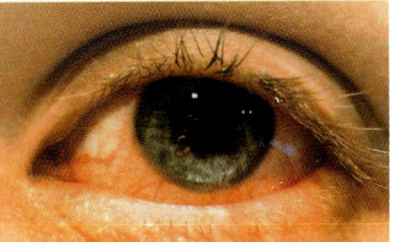

Fig. 33.8: Classic clinical triad of Reiter's syndrome.

PATHOPHYSIOLOGY

It involves the **activation of the immune system due to bacterial components**. Further **molecular mimicry** plays a role and causes damage to joints, eyes, skin, and the urinary system. **HLA-B27 association** is present in 25% of patients.

CLINICAL FEATURES

Usually, the patients of reactive arthritis are young (20–40 years) males. They present with **acute, asymmetric non-erosive oligoarthritis** (knee, ankle), which develops 3–4 weeks after a gastrointestinal/genitourinary infection episode. However, 30% of patients may not remember the history of any primary infection. Other features are:
- **Low back pain** due to sacroiliitis, which is usually unilateral
- **Urethritis**
- **Mucocutaneous lesions**: *Keratoderma blennorrhagicum* (pustular and scaling keratotic papules and plaques distributed over the extensor surfaces of the arms and legs as well as the palms and soles) **(Fig. 33.9A)** and *Circinate balanitis* (inflammation of glans or penile shaft) and can be seen in Reiter's syndrome **(Fig. 33.9B)**.
- **Enthesitis** (heel pain)
- **Ocular involvement:** Conjunctivitis, iritis, scleritis

INVESTIGATIONS

- Elevated ESR and CRP
- *Joint aspiration*: Gram stain and culture to rule out any infective pathology
- *HLA-B27*: It is positive in 25% of cases
- *Urine or stool analysis*: To assess any active urinary or GI infection
- *X-ray, MRI of the spine*: Sacroiliitis, bony erosion

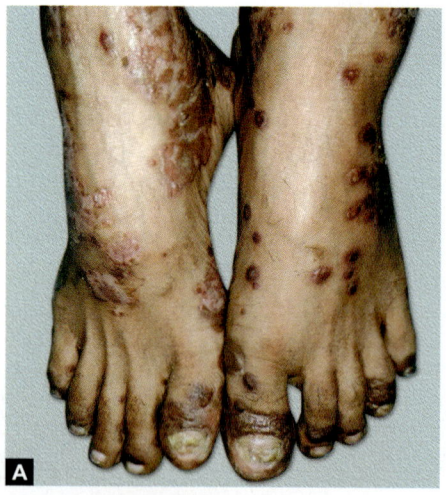
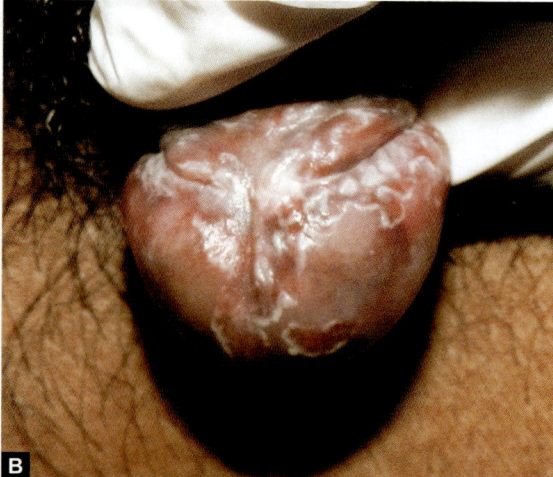

Figs. 33.9A and B: Mucocutaneous lesions in Reiter's syndrome: (A) Keratoderma blennorrhagicum; (B) Circinate balanitis.
(*Courtesy:* Professor Pratik Gahalaut, SKIMS, Bareilly and Professor Raghavendra Rao, KMC, Manipal)

- *X-ray of hand bones* may show fluffy periostitis
- Rheumatoid factor, antinuclear antibody (ANA) negative

TREATMENT

A majority of the patients are managed conservatively with NSAIDs and steroids. Few may require DMARDs. Antibiotics are needed to treat active infection, if any.
- **NSAIDs** reduce pain and inflammation of the involved joint.
- **Steroids:** Occasionally, *intra-articular injection* of steroids is required to reduce joint inflammation. *Systemic steroids* (if there is no infection) are reserved for severe cases.
- **Antibiotics** are required if there is an active infection in the genitourinary/gastrointestinal tract.
- **DMARDs** like sulfasalazine can be considered in chronic reactive arthritis, which is refractory to conservative treatment.

COMPLICATIONS

- Arrhythmias
- Aortic regurgitation.

ENTEROPATHIC ARTHRITIS

DEFINITION

Enteropathic arthritis is an inflammatory seronegative spondyloarthropathy associated with inflammatory bowel diseases (IBD) like ulcerative colitis and Crohn's disease.

PATHOPHYSIOLOGY

The interplay of *genetic predisposition, HLA-B27,* and *gut microbes* play a significant role in the pathogenesis of enteropathic arthritis **(Fig. 33.10)**.

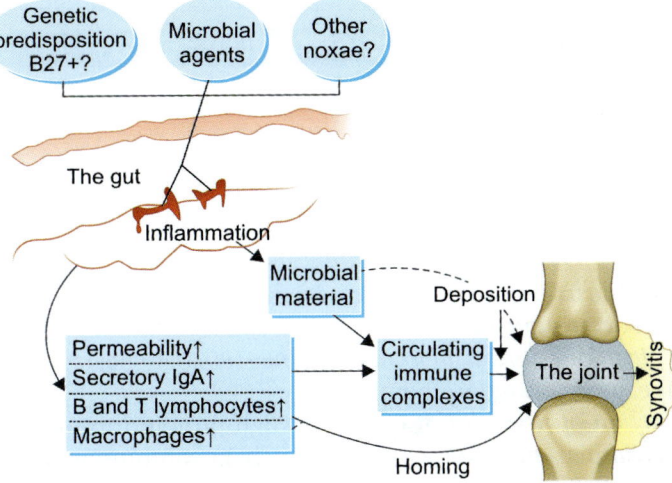

Fig. 33.10: Pathogenesis of enteropathic arthritis.

CLINICAL FEATURES

The characteristic complaints of patients with enteropathic arthritis are:
- **Features of inflammatory bowel disease (IBD):** Abdominal pain, diarrhea, altered bowel habits, and gastrointestinal (GI) bleed.
- **Low back pain** due to sacroiliitis
- **Peripheral arthritis**: It is a non-erosive, migratory type of arthritis. Usually, the knee and ankle are involved. They may have features of **enthesitis**—plantar fasciitis, tendo-Achilles tendinitis.
- **Mucocutaneous lesions:** *Erythema nodosum* **(Fig. 33.11)**, *pyoderma gangrenosum, aphthous stomatitis and anal fissures* are common mucocutaneous lesion observed in IBD.
- **Eye features:** Uveitis, iritis.

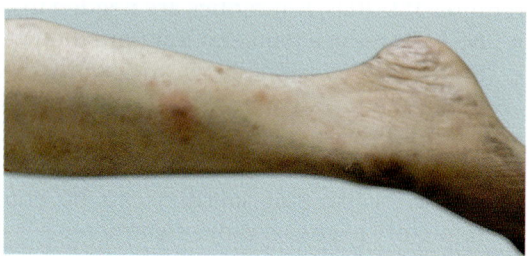

Fig. 33.11: Erythema nodosum.
(*Courtesy*: Professor Pratik Gahlaut, SKIMS, Bareilly)

INVESTIGATIONS

- Elevated ESR and CRP
- HLA-B27+
- *Colonoscopy*: Features of ulcerative colitis/Crohn's disease
- *X-ray and MRI of the spine*: Sacroiliitis.

TREATMENT

Apart from the treatment of IBD, the management of enteropathic arthritis is mainly symptomatic:
- **Analgesics:** NSAIDs should be avoided as they can exacerbate IBD.
- **DMARDs** such as sulfasalazine are useful due to their additional effect on IBD. TNF inhibitors can be tried in severe cases.

CRYSTALLINE ARTHRITIS: GOUT

DEFINITION

Gout is a disorder of purine metabolism characterized by hyperuricemia (>6.8–7 mg%) resulting in monosodium urate (MSU) deposition in the joints and periarticular tissues.

CLASSIFICATION

1. **Primary gout** is due to abnormal nucleic acid metabolism leading to hyperuricemia
2. **Secondary gout** occurs due to:
    - *Decreased filtration of uric acid from the kidney (90%)*: Renal failure, drugs like thiazide, cyclosporine, pyrazinamide, ethambutol
    - *High production of uric acid*: It occurs in high protein turnover conditions, such as tumors (leukemia, lymphomas), Paget's, hypoxanthine-guanine phosphoribosyl transferase (HPRT) disease (Lesch-Nyhan syndrome), chemotherapy of tumors, and skin disorders (psoriasis, exfoliative dermatitis).

RISK FACTORS OF GOUT

Hyperuricemia generally occurs due to either excess production of uric acid, under excretion, or a combination of both. The major risk factors are:
- Obesity and alcohol intake are major risk factors.
- **Dietary excess of purine-rich food:** Red meat, beans, peas, mushroom, cauliflower, alcohol
- **High cell turnover conditions:** Myeloproliferative disorders, chemotherapy, skin disorder such as psoriasis
- **Drugs:** Long-term use of diuretics, aspirin
- **Stress:** Post-traumatic, surgery

PATHOLOGY

The key to understanding gout pathology is that primarily *'fluctuations in serum uric acid level precipitate the attack of gout rather than the actual levels of serum uric acid.'* However, gouty attacks are directly correlated with the 'chronicity' of hyperuricemia and serum uric acid levels.

Pathology: The intermittent precipitation of monosodium urate (MSU) crystals in the joint results in foreign body reactions. Further, MSU crystals are engulfed by the macrophages, which initiate joint synovitis. Recurrent episodes of synovitis result in chronic gouty arthropathy.

CLINICAL FEATURES

- *Mostly, young individuals (20–50 years) are affected*
- **Acute gout:** Patients present with sudden onset, severe joint pain with red, warm, and shiny overlying skin with excruciating movements.
    - Typically, small joints of the foot are affected. **Classically first metatarsophalangeal (MTP)** joint of the great toe is involved, which is also known as **Podagra** (Fig. 33.12)
    - Sometimes, larger joints (ankle, knee) are involved.
- **Chronic gout:** Recurrent attacks present as chronic gout, wherein the involved joint becomes stiff, painful, and deformed. There may be **tophaceous chalky deposits** (MSU crystals) around the joint **(Fig. 33.13)**, bursae, tendons and ligaments. Tophi may also be

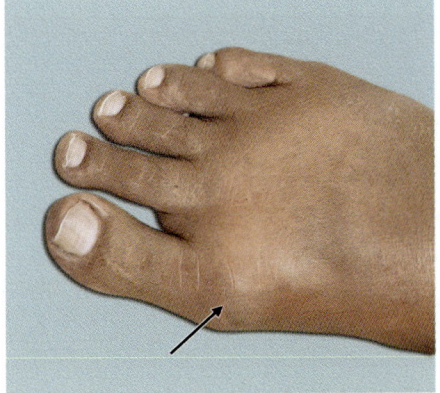

Fig. 33.12: Podagra of first metatarsophalangeal joint.

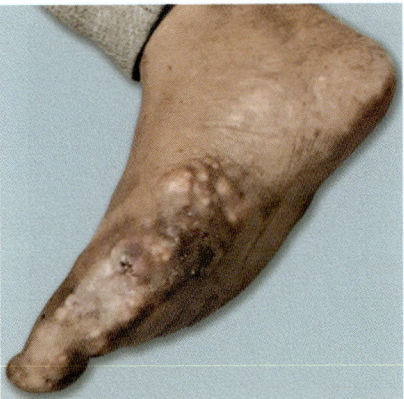

Fig. 33.13: Gout of the great toe with tophi around.

seen around the pinna and tendo-Achilles. Due to chronic hyperuricemia, there can be uric acid nephropathy resulting in *renal stone formation*.

INVESTIGATIONS

- **Serum uric acid:** It may or may not be elevated.
- **24-hour urine uric acid excretion:** More than 800 mg/day indicates excess uric acid production in the body.
- **X-ray:** Acute attack may show increased periarticular swelling
  Chronic gout may reveal
    - Periarticular erosions, joint space diminution
    - *G sign/Martel sign:* Punched out lesion of bone with overhanging edges **(Fig. 33.14)**
    - Soft tissue crystal deposition (tophi)
- **Joint aspiration:** It *could be diagnostic* if one can demonstrate uric acid crystals in the synovial fluid by polarized microscope. *MSU crystals are thin, needle-shaped, and negatively birefringent crystals* **(Fig. 33.15)**.

TREATMENT

- **General measures include dietary control, avoiding alcohol, hydration, and management of any underlying secondary cause of hyperuricemia**
    - Restrict high protein diet, especially red meat (bacon, beef, and pork) and seafood
    - Avoid beer or other alcoholic drinks
    - Plenty of water intake to avoid dehydration induced precipitation of uric acid (UA) and facilitate UA excretion.
    - Low-fat/fat-free milk
    - Management of underlying causes such as skin diseases/renal disorders, etc.
- **Medical treatment**
    - *Acute gout*: Rest and ice pack to the affected joint. Drugs such as:
        - *NSAIDs:* Indomethacin/Naproxen are effective in controlling acute episodes.
        - *Colchicine* is one of the best drugs to control acute episodes by inhibiting inflammatory mediators.
          Note: Colchicine can cause 'bloody diarrhea.'

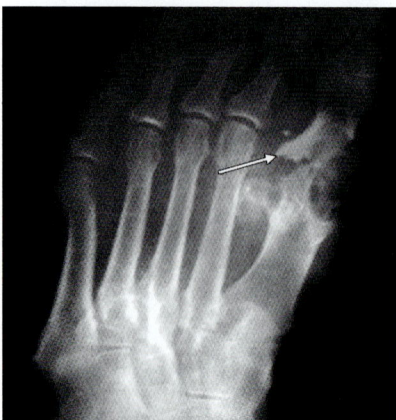

Fig. 33.14: Martel sign.

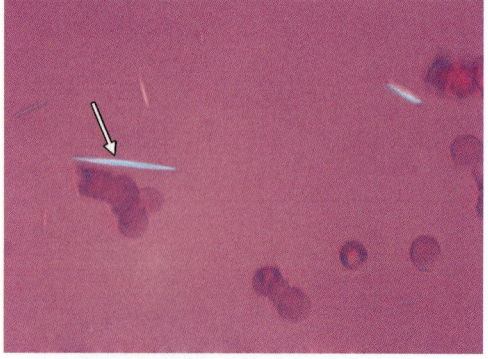

Fig. 33.15: Needle-shape negatively birefringent crystals of gout.
(*Source:* Wikimedia Commons)

- *Oral steroids* (prednisolone) can be added for 2–3 weeks if NSAIDs fail to control pain and inflammation.
  Once an acute gout episode is controlled, the patient can be started on uric acid-lowering drugs such as allopurinol or febuxostat.

  > Note: Uric acid-lowering drugs should not be given during an acute attack as they can precipitate gout by suddenly changing uric acid levels.

- **Chronic gout** is managed by uric acid-lowering drugs, initiated after an acute episode, and should be continued for 3–4 months. Various drugs used are:
  A. Xanthine oxidase inhibitors (XOI): Most preferred drugs in chronic gout.
     - *Allopurinol:* It is a purine based xanthine oxidase enzyme inhibitor.
     - *Febuxostat:* It is a non-purine based selective XOI. Currently, it is slightly preferred in cases of renal failure.
  B. Uricosurics: Probenecid has been used to lower uric acid by increasing uric acid excretion from the kidney. However, currently XOI are preferred over probenecid. Also, uricosuric is contraindicated if there are renal stones or 24-hour uric acid excretion >800 mg.
  C. Uricase: Pegloticase is a pegylated recombinant porcine uricase, the enzyme responsible for converting UA to allantoin, which is more soluble than uric acid and therefore more easily eliminated.

- **Surgical treatment**
  - Some cases might require tophi excision, especially if it is open or infected.
  - Arthroscopic synovectomy for persistent joint swelling and inflammation
  - Arthrodesis, joint replacement in arthritic joints.

DIFFERENTIAL DIAGNOSIS

- *Septic arthritis*: It cannot be ruled out even if there is MSU in the joint.
- Pseudogout
- Calcium oxalate deposition in the joint.

CRYSTALLINE ARTHRITIS: PSEUDOGOUT

DEFINITION

Recurrent monoarticular synovitis due to calcium pyrophosphate dihydrate (CPPD) deposition in the joints.

ASSOCIATED CONDITIONS AND PATHOLOGY

- Hemochromatosis and gout
- Hyperparathyroidism, systemic lupus erythematosus (SLE), and rheumatoid arthritis (RA)
- Wilson's disease

Most likely, pyrophosphate is secreted by the joint cartilage, which combines with calcium and forms calcium pyrophosphate crystal deposition (CPPD) **(Fig. 33.16)**. CPPD arthropathy can present as three distinct conditions—pseudogout, chondrocalcinosis, and chronic pyrophosphate arthropathy.

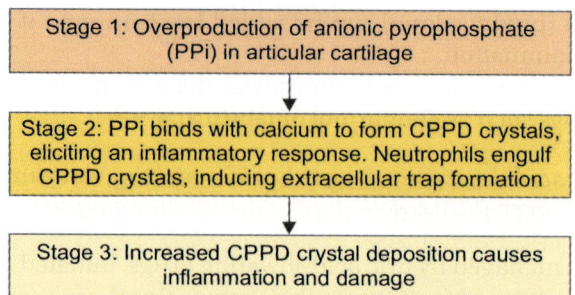

Fig. 33.16: Pathogenesis of calcium pyrophosphate crystal deposition (CPPD) arthritis.

1. **Pseudogout** is an acute synovitis of the joint due to CPPD crystal deposition.
2. **Chondrocalcinosis:** It is an asymptomatic condition characterized by the incidental radiological finding of calcification of cartilage, menisci, and intervertebral disc. Other disorders wherein chondrocalcinosis is observed are hyperparathyroidism, hypothyroidism, Wilson's disease, and alkaptonuria.
3. **Chronic pyrophosphate arthropathy:** These patients are older women who present with chronic arthritis of this section will discuss only pseudogout.

■ CLINICAL FEATURES OF PSEUDOGOUT

It mimics gout in clinical presentation, except that it occurs in *"older patients"* and affects *"larger joints"* (knee, wrist, shoulder, and ankle). These patients present with acute onset monoarticular joint pain and swelling.

Examination reveals:
- Increased local warmth, erythematous joint with effusion **(Fig. 33.17)**
- The ROM is painful and restricted.

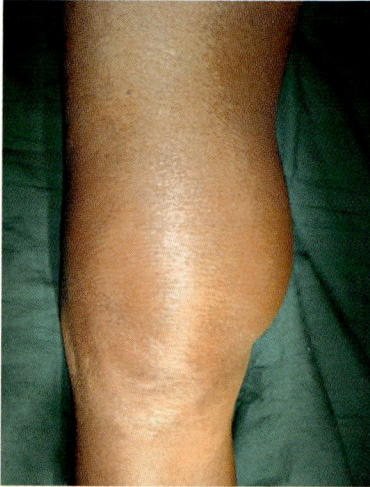

Fig. 33.17: Swelling of the knee joint in a patient with pseudogout.

Note that pseudogout may mimic septic arthritis due to its acute presentation. However, the latter can be ruled out by analysing the aspirated fluid.

■ INVESTIGATIONS

- **X-ray of the knee:** Calcification of menisci is quite frequent **(Fig. 33.18)**.
- **CT of the joint:** If X-rays are normal, a CT scan of the joint may help detect calcification of menisci or cartilage.
- **Joint aspiration: diagnostic**
    - Demonstrating CPPD crystals in the aspirated joint fluid by polarized microscope. *CPPD crystals are rhomboid-shaped and positively birefringent crystals* **(Fig. 33.19)**.
- Evaluate serum calcium, phosphorus, magnesium, thyroid stimulating hormone, and parathormone levels to rule out underlying disorders.

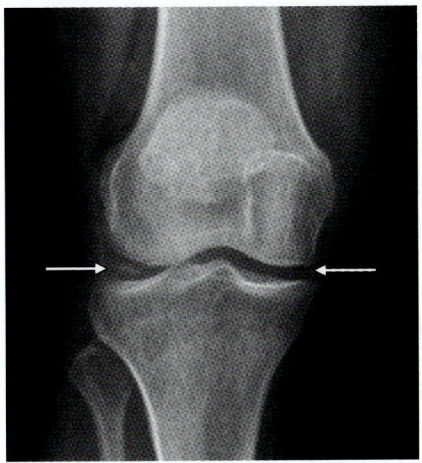

Fig. 33.18: Meniscal calcification in pseudogout (white arrows point over the calcified meniscus).

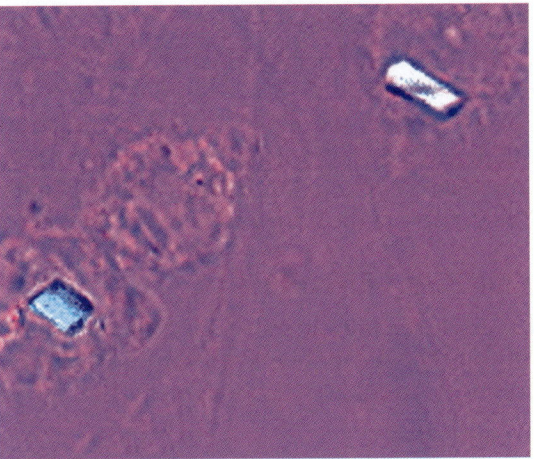

Fig. 33.19: Rhomboid shape positively birefringent crystals of pseudogout.
(*Source:* Wikimedia Commons)

TREATMENT

- **Medical management:** Control of associated causes (RA, SLE, etc.)
  - *Acute pseudogout*: The treatment is similar to gout using NSAIDs, steroids and colchicine. Rest and ice packs to the affected joint.
  - *Chronic pseudogout* is managed with optimal hydration and colchicine. For recurrent troublesome synovitis, radiosynovectomy can be performed with *intra-articular yttrium*-90 injections.
- **Surgical:** Arthroscopic debridement and synovectomy.

NEUROPATHIC/CHARCOT'S ARTHROPATHY

DEFINITION

Chronic, *progressive, painless destructive arthropathy of the joint* due to loss of pain sensation.

ETIOLOGY

Any condition which leads to loss of pain sensation might result in Charcot's arthropathy.
- **Diabetes mellitus:** It is the most common cause of Charcot's arthropathy. Typically, it involves the foot and ankle because *DM affects the longest neurons, most of which are relayed to the lower limb to the ankle and foot.*
- **Syringomyelia** is a common cause of Charcot's arthropathy, especially in the upper limb joints (shoulder and elbow).
- **Leprosy** (Hansen's disease)
- Arnold–Chiari malformation
- Syphilis
- Tabes dorsalis
- Alcoholism

PATHOPHYSIOLOGY

Two theories are implicated in the pathophysiology of Charcot's arthropathy—*neurogenic and vascular.*
- **Neurogenic:** Loss of pain sensation and proprioception leads to chronic perpetual micro-damage to the joint
- **Vascular:** Neuropathic limbs have dysregulated blood supply, which results in increased blood flow to the bones and consequent excess bone resorption and damage.

CLINICAL FEATURES

Painless, extensive destruction of the joint is the hallmark of Charcot's arthropathy.

Typically, the patients present with *gradually increasing swelling and painless joint deformity* **(Fig. 33.20A)**. Occasionally, there may be mild pain.

On examination:
- *Deformity* of the joint with gross swelling **(Fig. 33.20A)**.
- The skin may show *non-healing trophic ulcerations* **(Fig. 33.20B)**.
- There may be a slight increase in local warmth and erythema (due to increased blood flow), especially in the early stages of Charcot's, which can mimic an infection.
- *Movements at joint are painless and exaggerated* (due to gross bone-joint destruction).
- The *neurovascular examination* may reveal loss of pain, proprioceptive sensation and poor vascularity.
- *Features of instability* in various planes (due to gross bone-joint destruction) are present.

INVESTIGATIONS

- **X-ray of the affected joint (Figs. 33.21 and 33.22)**
    - Joint space narrowing
    - Gross destruction and dislocation of the joint

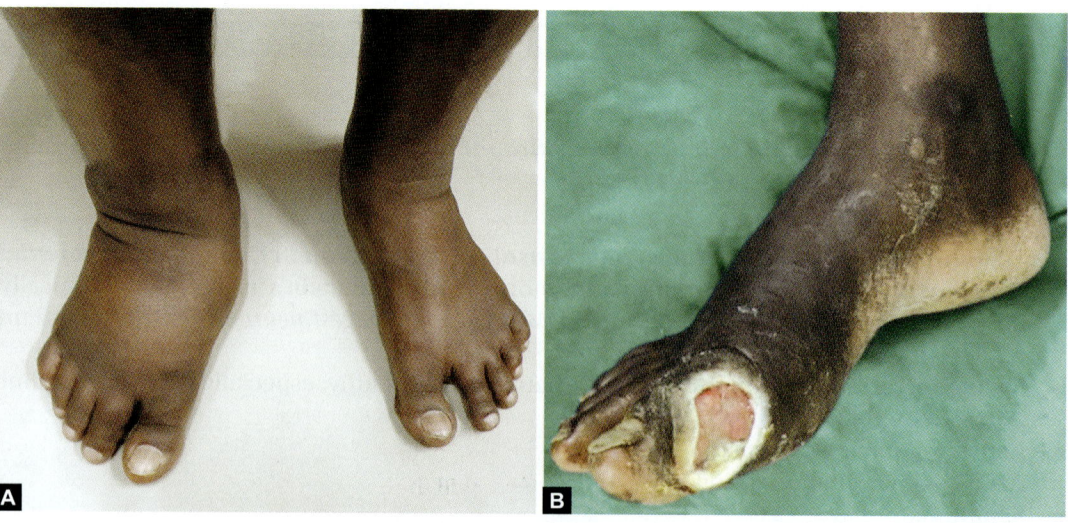

Figs. 33.20A and B: (A) Swelling and deformity of right foot with flattening of medial longitudinal arch; (B) Trophic ulcer over great toe.

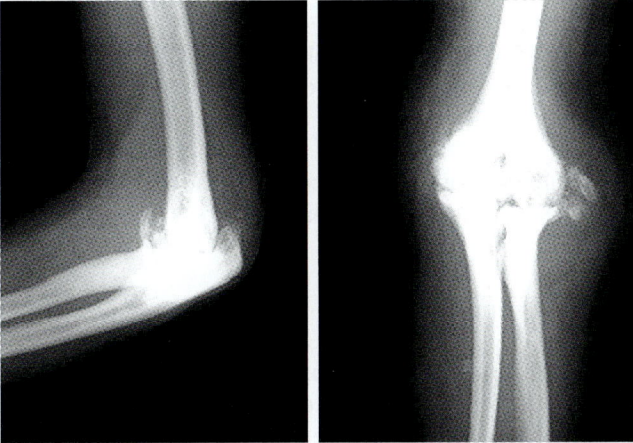

Fig. 33.21: X-ray of Charcot's elbow showing severe joint destruction, sclerosis, and loose bodies.

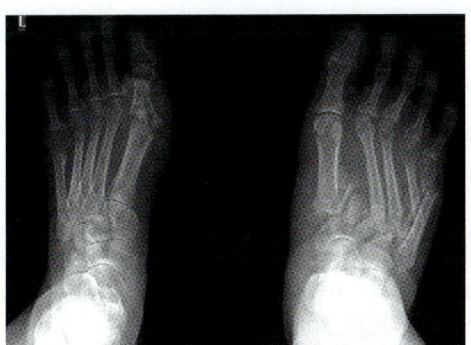 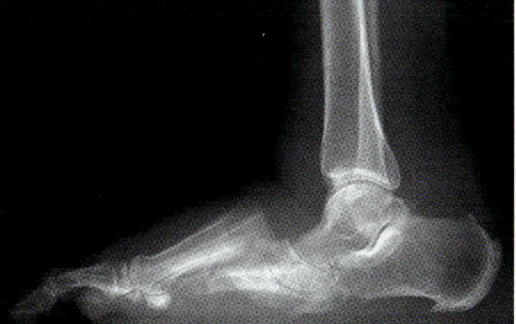

Fig. 33.22: Charcot's arthropathy of the right foot (AP and lateral views) showing dislocation of tarsometatarsal joints, debris, sclerosed bone, and fractures of metatarsals.

- ◆ Multiple, loose flakes of bone in the soft tissue space
- ◆ Dense sclerosed bone
- ◆ Heterotrophic ossification
- ◆ Occasional fractures
- **Magnetic resonance imaging (MRI)**
    - ◆ To rule out associated osteomyelitis in the affected region
    - ◆ In patients with upper limb Charcot's joint, syringomyelia of the cervical cord must be ruled out, which may show syrinx (a fluid filled cavity of central canal) **(Fig. 33.23)**.
- **Joint aspiration:** It should be done to rule out concomitant infection
- **Bone scan:** It is positive in both osteomyelitis and Charcot's arthropathy. A specific "Indium bone scan" will help in differentiating between the two as there will be cold spot in case of neuropathic arthritis, where osteomyelitis will have hot spots.

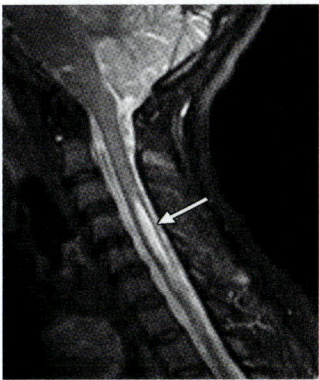

Fig. 33.23: MRI cervical spine showing syrinx in the central canal (white arrow).

TREATMENT

Typically, Charcot's arthropathy is an irreversible disorder. The mainstay of the treatment is to control the underlying condition and prevent complications such as ulcers and further injury to bones and joints.
- **General measures**
    - Treat/control the cause, if possible. For example, the diabetes mellitus should be strictly controlled. Hansen's disease must be treated aggressively.
    - Limb elevation
    - Treat infection
    - Functional bracing to support the joint.
- **Surgical treatment**
    - Debridement of ulcers and prominent exostosis excision
    - *Arthrodesis of unstable joint*: High chance of failure
    - *Total joint arthroplasty* is contraindicated due to high chance of failure as there is lack of proprioception, and poor neuromuscular control over muscles.

MISCELLANEOUS ARTHRITIS

SLE ASSOCIATED ARTHRITIS

- It is present in 95% of SLE cases. Typically, women are affected who are between 15 and 45 years.
- **Clinical features:** *Symmetrical polyarthritis* of small joints of the hand and foot, *serositis*, and *renal involvement* are common. Unlike RA, SLE arthritis is **migratory and non-erosive.** The deformities are similar to RA, but due to ligament laxity and muscle contracture and less due to joint destruction. There are **Malar rashes,** *which are discoid and photosensitive.*
- **Management:** CRP and ESR are high. ANA and Sm antigen are positive. Medical management is the key, with methotrexate, HCQ, and steroids.

HEMOPHILIC ARTHRITIS

It is characterized by repetitive hemarthroses and, ultimately, joint deformation in patients with bleeding disorders.

Etiology: It is an ***X-linked recessive disorder***, which manifests in men with females as the carrier of genes.

Types: There are three types of hemophilia:
1. ***Hemophilia A*** due to deficient factor VIII—85% of cases.
2. ***Hemophilia B*** (Christmas disease) due to deficient factor IX
3. ***von Willebrand disease*** is autosomal dominant with abnormal factor VIII and platelet dysfunction.

The severity of hemophilia: *If the factor VIII level is >40%, there is no bleeding tendency.*
A. ***Mild disease:*** *Factor VIII level 5–25%*
B. ***Moderate disease:*** *Factor VIII level 1–5% prolonged bleeding after injury/surgery*
C. ***Severe disease:*** *Factor VIII level <1%*

Clinical features: It starts manifesting in males 3–15 years old and presents with spontaneous bleeding in joints, muscles, and nerves.

- **Hemorrhages in the joint**: Typically, the knee is most commonly affected, followed by the ankle, elbows and hips. Initially, repeated bleeding causes chronic synovitis. Later, it results in joint destruction, fibrous ankylosis, and deformity.
- **Hemorrhages in muscle:** Quadriceps, triceps surae, iliacus, and deltoid is affected, resulting in deformity and contractures. Occasionally, there can be compartment syndrome followed by Volkmann ischemic contracture **(Fig. 33.24)**.
- **Hemorrhages in nerves** result in nerve palsy. The femoral nerve is most commonly affected, followed by the median nerve.
- **Hemophilic cysts/pseudotumor** is due to bleeding in a confined place. The most common site for pseudotumor formation is the thigh > abdomen (retroperitoneum), followed by the pelvis.
- **Other musculoskeletal features:** The *epiphyseal overgrowth* results in limb lengthening. There is *osteopenia* of bone, which results in pathological fractures.

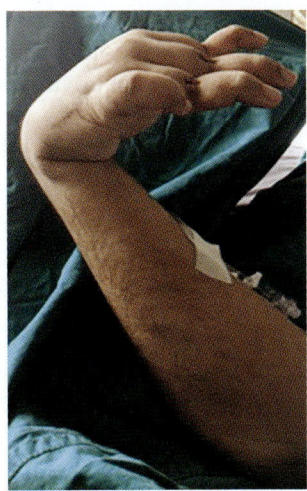

Fig. 33.24: VIC of hand in hemophilia.

Investigations

- *Clotting time is increased*, whereas bleeding time and prothrombin time are normal.
- *Deficient factor VIII*
- *Factor VIII antibody* is present in 5–25% of hemophiliacs. It is a *contraindication for surgery* as these antibodies neutralize the therapeutic factor VIII.
- **Radiology:** Bones and joints reveal generalized rarefaction, juxta-articular erosions, and subchondral cyst. *Epiphyseal overgrowth is one of the key signs.*

Knee joint findings are characterized by the widening of the intercondylar notch **(Fig. 33.25)**, squaring of the patella and femoral condyles **(Jordan's sign).**

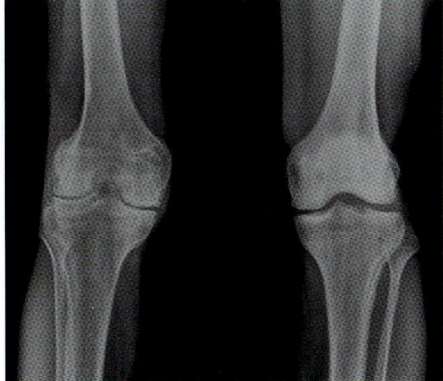

Fig. 33.25: Haemophilic knee. X-ray of right knee shows intercondylar notch widening, squared femoral condyles, and symmetric joint space reduction.

Treatment

The treatment of hemophilic arthropathy is to control bleeding, manage pain, prevent deformity, and treat existing painful synovitis and arthritis.

- **Control hemorrhage** by factor VIII replacement and FFP to increase factor level to 30–40%. In the case of an acute hematoma or hemarthrosis, increase the factor VIII level to 30–50%. If any surgery has to be performed, the factor VIII level should be 100% in 1st week, followed by maintenance to 50% in the next week.
- **Desmopressin** can be tried in mild-moderate hemophilia
- **Relieve pain** with ice packs, compression, and tramadol. Use NSAID with caution.
- **Preserve joint mobility and prevent deformity** through physiotherapy, braces, and traction.

- **Chronic synovitis** can be treated with arthroscopic synovectomy or radiation synovectomy (Yttrium, colloidal phosphorus-32 chromic phosphate).
- **Treatment of advanced arthritis** is by joint replacement/arthrodesis.

ALKAPTONURIC ARTHRITIS (SYN: OCHRONOSIS)

Alkaptonuria is a congenital disorder of amino acid **'tyrosine'** metabolism, in which amino acid tyrosine is not broken down beyond homogentisic acid due to a *lack of homogentisic acid oxidase enzyme*. Homogentisic acid gets deposited in soft tissues, cartilage, synovium, menisci, and intervertebral disc, affect the biomechanical properties of these structures.

Genetic: HGD gene has been implicated in ochronosis.

Clinical features: Initially, patients are asymptomatic, and only their urine turns black on exposure to air. Later, 'ochre' colored deposits occur in bone, cartilage, tendon sheath, ear pinna and sclera. The *joint symptoms appear after 40 years of age*. Generalized pain and stiffness of the spine and peripheral joints arthritis, especially the shoulder, is quite common.

Investigations
- Detection of **homogentisic acid in urine**—urine forms a yellowish precipitate on adding benedict solution (silver nitrate).
- Spine X-ray—*calcification of intervertebral disc* (**Fig. 33.26**).
- Peripheral joints: Arthritis, especially shoulders (**Fig. 33.27**).

Treatment: The treatment is symptomatic with analgesics and physiotherapy. The role of vitamin C is being evaluated. Recently, **nitisinone** (inhibitor of 4-hydroxy-phenyl-pyruvate-dioxygenase) has been tried, which reduces the level of homogentisic acid and can slow the progression of the disease. Joint replacement can be performed in severe cases of peripheral joint arthritis.

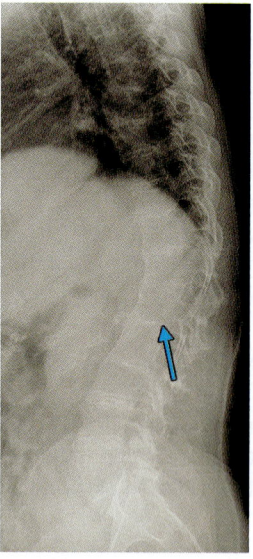

Fig. 33.26: Intervertebral disc calcification.

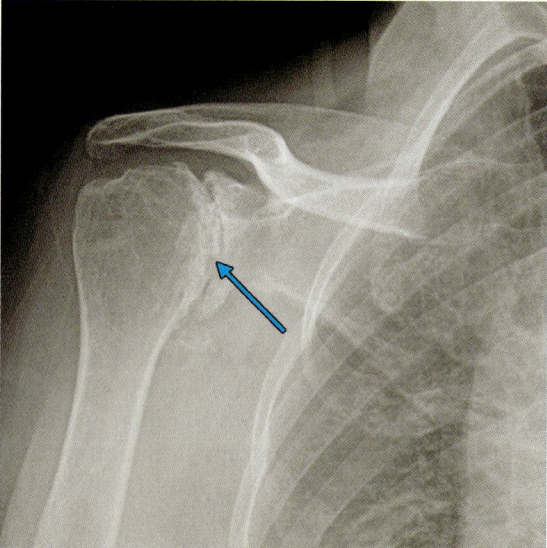

Fig. 33.27: Arthritis of shoulder joint (decreased joint space).

JUVENILE RHEUMATOID ARTHRITIS (JRA)/ JUVENILE IDIOPATHIC ARTHRITIS

Juvenile idiopathic arthritis (JIA) is a collection of chronic pediatric arthropathies *characterized by onset before 16 years of age and objective arthritis (in one or more joints) for at least 6 weeks. It is an autoimmune disorder which* typically affects the hand, wrist, knee, ankle and elbows. It may affect other joints too.

Risk factor: Female younger than 6 years, positive family history, HLA polymorphism

Pathology: It is characterized by chronic synovitis. Later, there is cartilage damage, resulting in arthritis and deformity.

Classification: It can present as *oligoarthritis* (4 or less joints), *polyarthritis* (5 or more joints) or *systemic disease*. In systemic disease, there is arthritis in one or more joints in addition to daily high-spiking fevers and evanescent, truncal, salmon-colored, macular rashes. Occasionally presentation could be of enthesitis or psoriatic arthritis.

Clinical features: Joint pain, morning stiffness, swelling, and fever are common. There can be enthesitis and Salmon rash. Uveitis or rheumatoid nodules are uncommon.

Investigations: ESR and CRP are elevated. RA factor and anti-CCP are positive in the polyarticular variant, whereas ANA is positive in the oligoarticular type.

Treatment is similar to rheumatoid arthritis with *analgesics, DMARDs (methotrexate), and steroids.* Biological agents are tried on patients who do not respond to DMARDs.

MSELENI JOINT DISEASE

It is a *crippling chondrodysplasia* of the *Mseleni tribe of Northern Kwazulu-Natal, South Africa.* Their rural population who speak 'Zulu language' is affected.

Clinical features: It presents as polyarthritis. The hip joint is most commonly affected with *hip dysplasia and protrusio acetabuli as the most common feature.*

KASHIN BECK DISEASE

It is a chronic disease of muscle and joints causing skeletal deformities and short stature, which is endemic in **North-Central China, North Korea, Tibet and South-East Siberia.**

Etiology: Idiopathic, *selenium deficiency, or mycotoxin contamination* have been implicated. Children and adolescent are most affected.

Clinical features: Symmetrical epiphyseal destruction and metaphyseal enlargement resulting in dwarfism. They also have polyarthritis, morning stiffness, short fingers, and growth retardation.

Notes

SECTION 6

Degenerative Conditions of the Spine

SECTION OUTLINE

34. Approach to Neck and Low Back Pain
    - Intervertebral Disc Prolapse
    - Cauda Equina Syndrome
    - Conus Medullaris Syndrome
    - Spondylosis (Spondylitis)
    - Spondylolysis and Spondylolisthesis
    - Lumbar Canal Stenosis

Degenerative Conditions of the Spine

34 CHAPTER

Approach to Neck and Low Back Pain

INTERVERTEBRAL DISC PROLAPSE (IVDP)

■ SURGICAL ANATOMY OF THE INTERVERTEBRAL DISC

There are 23 intervertebral discs (6 cervical, 12 thoracic, and 5 lumbar), almost constituting one-fourth of the spinal column. They are cushion-like structures sandwiched between the two vertebrae allowing spinal motion and providing stability. The intervertebral disc (IVD) has two parts—nucleus pulposus and annulus fibrosis **(Fig. 34.1A)**.

1. *Annulus fibrosus:* It is an outer encasing fibrous ring made of *type I collagen*, proteoglycan and water. The annulus fibrosus fibers are arranged in a specific pattern as 30° oblique fashion, reverse contiguous **(Fig. 34.1B)**. The oblique-reverse contiguous pattern of the annulus resists compressive forces exerted by the nucleus pulposus. It acts like a cage to protect the nucleus pulposus.
2. *Nucleus pulposus:* It is a central hydrated gel made of *type II collagen*, proteoglycan and 88% water. The nucleus transmits stress and weight to the adjacent vertebra. It is said to be the remnant of the notochord.

- **Endplates** are cartilaginous discs sandwiched between the vertebral body and the IVD, firmly supporting the entire intervertebral disc **(Fig. 34.2A)**. The end plate prevents disc herniating into the vertebral body and allows the diffusion of nutrients and oxygen between the disc and bone.
- **Supporting ligaments of IVD:** The anterior longitudinal ligament (ALL) and posterior longitudinal ligament (PLL), which stretch from the atlas to the sacrum, support the disc

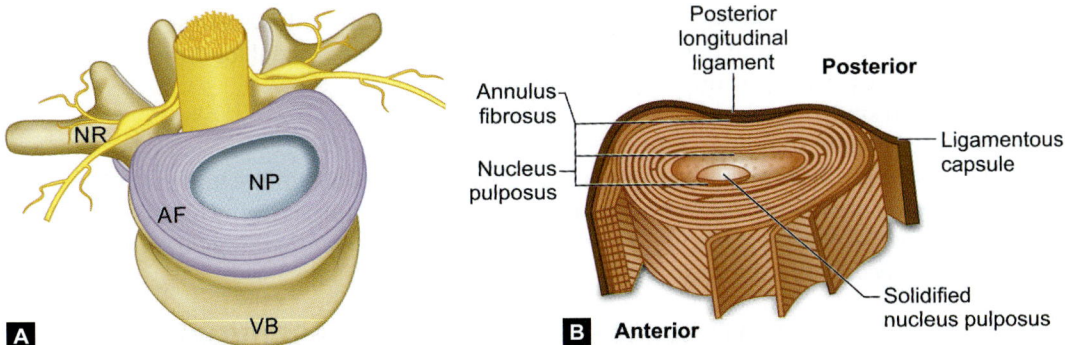

Figs. 34.1A and B: (A) Cross section of an intervertebral disc; (B) Structure of an annulus fibrosus showing reverse contiguous oblique pattern.
(NP: nucleus pulposus; AF: annulus fibrosus; VB: vertebral body; NR: nerve root)

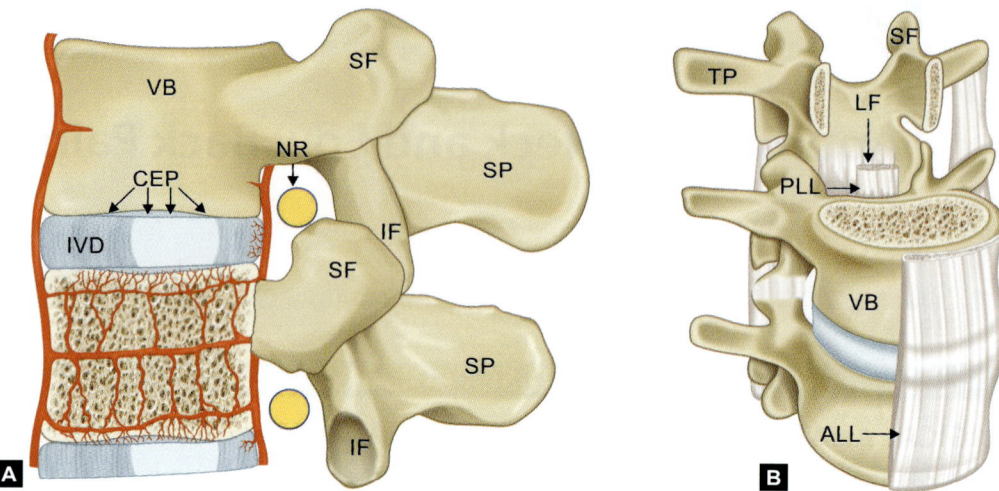

Figs. 34.2A and B: (A) Blood supply of the vertebral body, intervertebral disc and cartilaginous endplate; (B) Support to the intervertebral disc by anterior and posterior longitudinal ligament.
(VB: vertebral body; IVD: intervertebral disc; SF: superior facet; IF: inferior facet; NR: nerve root; CEP: cartilaginous endplate; SP: spinous process; ALL: anterior longitudinal ligament; PLL: posterior longitudinal ligament; TP: transverse process; LF: ligamentum flavum)

from the front and back, respectively **(Fig. 34.2B)**. In comparison to ALL, the PLL is weak. Therefore, the IVD tends to prolapse posteriorly.
- **Vascularity of IVD:** Most IVD is avascular except outer annulus fibrosus. IVD gets its nutrition through diffusion from the pores of the vertebral endplate, which are supplied by the vertebral blood vessel capillaries terminating at the endplate **(Fig. 34.2A)**.
- **Nerve supply of IVD:** The outer annulus fibrosus ring has nerve supply through the sinuvertebral nerve (via dorsal root ganglion). Hence, stretching the annulus fibrosus due to a disc bulge causes pain.

BIOMECHANICS OF THE IVD

- Annulus fibrosus has high "tensile stresses," whereas nucleus pulposus has high "compressive stresses".
- Intervertebral disc possesses viscoelastic properties (creep and hysteresis), allowing for deformation over time and energy absorption during repetitive axial loading.
  Intradiscal pressure is position dependent, which is:
    - *Lowest* in supine position
    - *Moderate* while standing
    - *Highest* while bending forward with load in hand, especially in the lumbar spine.
  Furthermore, the vertical stress on cervical spine increase while carrying loads on the head.
  Note: Hence, the chance of disc injury or prolapse is highest while leaning forward with load in hand, especially in lumbar spine.

RISK FACTORS FOR INTERVERTEBRAL DISC PROLAPSE (IVDP)

The disc herniation and prolapses are common in lumbar followed by cervical region as they are mobile segments prone for load concentrations. Disc herniations are uncommon

in thoracic region. There are several risk factors, which could result in disc degeneration and prolapses.
1. Aging
2. Jobs requiring repeated bending forward and heavy weight lifting, vibration, prolonged sitting or carrying overhead loads.
3. Obesity, smoking, sedentary lifestyle and lack of regular exercises.

PATHOPHYSIOLOGY OF IVDP

Commonly, disc herniation occurs in two situations—disc degeneration or traumatic.
1. **Degenerative:** It is the most common cause of disc herniation. The disc degeneration begins as the person ages, involving several pathological processes, such as gradual loss of water content of the disc, decreased proteoglycan content and consequent loss in the height of the disc. The cartilaginous endplates also starts calcifying affecting the disc nutrition. Furthermore, multiple episodes of microtrauma result in small tears in the annulus fibrosus, resulting in loss of support to nucleus pulposus causing gradual disc herniation. Any major trauma superimposed over this degenerated and weak disc can causes sudden disc herniation. Once the periphery of annulus is ruptured, the disc prolapses through the tear.
   A chronic disc degeneration (and or prolapse) gradually brings spondylotic changes in the spine.
2. **Trauma:** A major traumatic vertical load over the spine, such as fall over the buttock, lifting heavy weight while bending forward, or lifting heavy weight over the head could result in annulus rupture followed by disc herniation and prolapse. **Flowchart 34.1** briefly outlines the process of intervertebral disc prolapse.

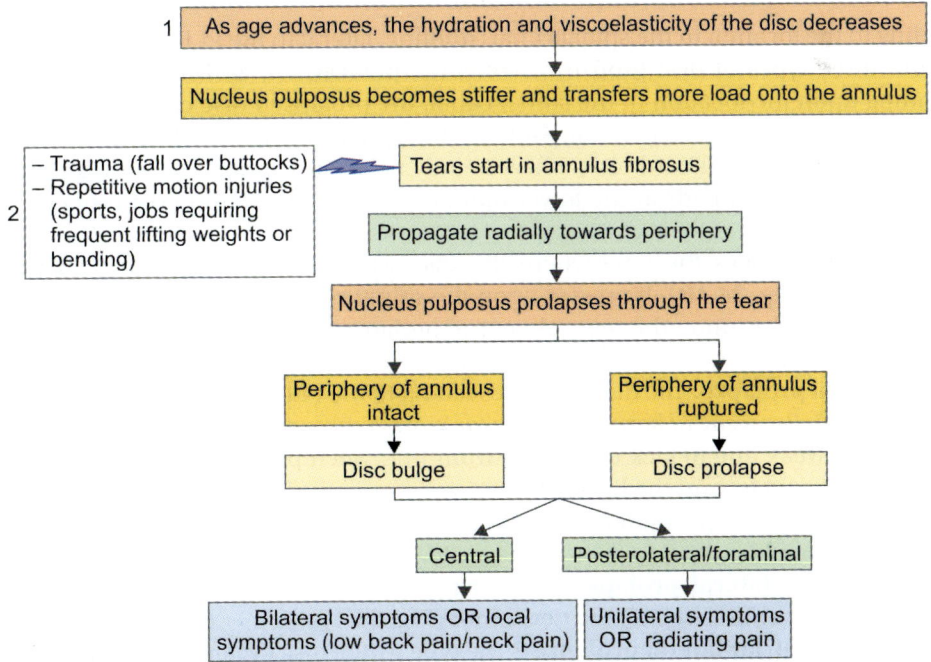

Flowchart 34.1: Pathogenesis of the intervertebral disc prolapse.

STAGES OF DISC HERNIATION (FIG. 34.3)

There are four stages in disc herniation:
1. Disc **degeneration:** Mechanochemical changes associated with aging causes discs to weaken, but without a prolapse.
2. Disc **prolapse or bulge or protrusion:** As the inner fibers of the annulus weaken and rupture, unable to contain hoop stresses, the nucleus pulposus bulges posteriorly.
3. Disc **extrusion:** A complete rupture of the annulus results in herniation of the nucleus pulposus. However, *extruded disc material remains continuous with the parent disc.*
4. Disc **sequestration:** Part of the *extruded disc (nucleus pulposus) is separated* from the parent disc and freely floats in the spinal canal.

Note: Although disc prolapse/bulge/protrusion and extrusion are different stages of disc herniation, these terminologies are often used synonymously. However, sequestration is a distinct term wherein extruded disc material is completely separated.

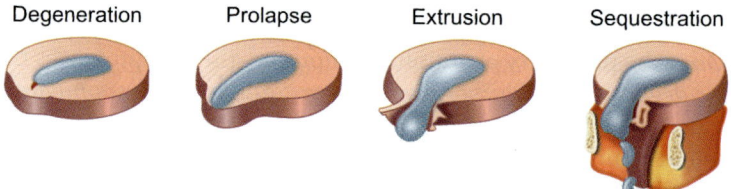

Fig. 34.3: Stages of disc degeneration.

TYPE OF DISC HERNIATION ACCORDING TO LOCATION WITH SYMPTOMS

According to the location in the spinal canal (midline, lateral to the PLL and neural foramina), there are three types of disc protrusion—central, paracentral, and foraminal **(Fig. 34.4A)**. Depending upon the location in the spinal canal, the prolapsed disc can compress upon the spinal cord or nerve roots. In cervical, thoracic and spinal canal upto L1 vertebra, a prolapsed disc can compress spinal cord also, whereas only roots are compressed in region below L1 vertebra as spinal cord ends at the lower border of L1 vertebra and nerve roots form cauda equina.

1. **Central prolapse** is the type where the disc which herniates into the middle of the spinal canal **(Fig. 34.4B)**. It presses upon the spinal cord (only upto L1 vertebra) and less frequently presses upon the roots. A central prolapse results in localized pain in the neck or back.
2. **Paracentral prolapse:** The disc herniates lateral to the PLL and compresses the nerve root **(Fig. 34.4C)**. *Paracentral herniations are far more common than central* as support over the annulus is weak due to lack of support from PLL. Such paracentral disc prolapses cause radiation of pain toward the limb.
    Further, paracentral/posterolateral prolapsed disc could be medial (axillary type) or lateral (deltoid or shoulder type) to the root **(Figs. 34.4D and E)**.
3. **Foraminal/far lateral prolapse** is the type where the disc herniates into the neural foramina directly pressing on the nerve root **(Fig. 34.4)**.
4. **Extraforaminal/far lateral prolapse** is the type where disc prolapse outside the foramina.

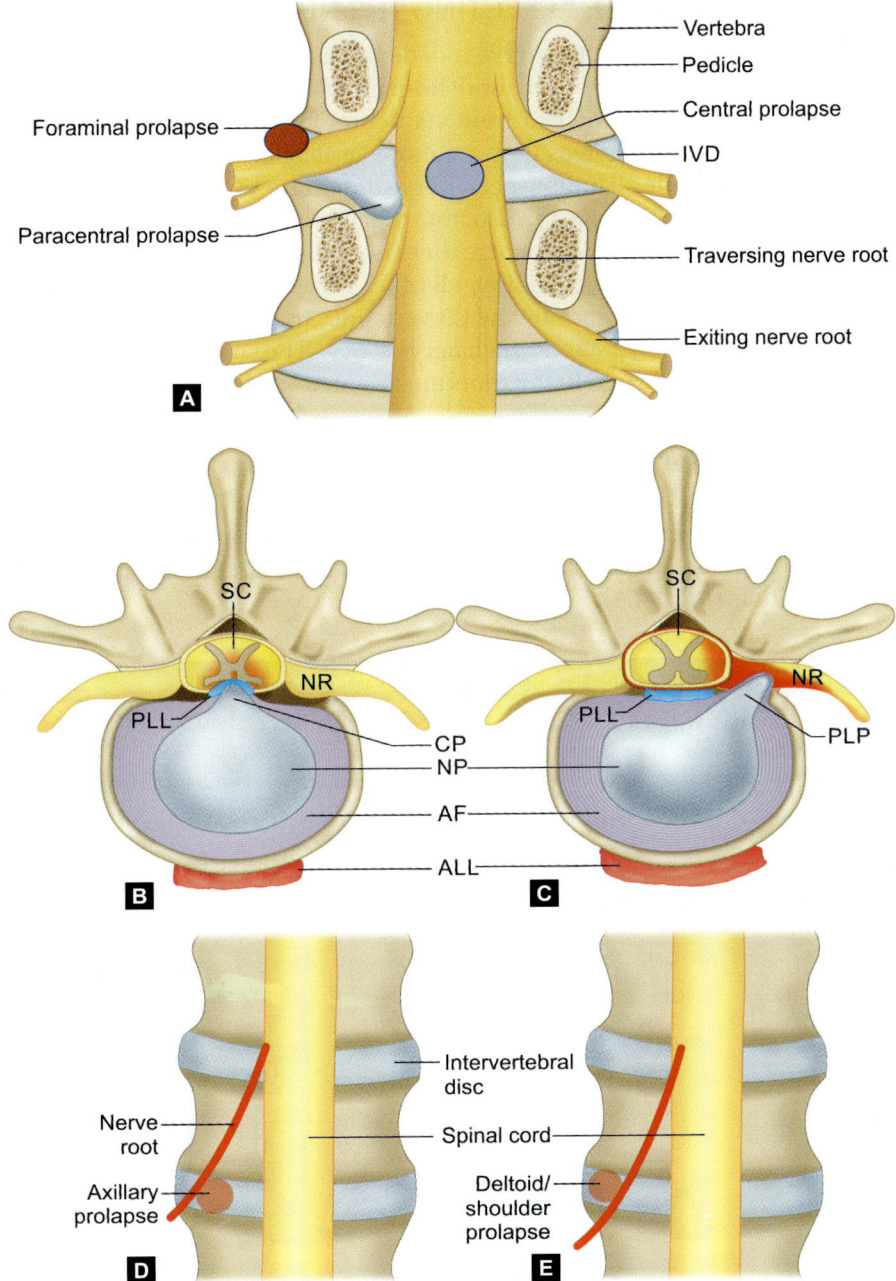

Figs. 34.4A to E: (A) Coronal section of lumbar spine showing central, paracentral/posterolateral and foraminal disc prolapse compressing nerve roots; (B) Axial section of the spine showing central prolapse of intervertebral disc compressing the spinal cord; (C) Axial section of the spine showing paracentral/posterolateral prolapse of intervertebral disc compressing the nerve root; (D) Axillary; (E) Deltoid type of paracentral disc prolapse with respect to nerve root.

(NP: nucleus pulposus; AF: annulus fibrosus; ALL: anterior longitudinal ligament; PLL: posterior longitudinal ligament; NR: nerve root; SC: spinal cord; CP: central prolapse; PLP: posterolateral prolapse)

LEVEL OF DISC PROLAPSE AFFECTING THE NERVE ROOT INVOLVEMENT

The level of disc prolapse and affected nerve root depends upon the orientation of nerve roots in the spinal canal, i.e., whether they are more horizontally or vertically oriented in the spinal canal. From the spinal cord till the exit from via neural forminal, the nerve roots are more horizontal in cervical region, whereas they are more vertical in lumbar region as spinal cord ends at L1 vertebra level while all lumbosacral nerve roots have to descend further downwards to exit via neural foramina **(Table 34.1)**. Also note that C1 root traverses above the C1 vertebra (between base of skull and C1 vertebra where there is no disc) and C2 root is passes below the C2 vertebra in horizontal fashion. Similarly, all other cervical roots pass horizontally below corresponding vertebra, e.g., C3 root below C3 vertebra. Another concept of 'traversing and exiting roots' is essential to understand which nerve root will be compressed in a disc prolapse. It is relevant in lumbar spine wherein the roots are oriented vertically.

Traversing root: It is the nerve root, which crosses the disc vertically/obliquely to 'exit' one level lower than the disc level **(Fig. 34.5A)**.

Exiting root: It is the nerve root, which exits the neural foramina **(Fig. 34.5B)**.

The paracentral discs are closer to traversing root, while foraminal discs lie adjacent to the exiting roots. Therefore, paracentral discs compress traversing root, while foraminal disc compress exiting roots **(Fig. 34.5)**.

	Root orientation and course in the spinal canal	Traversing root	Relation with pedicle while exiting the spinal canal
Cervical	Horizontally	No	Above the pedicle, e.g., (C4 root will cross above C4 pedicle)
Lumbar	Vertically	Yes	Below the pedicle, e.g., (L4 root will cross below L4 pedicle)

Table 34.1: Pattern of root orientation in spinal canal and relation with pedicles.

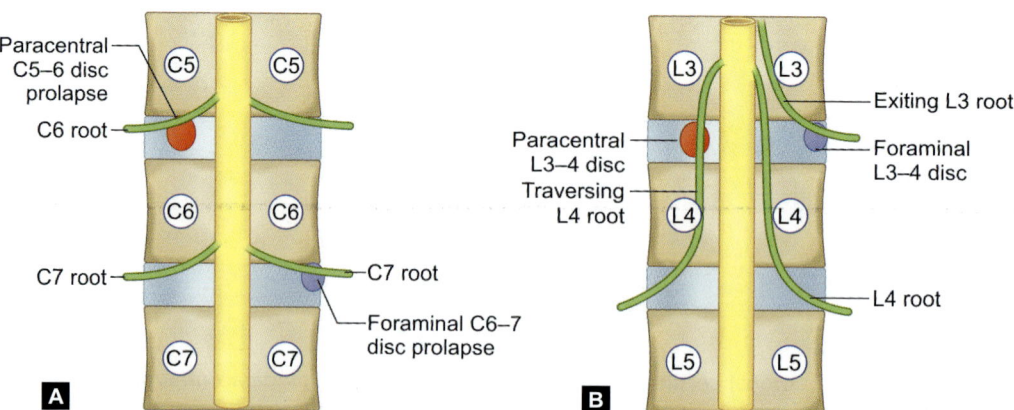

Figs. 34.5A and B: Compression of the nerve root by paracentral/foraminal herniated disc at cervical; (A) and lumbar spine (B). Note horizontal and oblique/vertical orientation of nerve roots in cervical and spine, respectively. The numbers in white circle on a vertebral body denote vertebral number and pedicle.

Combining above concepts, the nerve root compression in cervical and lumbar spine disc herniation corresponds to the *lower adjacent vertebra*. For example, in C4-5 disc herniation, the root involved is C5. In L4-5 disc herniation, the root involved is L5. In L5-S1 disc herniation, the root involved is S1. However, foraminal disc (of lumbar spine) will compress the superior level root. For example, foraminal disc prolapse of L4-5 level will compress L4 root, which is exiting at L4-5 level. **A sequestered disc may compress any root at any level** as it can migrate superiorly or inferiorly after sequestration.

GENERAL CLINICAL FEATURES OF IVDP

IVDP is one of the common causes of neck (cervical) and low back (lumbar) pain. It is uncommon in the dorsal region (<1%). *It is more common in cervical and lumbar regions* as these are more mobile regions of the spine leading to more stress concentration over these areas.
- Common region in the cervical spine for IVDP: C4-5, C5-6, C6-7
- Common region in the lumbar spine for IVDP: L3-4, L4-5, L5-S1

The patient with a disc prolapse presents with pain in the affected region with/without radiation to the limbs (depending upon the root compression). Severe prolapse results in ***sensorimotor deficit in the limb***.

- **Chronic multilevel disc prolapse in cervical spine** *(along with spondylotic changes) may result in cervical myelopathy due to chronic compression over the spinal cord.* Apart from features of cervical IVDP (neck pain, radiation to upper limbs), such patients develop upper motor neuron signs in limbs and gait disturbance.
- A massive disc prolapse at level of L1 vertebra could result in **conus medullaris syndrome**.
- Acute multilevel lumbar spine disc prolapse could result in **cauda equina syndrome**, whereas chronic multilevel disc prolapse along with spondylotic changes result in **lumbar canal stenosis**.

SPECIFIC CLINICAL FEATURES OF CERVICAL SPINE IVDP

Symptoms:
- ***Neck pain with/without radiation to the scapula and upper limb.***
- In the case of root compression, pain radiates toward the radial aspect of the shoulder, arm, forearm, and hand, as mostly C4-7 roots are involved. There may be paresthesia and numbness in the dermatome of the involved root. Occasionally, there may be motor weakness in the extremity.
- Neck pain increases while lying down on the same side (as roots are further compressed in the neural foramina due to laterally flexed spine narrowing the neural foramina).

Signs:
- Tenderness is present over the spinous process of the involved vertebra.
- Paraspinal spasm is present
- Movements are painful
- ***Spurling sign*** *is positive* (lateral tilt and neck rotation reproduces radiation in the limb)
- A complete neurological examination is a must to rule out sensory and motor deficits and bladder-bowel function. The sensory-motor assessment of commonly involved nerve roots C4-C8 is mentioned in **Table 34.2**.

Table 34.2: Clinical features of IVDP of the cervical spine occurring at various levels.

	IVDP C3-4	IVDP C4-5	IVDP C5-6	IVDP C6-7	IVDP C8-T1
Root compressed	C4	C5	C6	C7	C8
Region of pain and sensory deficit (if any)	Posterior neck, occiput, and trapezius pain	Suprascapular region and lateral upper arm	Radial aspect of the forearm and thumb	Pain in interscapular region, arm, posterior forearm, and middle finger	Inner aspect of the forearm and medial two fingers
Motor deficit in (weakness)		Shoulder abductor (deltoid)	Elbow flexion biceps), wrist extension (ECRL, ECRB)	Elbow extension (triceps), wrist flexion (FCR), finger extension	Interossei, FCU, and finger flexors (FDS, FDP)
Sluggish reflex		Biceps	Biceps and supinator	Triceps	None

(ECRL: extensor carpi radialis longus; ECRB: extensor carpi radialis brevis; FCR: flexor carpi radialis; FCU: flexor carpi ulnaris; FDS: flexor digitorum superficialis; FDP: flexor digitorum profundus)

- *Massive multilevel cervical disc herniation can cause spinal cord compression and cervical myelopathy leading to lower limb weakness.* It may reveal upper motor signs like the presence of Hoffmann sign, Finger fatigue sign, Lhermitte's sign and Clonus. The patient may have unstable gait.

SPECIFIC CLINICAL FEATURES OF LUMBAR SPINE IVDP

Symptoms:
- *Low back pain with/without radiation of the pain to the lower limb.* The pain is usually mechanical in nature, which increases with activity and decreases with rest.
- In case of the nerve root compression and level of the root, the pain radiates towards the front or back of the thigh, calf, and foot. Radiating pain is often described like a tingling/shock like sensation. Paresthesia and numbness in the 'dermatome of involved root' could be present. In L1–3 root involvement, patient complains of radicular pain over the front of the thigh. In contrast, the radicular pain is felt over gluteal region, back of thigh, leg and feet if L4–S1 roots are involved.
- Pain increases while bending forward, coughing, sneezing, or turning in the bed.
- There may be motor weakness in the lower limb. The area of weakness depends upon the nerve root involvement.

Signs:
- *Sciatic list or postural scoliosis* may be noted in acute lumbar IVDP. It is due to muscle spasm.
- Tenderness is present over the spinous process of the involved vertebra.
- Paraspinal spasm is present

Specific signs for lumbar nerve root compression:
- In case of lumbar IVDP of L1–2 and L2–3 disc with L1, 2 or 3 nerve root compression, *femoral nerve stretch sign may be positive*.
- In case of lumbar IVDP of L3–4, L4–5, L5–S1 disc with L4, 5, and S1 root compression, following tests may be positive:

- *Straight leg raising test* + (should be less than 60–70° to be positive)
- *Lasegue test* +
- *Bowstringing test* +
- *Crossed SLR or well leg raising test is positive* in the axillary type of disc herniation. It is specific for lumbar disc prolapse.
- Acute multilevel lumbar IVDP may also present as *cauda equina syndrome*, whereas chronic multilevel lumbar IVDP along with spondylotic changes may present with *lumbar canal stenosis*.
- A complete neurological examination must be performed to rule out sensory-motor deficit and bladder-bowel function. The sensory deficit assessment helps identifying the root involved.
    a. **Test L2, L3 nerve root integrity** by assessing sensation in the anteromedial aspect of thigh and motor strength of hip flexion, hip adduction, and knee extension. The knee jerk may be sluggish.
    b. The rest of the motor examination of nerve roots from L4-S1 is mentioned in **Table 34.3**.

Table 34.3: Clinical features of IVDP of lumbar spine occurring at various levels.

	IVDP L3-4	IVDP L4-5	IVDP L5-S1
Root compressed	L4	L5	S1
Region of pain and sensory deficit (if any)	Lower back, sacroiliac joint (SIJ), posterior thigh, and anteromedial aspect of leg	Lower back, SIJ, posterior thigh, anterolateral aspect of leg, and dorsum of foot	Lower back, SIJ, posterior thigh, lateral border of foot and plantar aspect
Motor deficit in (weakness)	Knee extension, ankle dorsiflexors (also)	<ul><li>Ankle dorsiflexors (TA), subtalar invertors (TA, TP)</li><li>Toe dorsiflexors [(EHL), (EDL)]</li><li>Hip abductors</li></ul>	<ul><li>Plantar flexion at the ankle (tendoachilles) and toes</li><li>Subtalar evertors (PL, PB)</li><li>Hip extensors (Gluteus maximus)</li></ul>
Sluggish reflex	Knee jerk		Ankle jerk

(TA: tibialis anterior; TP: tibialis posterior; EHL: extensor hallucis longus; EDL: extensor digitorum longus; PL: peroneus longus; PB: peroneus brevis)

INVESTIGATIONS

- **Plain X-ray of the spine:** AP and lateral view, lateral flexion-extension view (for instability of spine)
    - Loss of cervical/lumbar lordosis (if there is paraspinal spasm)
    - In chronic disc disease, the intervertebral disc space decreases **(Fig. 34.6A)**.
    - In chronic IVDP, spondylotic changes are observed, such as osteophytes.
- **Magnetic resonance imaging (MRI) of the spine:** *It is the diagnostic investigation for IVDP* **(Fig. 34.6B)**. Following changes are observed on MRI:
    - Disc dehydration and degeneration
    - Disc protrusion/prolapse/sequestration
    - Nerve root/cord/both compression
    - Myelopathy in chronic cervical spine disc herniation
    - Multilevel lumbar IVDP can cause lumbar canal stenosis.

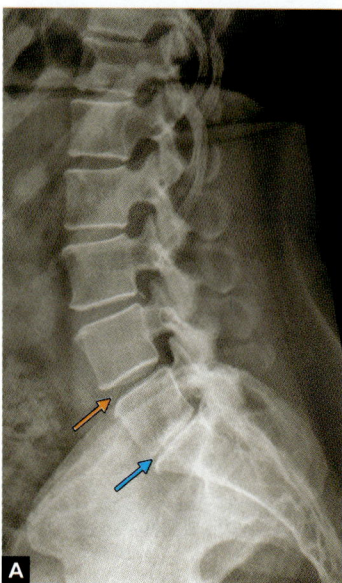 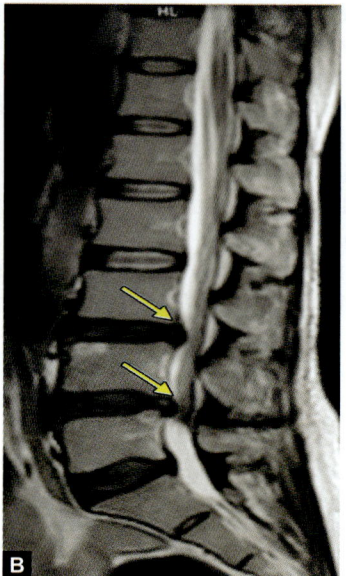

Figs. 34.6A and B: (A) Lateral X-ray of lumbar spine showing decreased disc space between L5–S1 vertebra (blue arrow) while orange arrow between L4–5 shows a normal disc space; (B) IVDP between L3–L4 and L4–L5 vertebra (yellow arrows).

(IVDP: intervertebral disc prolapse)

TREATMENT

The mainstay of treatment for disc disease/prolapse is conservative, except for certain specific situations where surgery is indicated. Most patients resume their normal activity within few weeks-months depending on severity of the prolapse and associated sensorimotor deficit.
- **General measures**
    - Rest for a few days
    - *Avoiding provocative movements*: Bending forward and lifting weight (in lumbar disc disease); prolonged working on computers (cervical disc disease).
- **Orthosis support**
    - Cervical collar (*in cervical disc disease*)/lumbosacral (LS) corset (*lumbar disc disease*)
- **Physiotherapy**
    - Pain relief by local application of moist heat, short-wave diathermy (SWD), interferential therapy (IFT), and transcutaneous electrical nerve stimulation (TENS).
    - Intermittent traction may also help.
    - Once pain decreases, mobilization and muscle-strengthening exercises (cervical isometrics/lumbar spinal extension) must be initiated.
- **Medical treatment**
    - Analgesics for pain relief
    - Muscle relaxant: Thiocolchicoside, tizanidine
    - Pregabalin, gabapentin for reducing neuralgic radiating pain.
- **Epidural steroid injection/selective nerve root block "in lumbar IVDP."**
    - Only *"patients with radicular pain"* with failed conservative treatment should be given a trial of epidural/selective nerve block
    - Not a popular option for cervical IVDP.

- **Surgery:** Indications for surgery
  - *Cauda equina syndrome* in lumbar IVDP is an *absolute indication of surgical intervention*
  - No pain relief despite 8–12 weeks of adequate conservative treatment
  - Increasing pain or neurological deficit.
    - ***In the lumbar spine, laminotomy and discectomy*** are performed (open discectomy/microdiscectomy/endoscopic discectomy).
    - ***In the cervical spine, anterior cervical discectomy and fusion*** of two vertebrae with bone graft and/cage.
    - ***Disc replacement*** has been tried in selected cases.

> The patient with radicular pain responds to surgery better than those who have only local pain.

CAUDA EQUINA SYNDROME (CES)

DEFINITION

Cauda equina syndrome (CES) is a type of lower motor neuron lesion, which results from the compression of multiple nerve roots in the lumbosacral (LS) region, causing variable sensorimotor symptoms.

It is considered *one of the emergencies in orthopaedics*.

ETIOPATHOLOGY

L1 to S5 roots lie in the lumbosacral region and are termed "cauda equina" (like horse tail). These multiple roots are responsible for sensorimotor innervation of the lower limb, bladder, and bowel. Compression of these roots at multiple levels results in cauda equina syndrome. Following are the common causes of CES:
- Multilevel lumbar disc prolapse
- Lumbar canal stenosis
- Tumor in the LS canal
- Traumatic vertebral # resulting in "retropulsion of vertebral body parts into the LS canal."
- Postsurgical hematoma.

CLINICAL FEATURES

- Low back pain
- Unilateral or bilateral radiating pain to the lower limbs
- Saddle anaesthesia
- Sensorimotor deficit in the lower limb
- Sluggish/absent bulbocavernosus reflex
- Bladder dysfunction-urinary retention

Rarely—bowel and sexual dysfunction.

INVESTIGATIONS

- Plain X-ray of the lumbosacral spine: AP, lateral view
- *Magnetic resonance imaging (MRI):* Diagnostic.

TREATMENT

Urgent surgical decompression of the canal.

COMPLICATIONS
- Residual sensorimotor deficit
- Sexual dysfunction
- Bladder or bowel dysfunction.

CONUS MEDULLARIS SYNDROME (CMS)

DEFINITION
The constellation of "sudden and bilateral" features due to compression of the conus medullaris, which is characterized by
- Acute, severe back pain ± radiation to the lower limb
- Bladder dysfunction
- Impotence

[Note: Read the chapter 16 on spinal injuries for conus medullaris syndrome and difference between conus medullaris and cauda equina syndrome].

SPONDYLOSIS (Syn: Spondylitis)

DEFINITION
Spondylosis is defined as a natural degenerative process of vertebral motion segment (vertebra, intervertebral disc and facet joints).

It is commonly known as spondylitis. However, spondylosis is a pathologically more appropriate term as there is no obvious inflammation in the degenerative disorder of the spine. It affects all the regions of the spine, but most commonly, the cervical and lumbar are involved as these are more mobile segments. The rate of progression of the degenerative process varies from person to person.

Cervical spondylosis: The increased movements in the area of the cervical spine lead to degenerative changes with increasing age that manifests with neck pain that may radiate to the scapula and the upper limbs.

Lumbar spondylosis: It manifests with mechanical pain in the low back during prolonged sitting, walking, standing, and lifting heavy weights. Occasionally, there may be radiation of pain in the lower limb.

ETIOLOGY
- Aging
- Repetitive strain
- Family history
- Smoking
- Occupational hazards: Repeated lifting, bending, driving, lifting weight on the head
- Post-traumatic, chronic disc disease/prolapse.

PATHOPHYSIOLOGY
There are three stages in spondylosis:
1. **Stage of disc degeneration and facet synovitis:** The process of disc degeneration starts with the nucleus pulposus losing hydration leading to gradual loss in disc height. Further,

there are microtears in annulus and localized synovitis of facet joints. Due to disc damage, there can be disc herniation.
2. **Stage of instability and arthritis:** Disc degeneration leads to increased stress, instability of vertebral motion segment and erosion of the cartilage end plates, resulting in rubbing of end plates of two adjacent vertebrae and facet joint arthrosis.
3. **Stage of stability:** As a protective mechanism for the 'instability' in vertebral motion segment, the vertebral body grows a new bone (bone spurs) around the facet or uncinate joints to provide extra stability to the vertebral motion segment. The presence of spurs, hypertrophied joint capsules, infolded ligaments and loss of disc height lead to vertebral canal and neural foraminal stenosis, resulting in compression over the nerve roots and/or spinal cord. Spinal cord compression occurs in cervical or thoracic regions, whereas lumbar region changes result in nerve root compression.

CLINICAL FEATURES (FOR CERVICAL, LUMBAR SPONDYLOSIS)

Symptoms:
1. Chronic pain and stiffness of the neck or back with periods of remissions and exacerbations. Typically, pain is mechanical in nature that increases with movement/loading (standing, walking, sitting, and neck movements).
2. In advanced spondylosis, there could be tingling and numbness in the upper limbs or lower limbs (depending on the region), which could be unilateral or bilateral. In severe cases of chronic cervical spondylosis with resulting severe stenosis, there can be *features of cervical myelopathy who present with unstable gait*. Severe chronic lumbar spondylosis results in *lumbar canal stenosis, which presents with neurogenic claudication*.

Signs:
1. Tenderness over the affected vertebra is present, and movements of the spine (cervical/lumbar) are decreased.
2. There may be a local muscle spasm.
3. Neurological deficits are rare in mild to moderate spondylosis of both cervical and lumbar region. Sometimes, there can be feature of nerve root compression.
   In patients with cervical myelopathy, there will be unstable gait, UMN signs in the limbs, and sensorimotor disturbance. Chronic lumbar spondylosis can result in lumbar canal stenosis.

INVESTIGATIONS

1. **X-ray of the spine (AP, lateral):** Osteophytes and decreased disc height are common findings **(Fig. 34.7)**. Late cases may show facet joint arthritis.
2. **Magnetic resonance imaging (MRI):** MRI helps evaluating disc disease, spinal cord and root compression, facet arthritis, and canal stenosis.
3. **Computed tomography (CT) scan** is useful in evaluating canal stenosis.

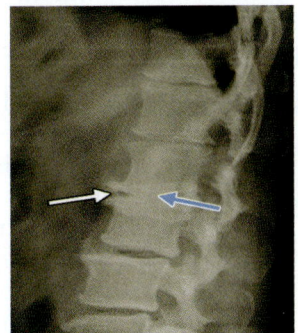

Fig. 34.7: Lumbar spondylosis X-ray shows osteophytes (white arrow) and narrow disc space (blue arrow).

TREATMENT

The treatment of spondylosis (cervical or lumbar) is largely conservative.
- **General treatment**
    - *Medication*: Analgesics, muscle relaxants (tizanidine, thiocolchicoside), and gabapentinoids (Pregabalin, Gabapentin) for radicular pain.
    - *Physiotherapy*: Heat or cold therapy, short-wave diathermy, TENS, intermittent local traction; and muscle strengtheninging exercises (low back and cervical spine)
    - *Lifestyle changes*: Stop smoking, avoid/minimize activities that exacerbate pain
- **Orthosis**
    - Soft cervical collar for cervical spondylosis
    - Lumbosacral corset for lumbar spondylosis
- **Surgery:** It is rarely required in spondylosis unless the neurological symptoms, such as radiating pain, motor weakness not responding to conservative treatment. It is also advocated in cervical myelopathy or lumbar canal stenosis with severe symptoms with short claudication distance affecting ambulation and activities of daily living. The surgery aims to decompress the spinal canal and neural foramina.
    Various surgical options in cervical and lumbar spine are:
    - **Cervical:** Anterior cervical discectomy with fusion OR corpectomy + discectomy and fusion.
    - **Lumbar:** Laminectomy is a procedure wherein the lumbar canal is decompressed by removing a part of lamina along with osteophytes, ligamentum flavum, and part of facets.

SPONDYLOLYSIS AND SPONDYLOLISTHESIS

INTRODUCTION

Spondylolysis: It is the *defect in the pars interarticularis of the lumbar vertebra*.

The pars interarticularis is a part of lamina and is the bony bridge between the two articular facets (superior and inferior). It is the weakest area in posterior elements of the spine, and is susceptible to fracture. Spondylolysis is almost always a precursor to spondylolisthesis.

Spondylolisthesis: *The forward translation (slip) of one vertebra over the other* in the sagittal plane. It is most commonly seen at the level of the L4-L5 vertebra **(Figs. 34.8A to C)**.

CLASSIFICATION OF SPONDYLOLISTHESIS

1. **Dysplastic:** Congenital malformation of posterior elements, such as facet anomaly or elongation of the pars result in decreased ability of the vertebra to resist anterior translation, leading to spondylolisthesis.
2. **Isthmic:** It is due to a defect in the pars interarticularis, which could be due to acute traumatic fracture or stress fracture **(Fig. 34.8C)**. *The stress fractures of pars are often seen in adolescent athletes, resulting in back pain*. Isthmic variety is most common in young patient, and the *most common location of isthmic listhesis is L5-S1*.
3. **Degenerative:** It is the most common type of listhesis occurring in adults. It is due to facet joint and disc degeneration. It *commonly occurs at L4-5 level*.
4. **Traumatic:** It is seen after a high velocity trauma resulting in damage to the neural arch, especially in pedicles or facets. Unlike isthmic variant, fracture is not through the pars interarticularis.

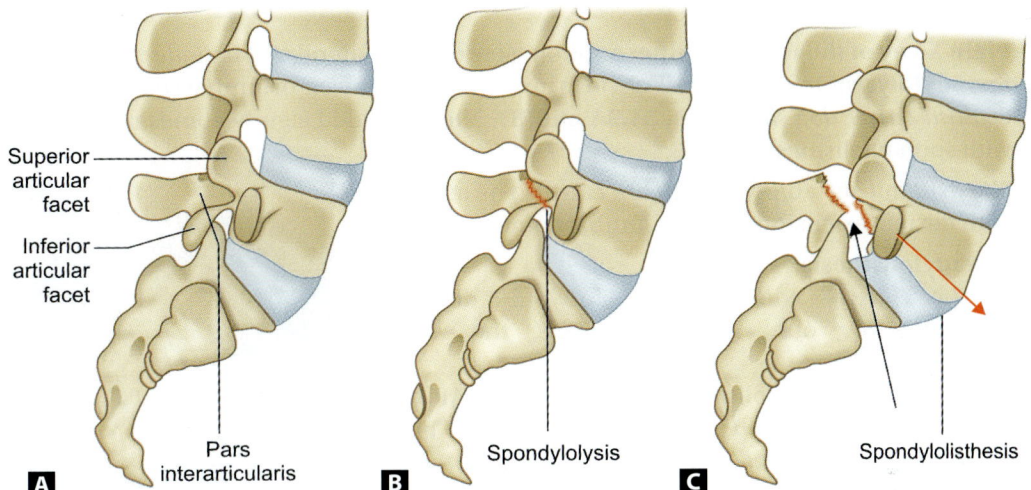

Figs. 34.8A to C: (A) Sagittal view of the spine showing normal relation of superior and inferior facets and pars; (B) Spondylolysis of L5 vertebra (red zigzag line in pars of L5 vertebra); (C) Spondylolisthesis of L5 vertebra (black arrow)—forward slippage of L5 vertebra over S1 vertebra (red arrow).

5. **Pathological:** Osteoporosis, Paget's, metastatic carcinoma destroying the pars articularis or facets.
6. **Iatrogenic**.

MEYERDING'S SCALE FOR CLASSIFYING GRADE OF SPONDYLOLISTHESIS

Meyerding classification is based upon degree of forward translation (slip) of the upper vertebra with respect to the lower vertebra:
- *Grade I*: Less than 25% slip
- *Grade II*: 25–50% slip
- *Grade III*: 50–75% slip
- *Grade IV*: 75–100% slip
- *Grade V*: Greater than 100% (*Spondyloptosis*)

CLINICAL FEATURES

Symptoms:

Mechanical low back pain is the most common presentation of spondylolysis and listhesis. Forwards slipping of vertebra results in traction over nerve roots, which may cause radiation of the pain to one/both lower limbs along the distribution of stretched nerve root.

Signs:

In patients with spondylolysis, there may not be any localising signs except painful extension. Most signs are observed in spondylolisthesis.
- Attenuated lumbar lordosis
- There may be vertebral tenderness in spondylolysis, while **a step is palpated** over the spinous process of the slipped vertebra (spondylolisthesis)
- **Lumbar spine extension is painful** (Note: *Painful extension of lumbar spine is also observed in lumbar canal stenosis, facet joint arthrosis*).

INVESTIGATIONS

1. **Plain X-ray of the lumbar spine:** Anteroposterior (AP), lateral and *oblique view*.
   Spondylolysis: Defect in pars is obvious in *lateral/oblique view* of lumbar spine—*Beheaded Scottish terrier dog sign* **(Figs. 34.9A and B)**. The beheaded sign becomes more obvious with spondylolisthesis.

   The dynamic instability of vertebra can also be assessed with flexion-extension views of lumbar spine.

   Spondylolisthesis:
   - The lateral view shows forward displacement of one vertebra over the other **(Fig. 34.9B)**.
   - In severe spondylolisthesis of L5 vertebra, AP view shows *Napoleon hat sign* **(Fig. 34.10)**. The "brim" of hat is formed by the caudal translation of the transverse processes and the "dome" of hat is formed by the body of L5.

2. **Computed tomography (CT) scan:** It helps identify covert bony pathology, such as defect in pars/facet anomaly/facet degeneration.

3. **Magnetic resonance imaging (MRI)** helps identify *compression of nerve roots, disc disease, and facet anomalies*.

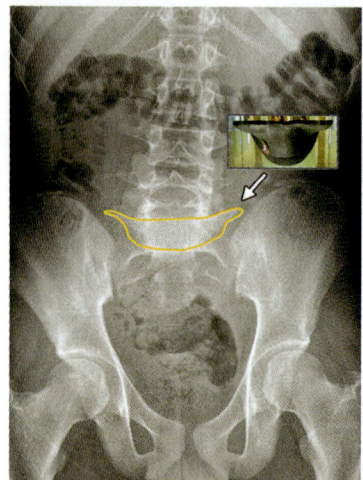

Fig. 34.10: Inverted Napoleon hat sign.

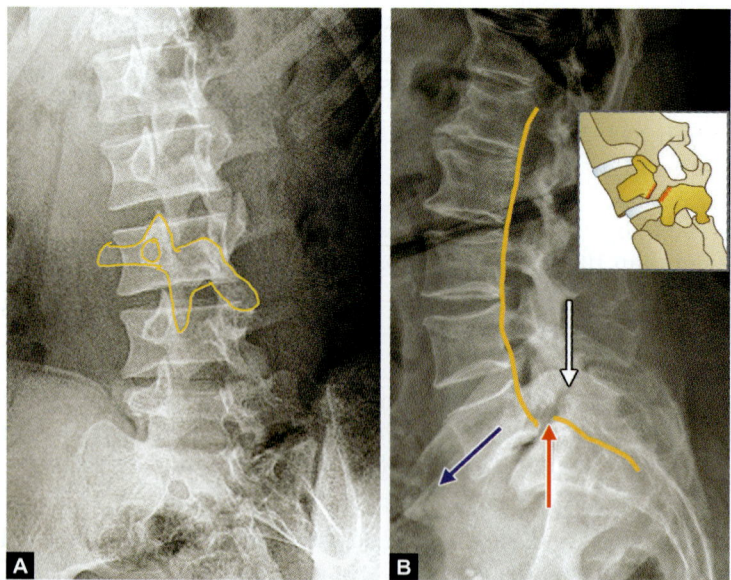

Figs. 34.9A and B: (A) Normal oblique view of the lumbar spine showing a standard Scottish dog silhouette formed by posterior spine elements with the transverse process forming the nose; (B) Spondylolisthesis showing a break in pars interarticularis (white arrow). Blue arrow shows forward slippage of L5 over S1 vertebra. Usually, the posterior border of all vertebrae and sacrum are in the same line. However, there will be a break in posterior body alignment in the case of spondylolisthesis (yellow line break shown with a red arrow). Inset picture shows a beheaded Scottish terrier dog sign observed in oblique views.

TREATMENT

Most cases of spondylolysis and spondylolisthesis are managed conservatively by:
1. **Lifestyle modification:** Correct posture, avoid smoking, and weight reduction
2. **Physiotherapy:**
   - Spinal flexion exercises
   - Pain relief by moist heat, short-wave diathermy (SWD), and interferential therapy (IFT)
3. **Orthosis:** Lumbosacral corset
4. **Medication**
   - Analgesics
   - Pregabalin/gabapentin to reduce neuralgic pain
5. **Epidural/facet injections** of steroid and local anesthetic to relieve neuralgic radiating pain
6. **Surgical options:** Major unstable spondylolisthesis *'not responding to conservative treatment'* may require spinal canal decompression, surgical stabilization of (slipping) vertebrae by spinal instrumentation and vertebral fusion of affected levels.

LUMBAR CANAL STENOSIS

DEFINITION

Lumbar canal stenosis (LCS) is defined as the **narrowing of the spinal canal, the nerve root canal or the vertebral foramina**.

ETIOPATHOGENESIS

It could be due to congenital or acquired causes. The common acquired causes are degenerative spondylosis, multilevel disc prolapse, post-traumatic, spondylolisthesis, metabolic (fluorosis) or systemic diseases like ankylosing spondylitis.

The **degenerative disease of the spine and disc is the most common cause of lumbar canal stenosis**. Chronic degenerative changes in the lumbar spine result in the narrowing of the spinal canal due to *arthritic facet joints, hypertrophied capsules of facet joints, prolapsed discs, stiff ligaments (PLL and ligamentum flavum), and bone spurs*. These multiple factors cause a reduction in space for the nerves to traverse the spinal canal and spinal foramen leading to pressure over the multiple nerve roots **(Figs. 34.11A and B)**.

Note that the lumbar spinal canal volume reduces in an extended spine. Therefore, activities which result in increased spine extension, such as standing erect, or descending stairs/ramp, further aggravate the symptoms. Therefore, bending forward relieves symptoms of LCS.

Stenosis can occur as per the location along the spinal canal: Cervical/thoracic/lumbar, of which *lumbar is the most common*.

CLINICAL FEATURES

Usually, diagnosis of lumbar canal stenosis (LCS) is clinical as there are no specific clinical features.

Symptoms:
- Typical LCS due to degenerative spine is common in the **elderly population >55–60 years**.

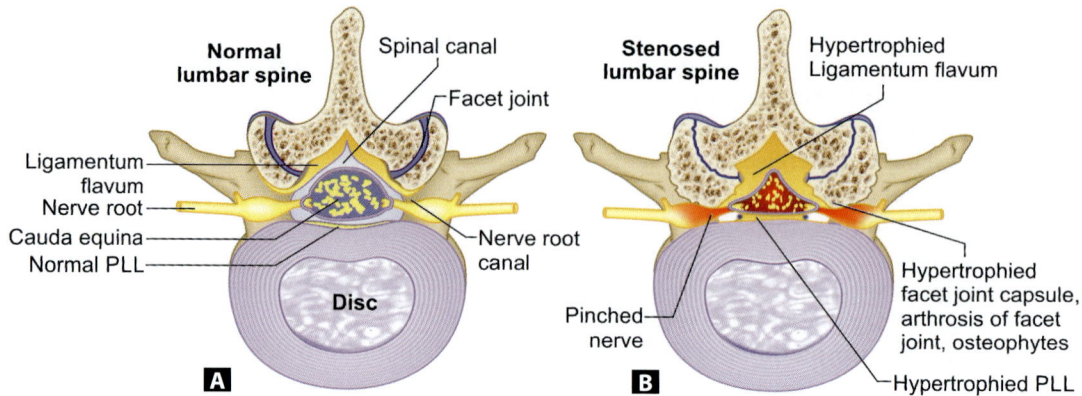

Figs. 34.11A and B: (A) Normal anatomy of a axial section of the lumbar spine elaborating the orientation of all structures in and around the spinal canal; (B) Pathological changes in lumbar canal stenosis.
(PLL: posterior longitudinal ligament)

- Classically, patients with LCS complain of **pain radiating to both lower limbs, more than the other**. The radiating pain may be associated with paresthesia/tingling in the lower limbs. The patients may also complain of **calf cramps**. The **neurogenic claudication** is *one of the classical clinical features of lumbar canal stenosis*. Neurogenic claudication pain increases while standing and walking and relieves during rest. The walking distance is variable and uphill walking is less painful.
- **Low back pain:** It is less frequent. The back pain increases during activities requiring spine extension as canal diameter decrease during spine extension. Therefore, low back pain is aggravated during standing, walking or bending backwards, and descending stairs/ramp. It improves with forward bending and ascending stairs/ramp.
(*Note: Differentiating neurogenic claudication from vascular claudication is important*).

Vascular claudication also increase while walking. However, the distances are fixed and uphill walking increases symptoms. Furthermore, distal pulses are feeble or absent.

Signs:
- Local spine examination is often normal or may reveal vertebral tenderness.
- The spine extension is painful. Other movements may be normal or decreased.
- Neurological examination of the lower limb may reveal sensory disturbance. The motor deficit is rare.
- Vascularity of the lower limb must be assessed to rule out vascular claudication.

INVESTIGATIONS

1. **X-ray of the lumbosacral spine (AP, lateral):** Spondylotic changes may be noted.
2. **Computed tomography (CT) scan** is useful to assess spinal canal diameter, which is decreased in canal stenosis.
3. **MRI:** It is the *investigation of choice* to assess the canal diameter and narrowing, disc prolapse, and compression over the roots.

TREATMENT

Most cases are managed conservatively. However, a disabling radiating pain or neurogenic claudication not responding to conservative treatment may require surgical decompression.

Conservative treatment:
1. **Lifestyle modification:** Correct posture, avoid smoking, and weight reduction
2. **Physiotherapy:**
    * Spinal flexion exercises
    * Pain relief by moist heat, SWD, IFT
3. **Orthosis:** Lumbosacral corset
4. **Medication**
    * Analgesics: for pain relief
    * Pregabalin/gabapentin to reduce neuralgic pain
5. **Epidural/facet injections** of steroid and local anesthetic to relieve neuralgic radiating pain

Surgical treatment: If conservative treatment fails, and symptoms are affecting the activities of daily living, spinal decompression (laminectomy) is the treatment of choice.

DIFFERENTIAL DIAGNOSIS

- Vascular claudication
- Peripheral neuropathy

COMPLICATIONS OF CERVICAL CANAL STENOSIS

Cervical cord myelopathy: In the case of chronic cervical spondylosis-induced cervical canal stenosis, it is observed in elderly patients. These patients present with chronic neck pain, gait disturbance and other upper motor signs in the limbs.

Notes

SECTION 7

Metabolic Diseases of the Bone

SECTION OUTLINE

35. Metabolic Diseases of the Bone
    - Brief Review of Role of Calcium, Phosphorus, Magnesium, Vitamin D and their Regulations
    - Rickets
    - Osteomalacia
    - Osteoporosis
    - Osteosclerosis Disorders
        – Osteopetrosis
        – Paget's Disease
        – Fluorosis
    - Hyperparathyroidism
    - Scurvy

CHAPTER 35

Metabolic Diseases of the Bone

BRIEF REVIEW OF ROLE OF CALCIUM, PHOSPHORUS, MAGNESIUM, VITAMIN D AND THEIR REGULATIONS

ROLE OF CALCIUM, PHOSPHORUS, MAGNESIUM

Calcium

- Normal body calcium (Ca) is about 1 kg. Almost 99% of the calcium is stored in the bone. It is obtained through the dietary sources, such as cheese, milk, almond, spinach, beans, lentils, and eggs. Normal serum calcium values range from 8.5 to 10.2 mg/dL in adults.
- Normal calcium Recommended Dietary Allowances (RDA): 1 g/day.
- *Calcium absorption from the gut is promoted* by Calcitriol (active vitamin D3).
- *Calcium absorption from the gut is inhibited* by the presence of phytates (grains, beans), oxalates (tea, coffee), excess intake of phosphates (common in soft drinks), fat and certain drugs (steroids, thyroxine, anticoagulants).
- **Function of calcium:** Serum Ca is essential for bone formation as required for hydroxyapatite $[Ca_5(PO_4)_3OH]$ formation, neuromuscular transmission, blood coagulation, muscle contraction, and cyclic-AMP pathway.
- **Serum calcium abnormalities:** Significantly low ionic serum Ca causes tetany, whereas excess Ca causes depressed neuromuscular transmission.

Phosphorus

- Serum phosphate normally ranges from 2.5 to 4.5 mg/dL in adults. Inorganic phosphate (iP) is regulated by parathyroid hormone (PTH) and 1,25-DHCC. If iP increases, there is reciprocal fall in Ca which stimulates PTH secretion, suppressing iP resorption from proximal renal tubules and promoting excretion.
- **Function of phosphate:** Phosphate is required for hydroxyapatite formation, cell signaling and energy transport in the cells.
- **Serum phosphate abnormalities:** Deficiency of phosphate results in rickets or osteomalacia, whereas hyperphosphatemia results in hypertension, cardiac failure, delirium, seizures, etc.

Phosphorus is an element, whereas phosphate is an anion which is formed after phosphorus combines with oxygen. Phosphates are present in the body.

Magnesium
- Magnesium is essential for the secretion and peripheral action of PTH. It also plays an essential role in mineral homeostasis.
- In the event of hypocalcemia and hypomagnesemia, the latter needs to be corrected to treat the former effectively.

CALCIUM AND VITAMIN D REGULATION IN THE HUMAN BODY

Calcium Regulation
The calcium levels are maintained in the body by the interaction of serum calcitonin and parathormone. The calcium regulation cycle is illustrated in **Figure 35.1**.
- ***High levels of calcium stimulate calcitonin release*** from the thyroid, which stimulates osteoblasts leading to calcium deposition in bone and increasing calcium excretion through the kidney, *thereby lowering serum calcium levels.*
- ***Low levels of calcium stimulate parathormone release*** from the parathyroid gland, which stimulates osteoclastic activity leading to calcium resorption from bone and decreased excretion of calcium through the kidney, *thereby increasing serum calcium levels.*

Vitamin D Synthesis, Regulation and Function
Vitamin D is synthesized from 7-dehydrocholesterol in the skin as cholecalciferol (vitamin D3) in the presence of ultraviolet rays-B (230–310 nm). Further, vitamin D3 is converted into 25-hydroxy cholecalciferol (25-HCC) in the liver. Under the influence of 1-α hydroxylase, 25-HCC is converted into 1,25-dihydroxy cholecalciferol (Calcitriol) in the kidney **(Fig. 35.2)**. The calcitriol (active vitamin D) has an essential role in calcium metabolism in intestine and bone.

Common terms of vitamin D
- ***Vitamin D3:*** Cholecalciferol
- ***Vitamin D2:*** Ergocalciferol
- ***Calcidiol-25:*** Hydroxycholecalciferol
- ***Calcitriol (active vitamin D):*** 1,25-DHCC

- **Intestine:** Calcitriol stimulates calcium and phosphate absorption from the gut.
- **Bone:** Calcitriol has several functions:
  - Promotes Ca transport across the osteoblast cell membrane and indirectly assist osteoid mineralization.
  - Promotes osteoclastic resorption of bone (in response to PTH).

RICKETS

DEFINITION
Rickets is characterized by ***inadequate mineralization of the bone matrix in a growing skeleton resulting in growth plate cartilage abnormality***. The effect of rickets are predominantly observed in long bone.

ETIOLOGY
There are two types of rickets, hypocalcemic and hypophosphatemic.
- **Hypocalcemic/calcipenic rickets:** It occurs due to vitamin D or calcium deficiency. It is of three types **(Table 35.1)**

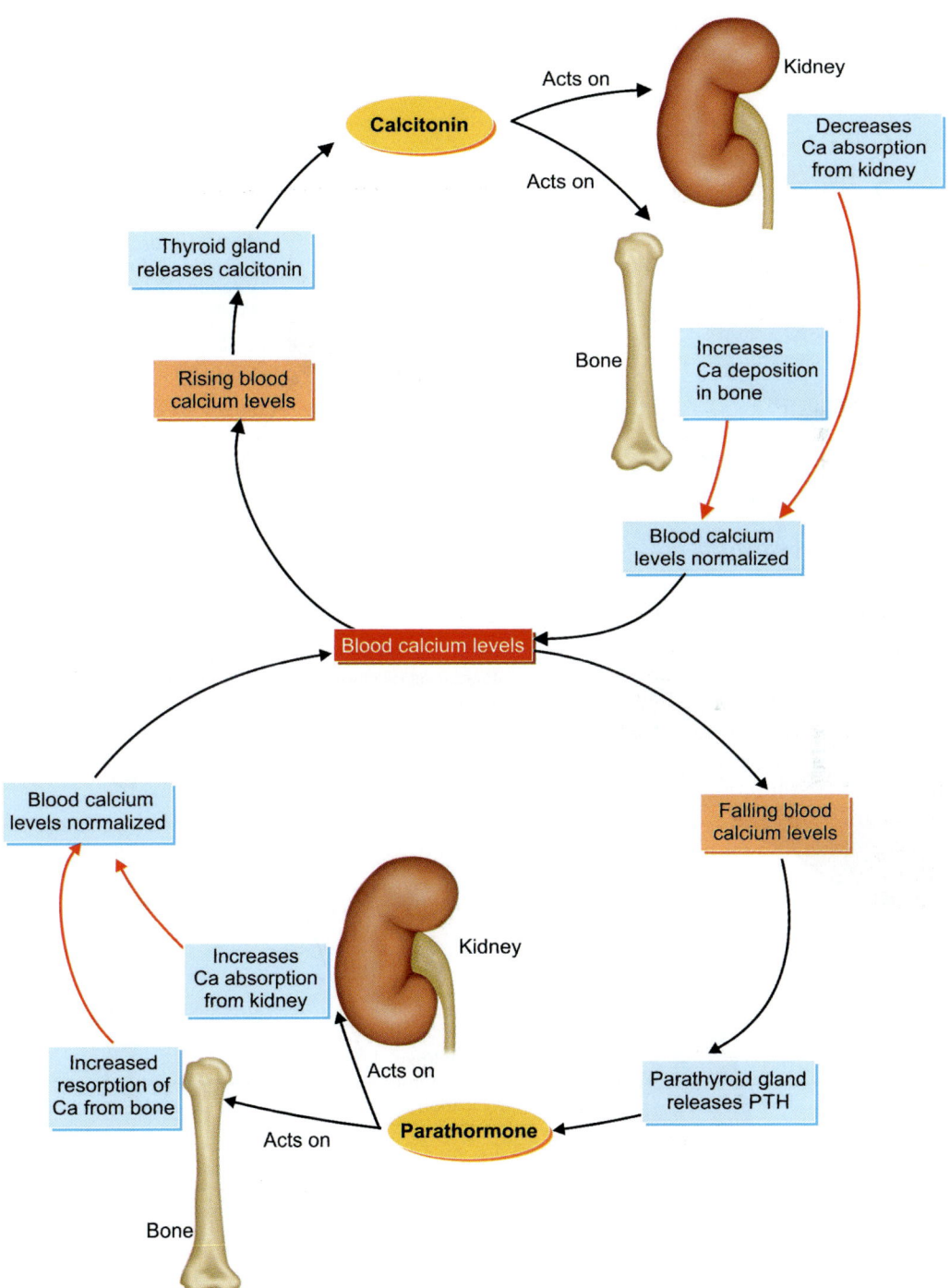

Fig. 35.1: Calcium homeostasis cycle in the human body.

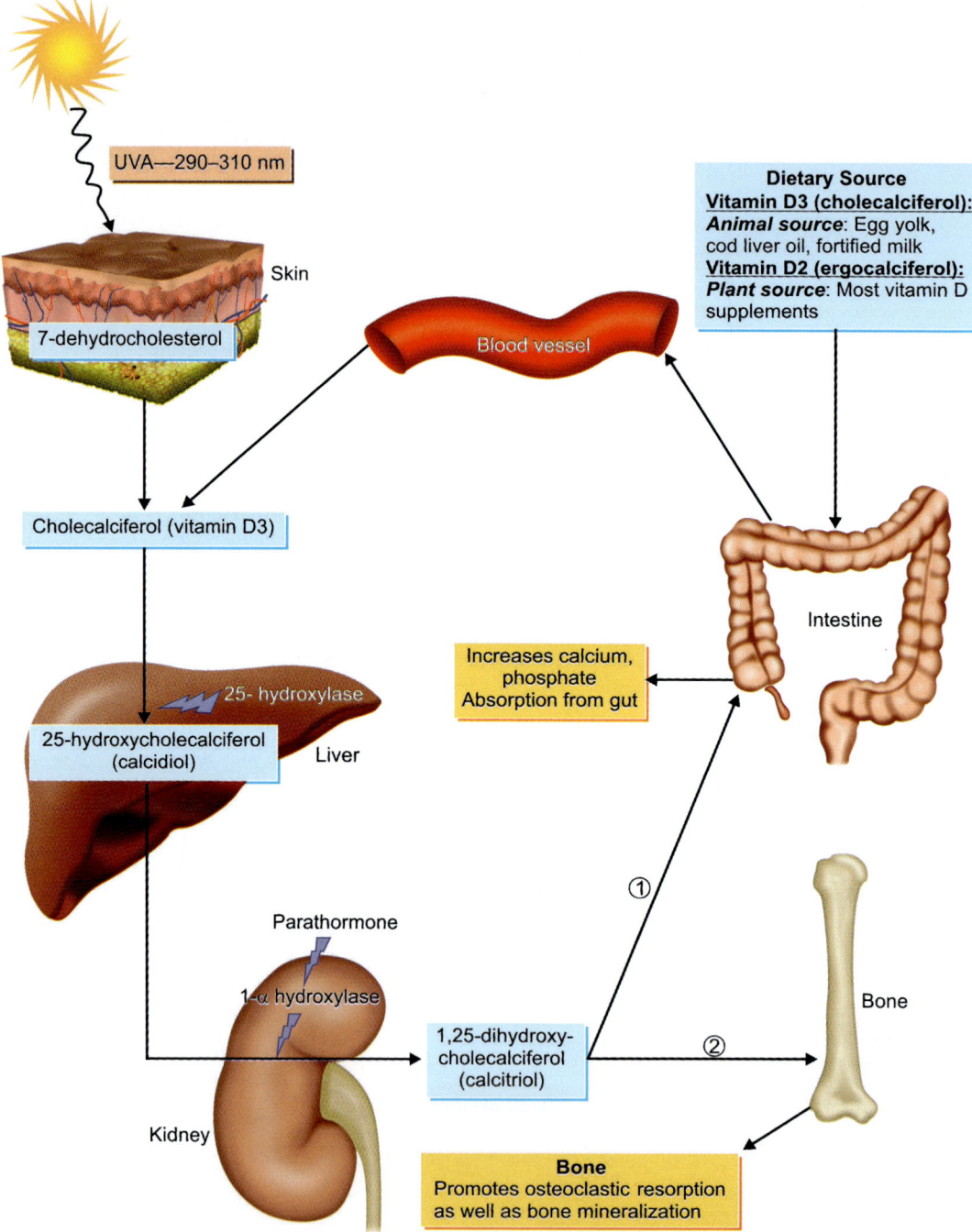

Fig. 35.2: Vitamin D regulation cycle in the human body. The zigzag blue lightening bolt indicates 'under influence of'.

1. ***Vitamin D/calcium deficiency rickets:*** Vitamin D deficiency remains the most common cause of rickets.
2. ***Vitamin D dependent rickets type I:*** It is an *autosomal recessive disorder* wherein active vitamin D is not formed in the kidney due to *lack of 1-hydroxylase enzyme*.
3. ***Vitamin D dependent rickets type II:*** It is an *autosomal recessive disorder* wherein active vitamin D cannot act over the receptors due to *end-organ resistance*.

- **Hypophosphatemic/phosphopenic rickets:** It occurs due to chronic phosphate deficiency, which can occur due to dietary deficiency or renal wasting. Note that dietary deficiency of phosphate is rare as phosphate is abundant in the diet, whereas *renal loss-related hypophosphatemia (genetic or acquired) is the most common cause of low phosphate level in the body* **(Table 35.1)**. Several important facts about phosphopenic rickets and their causes are mentioned below.

Table 35.1: Types and causes of rickets.

Calcium/vitamin D deficiency—calcipenic rickets	Phosphate deficiency—phosphopenic rickets

Vitamin D/Ca deficient
- Lack of sunlight exposure
- Lack of Ca/vitamin D3 in the diet
- Poor calcium absorption in "malabsorption syndrome" such as celiac disease
- *Drugs preventing absorption*: Phenytoin, rifampicin
- Chronic liver disease
- Chronic renal disease (renal osteodystrophy)
	Renal phosphate wasting
	- *Genetic hypophosphatemic rickets*
	  – X-linked hypophosphatemic rickets *or* familial hypophosphatemic rickets (*vitamin D resistant rickets*)
	  – Autosomal dominant hypophosphatemic rickets
	  – Autosomal resistant hypophosphatemic rickets
	  – McCune Albright syndrome
	  – Renal tubular acidosis (RTA)
	  – Fanconi syndrome: Proximal renal tubular absorption defect
	  – Drug-induced phosphate loss: Acyclovir, diuretics (thiazides, frusemide), theophylline, steroids, bronchodilators, bisphosphonates, alcohol, phenytoin
	- *Acquired*
	  – Oncogenic/tumors secreting phosphatonins (FGF)
	  – RTA

Type I vitamin-D-dependent rickets - Autosomal recessive disorder - Lack of 1-α hydroxylase enzyme in the kidney. Hence, no active vitamin D is synthesized. - Symptoms within 1st year of life - Normal calcidiol levels, low calcitriol levels	**Poor phosphate intake:** Rare
Type II vitamin-D-dependent rickets - Autosomal recessive disorder - Receptor resistance to "calcitriol/active vitamin D" - Symptoms of rickets start within 2 years of life: **Alopecia** is characteristic of this type of rickets. There can be other ectodermal anomalies, such as multiple milia, oligodontia, and ectodermal cysts.	

- **Most hypophosphatemic rickets** *are predominantly genetic, characterized by elevated fibroblast growth factor-23 (FGF), which inhibits phosphate resorption in the kidney. Certain tumors also secrete FGF-23 inhibiting phosphate resorption. Therefore, FGF-23 level assessment is an essential part of hypophosphatemic rickets evaluation.*
- **Fanconi syndrome** *is characterized by failure of resorption of certain substances, including phosphate, from proximal convoluted renal tubules.*
- **Renal tubular acidosis** *results in resorption defect arising out of the proximal or distal part of renal tubules.*

PATHOPHYSIOLOGY

- Rickets occurs due to disrupted calcium, vitamin D, and phosphate homeostasis resulting in several changes in the growth plate, such as:
  - Failure of apoptosis of chondrocytes of hypertrophic zone leading to **irregular, deformed cartilage growth**.
  - Poor calcification of cartilage matrix at the "zone of provisional calcification" results in *'large areas of unossified osteoid tissue in the growth plate'*.
  - Irregular, deformed, and unossified cartilage results in a **weak and deformable bone** under stress, which is a typical change in rickets.

CLINICAL FEATURES

The clinical features of florid rickets can be observed right from the skull to the lower limbs. The signs are musculoskeletal/osseous and non-osseous.

Osseous/Musculoskeletal Signs

- **Skull**
  - Craniotabes: Soft skull bone (parietal and occipital) which collapses on pressure and springs back to normal when the pressure is relieved (ping-pong skull).
  - Frontal bossing
  - Delayed closure of fontanelle
  - Poor dentition.
- **Chest**
  - Rachitic rosary (costochondral painless swelling)
  - Harrison's sulcus: Due to the pull of the diaphragm on 'soft' lower ribs
  - Pectus carinatum/pectus excavatum.
- **Spine:** Cat-back deformity/kyphosis, scoliosis.
- **Abdomen:** *Potbelly*—due to the poor tone of the abdominal muscle resulting in visceroptosis.
- **Wrist:** Widening of the wrist due to rachitic changes in metaphysis of the lower ulna and radius.
- **Pelvis:** Triradiate pelvis—it occurs due to protrusion of the acetabulum into the pelvis. *Note that it is a radiological sign.*
- **Lower limb**
  - Hip: Coxa vara
  - Knee: Genu varum/genu valgum/wind swept deformity (one knee in varum while other in valgum)
  - Double malleoli (Marfan's sign): It is due to metaphyseal widening.

- **Other signs**
  - Muscle hypotonia, proximal myopathy
  - Growth retardation: More common in hypophosphatemic rickets
  - Pathologic #
  - Bone pain and tenderness: More common in hypophosphatemic rickets.

Nonosseous Signs

Anemia, hypocalcemic convulsions, cardiomyopathy.

INVESTIGATIONS

- **Plain X-ray:** Plain X-ray of the wrist, knee and ankle shows **(Figs. 35.3A and B):**
  - *Epiphysis:* Decreased height (thinned) and delayed appearance
  - *Growth plate/physis:* Increased thickness/wide
  - *Metaphysis:* Widening, cupping, splaying, and fraying of edges
  - *Diaphysis:* Thinned cortex, osteopenia. Occasionally, one may find Harris arrest lines which indicate healing rickets.
  - Severe rickets may cause pathological fractures in bone. Pelvis may show *triradiate pelvis.*
- **Blood tests in calcipenic rickets (Table 35.2):**
  - **Ca, P, ALP and PTH levels:** Ca and P levels are low, whereas ALP and PTH levels are always high in hypocalcemic rickets.
  - **1,25-dihydroxycholecalciferol (DHCC):** Levels vary in different types of calcipenic rickets. 1,25 DHCC may be normal/high or low in nutritional rickets. However, 'serum vitamin D3 is low in nutritional rickets.' Furthermore, 1,25 DHCC is very low in type I vitamin D rickets, whereas very high in type II vitamin D rickets.
  - **24-hour urinary calcium and phosphate**: Urinary calcium and phosphate are low in all types of calcipenic rickets.
  - **Serum urea, creatinine:** Serum urea and creatinine are normal in calcipenic rickets, while elevated in renal rickets.

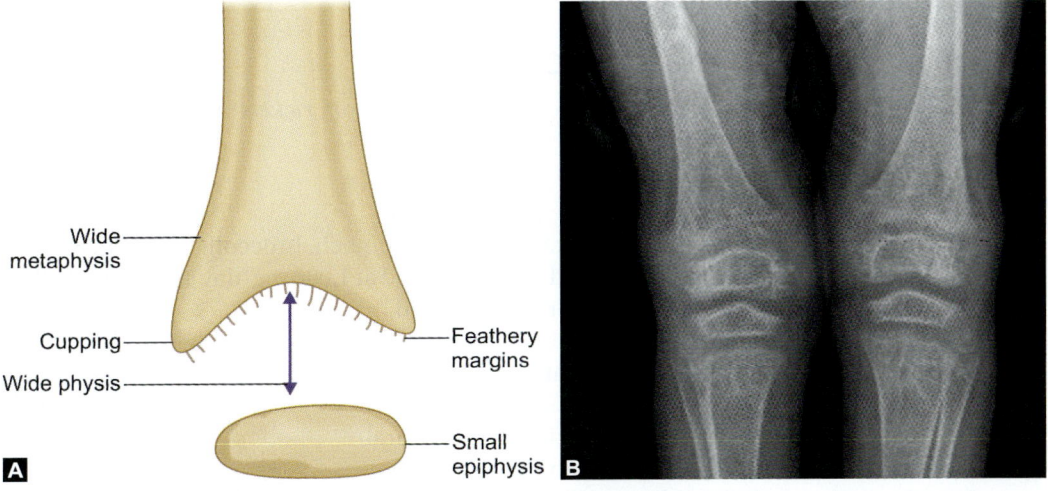

Figs. 35.3A and B: (A) Illustration of bony changes in rickets; (B) AP X-ray of the knee with characteristics ricket changes.

Table 35.2: Different investigations with their serum levels in rickets.

	Ca	P	ALP	PTH	1,25-DHCC	FGF-23
Nutritional rickets	↓	↓	↑	↑	Normal/high	Normal
Type 1 vitamin D dependent rickets	↓	↓	↑	↑	↓↓	Normal
Type 2 vitamin D dependent rickets	↓	↓	↑	↑	↑↑	Normal
Hypophosphatemic rickets	Normal	↓	↑	Normal	↓↓	↑↑

Note: In certain types of renal hypophosphatemic Rickets or rare phosphate dietary deficiency, FGF-23 may be normal. However, serum phosphate remains very low, while urinary phosphate levels are high.

Clinical Features and Investigations of Hypophosphatemic Rickets

- The onset of Phosphopenic Rickets is earlier than calcipenic rickets.
- Lower limbs are more affected than upper limb in phosphopenic rickets than calcipenic rickets.
- Enamel hypoplasia and tetany are absent in phosphopenic rickets, whereas dental abscess is more common in phosphopenic rickets.
- Growth retardation/stunted growth is more common in phosphopenic rickets than calcipenic rickets.

Investigations
- Serum phosphate is decreased, while calcium, PTH and 1,25-DHCC is normal
- ALP is moderately increased (less than what is seen in calcipenic rickets)
- Urine phosphate levels are high (due to decreased resorption)
- FGF is often elevated
- Serum urea and creatinine are elevated in renal failure rickets
- Glycosuria and bicarbonaturia in Fanconi syndrome
- RTA cases may show altered pH of urine.

In this chapter, the treatment of calcipenic rickets will be discussed in detail. The details of the rest of the type of Rickets are out of this chapter's scope.

■ TREATMENT OF NUTRITIONAL RICKETS

Treating nutritional rickets involves *medical management of rickets* and *management of deformities*.

Medical/Conservative Management
- **A healthy diet rich in calcium:** Milk, cheese, cereals, spinach, broccoli, egg yolk, fish
- **Dietary/supplemental calcium:** It should be maintained at 1,000 mg/day as the requirement for calcium increases after vitamin D therapy is started.
- **Adequate sunlight exposure**
- **Vitamin D3 supplementation:** There are two prevalent methods of vitamin D therapy.
    - *Stoss therapy:* Stoss therapy is a single dose (oral/intramuscular) 1–6 lakh IU of vitamin D3
    - *Low dose vitamin D for 2–3 months:* 1,000–10,000 IU/day for 2–3 months

Trivia: Stoss is a German word, which means- 'to push'.

Once the medical management is initiated, one must do a serial (monthly) clinical, serological and radiological follow-up to assess improvement.
- **Clinical:** Improvement in general well-being and deformities.
- **Serological:** Serum calcium and phosphate levels improve, and ALP and PTH levels start normalizing.
- **Radiological:** Observe for the *white line of calcification at the zone of calcification* in X-ray during the healing phase, which marks the radiological healing of rickets **(Fig. 35.4)**.

Treatment of type I vitamin D-dependent rickets: Since Calcitriol is not formed in this type, the supplement of the active form of vitamin D (calcitriol) to be given.

Treatment of type II vitamin D-dependent rickets: High dose of calcitriol is given to overcome the receptor resistance.

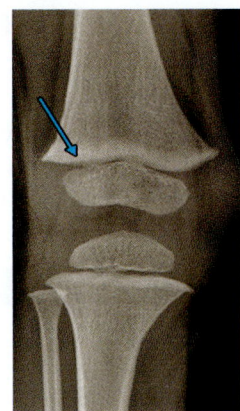

Fig. 35.4: White line of calcification (blue arrow) in healing phase of rickets.

Management of Limb Deformities
- **Mild to moderate deformities**
    - It may gradually improve with medical treatment.
    - Rarely, bracing (mermaid brace) can be used for lower limb genu varum/genu valgum deformities **(Fig. 35.5A)**.
- **Moderate to severe deformities**
    Residual moderate to severe deformities can be managed surgically by:
    - **Hemiepiphysiodesis:** It is a surgery wherein physical growth is temporarily arrested on one side of the growth plate to correct deformities **(Fig. 35.5B)**.
    - **Corrective osteotomy:** Corrective osteotomy is performed only after metabolic healing starts as osteotomy would not heal in presence of abnormal metabolism. The healing of rickets is indicated by:
        - Presence of 'White line of calcification' at the zone of calcification **(Fig. 35.4)**
        - Normalized serum ALP.

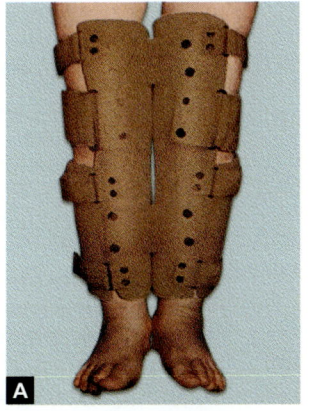 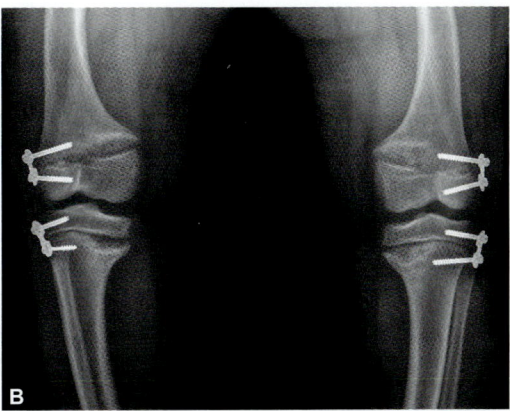

Figs. 35.5A and B: (A) Mermaid splint; (B) Hemiepiphysiodesis on distal femur and proximal tibia physis.
(*Courtesy:* Dr Upendra Kumar)

TREATMENT OF PHOSPHOPENIC RICKETS

- Oral phosphates
- Vitamin D3, if low
- Once the mesenchymal tumour causing oncogenic rickets is removed, the condition may significantly improve.
- Certain drugs causing phosphate loss, such as acyclovir, must be substituted with others.

OSTEOMALACIA

DEFINITION

Osteomalacia is characterized by ***defective mineralization of bone matrix in the adult bone*** resulting in large areas of the unossified matrix.

The pathological process of rickets and osteomalacia is the same.

ETIOLOGY

- Vitamin D deficient diet, poor replenishment in successive multiple pregnancies
- Poor exposure to sunlight
- Poor absorption of vitamin D and calcium from the gut
- Renal osteodystrophy or chronic renal disease
- Hypophosphatemia
- Chronic alcoholism
- *Drugs preventing Ca absorption*: Phenytoin, rifampicin, glucocorticoids, ifosfamide, etidronate, or aluminum. Even drugs limiting absorption of phosphate or increasing its excretion can cause osteomalacia (acyclovir, steroids, bronchodilators).

CLINICAL FEATURES

It affects adult patients who present with:
- Generalized bone pain, backache and generalized muscular weakness are the common presentations.
- Pathological fractures of long bones, ribs, and vertebrae can occur.
- Waddling gait.
- *Proximal myopathy*: It results in difficulty in getting up from squatting/sitting position.

INVESTIGATIONS

- **Plain X-ray**
    - ***Diffuse osteopenia***.
    - Spine: ***Codfish vertebra/biconcave vertebra*** are seen due to indentation on soft vertebral bodies by the intervertebral disc **(Fig. 35.6A)**.
    - ***Looser zone:*** It is observed in ribs, medial border of the scapula, and medial femoral cortex **(Fig. 35.6B)**.

Looser zone

These are cortical infractions or Milkman lines, 2–3 mm wide transverse lucencies traversing part way through a bone, usually at right angles to the involved cortex and are associated most frequently with osteomalacia and rickets. They are pseudofractures and considered a type of insufficiency fracture with sclerotic irregular margins and are often symmetrical.

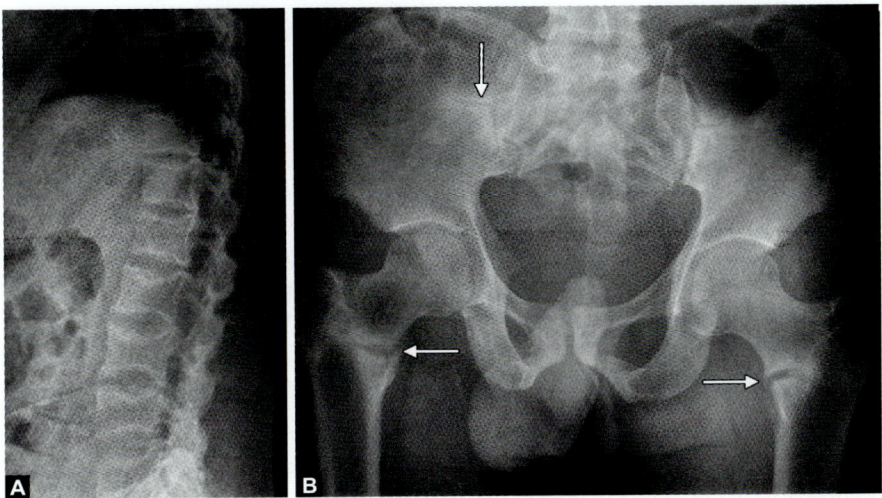

Figs. 35.6A and B: (A) X-ray of the lumbar spine showing biconcave/codfish vertebra; (B) X-ray pelvis and proximal femur showing looser's zone (white arrows) in proximal femur and ilium.

- Pelvis:
  - ***Protrusio acetabuli*** signifies a deeper acetabulum cavity protruding medial to ilioischial line
  - ***Trefoil pelvis:*** Softening of the innominate bone of the pelvis allows the acetabuli to indent laterally **(Fig. 35.7)**. Severe trefoil pelvis can cause cephalopelvic disproportion resulting in obstructed labor.
- Hips: ***Coxa vara*** (decreased femoral neck-shaft angle)
- Serological tests:
  - Low Ca, phosphate
  - Elevated ALP, parathormone
  - Low vitamin D.

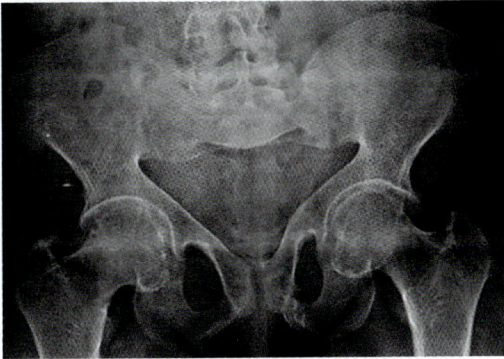

Fig. 35.7: Trefoil pelvis.

TREATMENT

- Calcium and vitamin D supplement (6 lakh IU stat or 1,000 IU daily)
- Hepatobiliary or chronic renal disease patients must receive calcitriol.

DIFFERENTIAL DIAGNOSIS

- Osteoporosis
- Multiple myeloma
- Fibromyalgia.

OSTEOPOROSIS

INTRODUCTION

Normal bone is composed of approximately 65% minerals and 35% matrix. Together matrix and minerals are known as bone mass.

Osteoporosis is defined as *'decrease in bone mass'* and *'micro-architectural deterioration of bone leading to bone fragility,'* and consequent increase in fracture risk.

World Health Organization (WHO) criteria of osteoporosis: Using dual-energy X-ray absorptiometry (DEXA) scan, which measures bone mineral density via T-score. *T-score "less than –2.5 and below standard deviation"* is considered to have osteoporosis.

Rickets and osteomalacia are qualitative disorders (quality of bone formed is poor), whereas osteoporosis is a quantitative disorder (quantity of bone remaining is deficient).

CLASSIFICATION

Osteoporosis is classified into two types, primary and secondary. Primary osteoporosis is associated with aging or menopause, whereas secondary osteoporosis is characterized as having a clearly definable etiology.

1. **Primary**
    - *Type I osteoporosis*: Postmenopausal osteoporosis
    - *Type II osteoporosis*: Senile osteoporosis, which occurs as a result of the aging process.
2. **Secondary**
    - *Endocrinal*: Cushing syndrome, hyperparathyroidism, hyperthyroidism
    - *Drug-induced*: Corticosteroid, heparin, anticonvulsants, frusemide, lithium
    - *Nutritional*: Malnutrition
    - *Disuse*: Nonambulatory patients
    - *Inflammatory diseases*: Rheumatoid arthritis

RISK FACTORS FOR OSTEOPOROSIS

The risk factors for osteoporosis are mentioned in **Box 35.1**.

Box 35.1: Risk factors for osteoporosis.

- Previous history of fragility fractures
- Old age (greater than 50 years in females; greater than 65 in males)
- Females
- Menopause
- Oophorectomy during reproductive years
- Smoking, excess alcohol consumption
- Low vitamin D and calcium intake
- Prolonged immobilization, inactivity
- Drugs: Heparin, steroid intake, especially if intake >7.5 mg for long duration, frusemide (*Note: Thiazide is protective for osteoporosis*), excess thyroxine.

PATHOPHYSIOLOGY

The crux of osteoporosis pathophysiology is the *"imbalance between bone resorption and bone formation"* during bone remodeling.

As the birth, bone growth continues increasing bone mass. The peak bone mass (PBM), which indicates density and strength of the bone is likely achieved by the age of 30 years. Note that PBM is higher in males as compared to females. After that age, the PBM is maintained by a regular remodeling process. Factors affecting PBM are mentioned in **Box 35.2**. Of *note: Remodeling is a lifelong process wherein matured, dead or damaged bone is removed by osteoclast followed by new bone laid by osteoblast.*

> **Box 35.2:** Factors affecting peak bone mass (PBM)
>
> - **Gender:** More in males
> - **Race:** African females have higher PBM than Caucasian females
> - **Physical activity:** Girls and boys with higher physical activity have higher PBM
> - **Hormonal:** Protective action of estrogen ensure adequate PBM
> - **Lifestyle:** Smoking, alcohol, sedentary lifestyle lead to lower PBM
> - **Nutrition:** Poor nutrition results in lower PBM.

- In females, minimal change in peak bone mass (PBM) occurs between the age of 30 and menopause. However, PBM reduction accelerates afterwards due to lack of protective action of estrogen, resulting in increased bone resorption and decreased bone deposition.
- *Inadequate PBM, increased osteoclastic bone resorption, and poor osteoblastic bone formation is the key to osteoporosis.*
- Furthermore, lack of Ca and vitamin D leads to impaired bone deposition and may reduce PBM formation. Also, low serum ionic calcium stimulates parathyroid hormone (PTH), which further removes calcium from the bone leading to poor bone mineral density (BMD).
- Trabecular/cancellous bone is more active and subjected to more remodeling than cortical bone. Hence, *more osteoporosis occurs in the trabecular bone* (spine, pelvis and metaphyseal area of long bones, especially hip and distal radius) than cortical bone.

CLINICAL FEATURES

A large majority of the patients are asymptomatic. **Generalized back pain** is the most common complaint, followed by **fragility fractures**. Fragility fractures are *common in the cancellous bone*, such as spine, distal radius, and bones around the hip joint (femoral neck, intertrochanter region, pubic rami).

The examination may reveal **dorsal spine round back kyphosis** (Dowager's hump) **(Fig. 35.8)**. There may be tenderness over the spine. The kyphotic deformity may be palpable. A summary of the clinical features is mentioned in **Box 35.3**.

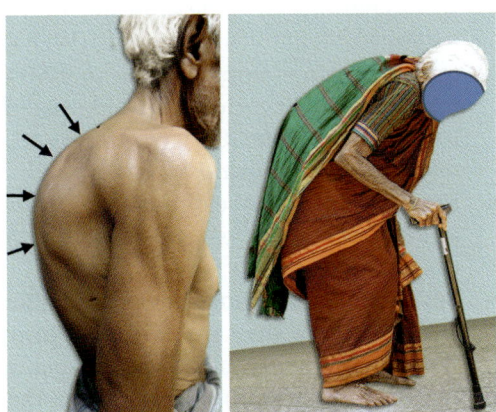

Fig. 35.8: Dowager's hump or round back kyphosis in a osteoporotic patient. Multiple black arrow suggest the exaggerated dorsal kyphosis. *(Courtesy:* Astro Mohan)

Box 35.3: Clinical features of osteoporosis.

- **Back pain:** Generalized
- **Pathological fractures** with trivial fall or minor trauma, observed in
   - *Spine*: Single or multiple vertebral fractures in dorsal and lumbar spine
   - Fracture neck and intertrochanteric femur
   - Fracture distal radius
- **Kyphosis:** Due to single or multiple osteoporotic fractures of dorsolumbar spine.

Presence of a single osteoporotic fracture is the most crucial evidence that patient is having osteoporosis!

INVESTIGATIONS

- **Plain X-ray of the spine (Fig. 35.9):** It is one of the essential X-rays required to assess osteoporosis.
   - Loss of trabeculae and vertebral height
   - Single or multiple vertebral fractures in the dorsal and lumbar spine
   - **Codfish vertebra**/fish mouth appearance
- **Plain X-ray of the hip:** Hip X-rays can be used to *grade osteoporosis based upon Singh's index* (grade six to zero), which is based on the visibility of primary and secondary trabeculae in the hip. Grade six is considered to be normal, whereas grade 0 is considered to be severe osteoporosis (Read chapter 18 on fracture neck femur to understand trabaculae).
- **Dual-energy X-ray absorptiometry (DEXA) scan:** Currently, *DEXA is the standard gold method to assess BMD and future fracture risk.* Typically DEXA scan is performed in the spine and pelvis. According to World Health Organization (WHO), based on t-score obtained from DEXA scan, BMD is classified into three categories—normal, osteopenia, and osteoporosis **(Box 35.4)**. *(Read Box 35.6 at the end of the chapter for details of BMD).*
- **Frax tool:** Frax tool estimates the *probability of an individual sustaining an osteoporotic fracture* over the next 10 years.
- **Serum calcium, phosphorus, and alkaline phosphate, PTH, Vitamin D levels**
   - Essentially, they are normal in primary osteoporosis. However, vitamin D can be low. They are performed to assess secondary causes of osteoporosis.
- **Serum biomarkers:** Various biomarkers for bone formation, resorption, and regulation are released during bone remodeling process of osteoporosis. Levels of *Procollagen type 1 N-terminal Propeptide (P1NP), bone-specific alkaline phosphatase, osteocalcin-C are* bone formation biomarkers; *hydroxyproline and hydroxylysine* are bone resorption biomarkers; and receptor activator of NF-κ B ligand (RANKL) and osteoprotegrin are bone regulation

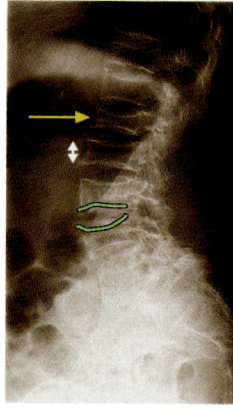

Fig. 35.9: X-ray of osteoporotic spine showing loss of vertebral height (white arrow), vertebral fracture (yellow arrow), and codfish vertebra (green lines)

Box 35.4: WHO criteria of BMD grading based upon t-score.

Normal: T-score between -1 and +1 standard deviation (SD)
Osteopenia: T-score between -1 and -2.5 SD
Osteoporosis: T-score less than -2.5 SD

biomarkers. In combination with the measurement of BMD, clinical applications of bone biomarkers may provide comprehensive information for diagnosis of osteoporosis. Nevertheless, they are not routinely performed in establishing the diagnosis of osteoporosis.
- **Calcaneal or distal radius ultrasound to assess BMD:** Not sensitive and specific as DEXA scan.
- **Computed tomography (CT) scan:** Not preferred due to radiation.
- **Transiliac biopsy to assess bone quality:** Rarely performed as it is invasive.

Figure 35.10 at the end of the osteoporosis discussion illustrates the difference between normal, osteoporotic, rickets and osteomalacic bone.

TREATMENT

Treatment of osteoporosis involves *preventing further bone loss, assisting new bone formation, and treating pain and deformity due to vertebral collapse or other fractures.* Various general and measures are fundamental basis to treat osteoporosis. Vertebral or other fractures may require conservative/surgical intervention.

General Measures

- Healthy protein-rich diet and regular exercise *(Note: New bone formation requires matrix, which requires adequate protein. Exercises induce adequate strain over the bone for remodeling)*
- Avoid smoking, alcohol intake
- Calcium and vitamin D supplements
- Braces to support osteoporotic spine or after a vertebral fracture.

Pharmacologic Treatment

The various drugs used in the treatment of osteoporosis are:
- Major drugs used are **osteoclast activity inhibitors** *or* **osteoblast activity stimulators** to restore the biological balance of osteoporosis.
    - *Osteoclast inhibitors:* Bisphosphonates, calcitonin
        - *Bisphosphonates are the drug of choice for managing both senile and post-menopausal osteoporosis.* They reduce the risk of vertebral and nonvertebral fractures.
        - Calcitonin acts as an osteoclast inhibitor, reducing vertebral fracture risk.
    - *Osteoblast stimulator:* Recombinant parathormone is used to treat severe osteoporosis as it helps in newborn formation by stimulating the osteoblast. It reduces the risk of both vertebral and non-vetebral fractures.
    (Read **Box 35.5** *about details of drugs in osteoporosis*).
- **Selective estrogen receptor modulator (SERM):** *Raloxifene*
    It is an estrogen receptor agonist that helps in *new bone formation*. It also *inhibits osteoclasts*. It is indicated in post-menopausal osteoporosis and reduces the risk of vertebral fracture. Side effects include hot flashes and calf cramps. Also, there is a risk of thromboembolism in the first few months of initiation of therapy.
- **Monoclonal antibody:** *Denosumab*
    It binds against the receptor activator of nuclear factor kappa-B ligand (RANKL) receptors and *inhibits osteoclast formation* resulting in decreased bone resorption. Decreased bone resorption results in increased bone density and reduced risk of fracture. It mimics the effect of the endogenous protein "osteoprotegerin."

> **Box 35.5:** Important facts about common drugs used in treating osteoporosis.
>
> - **Bisphosphonates**
>   - Osteoclast inhibitors
>   - **1st Gen:** Etidronate; **2nd Gen:** Alendronate, residronate; **3rd Gen:** Ibandronate, Zolendronic acid
>   - Given orally/injectable; daily/weekly/monthly/yearly preparations
>   - Gold standard for mild-moderate osteoporosis
>   - **Adverse effect:** Gastritis, esophagitis, and jaw osteonecrosis. *Long-term use of bisphosphonates could result in stress fracture of proximal femur in subtrochanteric area.* These fractures are prone for nonunion
>   - **Contraindications:** Hypocalcemia, known as hypersensitivity, esophageal atresia.
> - **Parathormone**
>   - It is an osteoblast stimulator.
>   - Given as daily subcutaneous injection as pulse therapy. Although parathormone is known to stimulate osteoclast, pulse therapy paradoxically stimulates osteoblast.
>   - **Indication:** Severe osteoporosis
>   - **Adverse effect:** Dizziness, nausea, and headache
>   - **Contraindicated:** Paget's disease.
> - **Calcitonin**
>   - Osteoclast inhibitor
>   - Given as nasal sprays/subcutaneous injections
>   - Also given in acute vertebral compression fracture for pain relief
>   - **Adverse effect:** Transient rhinitis, dizziness, and nausea.

> **Box 35.6:** Relevant facts about BMD scan.
>
> - Gold standard investigation to detect BMD is DEXA scan
> - *DEXA*: Dual energy X-ray absorptiometry
> - Performed for lumbar spine (L2-4 lumbar vertebra) and hip
> - Two scores can be calculated: T and Z score
> - *T score*: BMD is compared with a healthy 30-year-old person
> - *Z score*: BMD is compared with age and gender-matched normal person
> - Typically, T score is used to grade BMD and treat osteoporosis
> - *Normal BMD*: T score is between −1 and +1 SD
> - *Osteopenia*: T score is between −1 and −2.5 SD
> - *Osteoporosis*: T score is below −2.5 SD

Common side effects include muscular pain, infection, atypical hip fracture, and rarely jaw osteonecrosis.
- **Strontium ranelate:** It increases bone formation by *stimulating osteoblasts and inhibiting osteoclasts.*
- **Anabolic steroids:** Injection of 'Nandrolone acetate' helps in protein synthesis required for bone matrix formation.

Osteoporotic Fracture Treatment

Osteoporotic fractures occur both in spine (vertebral) and limbs (nonvertebral), which can be managed conservatively or operatively.

- **Vertebral fractures:** They can be managed conservatively with analgesics and braces, while some may require surgery (vertebroplasty, kyphoplasty).
    - *Osteoporotic vertebral collapse*: **Spinal braces** to support the spine **(Fig. 35.10A)**.
    - *Vertebroplasty or kyphoplasty*: It is performed for 'acute painful osteoporotic vertebral fractures'.
        - *In vertebroplasty*, bone cement is injected into the fractured vertebra, which stabilizes the vertebra, resulting in reduced pain. However, the *shape of the collapsed vertebra remains unaltered* **(Figs. 35.10B and C)**
        - *In kyphoplasty*, a balloon is inflated inside the collapsed vertebra to create a space, followed by the bone cement injection into the space created. Unlike vertebroplasty, *kyphoplasty improves kyphosis due to the vertebral collapse* **(Figs. 35.11A to D)**.

NONVERTEBRAL OR FRACTURES IN THE LIMBS

Most fractures require fixation while some can be managed with cast.

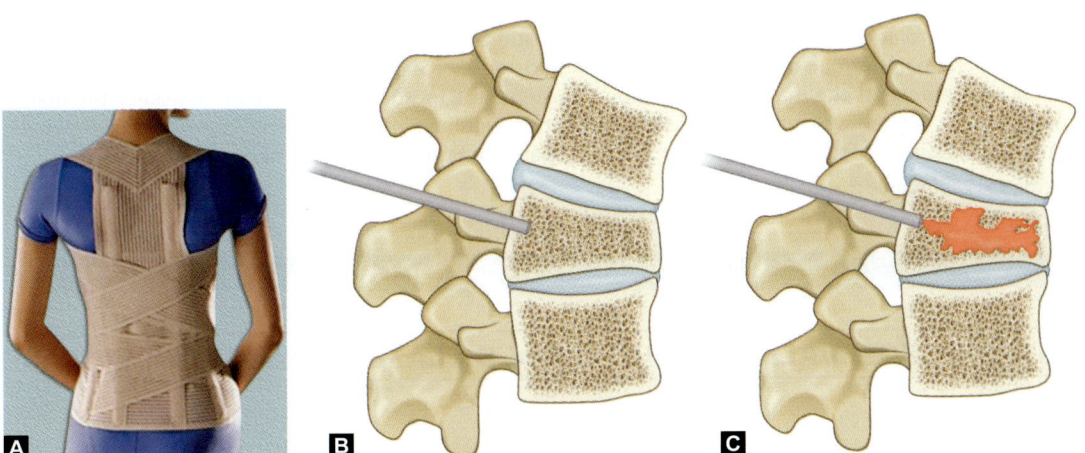

Figs. 35.10A to C: (A) Spinal brace for vertebral fracture; (B and C) Vertebroplasty-bone cement injection into a collapsed vertebra.

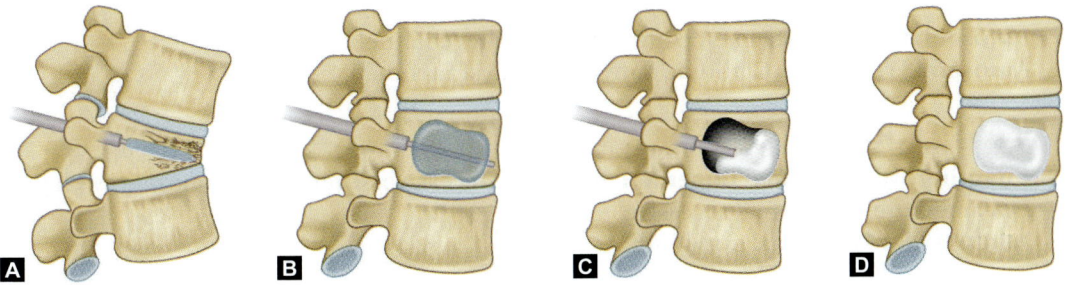

Figs. 35.11A to D: Kyphoplasty—showing correction of kyphotic vertebra with restoration of vertebral height with baloon inflation and bone cement injection.

Difference between Rickets, Osteomalacia, Osteoporosis, and Osteosclerosis

Figure 35.12 is self-explanatory, which shows that osteoporosis causes a decline in overall bone mass, including minerals and matrix. However, the ratio of mineral and matrix may remain same. In rickets/osteomalacia, the matrix component is more than minerals, whereas mineral component is higher than matrix in osteosclerosis.

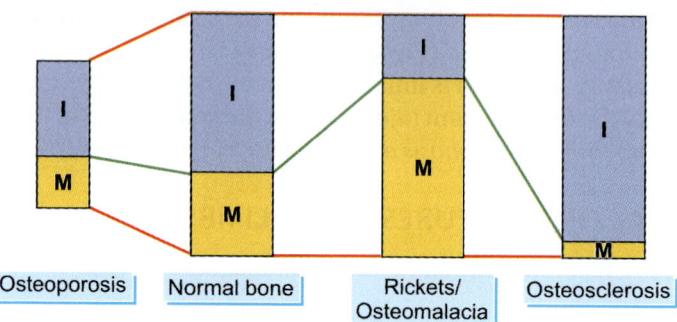

Fig. 35.12: Bar diagram showing the change in the ratio of bone matrix (M) versus minerals or inorganic material (I) ratio in normal, osteoporosis, rickets, and osteosclerosis (not to the scale: only illustrative). The yellow box represents the matrix and the blue represents the inorganic component. In rickets, the matrix component is higher, whereas osteosclerotic condition will have more inorganic components. However, osteoporosis will have a similar ratio of organic: inorganic but the overall mass of bone reduces.

(M: matrix; I: inorganic material).

OSTEOSCLEROSIS DISORDERS

OSTEOPETROSIS/ALBERS-SCHÖNBERG DISEASE/ MARBLE BONE DISEASE

■ DEFINITION

A metabolic disease of bone due to *"defective osteoclastic resorption of bone in immature bone"* leads to altered bone modeling and remodeling.

■ GENETICS

- **Autosomal dominant (most common):** Chloride channel dysfunction
- **Autosomal recessive:** Carbonic anhydrase II dysfunction.

■ CLASSIFICATION

- **Infantile/osteopetrosis congenita:** Autosomal recessive, severe form, bone marrow failure
- **Intermediate:** Autosomal recessive
- **Adult/tarda:** Autosomal dominant.

■ PATHOGENESIS

- The primary mechanism involved in all types of osteopetrosis is the *"failure of normal osteoclastic bone resorption."*

CLINICAL FEATURES

Clinical features vary in three different variants of osteopetrosis, which are mentioned in **Table 35.3**. The bones are brittle and, therefore, more prone to pathological fractures. Also, joints are predisposed to secondary OA.

Table 35.3: Clinical features in different variants of osteopetrosis.

Variant	Age of onset	Clinical features	Prognosis
Infantile	Infants	▪ *Bone marrow failure*: Pancytopenia ▪ Recurrent infections, bleeding ▪ Failure to thrive and growth retardation ▪ Blindness and hydrocephalus ▪ Often early death unless a bone marrow transplant is done	Poor
Intermediate	Childhood	▪ *No bone* marrow failure ▪ Growth retardation ▪ Sensorineural hearing loss ▪ Renal tubular acidosis	Poor
Adult/tarda	Adulthood	▪ Often asymptomatic ▪ Mandibular osteomyelitis ▪ Brittle bones and repeated fractures with normal fracture healing ▪ 2° degenerative joint disease	Good

INVESTIGATIONS

- **Plain X-ray**
    - Increased density of the bone and increased cortical thickening **(Fig. 35.13)**
    - Decreased medullary canal diameter
    - *Erlenmeyer flask deformity* of the proximal humerus and distal femur **(Fig. 35.14A)**
    - *Rugger jersey spine* **(Fig. 35.14B)**.

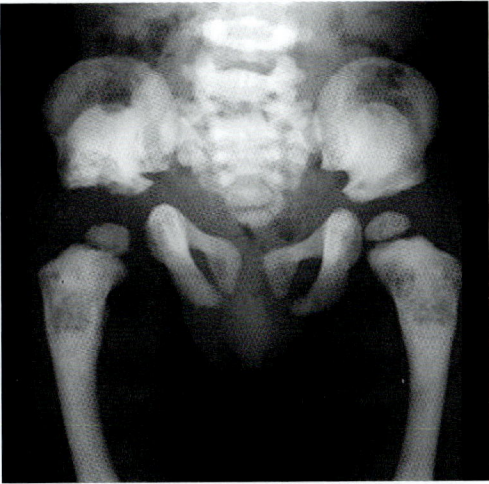

Fig. 35.13: Osteopetrosis of pelvis and femur.

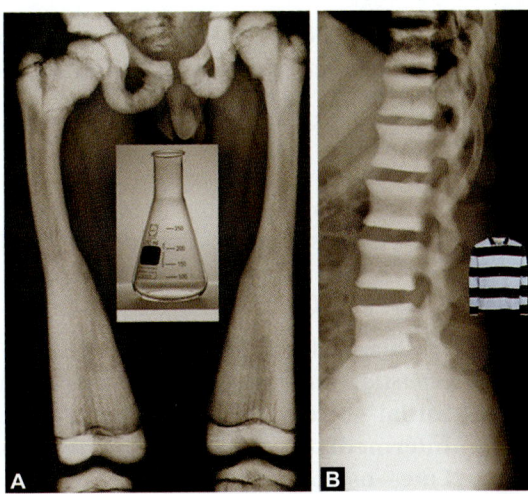

Figs. 35.14A and B: (A) Erlenmeyer flask deformity of femur; (B) Rugger jersey spine.

Note: Conditions causing osteosclerosis (radiological) are mentioned in **Box 35.7**.
- **Blood investigations:** Abnormal in autosomal recessive state
  - Increased acid phosphatase
  - Increased parathyroid hormone (PTH), calcium.

> **Box 35.7:** Conditions causing increased bone density/osteosclerosis.
> - Paget's disease
> - Marble bone disease
> - Fluorosis
> - *Secondaries from tumors*: Prostate, breast cancer.

ORTHOPAEDIC TREATMENT

- **Medical management**
  - For infantile/intermediate variants
    - Bone marrow transplant
    - High dose of calcitriol
  - For adult variant: Interferon gamma-1 beta
- **Treatment for fractures and joint disease**
  - *Conservative*: Casts
  - Open reduction internal fixation (ORIF)/closed reduction internal fixation (CRIF)
  - Joint replacement for degenerative joint disease.

COMPLICATIONS

- Degenerative joint disease
- Re-fractures
- Delayed unions
- Malunion
- Infection.

PAGET'S DISEASE/OSTEITIS DEFORMANS

DEFINITION

Paget's disease of bone (PDB) is a ***disorder of bone turnover*** characterized by *"defective bone remodeling wherein there is an initial increase in bone resorption followed by increased bone deposition".*

GENETICS

- Most cases are spontaneous. Few are familial, wherein 40% cases are autosomal dominant.
- SQSTM1 is the single most important predisposing gene for PDB.

PATHOPHYSIOLOGY

- The primary abnormality is *"increased osteoclastic resorption"* followed by increased osteoblastic bone deposition". It has three phases:
  1. **Initial—osteolytic phase:** Characterized by increased bond resorption
  2. **Intermediate—mixed phase:** Mixed; osteoclastic and osteoblastic
  3. **Late—osteoblastic phase:** In this phase, a disorganized "woven" type of bone is formed, which is weak and allows excess fibroblastic connective tissue and blood vessels resulting in a hypervascular bone state.

Note

Pnemonic to remember pathological phases of Pagets—'LMB'; **L**ytic, **M**ixed, and **B**lastic.

In the late osteoblastic phase, there is gradual enlargement of the bones resulting in deformity, pathological fractures, compression of the structures inside the bone tunnels or canals, and hypervascular, resulting in a high cardiac output failure state.

Clinical types: It could be *monostotic (single bone)* or *polyostotic (multiple bones)* type.

CLINICAL FEATURES

Paget's disease of bone (PDB) affects patients older than 50 years of age. Men are more affected than women. *The pelvis, followed by the tibia, is the most commonly involved bone.* Other bones involved are the skull, spine, femur, and clavicle.

Symptoms: PDB is often asymptomatic and diagnosed incidentally with high alkaline phosphatase. Symptomatic ones present with:
- **Bone pain** is the most common symptom.
- There may be an **obvious deformity in the long bones and spine** (Fig. 35.15).
- Patients may also present with **pathologic or stress fractures** due to weak "pagetic bone."
- There may be skull enlargement leading to headaches and a change in hat size **(Fig. 35.15)**.
- Others—**tinnitus and hearing loss.**

Signs
- The **deformity** may be noted in the involved parts, such as *progressive bowing of tibia and femur and kyphosis of the spine.* The neck may be short due to a flat skull and lion face (Leontiasis ossea due to overgrowth of face and cranial bones).
- There may be *features of spinal canal stenosis,* such as back pain with radiation to lower limbs, and neurogenic claudication.

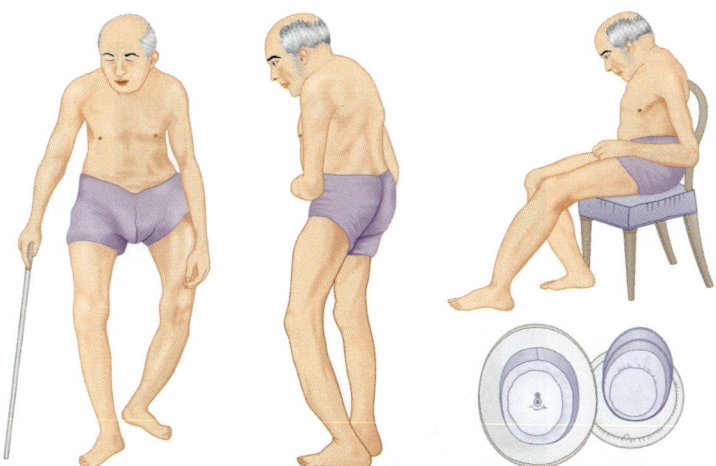

Fig. 35.15: Deformities in spine and leg of a pagetic patient. There may be progressive hat size increase due to enlarging skull.

- There may be *excessive warmth* of a part due to increased vascularity. Further, there may be a *high-output cardiac failure*.
- *Hearing impairment* may occur due to VIII cranial nerve compression resulting from otosclerosis
- Bones may show *secondary osteosarcomatous change, especially flat bones*.

INVESTIGATIONS

- **Plain X-ray**
    - Both increased and decreased density of bone may be seen depending upon the pathologic state of the disease.
    - Pelvis: *Coarse trabeculae and brim sign* (iliopectineal line sclerosis) are noted **(Fig. 35.16)**
    - Long bones: *Bowing and thickening of the femur and tibia* **(Fig. 35.17)**. Loss of distinction between cortex and medulla, blade of grass appearance
    - Skull: *Osteitis circumscripta*—cotton wool exudate in the skull **(Fig. 35.18)**
    - Spine: *Picture frame vertebra* (peripheral sclerosis, central lucency) **(Fig. 35.19)**
    - *Pathologic fractures.*
- **Bone scan:** Intense hot spots in initial lytic and mixed phases, later less intensity.
- **Serum investigations**
    - Serum alkaline phosphatase (ALP): Elevated
    - *Elevated urine markers*: Hydroxyproline, deoxypyridinoline, and C- and N-telopeptide
    - Elevated procollagen I N-terminal peptide
    - *Hyperuricemia*: Due to high collagen/nucleic acid turnover
    - Rarely associated high PTH levels in 10–15% of cases.
- **Bone Biopsy**: It reveals a *mosaic pattern*. However, it is rarely required.

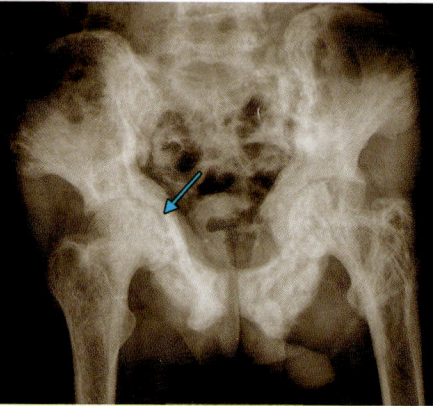

Fig. 35.16: Coarse trabeculae in pelvis and hips in Paget's disease. Brim sign is noted (blue arrow).

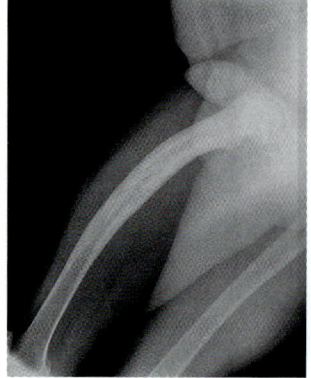

Fig. 35.17: Bowing of femur in Paget's disease.

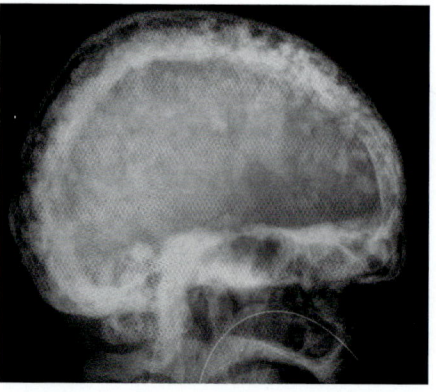

Fig. 35.18: Cotton wool appearance of the skull in Paget's disease.

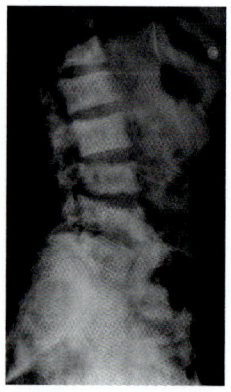

Fig. 35.19: Picture frame vertebra in Paget's disease.

TREATMENT

- **Medical treatment** remains the mainstay of the treatment.
    - Mild pain can be managed with nonsteroidal anti-inflammatory drugs (NSAIDs).
    - **Bisphosphonates** (osteoclast inhibitors) are the *first line of management in patients with Paget's disease*. Various bisphosphonates used are oral (alendronate/risedronate) or intravenous (zoledronic acid/pamidronate) formulations.
    - **Calcitonin** has been found very effective in pain relief due to its osteoclast inhibitor action. It is available as a nasal spray/subcutaneous injection.
    - **Surgical treatment:** Pathological fractures may require internal fixation, while an arthritic joint may require replacement.

COMPLICATIONS

- Pathological fractures
- Nonunion, delayed union
- Degenerative joint disease
- Secondary osteosarcoma.

> **Important**
> Teriparatide or parathormone is *contraindicated in Paget's disease* as it can lead to the development of osteosarcoma.

FLUOROSIS

DEFINITION

Fluorosis is a condition wherein fluorapatite crystals are deposited in the bone due to increased serum fluoride content.

ETIOLOGY

Fluorosis occurs due to the consumption of water contaminated with high fluoride concentrations. The normal concentration of fluoride in water is 1 ppm. *An excess of 2–4 ppm of fluoride in water results in fluorosis*. It is common in certain parts of India, such as Andhra Pradesh, Tamil Nadu and Punjab.

PATHOPHYSIOLOGY

Fluoride is essential for *dental enamel formation and bone mineralization*. Inadequate intake of fluoride results in dental caries, whereas excess fluoride is deposited in bones, teeth, and other soft tissues resulting in various pathologies.

Excess fluoride results in the stimulation of osteoblasts and is deposited in bones along with hydroxyapatite crystals as fluorapatite crystals, which *alters the mechanical performance of the bone*, making it more brittle and sclerotic. It also gets deposited in ligaments and cartilage, affecting the *flexibility of the structures* and mechanical properties of cartilage.

CLINICAL FEATURES

Fluorosis has *dental, musculoskeletal and neurological* manifestations.
- **Dental fluorosis**
    - *Dental mottling* is the first manifestation of fluorosis **(Fig. 35.20)**. Also, there is a loss of shiny appearance.

- **Skeletal fluorosis**
  - *Back pain, joint pain and stiffness* are common symptoms. Muscle weakness and fatigue are also common.
  - *Joint pain and secondary osteoarthritis* (due to effect on joint cartilage).
  - *Increased incidence of pathological fractures* (due to increased brittleness of the bone).
- **Neurological manifestations**
  - Fluorosis of the spine (ligament calcification) results in *spinal canal stenosis*, which can result in neurogenic claudication. *Spastic paraparesis* in extreme cases due to canal stenosis resulting from osteophytes, ossified ligaments, and soft tissues.

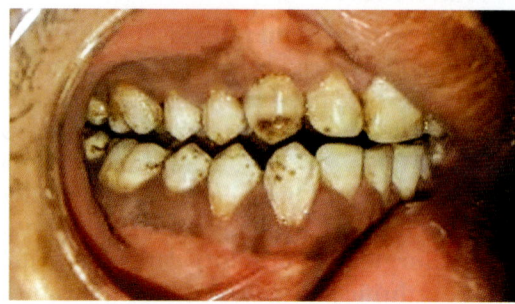

Fig. 35.20: Dental fluorosis showing mottling and loss of shine.
(*Courtesy:* Dr Vatsala, Senior Reader, MCODS, Manipal)

INVESTIGATIONS

- **X-ray**
  - Increased density of bone, especially in spine and pelvis).
  - *Calcification of the interosseous membrane* of the forearm, leg, and obturator membrane is characteristic **(Fig. 35.21)**.
  - *Calcification of ligaments of the spine,* spinal canal stenosis.
- **Estimating fluoride levels in drinking water, blood, and urine** will help clinch the diagnosis.

TREATMENT

- Drinking defluorinated water is a must. Avoid fluoride-rich food such as black tea, fish, wine
- No specific treatment is available for fluorosis. Symptomatic treatment is provided.

Nalgonda technique: Water deflorination technique developed by National Environmental and Engineering Research Institute (NEERI).

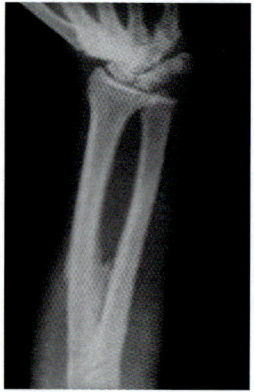

Fig. 35.21: Forearm interosseous membrane calcification.

HYPERPARATHYROIDISM

■ DEFINITION

Hyperparathyroidism is characterized by excess parathormone secretion, either by the parathyroid glands or another focus (malignant tumor like breast, lung), resulting in multi-system manifestation.

■ FUNCTION OF PARATHORMONE (PTH)

The primary action of normal PTH is to ensure optimal serum calcium levels in the body. Parathormone is secreted from parathyroid glands, which act on renal tubules, renal parenchyma, and bone to maintain the serum calcium levels. The important functions of PTH are as follows:
- **On renal tubules:** Calcium resorption, phosphate excretion.
- **On renal parenchyma:** It helps convert 25-DHCC into 1,25-DHCC under the influence of 1-α hydroxylase enzyme.
- **On bone:** It stimulates osteoclastic resorption of bone, and thereby calcium and phosphates are released in the blood.
- **On gut:** It enhances calcium resorption.

Decreased calcium level in the serum stimulates the secretion of parathormone from the parathyroid glands, which act on renal tubules, renal parenchyma, and bones to increase the calcium levels in the body **(Fig. 35.1)**.

■ CLASSIFICATION OF HYPERPARATHYROIDISM

There are three types of hyperparathyroidism: Primary, secondary, and tertiary.
1. **Primary:**
    - It is due to increased PTH secretion from primary parathyroid adenoma.
    - It is common in middle age women (40s–60s)
    - It results in *"osteitis fibrosa cystica".*
2. **Secondary:** Secondary hyperparathyroidism is due to conditions responsible for chronic hypocalcemia, such as vitamin D deficiency, chronic renal failure, which stimulates parathyroid glands to secrete more PTH, resulting in high levels of circulating PTH.
3. **Tertiary:** Due to chronic secondary hyperparathyroidism, the parathyroid glands become hyperplastic and dysregulated, free from negative feedback control (irrespective of calcium levels), and continuously secrete PTH.

■ PATHOPHYSIOLOGY

The principal action of high PTH levels is to stimulate bone osteoclasts, resulting in extensive bone resorption and causing the release of high levels of calcium and phosphate in serum. ***Also, PTH enhances tubular resorption and intestinal resorption of Calcium.*** Increased bony resorption and renal conservation of calcium results in high serum calcium levels, causes increased calcium filtration across renal tubules causes nephrocalcinosis and renal stones. Hyperosteoclastic activity results in extensive bone resorption, subperiosteal erosions, endosteal cavitations and marrow replacement creating large hollows filled by granulation and fibrous tissue ***(Osteitis fibrosa cystica—OFC or Von-Recklinghausen disease of bone)***. Further, extensive bone resorption results in hemorrhage and giant cell reaction within the fibrous stroma, giving rise to a brownish, liquified tumor-like mass known as *"Brown tumor"*. The OFCs or brown tumors are common in the mandible, maxilla, ribs, clavicle, spine, and pelvis. They are expansile lesions that can rarely have compressive features. Further, the lytic bone is prone to pathologic fracture. **Figure 35.22** outlines the pathophysiology of hyperparathyroidism.

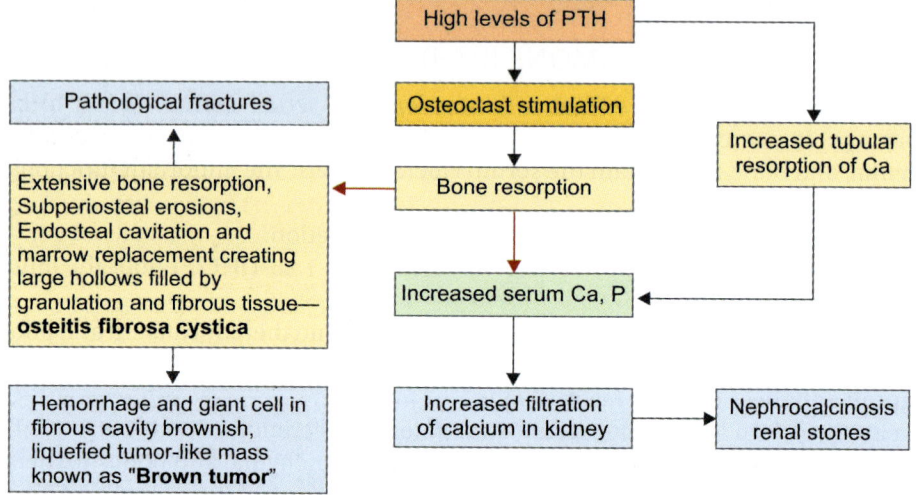

Fig. 35.22: Pathophysiology of hyperparathyroidism.

CLINICAL FEATURES

The clinical features of hyperparathyroidism depend upon the type, primary, secondary or tertiary.
- The **primary hyperparathyroidism** is characterized by *"bones-stones-groans and psychic moans."*
    - *Bones:* Bone pain, pathological #
    - *Stone*: Renal stones
    - *Abdominal groans*: Constipation
    - *Psychic moans:* Often may present with psychiatric symptoms.
    - Weakness and malaise, features of proximal myopathy.
- The clinical features of **secondary hyperparathyroidism** depend upon the underlying cause, such as vitamin D deficiency. There can be *tetany* due to hypocalcemia.

INVESTIGATIONS

- **Blood test:** *In primary hyperparathyroidism,* both serum PTH and calcium levels are raised, while phosphate levels are low. In secondary hyperparathyroidism, the PTH and ALP levels are high, while calcium and phosphates are low.
- **USG and sestamibi scan for parathyroid adenoma assessment**
- **X-ray of bones:**
    - Generalized osteopenia, *osteitis fibrosa cystica, brown tumor* (**Fig. 35.23A**), and pathological fracture.

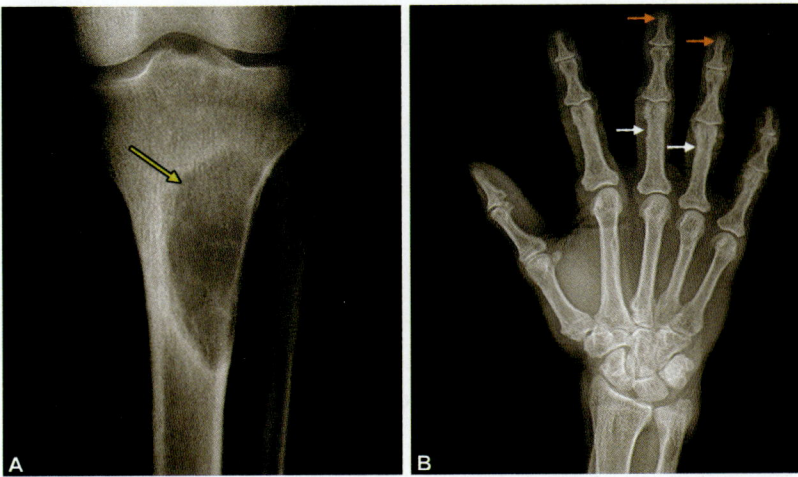

Figs. 35.23A and B: (A) Brown tumor in proximal tibia (yellow arrow); (B) Subperiosteal resportion of radial side of middle phalanx (white arrows) and terminal phalanx bone resorption (orange arrows).

- X-ray of hand in hyperparathyroidism: Subperiosteal resorption of the radial side of the middle phalanx is characteristic of hyperparathyroidism. Bony erosion of the terminal phalanx (acrosteolysis) is also seen **(Fig. 35.23B)**
- *Salt and pepper appearance of the skull*
- *Loss of lamina dura* of the teeth
- *Rugger jersey spine:* It is seen in renal osteodystrophy (also in osteopetrosis), wherein there are alternate bands of osteosclerosis and osteolysis in the vertebra.
- **Urine analysis:** Hypercalciuria.

TREATMENT

- **Primary hyperparathyroidism:** Proper hydration, symptomatic treatment for constipation, and treatment of renal stones. The calcium intake must be decreased in primary hyperparathyroidism. Further, surgical removal of parathyroid adenoma is required in primary hyperparathyroidism. Post-adenoma excision, *watch for Hungry bone syndrome* **(Box 35.8)**.
- **Secondary hyperparathyroidism:** It must be treated with the treatment of the underlying cause. Supplementations of calcium and vitamin D are required.

Box 35.8: Hungry bone syndrome.

Hungry bones syndrome is seen in patients of primary hyperparathyroidism who undergo parathyroid adenoma excision. After the parathyroid adenoma excision, the PTH levels drastically reduce, resulting in hypocalcemia, hypomagnesemia, and hypophosphatemia. It occurs due to sudden influx of calcium into the bone from the blood due to drop in PTH levels, as high level of PTH was responsible for mobilization of calcium from the bone. This is a dangerous condition as it can lead to severe tetany, an other metabolic malfunction. It must be treated with high dose of calcium, magnesium, supplemented with active vitamin D.

SCURVY

■ DEFINITION

Scurvy is characterized by skeletal manifestations due to vitamin C deficiency.

■ ETIOLOGY

Vitamin C deficiency is seen in:
- Children older than 6–12 months
- Elderly greater than 60 years.

■ RISK FACTORS

- Children fed with condensed milk, elderly on bread diet
- Chronic alcoholics
- Malabsorption syndromes
- Smokers
- Overcooked food.

■ PATHOPHYSIOLOGY

Vitamin C is required for the synthesis of collagen. And therefore, vitamin C deficiency leads to the poor synthesis of collagen and chondroitin sulfate. *A defective collagen results in a fragile basement membrane of capillaries leading to bleeding tendency and defective bone. Since type 1 collagen is required at the metaphysis of growing bone, the bone formation at metaphysis and spongiosa is also affected.* Furthermore, carnitine production is also affected.

■ CLINICAL FEATURES

Since breast milk is rich in vitamin C, breast milk fed infants are usually spared from vitamin C deficiency. The clinical features of scurvy are osseous and non-osseous.

General Features

Lethargy, malaise, anemia.

Osseous Features

Scurvy affects areas of rapid growth: Wrist, knees and sternal end of ribs
- Exquisite multiple *painful bony swelling* over the metaphyseal area of the long bone (due to subperiosteal hemorrhage) may result in pseudoparalysis. Pathologic fractures are also reported.
- *Scorbutic rosary:* Painful step-off deformity at the costochondral junction due to costochondral separation. *(cf. Scorbutic rosary, the Rachitic rosary is rounded and nodular and painless).*
- *Joint effusion* (hemarthrosis)
- *Myalgia* may be present due to reduced carnitine production.

Nonosseous Features

Bleeding gum, hematuria, hematemesis, loss of teeth, mucocutaneous petechiae, ecchymosis, and hyperkeratosis.

INVESTIGATIONS

- **X-ray of the wrist, knee (Fig. 35.24)**
    - *White line of Frankel:* Widened zone of provisional calcification between epi- and metaphysis
    - *Trummerfeld zone:* Transverse radiolucent adjacent to Frankel line (scurvy line)
    - *Wimberger ring:* Ring of increased density around epiphysis
    - *Pelkin spur:* Metaphyseal spur
    - *Subperiosteal elevation and periosteal reaction*
    - *Pencil thin cortex*
    - *Ground glass osteopenia*
    - Fractures and epiphyseal separation.
- **Serum ascorbic acid:** Low.

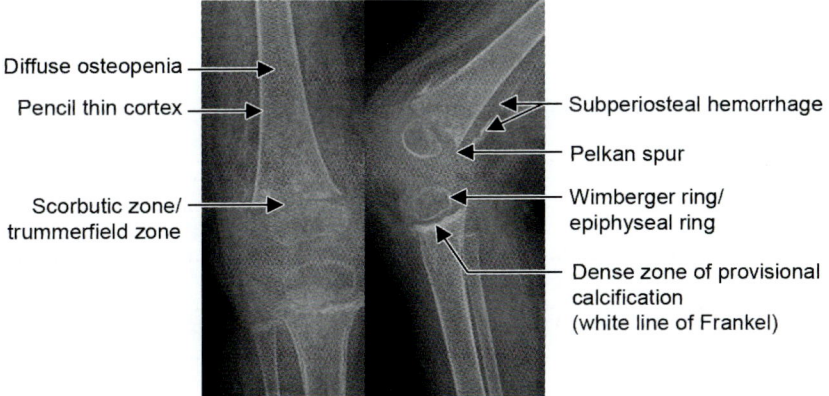

Fig. 35.24: X-ray of a scorbutic knee with characteristic features.

TREATMENT

Oral vitamin C supplementation. 100–250 mg vitamin C four times a day for few days.

SECTION 8

Neuromuscular Disorders

SECTION OUTLINE

36. Neuromuscular Disorders
    - Poliomyelitis
    - Duchenne Muscular Dystrophy

CHAPTER 36

Neuromuscular Disorders

POLIOMYELITIS

DEFINITION

It is an *enterovirus infection* caused by poliovirus types 1-3 (picornaviridae family), which affects the anterior horn cell (AHC) in the spinal cord.
- About 90% of the polio infections are asymptomatic
- Vast majority affected are children less than 3 years
- Mostly affects nonimmunized children.

ETIOPATHOGENESIS

- Poliovirus is an *enterovirus and RNA type of virus*.
- It has three serotypes, 1-3. Type 1 is most commonly implicated in polio infection.
- *Fecal-oral route* is the common route of infection.
- Poliovirus enters gastrointestinal tract (GIT), and multiplies in tonsils, lymph nodes of neck and Peyer's patches of intestine. Its incubation period may vary from 2-21 days.

Risk factors
- Lack of vaccination
- Poor sanitation
- Endemic area

During this period, patient may remain asymptomatic or may have features of self-limiting mild gastroenteritis or respiratory tract infection. The viremia may subside or it may enter the central nervous system where virus attacks anterior horn cells in the spinal cord or rarely brainstem. AHC affection results in muscle palsy whereas brainstem affection causes respiratory palsy. The brief pathogenesis is described in **Flowchart 36.1**.

CLINICAL FEATURES

More than 95% patients affected by the Poliovirus remain asymptomatic. About 3-4% may have abortive poliomyelitis wherein patients suffer from mild self-limiting gastroenteritis or influenza like symptoms, which subsides within one week. Few may have aseptic meningitis. Less than 1% suffer from most clinical poliomyelitis. There are three stages of poliomyelitis:
1. **Stage 1:** Acute poliomyelitis—may last for 1-2 weeks
2. **Stage 2:** Recovery stage—may last for 3 months to 2 years
3. **Stage 3:** Postpolio residual palsy (PPRP) is seen after 2 years of disease onset

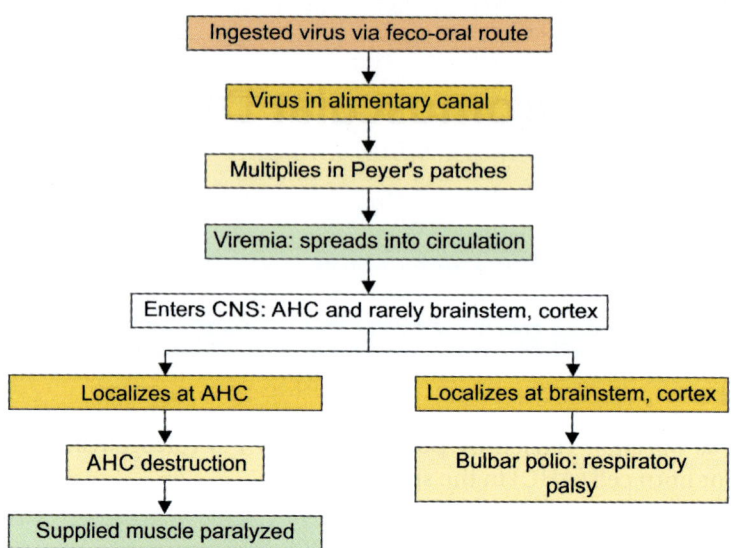

Flowchart 36.1: Pathogenesis of poliomyelitis.

(AHC: anterior horn cell; CNS: central nervous system)

Acute Poliomyelitis Stage
- Fever, malaise, and GIT prodrome
- Neck stiffness, irritability, nausea, vomiting (features of meningitis)
- Acute flaccid asymmetric motor palsy with **no sensory loss**
- Tender muscles
- Bladder bowel normal
- Respiratory muscle palsy (rare)
- In bulbar poliomyelitis, the cranial nerves are also affected. Nasal intonation and respiratory obstruction may occur. In severe cases, bulbar palsy may result in death due to respiratory palsy.

Differential diagnosis
- Guillain–Barré syndrome
- Traumatic neuritis
- Postdiphtheria palsy

Recovery Stage
It may last from 3 months to 2 years
- No tenderness
- Paralyzed muscle start recovering.

Residual Palsy Stage
After 2 years of onset of disease
- No return of power
- Deformities
- Disuse atrophy
- Limb shortening.

- Muscle most commonly affected: *Quadriceps*
- Complete palsy in foot: *Tibialis anterior*
- Complete palsy in hand: *Opponens pollicis*

INVESTIGATIONS

It is mandatory to notify local health authorities about a suspected case of acute flaccid palsy or polio.

- Virus can be detected by *PCR or culture from stool*, pharynx, or cerebrospinal fluid (CSF). The patient keeps excreting virus intermittently for 2 months. The load is quite high in 1st two weeks of infection.
- *Magnetic resonance imaging (MRI) of the spine:* It is not routinely performed. However, it may reveal anterior horn changes.
- *Poliovirus antibodies* are present in serum.

TREATMENT

- **Acute stage*:*
  - *Supportive care:*
    - Intravenous (IV) fluids
    - Antipyretics
    - Ventilatory support if bulbar poliomyelitis resulting in respiratory paralysis.
  - *Splint the affected limb to:*
    - Decrease pain and spasm
    - Prevent deformity
- **Stage of recovery:** The aim in this stage is to—
  - Assist recovery of paralyzed muscles by extensive physiotherapy
  - Prevent deformities by the use of orthotic devices
- **Residual palsy:** *No further recovery is possible* in muscle power
  - Make use of available muscle power
  - Make limb as functional as possible with help of *orthosis and surgery*
  - *Rehabilitation*: Educational and vocational

The role of surgery in poliomyelitis is explained in **Box 36.1**.

Mainstay of treatment in recovery stage is "physiotherapy"
- Passive mobilization of joints affected
- Active physiotherapy
- Hydrotherapy

Box 36.1: Role of surgery in poliomyelitis.
- Correct established deformities
- *Improve muscle balance*: Tendon transfer
- *Joint stabilization*: Arthrodesis
- Spinal fusion and instrumentation for spinal deformities
- Corrective osteotomies
- Limb lengthening

MYOPATHIES

DEFINITION

Disease of muscle unrelated to neuromuscular junction or nerves.

ETIOLOGY

- **Congenital:** Duchenne, facioscapulohumeral
- **Metabolic:** Periodic hyper- or hypokalemic paralysis, hypo- or hypercalcemia

- **Drug induced:** Steroids, lipid lowering agents, and retroviral therapy
- **Toxic:** Alcoholic
- **Inflammatory:** Dermatomyositis, polymyositis, systemic lupus erythematosus (SLE), and rheumatoid arthritis (RA)
- **Endocrinal:** Addison's, hypo/hyperthyroidism
- **Infectious:** HIV and cysticercosis.

COMMON CLINICAL FEATURES

- Bilateral symmetric proximal weakness
- Malaise and fatigue.

DUCHENNE MUSCULAR DYSTROPHY

Duchenne muscular dystrophy (DMD) is a *X-linked recessive* congenital muscular dystrophy characterized by early onset progressive muscle wasting, scoliosis and cardiomyopathy.

It is more common in males.

- **Genetics:** It is a *X-linked recessive disorder (Xp21)* with *dystrophin gene mutation*.
- **Pathophysiology:** The absence of dystrophin results in lack of muscle fiber regeneration followed by replacement with fibro-fatty tissue.
- **Clinical features:**
  - The age of onset is 2–6 years
  - It is characterized by *Proximal muscle weakness* (difficulty in lifting arms up) or getting up from a squatting position, difficulty in climbing stairs, hopping and jumping
- **Examination reveals:**
  - *Calf pseudohypertrophy*
  - *Gower's sign:* The patient climbs on himself when made to get up from a sitting position **(Fig. 36.1)**.
  - *Scoliosis*
  - Gait abnormality: Trendelenburg gait
  - Cardiomyopathy
- **Investigations:**
  - Elevated creatine phosphokinase (CPK) enzyme level
  - Muscle biopsy reveals absent dystrophin
  - Electromyography (EMG) shows myopathic pattern
- **Treatment:** Oral steroids, pulmonary and cardiac care, contracture releases, and rehabilitation
- **Prognosis:** Most are unable to ambulate independently by the age of 10, wheelchair bound by 15, and die due to cardiorespiratory problems by the age of 20.

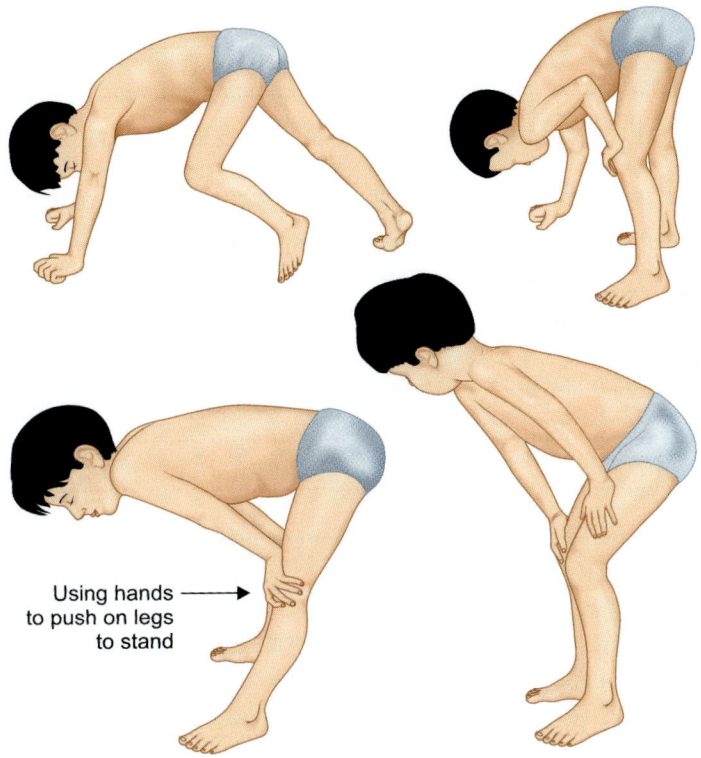

Fig. 36.1: Gower's sign.

SECTION 9

Cerebral Palsy

SECTION OUTLINE

37. Cerebral Palsy

CHAPTER 37

Cerebral Palsy

DEFINITION

Cerebral palsy (CP) is a **nonprogressive, upper motor neuron disease** primarily affecting motor function and muscle coordination caused by damage to the **"developing immature brain"** before, during, or just after birth within two years.

ETIOLOGY/RISK FACTORS

- **Antenatal:** Prematurity, maternal infections [toxoplasmosis, others (syphilis, hepatitis B), rubella, cytomegalovirus, herpes simplex (TORCH)], multiple gestations, and pregnancy complications in the mother (eclampsia)
- **Perinatal:** Birth anoxia/asphyxia, birth trauma
- **Early neonatal:** Encephalitis, meningitis, and kernicterus.

PATHOGENESIS

Most of the etiological factors causing cerebral palsy affect the *periventricular motor fibers of the cerebral cortex and its myelination resulting in "periventricular leukomalacia."* The periventricular area carries the motor fibers to the muscle and controls the tone. Hence, most clinical effects of cerebral palsy are motor in nature **(Flowchart 37.1)**.

Flowchart 37.1: Pathogenesis of cerebral palsy.

```
  Prematurity     Birth trauma    Maternal infection,    Other causes
                                       TORCH
        │              │                │                    │
        └──────────────┴────────┬───────┴────────────────────┘
                                ▼
   • Intraventricular hemorrhage
   • Severe compromise in O₂/cerebral perfusion
   • Altered biochemical parameters (cytokines, reactive O₂ species, excitotoxicity)
                                │
                                ▼
   Periventricular motor fibers are damaged and their myelination by oligodendrocytes is affected
                                │
                                ▼
                   Periventricular leukomalacia
                                │
                                ▼
                        Cerebral palsy
```

[TORCH: toxoplasmosis, others (syphilis, hepatitis B), rubella, cytomegalovirus, herpes simplex]

RELEVANT PATHOANATOMY: STRUCTURES/AREAS AFFECTED

- **Primary effect:** The primary effect is on the brain (static encephalopathy), leading to manifestation in the musculoskeletal system and other functions.
  - *Musculoskeletal effects*
    - Abnormal tone (spasticity/hypotonia)
    - Abnormal balance
    - Loss of motor control
    - Loss of coordination.
  - *Others*
    - Mental retardation
    - Epilepsy
    - Hearing and speech disturbance
    - Behavioral disorders.
- **Secondary effects on the musculoskeletal system**
  - Growth disturbance
  - Dislocations
  - Contractures
  - Gait disturbances
  - Deformities in the foot, ankle, knee, hip, hand, and spine.

CLASSIFICATION OF CEREBRAL PALSY

- **Neurological types**
  1. *Spastic:* It occurs due to cerebral cortex damage and corticospinal tract involvement.
  2. *Athetoid:* It occurs due to basal ganglia damage.
  3. *Ataxic:* It occurs due to cerebellum damage.
  4. *Atonic* or *hypotonic*
  5. *Mixed.*
- **Motor anatomical types (Fig. 37.1)**
  1. *Monoplegia*: Any one limb is involved.
  2. *Hemiplegia:* One half of the body is involved.

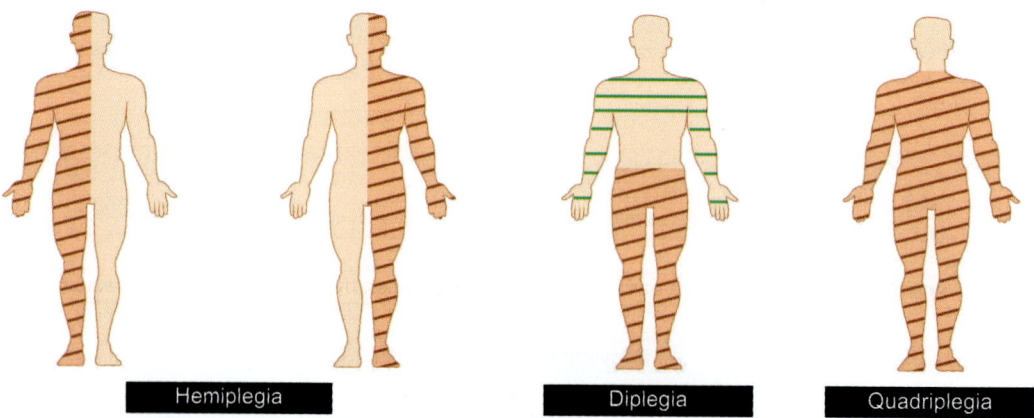

Fig. 37.1: Various types of motor anatomical cerebral palsy. Light green hash in diplegia suggests lesser involvement of upper limb compared to lower limb.

3. *Double hemiplegia:* Upper limbs more involved than lower limb
4. *Diplegia:* Lower limbs more involved than upper limb
5. *Quadriplegia:* All four limbs are involved
6. *Athetoid/extrapyramidal type.*

CLINICAL FEATURES

The clinical feature depends upon the type of CP. Most kids have gait abnormality and delayed developmental milestones.

- **Spastic CP:** It is the most common type of CP (70%). It is classified as per limb involved. Common features are:
  - *Spasticity* and brisk reflexes
  - *Scissoring gait* **(Fig. 37.2)**
  - *Spastic diplegia/hemiplegia/quadriplegia*
  - *Pseudobulbar palsy:* It is due to bilateral corticobulbar tract lesion causing dysarthria, dysphagia, tongue and facial weakness and emotional lability.
  - *Persistent neonatal reflexes*
  - *Opisthotonus:* It is an abnormal rigid position of the body wherein the person holds their body in an arched position with only an extended head and heel touching the couch, while rest of the back is above the couch.
  - *Mental retardation and speech and hearing disturbance*
  - Various *deformities and contractures* in the lower and upper limbs are observed such as:
    - **Hip:** Flexion, adduction, internal rotation; hip dislocation/subluxation
    - **Knee:** Flexor/extensor spasticity
    - **Ankle:** Equinus
    - **Foot:** Pes valgus
    - **Shoulder:** Adduction and internal rotation contracture
    - **Elbow:** Flexion contracture, pronated forearm
    - **Wrist:** Palmar flexed, finger flexed at metacarpophalangeal joint
    - **Spine:** Scoliosis.
- **Atonic CP:** Hypotonia
- **Athetoid CP:** It is characterized by involuntary movements of hands and legs such as:
  - Athetosis
  - Chorea
  - Dystonia
  - Tremor.
- **Ataxic CP:** Ataxic gait
- **Mixed CP:** Combination of spastic, athetoid, and ataxic types.

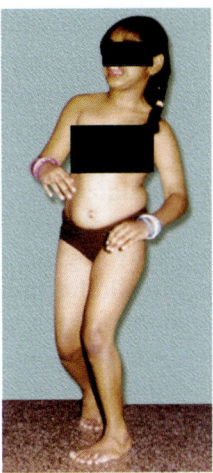

Fig. 37.2: A patient with spastic CP.

INVESTIGATIONS

The diagnosis is primarily based upon history and clinical examination.
- **Brain MRI:** *Periventricular leukomalacia (56%) is the most common finding,* followed by white or gray matter lesions.

- Hearing and vision test
- Genetic screening is required if there is evidence of a genetic disorder.

TREATMENT

It is important to understand the priorities in managing a CP child. The priorities in the management of CP are **CSDTW** (**C**ommunicate, **S**it, **D**ress, **T**oileting, and **W**alk in the order of preference).
- Ability to ***communicate***
- Ability to ***sit***
- Ability to ***dress and toileting***
- Ability to ***walk***.

Children with CP require ***a multidisciplinary approach*** with professionals from various specialties. The role of the different specialists is mentioned below:
- **Orthopaedician:** For various preventive and corrective measures for deformities and contractures of bones and joints.
- **Pediatrician:** Monitor growth
- **Psychologist**
- **Neurologist**
- **Physiotherapist (PT):** To assist with the development of neuromuscular control, prevent contractures, gait training, and minimize spasticity
- **Occupational therapist (OT):** Assist in implementing the use of assistive devices like ankle-foot orthosis (AFO), wheelchairs, and walkers
- **Speech and hearing specialist**
- **Nutritionist:** For a balanced nutritious diet
- **Social worker**.

Treatment Options and Modalities for Musculoskeletal Pathologies
- **Occupational therapy (OT)/physical therapy (PT)/speech therapy**
- Various **orthosis and adaptive equipment:** AFO, splinting, casts, braces, walkers, and wheelchair
- **Various therapeutic measures** are applied to reduce spasticity, such as:
    - *Injection therapy:*
        - **Botulinum toxin/Ethyl alcohol** is injected into spastic muscle belly, which helps reduce spasticity to facilitate OT, PT, and further casting or bracing to improve the deformity. Note that these injections are avoided in upper limb due to proximity of neurovascular bundle to the muscle bellies.
    - *Pharmacologic therapy:* Baclofen, diazepam, clonazepam are used to reduce muscle spasm.
- **Orthopaedic surgery:** The goal is to prevent or minimize deformity and surgically correct pathological causes to maximize mobility and function.

    Single event multilevel surgery (SEML) is recommended to minimize total recovery time rather than yearly birthday surgery (i.e., a yearly procedure). The various procedures which could be performed are:
    - *Tendon transfer:* Distal rectus transfer for stiff knee gait
    - *Neurectomy:* Obturator neurectomy to improve adductor spasm

- *Contracture release, tendon lengthening.* Note that tendoachilles lengthening is contraindicated in equinus contracture of ankle. However, gastrocsoleus aponeurotic lengthening is performed, whenever indicated.
- *Corrective osteotomies:* Distal femoral extension osteotomy for crouch gait
- *Joint stabilization*: Correction of hip dislocation, triple arthrodesis of the foot.
- **Neurosurgical options:** Selective posterior rhizotomy.

COMPLICATIONS OF CEREBRAL PALSY
- Feeding difficulty
- Drooling
- Hearing impairment
- Behavioral problems
- Growth impairment
- Aspiration
- Epilepsy
- Osteoporosis
- Visual impairment
- Incontinence.

SECTION 10

Bone Tumors

SECTION OUTLINE

38. Basics of Bone Tumors
39. Benign Bone Tumors and Tumor-like Lesions
40. Malignant Bone Tumors

CHAPTER 38

Basics of Bone Tumors

■ INTRODUCTION
- Malignant bone tumors are less than 1% of all malignancies of the body.
- They occur in all age groups.
- Bone tumors are true tumors (benign and malignant) and tumor-like lesions.

■ TYPES OF BONE TUMORS
Flowchart 38.1 shows types of bone tumors.

■ CLASSIFICATION OF BONE TUMORS
Bone tumors can be classified in several ways.
- **The World Health Organization (WHO) classification:** It is the most commonly used classification of bone tumors, which is based on the *cell of origin* of the bone tumor **(Table 38.1)**.
- **Based upon type:** Benign or malignant.

Apart from the classification according to the cell lines, it is essential to understand the occurrence of various tumors in *different age groups* **(Table 38.2)** and *locations* (epiphyseal/metaphyseal/diaphyseal) in a long bone **(Fig. 38.1)**, which helps in the differential diagnosis.

Occurrence of various bone tumors in different parts of the body (skeleton) is shown in **Figure 38.2**.

■ CLINICAL FEATURES AND INVESTIGATIONS OF A BONE TUMOR
The diagnosis of a bone tumor depends upon a thorough history and examination. **Table 38.3** helps in differentiating between benign and malignant tumors.

Flowchart 38.1: Types of bone tumors.

```
                        Bone tumors
                       /           \
              True bone tumors    Tumor-like lesions
              /        \                |
          Benign     Malignant      • Bone cyst
         • Latent    /      \       • Fibrous dysplasia
         • Active  Primary Secondary • Eosinophilic granuloma
         • Aggressive                • Brown tumor
```

Table 38.1: World Health Organization classification of bone tumor.

Cell type	Benign	Malignant
Osteoblast (Bone-forming cell)	• Osteoblastoma • Osteoid osteoma • Osteoma	Osteosarcoma
Chondroblast (Cartilage-forming cell)	• Chondroblastoma • Enchondroma • Osteochondroma	Chondrosarcoma
Osteoclast-like cells/unknown cells	Giant cell tumor	Adamantinoma
Vascular cells	Hemangioma	Hemagiosarcoma
Marrow cells		Multiple myeloma
Fibrous	• Fibroma • Nonossifying fibroma	Fibrosarcoma
Lipid cell	Lipoma	Liposarcoma
Nerve cell	Schwannoma, neurofibroma	Malignant peripheral nerve sheath tumor (MPNST)

Table 38.2: Differentials of bone tumor based upon age.

Age group	Benign	Malignant
5–20 years	Chondroblastoma and osteoid osteoma	Ewing's sarcoma, osteosarcoma
10–30 years	Osteochondroma and chondromyxoid fibroma	Osteosarcoma
20–45 years	Giant cell tumor	Chondrosarcoma (20–60)
20–60 years	Benign fibrous histiocytoma	Malignant fibrous histiocytoma (currently known as pleomorphic sarcoma)
30–80 years	Hemangioma, osteoma, lipoma	Chordoma

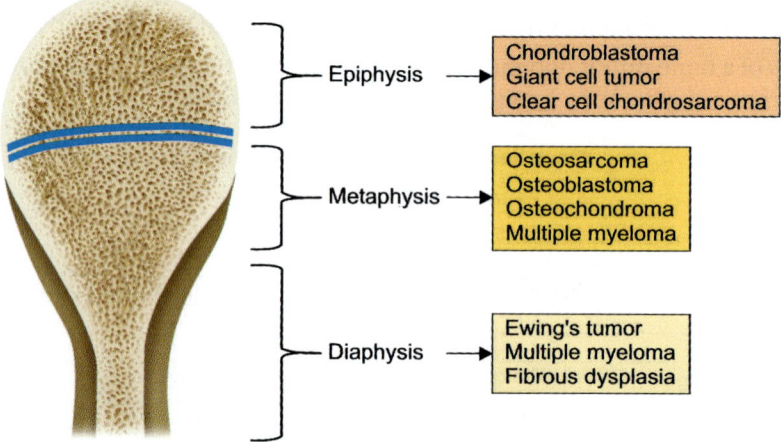

Fig. 38.1: Occurrence of specific tumors in a various part of a long bone.

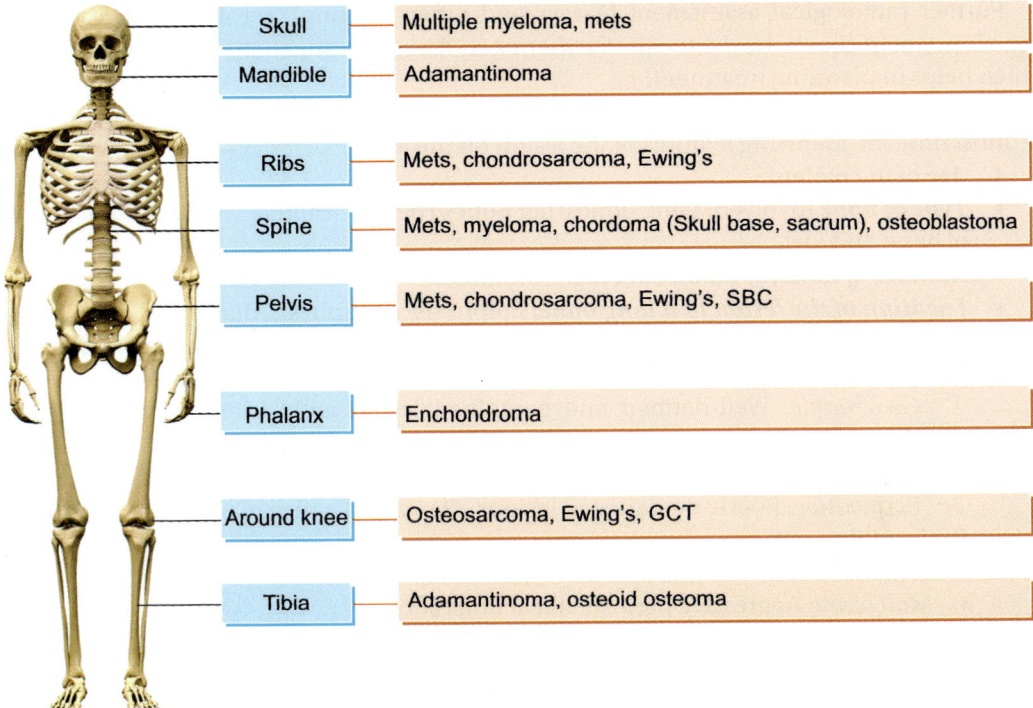

Fig. 38.2: Occurrence of various bone tumors in different parts of the skeleton.
(mets: metastasis; GCT: giant cell tumor; SBC: simple bone cyst)

Table 38.3: Differences between benign and malignant bone tumors.		
Characteristics	**Benign**	**Malignant**
Growth	Slow, may stop at maturity	Rapid
Duration	Long	Short
Pain and swelling appearance	Swelling followed by pain	Pain followed by swelling
Pain character	Localized, subsides with rest	Constant, present even on rest and at night
Systemic features (weight and appetite loss, fever)	Rare	Weight loss and loss of appetite are common in large tumors/with systemic involvement. However, it is not a routine finding
Spread	Commonly, local only	Infiltrative in adjacent bone/tissue
Swelling surface	Smooth	Irregular
Local temperature	Normal/raised	Raised
Consistency	<ul><li>Firm/hard</li><li>Sometimes, tumors like GCT can have variable consistency</li></ul>	Variable
Metastasis	<ul><li>Not common. However, GCT can rarely metastasize!</li></ul>	Yes
Radiograph	<ul><li>Limited "geographic growth"</li><li>Well-defined margins</li></ul>	<ul><li>"Moth eaten" or "permeative" appearance</li><li>Ill-defined margins</li></ul>

Further radiological assessment (X-rays and other imaging), serological investigations, and biopsy help clinch the diagnosis. Furthermore, these investigations help stage the tumor, which helps in planning treatment.

- **Plain radiograph assessment** is vital in establishing a primary working diagnosis. One must note the following features of the lesion on the X-ray.
    - *Age* of the patient.
    - *Type of bone* involved: Long bones/flat bones (pelvis, scapula, vertebrae)/small bones of hand and feet.
    - *Number of bone(s) involved:* Single/multiple.
    - *Location of the lesion in a long bone*: Epiphysis/metaphysis/diaphysis.
    - *Location of the lesion in a vertebra:* Anterior element (body)/posterior element.
    - *Margins of lesion*: **Lodwick classified tumor margins into three types**—
        1. *Geographic:* Well-defined and contained lesion with sclerotic margin (benign lesions)
        2. *Moth-eaten:* Multiple scattered 2–5 mm lytic lesions (Ewing's)
        3. *Permeative:* Poorly demarcated lesions <2 mm indicative of high-grade tumor.
    - *Periosteal reaction*:
        - *Benign*: Absent/solid buttressing type
        - *Malignant*: Aggressive periosteal reactions such as:
            - *Ewing's*: Interrupted onion peel appearance
            - *Osteosarcoma*: Sunburst appearance and Codman's triangle.
    - *Tumor matrix:*
        - *Calcification*
            - Benign tumors, such as chondroblastoma can show punctate calcification
            - Rings and arcs, popcorn calcification is seen in small lesions such as enchondroma and large malignant lesions such as chondrosarcoma
        - *Osseous (bony) matrix:* Seen in bony forming tumors such as osteoblastoma (benign) and osteosarcoma (malignant)
        - *Ground glass (fibrous matrix/woven bone):* It is typically seen in fibrous dysplasia of the bone.
    - *Specific findings (if any):*
        - *Soap bubble appearance*: Giant cell tumor
        - *Fallen leaf sign*: Simple bone cyst
        - *Finger in balloon sign*: Aneurysmal bone cyst
        - *Shephard crook deformity* (in the proximal femur): Fibrous dysplasia
        - *Punched out lesion*: Multiple myeloma
        - *Onion peel appearance*: Ewing's sarcoma.
- **Further imaging** is performed to detect the soft tissue invasion, proximity/involvement of the neurovascular bundle, and metastasis with the help of MRI, CT, Bone, and/PET scan.
    - *MRI scan*: Soft tissue invasion, bone marrow involvement as a skip lesion, proximity to the neurovascular bundle

Mirel's score

Mirel score predicts the risk of pathological fracture in a long bone due to the metastatic lesion. It is based on clinical and radiological criteria mentioned in **Table 38.4**. If the Mirel score ≥8, the possibility of pathologic fracture is increased. If the diagnosis of tumor is already established, the prophylactic fixation can be performed.

Table 38.4: Mirel's score criteria.

Score	Site of lesion	Ratio of the lesion to the diameter of bone	Nature of lesion	Pain
1	Upper limb	<1/3rd of the cortex	Blastic	Mild
2	Lower limb	1/3–2/3 of the cortex	Mixed	Moderate
3	Peritrochanteric	>2/3rd of the cortex	Lytic	Severe

- *CT scan:* For better bone delineation, matrix calcification
- *Bone scan:* It is performed to detect skeletal metastasis using Technetium-99m (99mTc) radioisotope. It is useful only in bony metastasis and not soft tissue. The Tc-99 isotope is taken up by the bony areas with increased new bone formation/high bone turnover. Therefore, its uptake is higher in tumors, trauma, and infection.
- *PET scan:* PET scan is performed using fluorodeoxyglucose (F18–FDG). Its uptake is higher in areas with a higher cellular metabolism (bony and soft tissue both). It can be combined with CT or MRI (PET-CT/PET-MRI). PET scan has the following advantages over bone scan:
  - It helps the select area of the appropriate biopsy
  - Helps staging malignancies
  - It helps in monitoring the effect of therapy (chemo/radio)
  - It helps detect recurrences
  - It may help differentiate between benign and malignant lesions.
- *Plain CT scan of the chest:* To detect metastasis in lung parenchyma.
- **Serological investigation:**
  - *Increased alkaline phosphatase (ALP):* Osteosarcoma, Ewing's sarcoma
  - *Increased prostate-specific agent:* Prostate metastasis
  - *Increased serum LDH:* Ewing's sarcoma, lymphoma, leukemia
  - *Presence of M-band on serum protein electrophoresis:* In multiple myeloma
  - Low Hb and elevated ESR in multiple myeloma.
- **Genetic analysis:** t(11:22) translocation in Ewing's sarcoma
- **Biopsy:** The gold standard for establishing the tumor diagnosis is by the "biopsy" of the lesion. The biopsy can be performed on the primary bone tumor/metastasis in several ways:
  - Core biopsy using Jamshidi (J) needle: *Currently preferred method*
  - Incisional biopsy using a small planned incision over the tumor
  - Excisional biopsy.

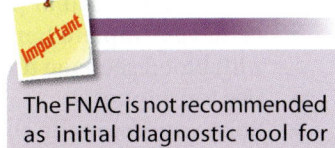

The FNAC is not recommended as initial diagnostic tool for bone sarcomas.

1. **Core biopsy (TRU cut):** Currently, it is the *most preferred method of biopsy in bone tumors* as it is a safe and reliable method to establish the diagnosis of bone tumors.

   It is performed through a small stab using a Jamshidi needle and taking multiple cores from the representative part of the tumor. There is minimal soft tissue trauma with less contamination of normal tissue by the tumor cells around the tract of the needle, which is easily excisable during limb salvage surgery. It is less invasive, easier for deeper areas such as the spine and pelvis, cheaper, and can be performed under local anesthesia.

2. ***Incisional biopsy:***
   - Carefully planned incision over tumor to take a piece of tissue from the margin of the tumor without spillage. The biopsy scar must be excised during the definitive tumor surgery to prevent a recurrence.
   - *Currently, it is no longer favored as similar results are obtained with a core needle biopsy.*
3. ***Excisional biopsy:*** It is planned for small/completely excisable benign tumors smaller than 5 cm, which are entirely excised and submitted for biopsy.

While performing the biopsy, there are certain principles to be followed.

Principles of biopsy: One must follow certain principles while performing the biopsy:
- Perform all investigations, especially MRI, before the biopsy to avoid artefacts in imaging post biopsy.
- *Most importantly, the biopsy must be performed by the surgeon who will eventually perform the definitive surgery as a poorly planned biopsy incision, and the technique would jeopardize the limb salvage procedure.* An improperly performed biopsy can compromise future limb salvage.
- If using a tourniquet, do not exsanguinate the limb.
- To get representative tissue, take the sample from the periphery, not the central necrotic area, especially in bone sarcomas.
- Select shortest route to the tumor
- To violate only single compartment and not multiple compartment
- Through a muscle rather than intermuscular plan (to contain any hematoma from tumor and hence reduce contamination/seeding of tumor cells)
- Pressure at biopsy entry point after biopsy to achieve hemostasis
- If a bony tumor with large soft tissue component is present, sampling from soft tissue is sufficient as it is representative.

In the case of open biopsy,
- Do not place transverse incisions over the limb.
- One single deep incision must be given, reaching up to the lesion without creating side flaps to avoid sideways tumor contamination.
- Avoid intermuscular planes and stay away from the neurovascular bundle.
- Achieve complete hemostasis before wound closure to avoid contamination of tissues with blood seepage under tissue planes.
- Use tourniquet
- Bony window made should be circular to avoid stress risers and pathologic fractures
- Drain if used, to be placed along the line of incision rather than parallel to it (reduces skin loss which biopsy track is being excised during limb salvage)

The histopathology characteristics of various tumors are listed in **Table 38.5**.

After complete clinical and radiological evaluation, and biopsy findings, the tumor is staged, which is essential for management. **Enneking** developed the tumor staging, both benign and malignant.

- **Staging of the bone tumor:**
   - The benign lesion is staged using Arabic numerals (1, 2, 3) **(Table 38.6)**. It is based on the stage, capsular involvement, and radiological appearance.
   - The malignant lesion is staged using the Roman numerals (I, II, III) **(Table 38.7)**. It is based on the histological grade, involved site (compartments), and metastasis.

Table 38.5: Characteristic biopsy findings of the common tumors.

Tumor	Characteristic histopathological feature
Giant cell tumor	Numerous *Mononuclear stromal cells and osteoclast-type giant cells*
Fibrous dysplasia	Irregular, curvilinear bony trabeculae **(Chinese letter pattern)**, lack of osteoblast rimming, and woven bone
Chondroblastoma	Sheets of *compact polyhedral chondroblast*. When the matrix calcifies, it produces a characteristic **chickenwire pattern** of mineralization
Enchondroma	Well-circumscribed nodules of benign hyaline cartilage containing bland-appearing chondrocytes
Osteosarcoma	Formation of **large lacy osteoid areas**, malignant spindle cells forming new bone
Ewing's sarcoma	Uniform **small blue round cells** with scanty cytoplasm, **Homer Wright rosettes**
Multiple myeloma	*Plasma cells with an eccentric nucleus and perinuclear halo*. Sometimes Bizarre cells, Mott cells, and flame cells

Table 38.6: Enneking's staging for benign tumors.

Stage		Radiologically
Stage 1	Latent	Well-defined, sclerotic margin
Stage 2	Active	Well-defined, lack of sclerotic rim
Stage 3	Aggressive	Blurred margins or broken cortex

Table 38.7: Enneking staging for malignant bone tumors.

Stage	Grade	Site	Metastasis
IA	Low	Intracompartmental (T1)	No
IB	Low	Extracompartmental (T2)	No
IIA	High	Intracompartmental (T1)	No
IIB	High	Extracompartmental (T2)	No
III	Low/high	Any	Yes

Compartment, in terms of bone tumor, is an area within its fascial envelope. However, bone, with its periosteum itself, is a compartment, e.g., a bone tumor breaching the cortex and entering neighboring soft tissue is an 'extra compartmental tumor'. A tumor within the muscle group is intracompartmental, whereas breaching the fascia outside the muscle group and entering into another group becomes extracompartmental.

■ TREATMENT

The treatment of the bone tumor depends upon whether it is benign or malignant. While Benign latent lesions are observed, benign active and aggressive lesions are managed with surgical intervention after confirmation of diagnosis. **Flowchart 38.2** outlines the basic principle of treatment of a symptomatic tumor.

Flowchart 38.2: Treatment of symptomatic tumors.

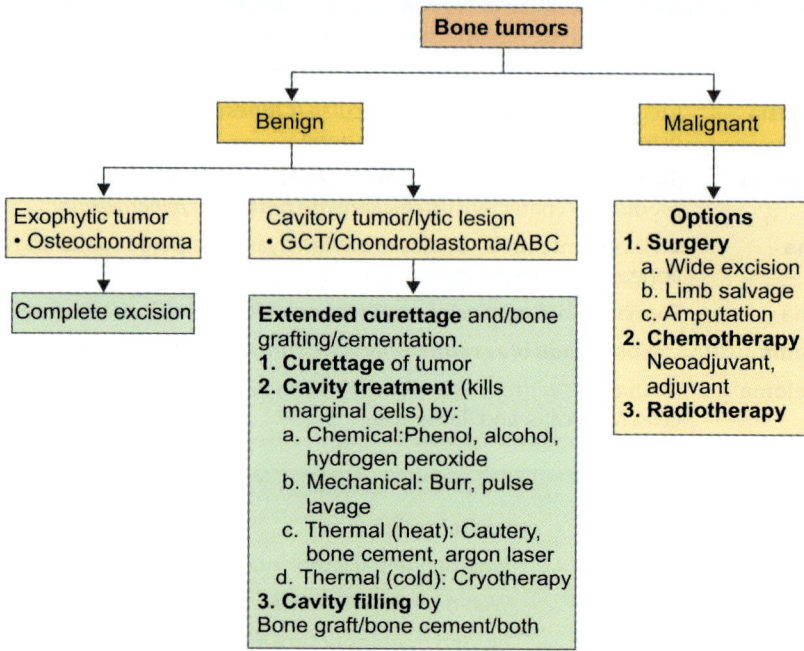

(GCT: giant cell tumor; ABC: aneurysmal bone cyst)

The surgery performed on the tumor could be of five types.
1. **Intralesional excision:** The tumor is excised within the lesion; the microscopic tumor remains.
2. **Marginal excision:** The tumor is excised through the reactive zone; microscopic tumor can be left behind in the reactive zone.
3. **Wide excision:** The tumor is excised outside the reactive zone along with normal cuff of the tissue.
4. **Radical excision:** It involves the removal of an entire anatomic compartment, which includes the tumor, tumor capsule, and all other structures of the compartment. However, due to poor functional outcome, radical excision is no more practiced.
5. **Limb salvage:** 'Limb salvage' is a term used in malignant tumor surgery, wherein *it aims to eradicate the tumor, restore the musculoskeletal integrity of the limb, and restore limb function.*
   More than 90% of patients with osteosarcoma, Ewing's sarcoma, and chondrosarcoma are amenable to limb salvage.
   Limb salvage is preferred over amputations if local recurrence, survival and functional outcomes are similar/better than amputations. However, problems associated with limb salvage surgery are—higher cost, infection, and prosthesis-related problems (infection, loosening).
   Indication of limb salvage surgery: Wide resection of the tumor should be feasible, and the reconstruction performed should provide functional outcome better than the amputation.
   Relative contraindication for limb salvage: (NIPF)
   - Neurovascular involvement
   - Infection

- **P**athological fracture
- **F**ungation of tumor.

Technique: Wide excision of the tumor, including biopsy site, followed by reconstruction of the gap created by the tumor, if required. The surgical options for limb salvage reconstruction are biological, nonbiological or both.
1. *Biological options:*
   - Massive structural allograft
   - Autografts: Vascularized and nonvascularized fibula
   - Tumor bone recycling by extracorporeal radiotherapy (ECRT) or cryotherapy:
     - ***In ECRT***, the bone tumor is excised, cleaned of all soft tissue attachments, and irradiated with 50Gy of radiation, which kills all tumor cells, rendering the bone specimen tumor free. It is then returned to the operating theater and re-implanted by stabilizing it with an appropriate internal fixation device. This method cannot be used in cases of malignant tumor with pathological fracture.
     - ***In cryotherapy***, the bone is exposed to liquid nitrogen, which kills tumor cells by freezing/cold effect and thawing. During cryotherapy, the rapid freeze causes formation of intracellular ice crystals. As the temperature rises during thawing, these crystals coalesce and mechanically disrupt the cell membrane, causing cell death. In malignant tumors, the involved bone is resected and dipped in liquid nitrogen for 20 minutes, wherein the temperature could be as low as -194°C. Freezing is followed by slow thawing. Then, the bone is replaced in original position and stabilized with internal fixation.
     Note: Cryotherapy can also be performed for giant cell tumor of the bone, wherein the liquid nitrogen is poured into the tumor cavity. Repetitive three freeze-thaw cycles increase the area of necrosis of tumor cells. However, there is a risk of adjacent soft tissue necrosis in case of spillage of liquid nitrogen.
   - Arthrodesis.
2. *Nonbiological options:*
   - Arthroplasty
   - Modular endoprosthesis
   - Custom-made/3D printed custom implant.

In the pediatric age group:
1. **Physis sparing procedure:** Canadelle technique is a two stage physiolysis. It is performed when physis is not involved by tumor.
2. **Van ness (rotationplasty):** It provides one time stable reconstruction. In this technique, the foot is rotated by 180° so that the heel faces forward (acting as knee) and foot faces backward (acting as below knee stump) over which an modified exoprosthesis is created **(Fig. 38.3)**.
3. **Amputations:** It is performed whenever wide resection cannot be performed.

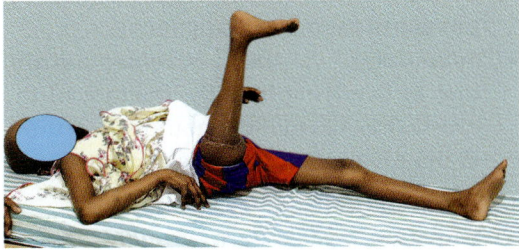

Fig. 38.3: Van ness (rotationplasty).
(Courtesy: Dr Navaneeth Kamath, Mangalore)

CHAPTER 39

Benign Bone Tumors and Tumor-like Lesions

OSTEOCHONDROMA (SOLITARY EXOSTOSIS)

■ INTRODUCTION

Although osteochondroma is considered a benign bone tumor, it is a hamartoma wherein the growth plate cells are displaced horizontally, continuing to grow and forming a bony swelling.

- **Age group:** 10–30 years
- **Location of tumor:** *Metaphysis*. Typically, it grows away from the joint
- **Cell of origin:** It is an extension or growth from an herniated growth plate subperiosteally.
- **Common site:** Fast-growing ends of bone—distal femur, proximal tibia, proximal humerus, distal radius, distal tibia, and fibula.

Always remember that *the actual tumor is bigger than what appears in the X-ray due to the radiolucent cartilage cap.*

Pathologically: It is a hamartoma. During the growth period, cartilage cells are displaced from the physeal plate, grow in the transverse direction rather than vertically, and form a bone lump on the side. It stops growing once the growth is complete. Even after maturing into bone, it continues to have a cartilage cap, and may continue to have a thin growth plate.

■ CLINICAL FEATURES

- It is a *slowly growing, painless bony swelling* at the metaphysis in patients between 10 and 30 years **(Fig. 39.1)**.
- The *swelling always grows away from the joint. It stops growing in size after skeletal growth is complete.* However, a sudden increase in size should raise suspicion of transformation into malignancy.
- *Sometimes, it may become painful due to* overlying bursitis, fracture of the exostosis stalk, malignant transformation, or neurovascular structure compression.

On examination:
- Palpation reveals hard, immobile swelling which is continuous with underlying bone. The skin overlying the lesion is free.

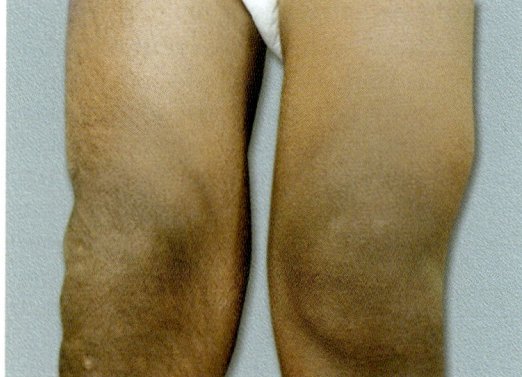

Fig. 39.1: Osteochondroma of the lower end of the left femur.

- Joint movement is normal unless it causes a mechanical block or becomes painful
- Rarely, there may be features of neurovascular compression.

INVESTIGATIONS

- **Plain X-ray (Fig. 39.2):**
  - Sessile or pedunculated growth, which is growing away from the joint
  - Outpouching of tubular bone at the metaphysis. There is classic *"corticomedullary continuity of tumor with the rest of the bone."*
- **MRI:** It helps assess malignant change, cartilage cap thickness, or bursitis. *If the thickness of the cartilage cap is >2 cm, it may indicate malignancy.*

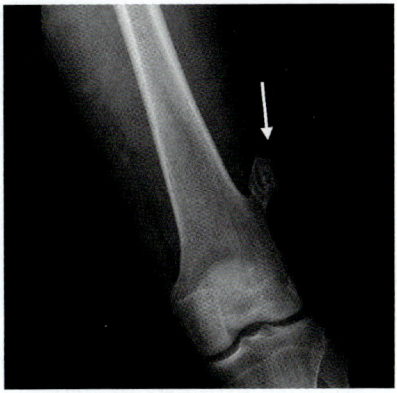

Fig. 39.2: X-ray of the left thigh shows a pedunculated exostosis (arrow) arising from the distal femur growing away from the knee joint.

HISTOPATHOLOGY

- Presence of a cartilage cap
- Cartilage resembles a disorganized growth plate with ossification toward the base
- The medullary cavity merges with that of the underlying bone.

TREATMENT

- **Solitary asymptomatic** lesions are managed *conservatively* and are kept under observation, and it must be watched for any increase in size or appearance of pain.
- **Symptomatic exostosis** must undergo *extraperiosteal excision*, in which the *tumor is excised along with a sleeve of periosteum* to avoid leaving any abnormal cells to reform the tumor. The excised tumor must be sent for biopsy to rule out malignant transformation (Figs. 39.3A and B).

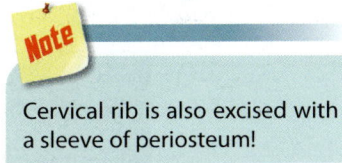

Cervical rib is also excised with a sleeve of periosteum!

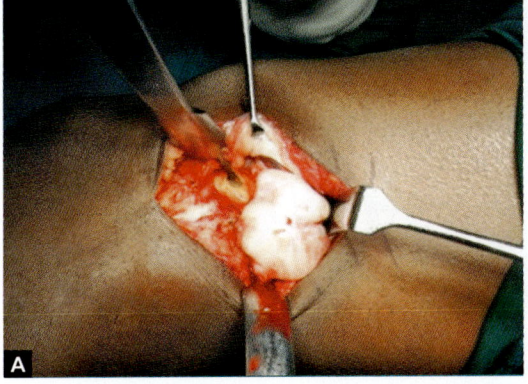
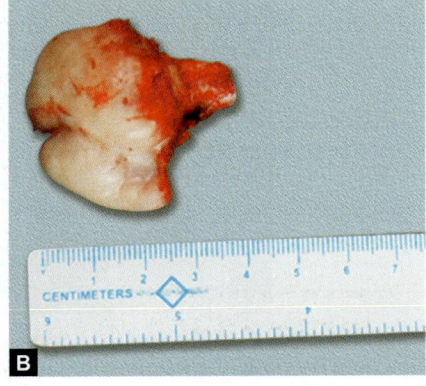

Figs. 39.3A and B: (A) Exostosis of distal femur; (B) Completely excised exostosis.

COMPLICATIONS

- Painful bursitis over the osteochondroma
- Fracture of the pedunculated stalk
- Mechanical block of the joint movement
- Neurovascular compression
- ***The chance of malignant transformation (chondrosarcoma) of solitary exostosis is <1%.***

MULTIPLE EXOSTOSES/DIAPHYSEAL ACLASIS/ HEREDITARY MULTIPLE EXOSTOSIS

INTRODUCTION

- Multiple exostosis or hereditary multiple exostosis (HME) is an ***autosomal dominant disorder***, wherein there is mutation in ***EXT1 and EXT2*** (tumor suppressor genes).
- It carries a ***higher chance of malignant transformation into chondrosarcoma*** (5%) compared to solitary exostosis (1%).

CLINICAL FEATURES

- The patient presents with multiple bony swellings (exostosis) all over the body. *Occasionally, patients are "short-statured."*
- Deformities are noticed in many parts of the body, such as:
    - Femoral shortening, coxa valga, and genu valgum
    - Ulnar shortening, radial bowing, and radial head dislocation

INVESTIGATIONS

- Plain X-ray **(Figs. 39.4A to C)**.
- **MRI:** In case of malignant transformation, the cartilage cap may be thickened >2 cm.

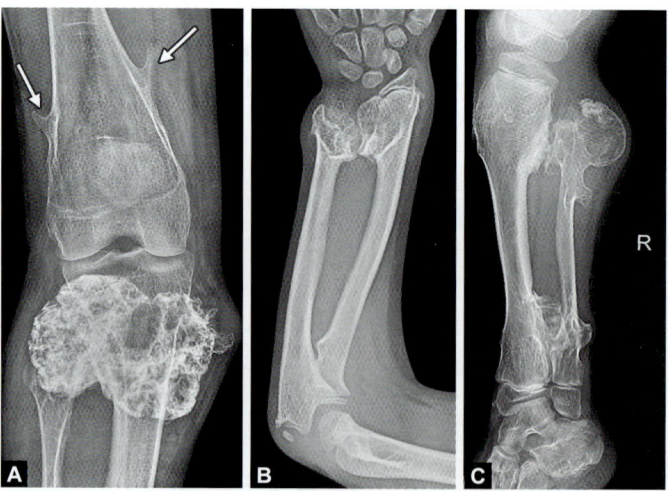

Figs. 39.4A to C: (A) HME with chondrosarcoma of proximal tibia; (B and C) Diaphyseal aclasis of radius-ulna and tibia-fibula.

(*Courtesy*: Dr Navaneeth Kamath, Mangaluru)

TREATMENT

- Similar to the solitary exostosis, the **symptomatic ones** should be excised. The biopsy must be performed to rule out malignancy.
- Other ones should be strictly observed for any sudden increase in pain and swelling, which may indicate malignant transformation.

UNICAMERAL BONE CYST/SIMPLE BONE CYST

INTRODUCTION

A simple bone cyst (SBC) is a benign, **tumor-like lesion.** It is the only true bone cyst.
- **Age group:** 8–15 years
- **Site of SBC:** *Metaphysis of a long bone*—the proximal humerus (65–70%) and proximal femur (30%). *Note that it rarely crosses physis (<1–2% of cases).*
- **Pathologically:** Simple bone cyst contains yellow serous fluid lined by a thin epithelial membrane. The membrane comprises connective tissues with scattered giant cells.
  There are two theories of SBC formation—synovial cell rest and venous obstruction theory; Former is accepted more than latter. Since the cyst fluid resembles synovial fluid, it supports synovial cell rest theory. Venous obstruction theory states that venous blockage of the drainage of the local interstitial fluid results in increased local pressure forming the bone cyst.
- **Active and latent lesion:** If the lesion is within 1 cm of the physis, it is known as an active lesion. In contrast, a lesion towards the diaphysis is considered to be a latent lesion.

CLINICAL FEATURES

- Usually, mild pain and swelling over the affected part.
- Occasionally, pathological fracture.

DIAGNOSIS

Plain X-ray shows (Fig. 39.5)
- Central, metaphyseal lesion
- Symmetrically expansile, thinned-out cortex but no cortical breach
- *Fallen leaf sign:* Fractured bone fragment settles in the dependent part of the cyst
- *Trapdoor sign:* The fractured piece of bone remains attached to the periosteum
- Sometimes, there can be a pathological fracture.

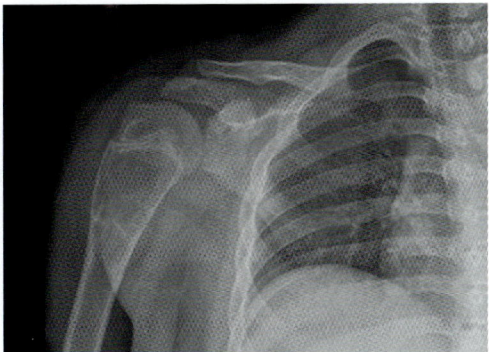

Fig. 39.5: X-ray of proximal humerus shows a simple bone cyst in the metaphysis.

TREATMENT

- **Conservative, if asymptomatic:** It should be kept under observation.
- **For active lesions:** *Cyst aspiration and intracystic injection of methylprednisolone.*
- **For larger lesions at risk of pathological # or enlarging after injection:** Internal fixation with the ender's nail helps drain and decompress the cyst **(Figs. 39.6A and B)**. The cyst in

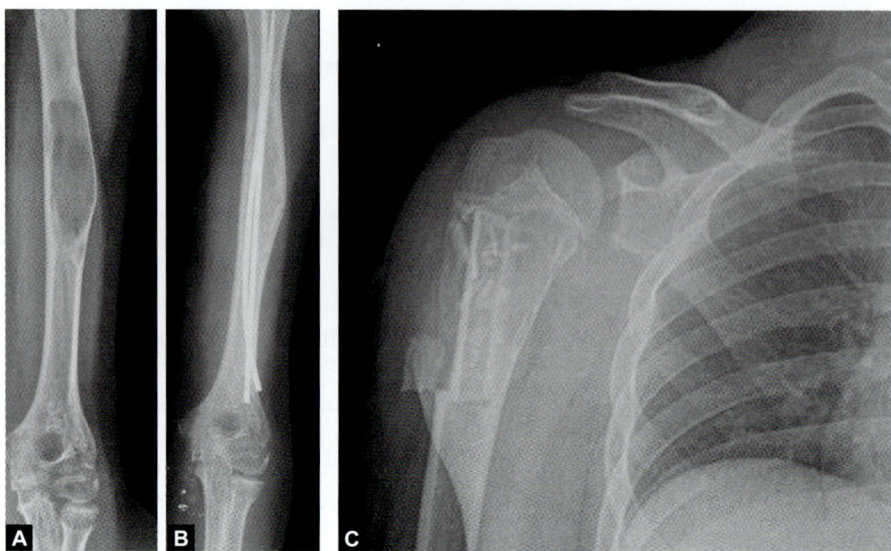

Figs. 39.6A to C: (A) SBC of humerus shaft; (B) Healed lesion after enders nailing; (C) X-ray showing curettage of the lesion with fibular strut grafting.

weight-bearing bones with a risk of pathological fracture can be managed with *curettage, bone grafting and internal fixation* **(Fig. 39.6C)**.

ANEURYSMAL BONE CYST (ABC)

INTRODUCTION

Aneurysmal bone cyst (ABC) is an aggressive ***tumor-like lesion***, which is highly vascular filled with multiple blood-filled cavities.
- **Age group:** First two decade
- **Site:** 65–70% of cases of primary ABC occur in the ***metaphysis of a long bone,*** whereas 25% occur in the spine.
    - ***Metaphysis of long bone:*** Proximal humerus, distal femur, proximal tibia are commonly involved.
    - ***Vertebra:*** It is common in posterior elements (pedicle, lamina, transverse and spinous process).
- **Types of ABC:** ABC could be **primary** (occurring in an erstwhile healthy bone) or **secondary** (occurs in bone affected by other primary lesions). Secondary ABC is associated with Giant cell tumors, chondroblastoma, simple bone cysts, fibrous dysplasia, and telangiectatic osteosarcoma.

CLINICAL FEATURES

- Usually, patients present with mild swelling and pain over the involved bone
- There can be a pathological fracture
- In the case of ABC of a vertebral body, the neurological deficit can occur if the lesion is large enough to compress the spinal cord.

INVESTIGATIONS

- **Plain X-ray (Fig. 39.7)**
  - Metaphyseal, expansile (ballooned), multiloculated lesion
  - Often eccentric
  - Honeycomb appearance (due to septation)
  - Large lesions have a *'finger in balloon'* appearance
- **MRI:** Characteristic *multiple fluid-fluid levels due to blood sedimentation*, septations along with a sclerotic rim
- **Aspiration** of the cyst shows hemorrhagic fluid
- **Needle biopsy:** Cavernous blood-filled space without endothelial lining. There are numerous giant cells and reactive fibroblasts.

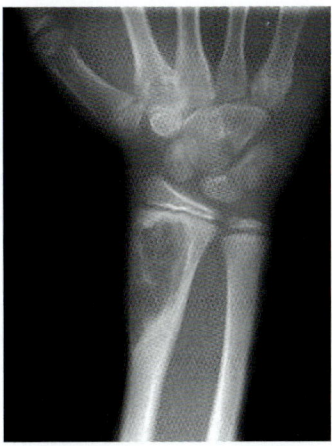

Fig. 39.7: Aneurysmal bone cyst of the radius metaphysis.

DIFFERENTIAL DIAGNOSIS

- **Giant cell tumor (GCT):** Located in the epiphysis
- **Simple bone cyst (SBC):** Central, metaphyseal, well-defined margins, and fallen fragment
- **Telangiectatic osteosarcoma:** Quite similar radiological appearance to ABC. Biopsy can establish the diagnosis.

TREATMENT

Almost all primary ABCs are symptomatic and therefore need treatment.
- The current standard treatment is *percutaneous curopsy with/without intralesional sclerosant*.
- Extended curettage with bone grafting of the cavity should be performed in large lesions with suspected mechanical instability. Internal fixation can be added in weight-bearing areas with a risk of pathological fracture after a curettage. Serial angioembolization is performed in large, surgically inaccessible sites.

What is curopsy?

Curopsy is a procedure is similar to a biopsy but uses a larger instrument to collect a sample of the tumor and its lining. Curopsy is thought to cause initiation of coagulation cascade locally which leads to healing of the lesion.

FIBROUS DYSPLASIA

INTRODUCTION

Fibrous dysplasia (FD) is a developmental bone **tumor-like lesion** caused by the failure of normal lamellar bone formation and replacement by woven bone and fibrous tissue.

The replacement of bone with fibrous tissue may lead to fractures, uneven growth, and deformity.

- **Age group:** Onset less than 30 years
- **Gender:** More common in *females*
- **Site:** *Usually, meta-diaphyseal region of long bones are affected.*
    - Proximal femur (most common site), tibia, humerus, ribs and facial bones.
- **Genetics:** FD is a non-familial disorder caused by **mutation of the GNAS (guanine nucleotide binding protein, alpha stimulating) gene**, which replaces normal bone with fibrous tissue and woven bone.
- **Types**
    - Monostotic (80%): Fibrous dysplasia of a single bone
    - Polyostotic (20%): Fibrous dysplasia of multiple bones
        - *Generalized fibrous dysplasia of facial bones*—'Leontiasis ossea.'
- **Often associated with McCune-Albright syndrome** whose features are as follows:
    - *The triad* of *polyostotic fibrous dysplasia, precocious puberty, and cafe-au-late spots* characterizes McCune-Albright syndrome.
    - *Pathogenesis of McCune-Albright syndrome*: Mutated GNAS results in increased intracellular cAMP signaling, which is responsible for the clinical manifestations of McCune-Albright syndrome. Other endocrine disorders, including hyperthyroidism, acromegaly, renal phosphate wasting, and Cushing syndrome, are also part of this disorder.

How café-au-lait spots of McCune-Albright syndrome and Neurofibromatosis are diffferent?

The irregular/jagged borders of the café-au-lait spots in *McCune-Albright syndrome* are often compared to a *map of the coast of Maine*, which is irregular. By contrast, smooth borders of café-au-lait spots of *neurofibromatosis* is compared to the *coast of California*, which is smooth.

CLINICAL FEATURES

- Usually incidental finding
- Mild swelling and occasional pain
- Pathological fracture.

DIAGNOSIS

- **Plain X-ray (Fig. 39.8A)** *is diagnostic*
    - The lesion is typically seen in metaphyseal-diaphyseal area of long bone
    - Expansile, lytic lesion in the medullary canal of long bone
    - *Ground-glass appearance*/opacity of lesion (due to septation). Sometimes, the lesion is surrounded by a thick sclerotic rim—'Rind sign.'
    - *Shepherd crook deformity* of proximal femur due to healing after multiple fractures **(Fig. 39.8B)**.
- **CT, MRI:** If required
- **Needle biopsy** is confirmatory. It shows
    - *Alphabet soup/Chinese letter appearance*
    - Fibroblast proliferation around the woven bone
    - Absence of osteoblast rimming.

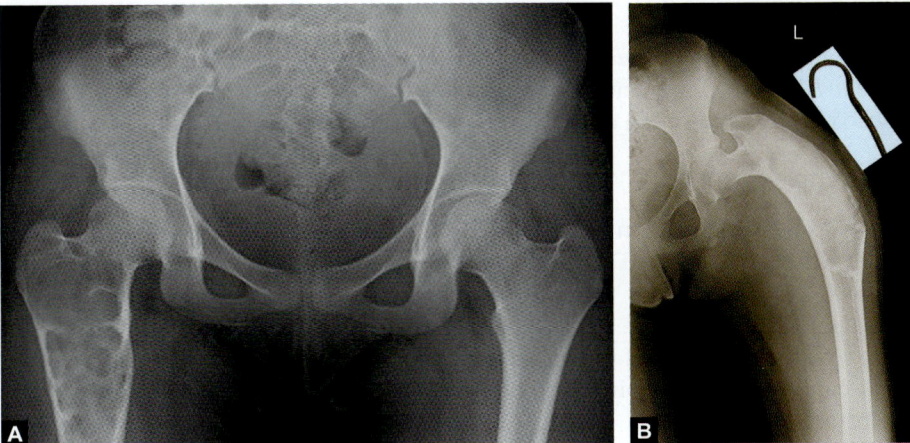

Figs. 39.8A and B: (A) Fibrous dysplasia of proximal femur. Note septated, expansile lesion with ground glass appearance; (B) Fibrous dysplasia of left proximal femur (note ground glass appearance of lesion) with shepherd crook deformity (inset picture shows a shepherd crook).

TREATMENT

- **Asymptomatic lesion in non-stress zones:** Observation
- **Symptomatic lesion:**
    - *In most cases, internal fixation is sufficient.* Curettage and bone grafting is added if there is cystic degeneration **(Fig. 39.9)**.
    - Bisphosphonate therapy: To reduce pain, especially in polyostotic fibrous dysplasia.

> **Note**
>
> **Mazabraud syndrome**
> Polyostotic fibrous dysplasia with intramural myxomas.

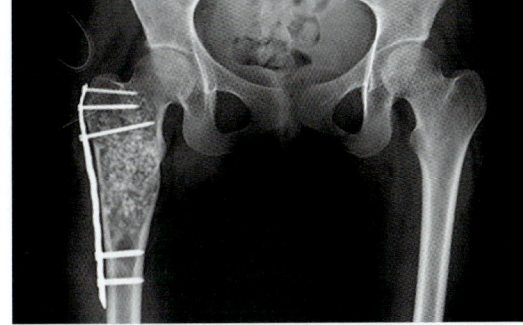

Fig. 39.9: Curettage of proximal femur fibrous dysplasia, bone grafting and internal fixation.

OSTEOID OSTEOMA

INTRODUCTION

Osteoid osteoma is a small painful benign tumor, which typically occurs in the diaphyseal cortex of the long bone.
- **Age group:** 2nd to 3rd decade
- **Gender:** It is more common in males.
- **Site:** Diaphysis/metaphysis of a long bone is the common location. Primarily the lower limb (50%) bones are involved, such as femur, and tibia. It is also seen in:
    - Spine in posterior elements
    - Scaphoid, proximal phalanx, and talus.

PATHOANATOMY

Osteoid osteoma has a **central nidus with surrounding reactive bone** with *increased prostaglandin E2 (PGE2) and cyclooxygenases (COX1/2) levels and increased unmyelinated nerve fibers.* Therefore, there is a dramatic response to NSAIDs/aspirin.

CLINICAL FEATURES

- Patients present with pain in the involved limb, which is worse at night. Typically, pain decreases with aspirin/NSAIDs, which also serve as a diagnostic test.
- Sometimes, there may be a tender swelling on the surface of the bone due to a solid periosteal reaction.
- There can be joint stiffness if the lesion is near a joint. Intracapsular femoral neck osteoid osteoma can result in hip joint synovitis and effusion, resulting in decreased movement and deformity.
- *List or postural scoliosis* if the lesion is in the spine (tumor on the concave side of the curve).

DIAGNOSIS

- **Plain X-ray**
    - Characteristic nidus with surrounding sclerotic zone **(Fig. 39.10)**
    - Solid buttressing type of periosteal reaction
- **CT scan (thin sliced):** Confirmatory **(Fig. 39.11)**. The nidus is <2 cm in size. If the nidus >2 cm, it is called osteoblastoma.
- **Bone scan:** Double-density sign

TREATMENT

- ***CT-guided radiofrequency ablation/cryoablation/CT-guided drilling*** is the current treatment of choice of osteoid osteoma.

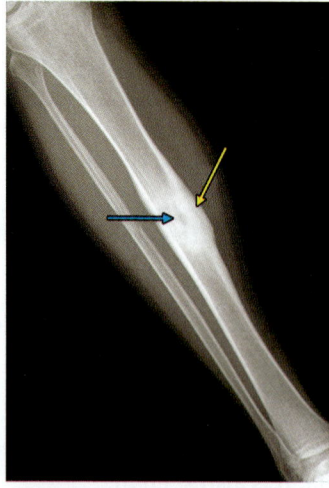

Fig. 39.10: Osteoid osteoma showing nidus (blue arrow) with periosteal thickening (yellow arrow).

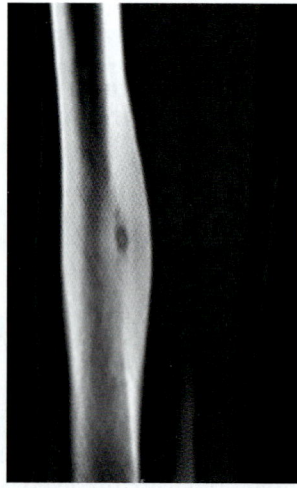

Fig. 39.11: CT scan tibia shows osteoid osteoma of tibia with a nidus in the center.

CT-guided drilling through the reactive bone is sometimes performed using the burr-down technique.
- **Surgical excision:** Rarely, complete excision of tumor (nidus) is performed if radiofrequency ablation is not possible. However, it is a morbid procedure and can miss a nidus.

DIFFERENTIAL DIAGNOSIS

Osteoblastoma: Osteoblastoma is a more aggressive lesion than osteoid osteoma and is characterized by
- Larger in size (>2 cm), a predilection for spine
- Inconsistent pain which is not relieved by NSAIDs
- X-ray shows a lesser degree of sclerosis around osteoblastoma.

OSTEOMA

- **Definition and cell of origin:** A benign neoplasm of osteoblasts
- **Site:** Flat bones of the skull and face. Often, it occurs near the paranasal sinuses **(Fig. 39.12)**.
- **Clinical features:** Mostly asymptomatic painless swelling of the skull bones. Occasionally, proximity to the sinus can block the sinus openings and cause sinusitis.
- **Treatment:** Symptomatic once can be excised.

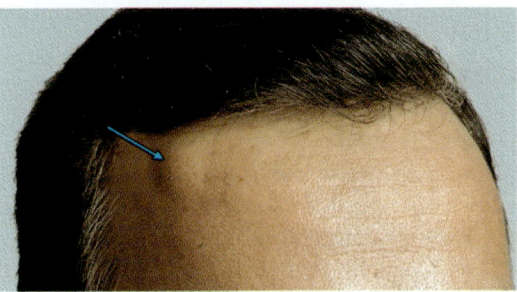

Fig. 39.12: Osteoma of the frontal bone (blue arrow).

GIANT CELL TUMOR OF BONE (GCTB)

INTRODUCTION

Giant cell tumor, previously addressed by the term 'osteoclastoma' is currently considered to be a misnomer. Osteoclastoma terminology can make the reader assume it is a neoplasm of osteoclasts (giant cells). However, a giant cell tumor of the bone (GCTB) consists of **true neoplastic stromal cells**, which recruit giant cells to cause bony destruction.

Definition: It is a benign tumor from a **cell of unknown origin** or **mononuclear cell of unknown origin**.
- **Age group:** 20–40 years
- **Gender:** It is one of the bone tumors, which is *slightly more common in females*
- **Location:** *Epiphysis* is the common location. Occasionally, it is present in apophysis.
- **Common sites of GCTB:**
  - The lower end of the femur
  - The upper end of the tibia
  - Distal radius
  - The proximal humerus and proximal fibula.
- Usually benign but has a tendency for local recurrences up to 25% of cases. The risk of metastatic lesions is 2%. However, the metastatic lesions are also benign.

CLINICAL FEATURES

- *Age*: 20–40 years
- Usually, chronic slow-growing eccentric swelling followed by pain in the epiphyseal region **(Fig. 39.13)**
- Occasionally, it presents with pathological #.

On examination:
- Bony tenderness may be present.
- Large swellings can show stretched skin.
- *Eggshell crackling* on deep palpation. However, it should always be avoided as this maneuver breaks the cortex.
- Joint involvement is rare.

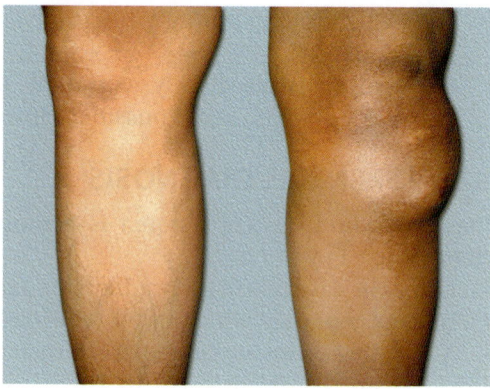

Fig. 39.13: Giant cell tumor of the left upper-end tibia.

INVESTIGATIONS

- **Plain X-ray (Fig. 39.14):**
  - *Epiphyseal lytic lesion*
  - *Eccentric*
  - *Expansile, cortical thinning*
  - Geographic *"soap bubble appearance"*
  - No calcification
  - Cortical erosion occurs with the expansion of lesions

  The Campanacci grading system of GCTB is based upon the radiological appearance of the tumor.
  - *Grade 1:* It has well-defined margins and an intact cortex.
  - *Grade 2:* It has relatively well-defined margins but cortical thinning and expansion but no breach of cortex.
  - *Grade 3:* The tumor borders are indistinct, there is a cortical breach and tumor extends into the soft tissue

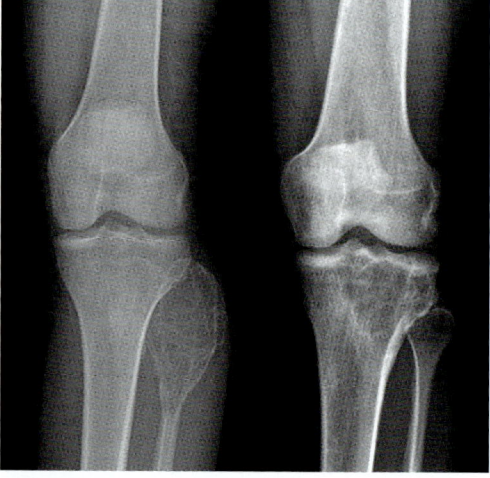

Fig. 39.14: X-ray knee shows giant cell tumor (GCT) of the upper-end fibula (left image) and upper-end tibia (right image).

- **Magnetic resonance imaging:** It is required to assess local invasion.
- **Chest X-ray:** It is required to look for any metastasis.
- **CT scan of the chest** is performed if metastasis is suspected on chest X-ray
- **True cut needle biopsy** is the confirmatory investigation, which must be performed to establish the diagnosis.

Histopathology: Hallmark multinucleated giant cells lying in the background of mononuclear stromal cells resembling macrophages.

TREATMENT

The intent of GCT treatment should be complete clearance of the disease. The most common option of GCTB treatment is extended curettage and bone grafting/cementation/both.

If disease clearance is possible by extended curettage, the same should be performed. However, if extended Curettage cannot achieve disease clearance, lesion resection and reconstruction is performed. Several options are possible for the treatment of GCT **(Flowchart 39.1)**.

- **Complete excision if possible,** especially when the function is not hampered after excising the tumor, e.g., GCT of the upper-end fibula.
- **Extended curettage of the cavity with bone grafting and/or bone cement filling of cavity (Fig. 39.15).** Extended curettage implies curettage and treatment of the cavity lining, wherein *thermal* (heat with cautery; cold with liquid nitrogen), *mechanical* (burr), and *chemical* (phenol) methods are applied to achieve tumor cell free margins. *It is the most common treatment done for GCT.*
- **Excision of the lesion with reconstruction (arthrodesis/arthroplasty/turn-o-plasty) (Figs. 39.16A to D):** In case of lesions where disease clearance is not possible.

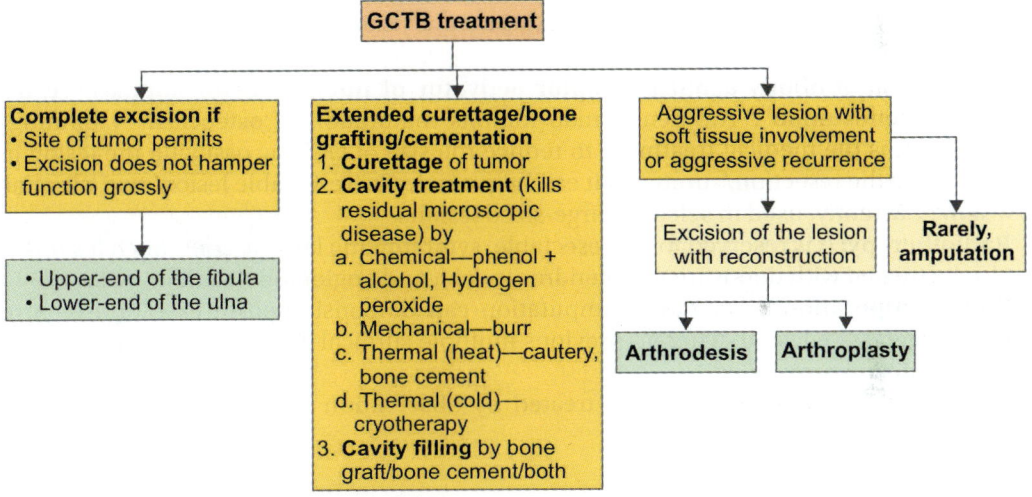

Flowchart 39.1: Treatment algorithm of giant cell tumor (GCT).

(GCTB: giant cell tumor of the bone)

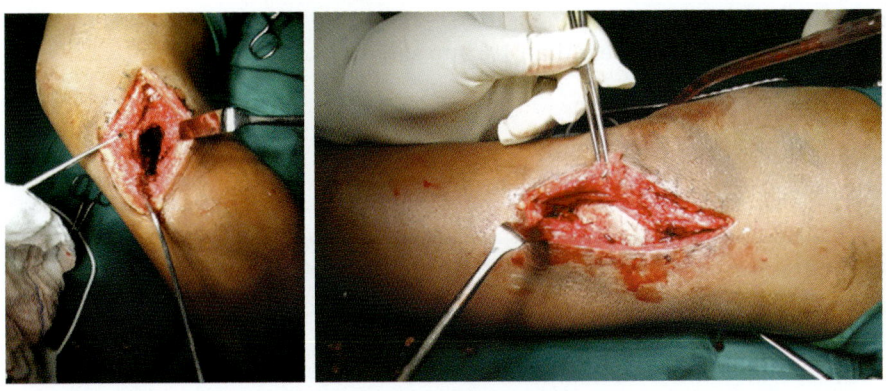

Fig. 39.15: Intraoperative picture showing curettage of the cavity and filling with bone graft and bone cement.

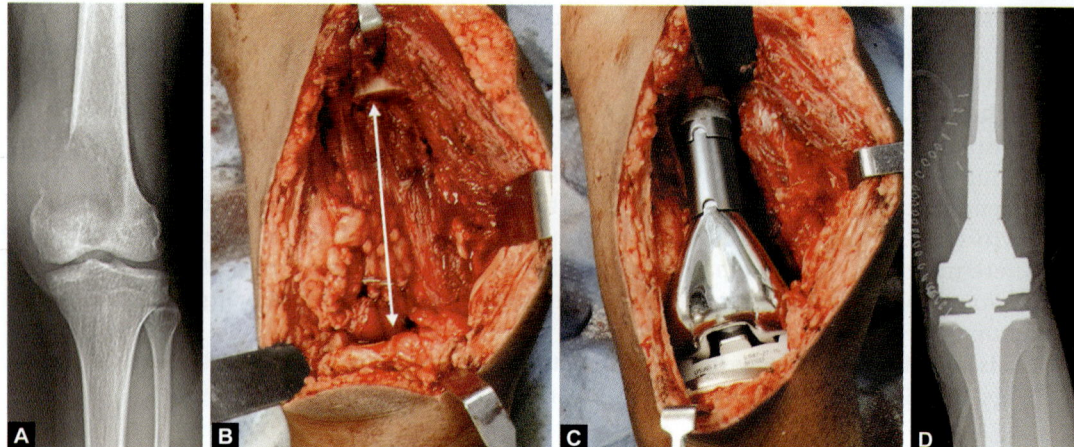

Figs. 39.16A to D: (A) GCT of distal femur; (B) Lesion resected (white arrow); (C) Megaprosthesis in situ; (D) Postoperative X-ray showing distal femur megaprosthesis.

- **Monoclonal antibody against receptor activator of nuclear factor kappa-B (RANK) ligand "denosumab":** The denosumab inhibits maturation of osteoclast by binding to RANKL. It is the medical treatment to reduce the size of GCT by ossifying the lesion and facilitating the resection/curettage. It can help convert a 'resectable lesion' to a 'curettable lesion'! Currently, used in selected large-sized lesions.
- **Radiotherapy:** It is reserved for unresectable, symptomatic large lesions. Such lesions can also be treated with denosumab, zolendronic acid, and angioembolization.
- **Rarely amputation:** Very rarely, amputation can be considered in case of a recurrent highly aggressive lesion, wherein previous multiple surgical attempts of curettage or limb reconstruction have failed.
- **Pulmonary metastasis:** It can be treated by observation or resection, denosumab or radiotherapy if above method fails.

COMPLICATIONS

- Pathological fractures
- Recurrences
- *Malignant transformation*: Less than 1% into sarcomas.

DIFFERENTIAL DIAGNOSIS

- Aneurysmal bone cysts (ABC)
- Telangiectatic osteosarcoma (in large lesion).

ENCHONDROMA (CHONDROMA)

- **Definition:** The benign neoplasm of cartilage cells lies inside a medullary canal (enchondroma).
- *It is the most common benign tumor of the hand.*
- **Site:** Clinically, it is commonly noticed in the phalanges of the hand and feet **(Fig. 39.17)**. However, the *most common location of enchondroma is femur*, where it is often an incidental X-ray finding.

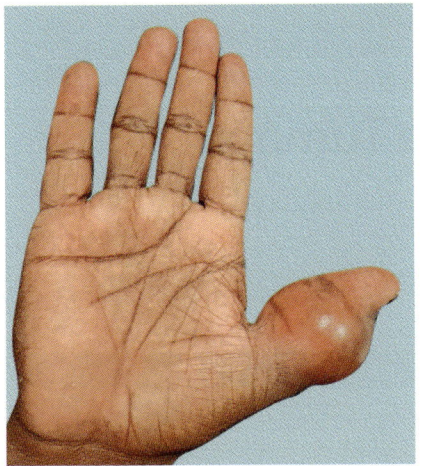

Fig. 39.17: Enchondroma of the thumb.

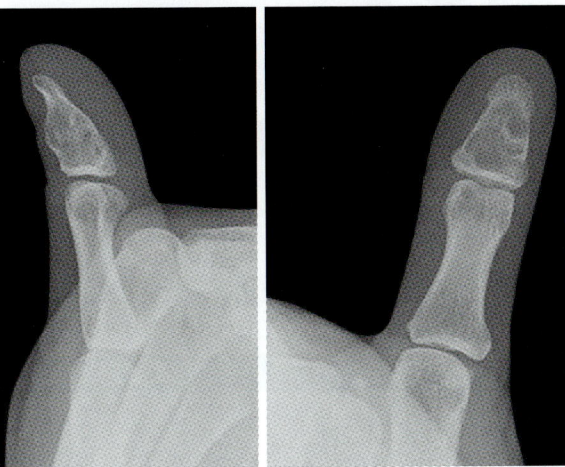

Fig. 39.18: Enchondroma of the distal phalanx of thumb.

- **Clinical features:** Patients present with painless/painful gradually increasing swelling of the bone, especially in hand. Occasionally, pathological fracture may occur.
- **X-ray:** Expansile lesion in the metaphysis of bone with stippled calcification **(Fig. 39.18)**
- **Treatment:** Symptomatic lesions require curettage with grafting.
- **Complications:** Pathological fracture, risk of chondrosarcoma (<1%)
- **Associated syndromes**
    - *Ollier's disease* is multiple enchondromas. The risk of malignant transformation into chondrosarcoma is 25–40%.
    - *Maffucci syndrome* is multiple enchondromas with cavernous hemangiomas and pheboliths. Enchondromas of Maffuci syndrome also carry high risk malignant transformation into chondrosarcoma (25–40%).

CHONDROBLASTOMA/CODMAN'S TUMOR

- **Definition**: It is a benign neoplasm of cartilage cells in the epiphysis of a growing skeleton.
- **Site**: *Epiphysis* of long bones in a growing skeleton
- **Clinical features:** Pain over the involved bone is the common symptom. There can be be *joint effusion* as epiphysis is involved.
- **X-ray:** Eccentric lytic lesion in the epiphysis, faint sclerotic rim, and matrix calcification **(Fig. 39.19)**
- **Histopathology:** Chondroblasts, *Chicken wire appearance* of cells with dystrophic calcification, and giant cells
- **Treatment:** The symptomatic lesions require curettage with grafting. Smaller lesions (<2.5 cm), which are close to physis or in inaccessible areas can be treated with radiofrequency ablation/cryotherapy.

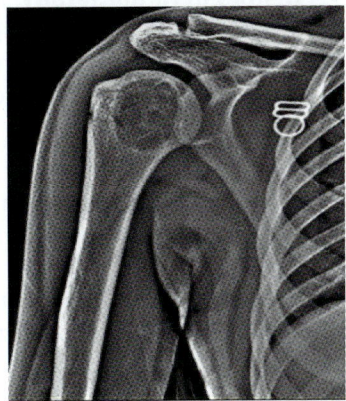

Fig. 39.19: Chondroblastoma of upper-end of the humerus.
(*Courtesy:* Dr Rajeev Reddy)

CHAPTER 40

Malignant Bone Tumors

OSTEOSARCOMA

■ INTRODUCTION

Osteosarcoma is a primary malignant bone tumor of mesenchymal origin characterized by osteoid formation. It is the *most common nonhematological malignancy of the bone*.
- **Age:** It affects individuals **between 10 and 20 years of age** due to maximal activity of osteoblast. Osteosarcoma has **bimodal distribution**, i.e., it is common between 10 and 20 years and also observed between 50 and 60 years.
- **Site:** It is most commonly observed around the area of maximal growth potential—60% around the knee (distal femur and proximal tibia), and proximal humerus.
- **Gender:** Males have a higher predilection.
- **Location:** Metaphysis.

■ PREDISPOSING FACTORS

- **Genetic predisposition**
  - Retinoblastoma gene
  - P53 gene
  - Increased risk in Rothmund-Thomson syndrome, Li-Fraumeni syndrome.
- **History of radiotherapy:** For secondary osteosarcoma
- **Finkel-Biskis-Jinkins (FBJ) murine virus**
- **Chemicals:** It was common in watchmakers who used radium to paint dials (for fluorescence). It is no more observed as radium is no more used for dial painting.

■ CLASSIFICATION

Osteosarcoma is classified into two types—primary and secondary. Primary osteosarcoma arises from (previously) healthy bone, whereas secondary osteosarcoma arises from a diseased or abnormal bone.
1. **Primary osteosarcoma:** It is of two types—central and peripheral/surface.
   - *Central/intramedullary osteosarcoma*: From de novo bone, mostly in long bones.
     - Intramedullary/central high-grade osteosarcoma. Depending upon the predominance of the cell type, it is further subclassified as:
       - Osteoblastic (50%)
       - Chondroblastic (25%)
       - Fibroblastic (25%).

- Telangiectatic
- Small cell
- Low-grade central
- **Surface (juxtacortical type) osteosarcoma**
  - Parosteal low grade *(distal femur posterior aspect is most common site)*
  - High-grade surface.
2. **Secondary osteosarcoma** arises from the diseased bone. Mostly flat bones are affected. Various predisposing factors for secondary osteosarcoma are:
   - Irradiated bone
   - Paget's disease
   - Bone infarct
   - Preexisting bone tumors—fibrous dysplasia
   - Preexisting infection—chronic osteomyelitis.

CLINICAL FEATURES

- **Age:** Second and sixth decade
- **Location:** Metaphysis
- *Patients with osteosarcoma present with pain and swelling of short duration in the metaphyseal region of a long bone. Usually, pain is felt first, followed by swelling.*
- **Pain:** Deep boring pain which is often present at rest or night.
- **Swelling:** Swelling of the affected bone with a rapid increase in size **(Fig. 40.1)**
- **Constitutional features:** Loss of weight and appetite is observed in the case of large tumors.
- **Metastasis:** It spreads by the hematogenous route. The most common site of metastasis is the lungs.

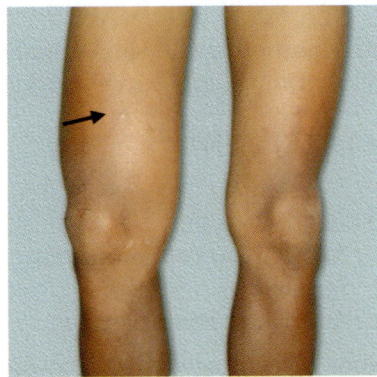

Fig. 40.1: Swelling of the right distal femur metaphysis (arrow).

On examination
- Diffuse swelling is noted over the affected part
- Skin appears stretched, shiny along with dilated veins
- Local rise in temperature is often present
- Bony tenderness is present over the affected bone
- Variable consistency
- Decreased range of movement (due to pain and spasm)
- Occasionally, pathological fracture
- *Late stage*: Tumor progresses to cause local fungation through the skin.

INVESTIGATIONS

- **Plain X-ray (Fig. 40.2)**
  - *Metaphyseal lesion*
  - *Permeative bone destruction* with new bone formation (lytic and sclerotic areas)
  - *Sunburst appearance*: When the tumor grows beyond the cortex and grows along the lines of new vessels

- **Codman's triangle:** Reactive new bone formation under the periosteum
- Cloud-like densities suggestive of new bone formation
- The cortex may be eroded, and there may be a pathological fracture.
  - Increased soft tissue shadow.
- **MRI-scan:** It is a must for the staging of the tumor, soft tissue invasion, marrow involvement, and relation to surrounding compartments and neurovascular structures
- **Bone scan:** To identify skeletal metastasis
- **X-ray and non-contrast CT scan chest:** To detect chest metastasis
- **Serology:** Serum alkaline phosphatase is raised (indicates increased osteoblastic activity)
- **J Needle biopsy:** It confirms the diagnosis.

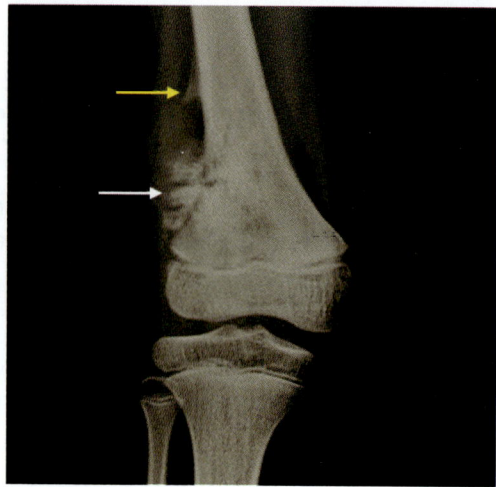

Fig. 40.2: Osteosarcoma of distal femur shows sunburst appearance (white arrow) and Codman's triangle (yellow arrow).

Histopathology: It shows malignant spindle cells forming *large "lacey" osteoid areas.*

TREATMENT

The treatment of osteosarcoma involves three steps (Flowchart 40.1):
1. **Neoadjuvant chemotherapy**
2. **Surgery**
3. **Adjuvant chemotherapy.**

Note: *Osteosarcoma is a highly radioresistant tumor; therefore, radiotherapy is not routinely used in treating osteosarcoma.*

Neoadjuvant chemotherapy (NACT): The goals are—
- Reduce vascularity of the tumor
- Reduce the chance of micrometastasis.
  The drugs used in NACT are:
  - Ifosfamide
  - Cisplatin
  - Methotrexate
  - Adriamycin.

Flowchart 40.1: Treatment algorithm of osteosarcoma.

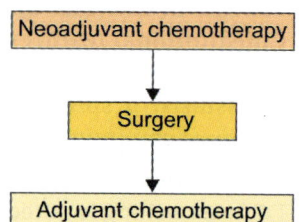

Surgery: Various options are:
- *Limb salvage:* It entails wide excision of the tumor and reconstruction with biological (massive allograft, arthrodesis), nonbiological (endoprosthesis) or both options.
- *Wide excision:* It can be performed in parosteal osteosarcoma. Chemotherapy is not required in parosteal osteosarcoma.
- *Amputation:* Wherever wide excision/limb salvage is not possible, amputation may be performed, followed by exoprosthesis application.

Various types of osteosarcoma

- **Intramedullary osteosarcoma:** Described above
- **Parosteal osteosarcoma:** More common in females; 30–40 years
  - Arises from surface of metaphysis
  - Often painless
  - Wide excision is choice
  - Routine chemo not indicated
  - Better prognosis than intramedullary/periosteal osteosarcoma
- **Periosteal osteosarcoma:** More common in females; 15–25 years
  - Occurs in diaphysis
  - p53 mutation
  - Surgical excision with/without chemo is the treatment of choice
  - Intermediate prognosis between intramedullary and parosteal osteosarcoma
- **Telengiectatic osteosarcoma:** Common in males
  - Locations of aneurysmal bone cyst (ABC)
  - Similar radiologic appearance as ABC

Adjuvant chemotherapy to continue for 3–4 months.
- Five-year survival: Currently, the 5-year survival rate after adequate therapy is approximately 50–70%.

EWING'S SARCOMA

INTRODUCTION

Ewing's sarcoma is a distinctive primary bone high-grade malignant neoplasm composed of small round blue cells
- **Age:** 5–25 years. It is most common in children <10 years
- **Site:** *Diaphysis* of long bone, pelvis (ilium), and ribs
- **Gender:** More common in males
- **Genetics:** t(11:22) translocation.

CLINICAL FEATURES

Patients with Ewing's sarcoma present with pain and swelling of short duration in the diaphysis of the affected bone.
- **Pain:** It is constant and deep boring type.
- **Swelling:** Swelling is diaphyseal **(Fig. 40.3)**. Often a rapid increase in size is observed.
- **Constitutional symptoms** are observed in large or disseminated disease. There can be intermittent fever, weight loss, and loss of appetite.
  Note that C-reactive protein (CRP), erythrocyte sedimentation rate (ESR), and leucocyte count are often raised in Ewing's, and *needle biopsy aspirate*

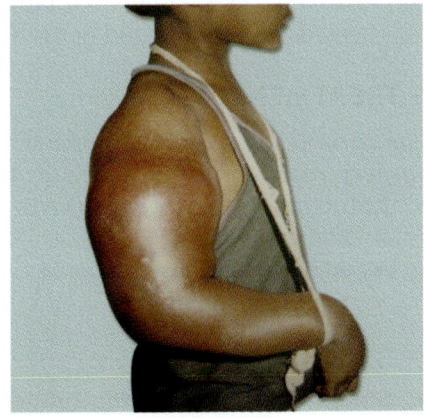

Fig. 40.3: Gross swelling of midshaft humerus.

may show necrotic material which can resemble pus, mimicking osteomyelitis! Therefore, the diagnosis must be confirmed with biopsy.
- **Metastasis** is most common in the lungs, followed by marrow and skeletal metastasis.

On examination
- Diffuse swelling is noted over the diaphysis of the affected bone
- *Skin*: Stretched and shiny, dilated veins
- Bony tenderness is present over the affected bone
- Soft to firm tumor.

Always remember
The differential diagnosis of Ewing's sarcoma is osteomyelitis and vice versa.

DIAGNOSIS

- **Plain X-ray (Fig. 40.4)**
    - It is a diaphyseal tumor with osteolytic areas. Often large soft tissue shadows.
    - Permeated/moth-eaten appearance
    - Lamellated, interrupted periosteal reaction classically known as *"onion peel appearance"*.
  In Ewing sarcoma of flat bone—lytic lesion with no periosteal reaction.
- **Serology:** Elevated ESR, alkaline phosphatase, and lactate dehydrogenase.
- **MRI:** To assess marrow involvement, local disease extent, relation with surrounding compartment, and neurovascular structures
- **F-fluorodeoxyglucose (FDG) PET/CT scan:** For metastasis
- **CT chest:** For metastasis
- **J needle biopsy:** Histopathology shows—
    - Sheets of monotonous small round blue cells with Homer Wright rosette formation
    - Immunostaining positivity for cells—*CD99 is positive in 95% of cases*. Others are FLi1, S100, NKX 2.2, periodic acid Schiff (PAS), and neuron specific enolase.

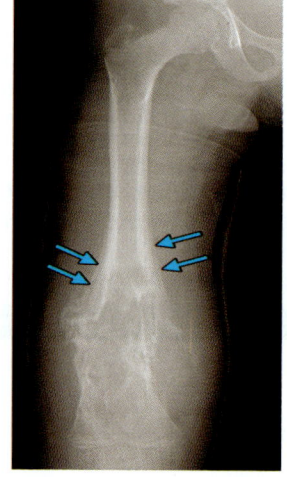

Fig. 40.4: Ewing's sarcoma of the femur diaphysis. Multiple blue arrows indicate interrupted lamellated periosteal reaction.

TREATMENT

The current treatment of choice is "induction chemotherapy followed by local control by surgery/radiotherapy." Thereafter, *adjuvant chemotherapy.*
- **Induction chemotherapy (VAC/IE):** First 8–12 weeks
    - Vincristine
    - Actinomycin-D
    - Cyclophosphamide
    - Ifosfamide
    - Etoposide
- **Surgery:** After multidrug induction chemotherapy, limb salvage surgery is preferred. Amputation is performed if limb salvage is not possible.
- **Adjuvant chemotherapy:** Maintenance chemotherapy for 6–12 months.

- Radiotherapy is used as adjuvant along with surgery in selected cases, and inaccessible/unresectable lesions of axial skeleton.

DIFFERENTIAL DIAGNOSIS
- Osteomyelitis
- Leukemia, lymphoma.

MULTIPLE MYELOMA/KAHLER'S DISEASE

INTRODUCTION
- **Definition:** Malignant bone tumor due to the proliferation of plasma cells producing an excess of monoclonal immunoglobulins.
- *It is the most common primary bone malignancy*
- **Age:** It is commonly observed in adults older than 40 years
- **Gender:** More common in **males**
- **Site:** *Commonly involves flat bones*—pelvis, ribs, skull, and vertebra; rarely long bone.

CLASSIFICATION
- Multiple myeloma
- *Solitary plasmacytoma*: Plasma cell tumor in a single location
- Osteosclerotic myeloma.

PATHOLOGY
The neoplastic plasma cells produce heavy and light-chain immunoglobulins. Among the heavy chains, IgG is most common.
- *Heavy chains*: IgG (52%), IgA (21%), and IgM (12%)
- *Light chains*: Kappa and lambda. *Lambda is also known as Bence-Jones protein.*

The rapidly multiplying plasma cells, overproduced immunoglobulins, and bone destruction cast manifold local (bone) and systemic problems **(Flowchart 40.2)**.
- *Marrow and bone:* The rapidly multiplying plasma cells cause the replacement of normal hematopoietic cell lines resulting in anemia, infections, and increased bleeding tendency. Further, the osteolysis of the bone by rapidly multiplying plasma cells causes bone weakening, pathological fractures, and an increase in serum calcium (hypercalcemia). Hypercalcemia cause anorexia, nausea, vomiting, polyuria, polydipsia and confusion.
- *Serum:* The increasing number of immunoglobulins in the serum causes an increase in viscosity of the serum resulting in hyperviscosity syndromes.
- *Kidney:* The deposition of light chain proteins in the kidney causes renal failure.

CLINICAL FEATURES
- It is commonly observed in patients who are aged >40 years
- The most common clinical feature is *localized* or *generalized bone pain*. The affected areas are ribs, spine, sternum, or long bones. Some patients develop *pathological #* due to weakened bone

Flowchart 40.2: Systemic and local effects of rapidly multiplying malignant plasma cells.

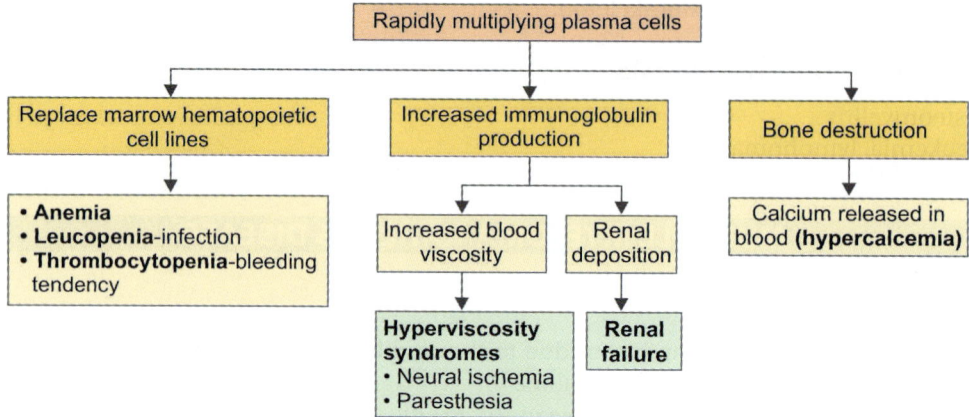

- Features of *fatigue and other constitutional features are present* due to:
    - Anemia
    - Renal failure (uremia)
    - Hypercalcemia—anorexia, nausea, vomiting, polyuria, polydipsia, depression or confusion.
- Some patients may develop amyloidosis.

DIAGNOSIS

- **Plain X-ray (Fig. 40.5)**
    - *Multiple punched-out lesions* without a reactive zone throughout the skeleton. They are commonly seen in spine > pelvis > ribs > upper limb > skull > femur and sternum
    - Wedge collapse of the vertebra (pedicle spared)
    - Rib border erosion
    - Diffuse rarefaction of bone.
- **Serological**
    - *Low hemoglobin and significantly elevated ESR* are common in multiple myeloma.
    - *Altered albumin: globulin ratio.* The normal ratio is 3:2. However, increased globulins in multiple myeloma reverse the ratio.
    - *Prominent M band* is present in serum protein electrophoresis. *Increased serum β2 globulins in electrophoresis indicates poor prognosis.*
    - Others are elevated serum calcium, urea, creatinine and uric acid.
- **Urine:** 50–80% of patients may show the presence of Bence-Jones protein (kappa and lambda light chains).

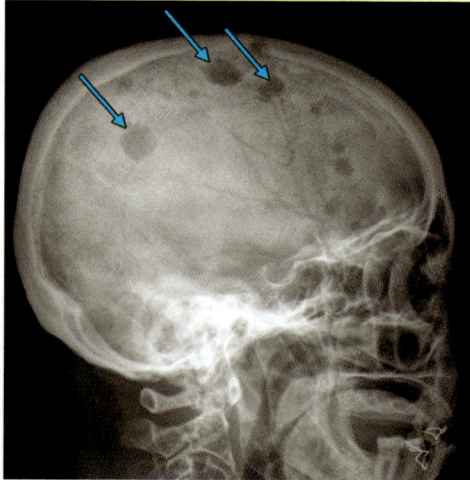

Fig. 40.5: Multiple punched-out lesions in the skull (blue arrows).

- **Bone scan:** It is not helpful as it shows a cold spot in 30% of cases.
- **Biopsy:** *Histopathology* shows.
  - Plasma cells with an *eccentric nucleus and chariot/cartwheel or clock face chromatin with clear area (Hoffa's zone)* adjacent to the nucleus
  - Plasma cells are CD56 and CD38 positive (normal plasma cells are negative for these CD types).
- **Bone marrow aspirate**
  - *Multiple myeloma*: Greater than 30% plasma cells.
  - *Solitary plasmacytoma*: 10–30% cells.

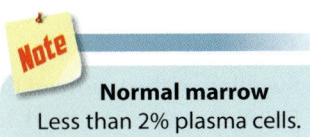

Normal marrow
Less than 2% plasma cells.

TREATMENT

- **Multidrug chemotherapy and steroid is the mainstay of the treatment.** It comprises:
  - Melphalan/bortezomib + dexamethasone + thalidomide/lanalidomide
  - Bisphosphonates are used to reduce bone pain and control hypercalcemia.
- *Stem cell transplantation:* Not curative but improves disease-free survival by 3–4 years. It is an option in patients fit for bone marrow transplant.

Operative treatment

- Impending fractures (Mirel score >8) should be treated with prophylactic internal fixation (intramedullary nail)
- Kyphoplasty can be added for acute painful vertebral compression fractures
- Pathological fractures should be treated with internal fixation.

CHONDROSARCOMA

INTRODUCTION

- **Definition:** Malignant tumor from mesenchymal cells forming malignant cartilage
- *Third most common bone tumor* (most common—multiple myeloma, second most common—osteosarcoma)
- Peak incidence: 4th to 6th decade
- Metastasis is via hematogenous route and most commonly occurs to the lungs.

TYPES

Chondrosarcoma occurs denovo in an otherwise healthy bone (primary chondrosarcoma) or in a diseased bone with preexisting lesions like enchondroma (secondary).

- **Primary chondrosarcoma**
  - Central
  - Surface
  - Clear cell chondrosarcoma
  - Mesenchymal
  - Dedifferentiated.
- **Secondary chondrosarcoma:** From existing lesions like enchondroma, exostosis, Ollier's disease, and Maffucci's syndrome.

CLINICAL FEATURES

- **Age:** Typically, it is seen after 40 years of age.
- **Location:** The most common site is *flat bones* such as the pelvis, and scapula, followed by the proximal femur. Also, it is the most common malignancy of the chest wall.
- **Clinical features:** It presents as gradually increasing pain and swelling of the involved bone. Constitutional features are uncommon.

On examination

- Swelling of the involved bone is noted **(Fig. 40.6)**.
- Palpation reveals a hard, lobulated surface with tenderness over the bony swelling.

DIAGNOSIS

- **Plain X-ray:** *Popcorn type of densities*, cortical destruction, mixed lytic sclerotic appearance **(Fig. 40.7)**.
- J needle core biopsy confirms the diagnosis. **High-grade chondrosarcomas** show hypercellular stroma consisting of characteristic *"blue-balls" of a cartilage lesion permeating the bone trabeculae*. **Low-grade chondrosarcomas** show features similar to enchondroma, few mitotic figures, hypercellularity, disorganization and enlarged chondrocytes with plump multinucleated lacunae.

TREATMENT

- Treatment of choice for a chondrosarcoma is *'wide local excision'* whenever feasible according to local disease extent, followed by limb salvage surgery. If limb salvage is not possible, amputation can be performed.
- Typically, chemo or radiotherapy has no role except chemotherapy in selected cases of dedifferentiated and mesenchymal chondrosarcoma.

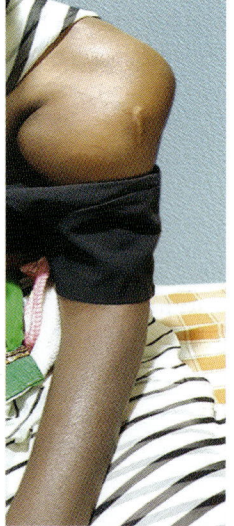

Fig. 40.6: Gross swelling of the proximal humerus.

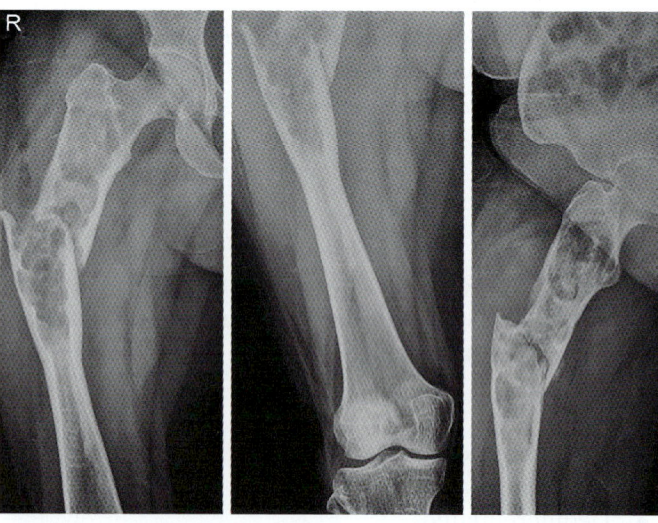

Fig. 40.7: Chondrosarcoma of proximal femur. Large lytic lesion affecting proximal femur with gross endosteal scalloping, with focal areas of matrix calcification and pathologic fracture.

SECTION 11

Peripheral Nerve and Brachial Plexus Injuries

SECTION OUTLINE

41. Approach to Peripheral Nerve Injuries
42. Specific Nerve Injuries
43. Brachial Plexus Injury

41 CHAPTER

Approach to Peripheral Nerve Injuries

SURGICAL ANATOMY OF A PERIPHERAL NERVE

- There are a total of 31 pairs of nerve roots: 8 cervical, 12 thoracic, 5 lumbar, 5 sacral, and 1 coccygeal.
- A mixed spinal nerve is formed with the union of the **ventral root (motor)** and **dorsal root (sensory),** which arise from the spinal cord. Further, each spinal nerve divides into *ventral (anterior division) ramus and dorsal ramus (posterior division)*. Each ramus is 'mixed in nature' having both sensory, motor, and autonomic components **(Fig. 41.1)**. Dorsal ramus collects sensory feeds from the dorsal trunk (skin and muscles of the back), while the ventral ramus feeds the ventral trunk and limbs.

Root: Either sensory/motor **Ramus:** Mixed (sensory, motor, autonomic)

- **Sensory fibers of dorsal and ventral rami:** It collects all somatic perceptions (touch, pressure, proprioception, vibration, pain, temperature) of the body. All sensory branches

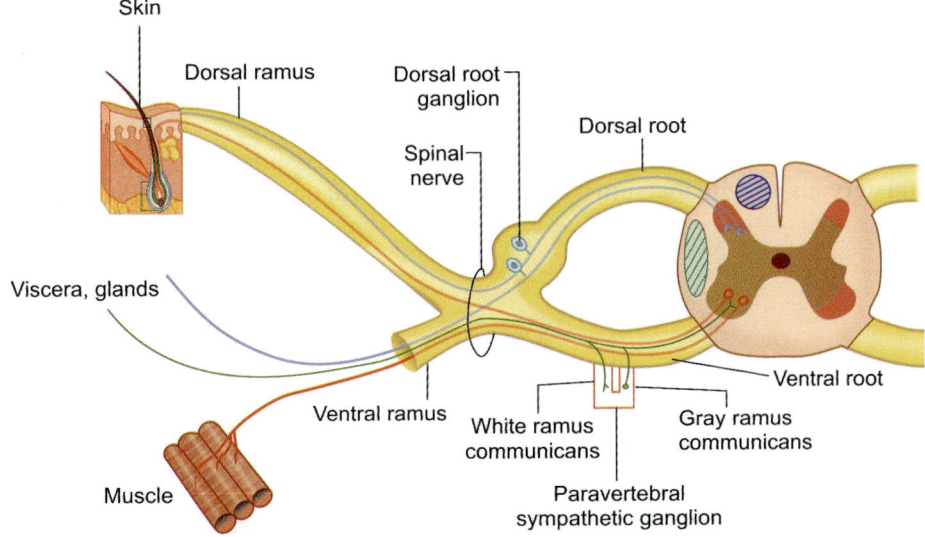

Fig. 41.1: Formation and supply of a peripheral nerve.

via dorsal and ventral rami finally enter the "dorsal root" of the spinal cord. Then, they are distributed into their respective tracts [spinothalamic tract (anterior and lateral) and posterior column tract] according to the type of sensation carried to be further relayed to the brain.
- **Motor fibers of dorsal and ventral rami:** It supplies all skeletal muscles of the body.
- **Autonomic fibers of dorsal and ventral rami:** It supplies all glands of skin and vessels.

BASIC UNIT OF A NERVE: AN AXON

The basic unit of a peripheral nerve is an axon comprising a cell body, an axonal cylinder and a terminal axon. The cell body lies in the anterior horn of the spinal cord. The neurilemmal sheath covers the axonal cylinder. The axonal cylinder terminates at the neuromuscular junction in the case of a motor fiber or a sensory organ in the case of a sensory nerve **(Fig. 41.2A)**. The axonal cylinder is responsible for ante- and retrograde conduction from the cell body to the axon terminal and reverse.

Microanatomy

Each nerve fiber is surrounded by a neurilemmal sheath, which is the outer cytoplasmic covering of the Schwann cell. Further, each nerve fiber is surrounded by loose connective tissue known as endoneurium. A group of many nerve fibers forms a fascicle surrounded by perineurium. Multiple fascicles form a nerve that is surrounded by epineurium **(Fig. 41.2B)**.

PATHOLOGIES AFFECTING NERVES

The peripheral nerve affection can affect the sensory and motor function of the extremity. Nerve affection/injury could be mononeuropathy/polyneuropathy.
- **Mononeuropathy:** Mostly traumatic, compressive (carpal tunnel syndrome, tumor compression), or infective (Hansen's disease).
- **Polyneuropathy:** Generalized causes like metabolic and endocrinal (diabetes mellitus, vitamin B complex deficiency), chemical exposure, inflammatory diseases [rheumatoid arthritis, systemic lupus erythematosis (SLE)], vasculitis, chronic alcoholism, and medications.

Clinically, one must differentiate between peripheral nerve affection (lower motor neuron) or central nervous system affection (brain and spinal cord; upper motor neuron).

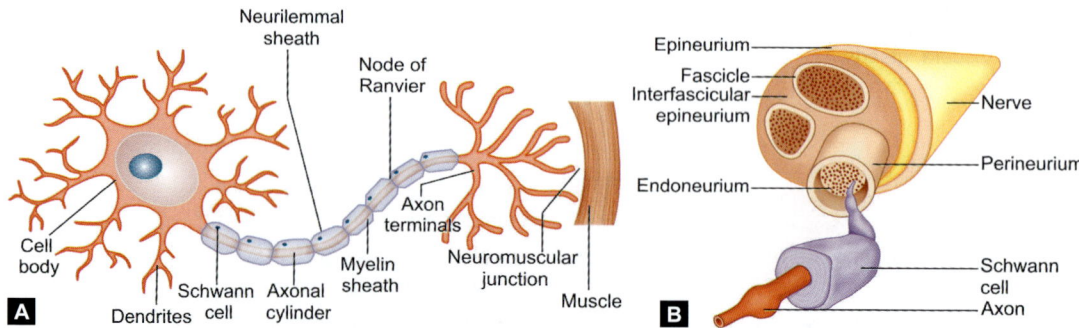

Figs. 41.2A and B: (A) Structure of an axon; (B) Microanatomy of a nerve.

Common conditions affecting nerves (mono/polyneuropathy)
Traumatic: Mechanical, thermal, chemical, surgical (iatrogenic)
Metabolic and endocrinal: Diabetes, vitamin deficiency: B_1, B_6, B_{12} deficiency
Infection: Hansen's disease, Lyme's disease, HIV, herpes simplex
Compressive neuropathy: Malunited #, carpal tunnel syndrome, tumor compressing nerves
Autoimmune diseases: Rheumatoid arthritis (RA), systemic lupus erythematosus (SLE), sarcoidosis, Guillain-Barré syndrome
Alcohol, chemicals: Chronic alcoholism, lead, exposure to glue, solvents, insecticides
Genetic: Friedreich's ataxia, Charcot-Marie-Tooth disease, Fabry's disease
Others: Medication (anticonvulsant, anti-HIV), radiation

MECHANISMS OF INJURY TO A PERIPHERAL NERVE

Peripheral nerves are susceptible to be injured by various mechanisms.
- **Acute compression** is usually by *crutches/faulty posture/tourniquets*. Usually, neuropraxia, and occasionally axonotmesis occurs in such injuries.
- **Traction** during *closed fractures/dislocations*. Usually, neuropraxia/axonotmesis type of injury to the nerve happens during traction.
- **Laceration/crush injury** usually results in neurotmesis.
- **Ischemic injury** during *Volkmann's ischemia*. It causes extensive fibrosis of the nerves, resulting in multifocal injury.
- **Chemical injury** by *local injection*. It causes extensive fibrosis of nerves and carries a poor prognosis.
- **Electrical injury** results in extensive longitudinal fibrosis and carries a poor prognosis.
- **Infection** *such as Hansen's disease* causes nerve inflammation and fibrosis.
- **Toxins** *such as lead* cause nerve inflammation and fibrosis.
- **Radiation and thermal injury** cause nerve fibrosis and carry a poor prognosis.
- **Metabolic** *such as vitamin B_{12} deficiency*, causes demyelination.

CLASSIFICATION OF NERVE INJURIES

The nerve injury classification helps plan the treatment and prognosis **(Table 41.1)**.
- **Seddon's classification:** Described by Sir Herbert Seddon in 1943. Seddon classified nerve injury into three types—neuropraxia, axonotmesis, and neurotmesis.
  - **Neuropraxia:**
    - It is the *mildest type* of nerve injury and occurs as a result of compression.
    - Structurally, there is a *"focal conduction block to nerve impulses in the axonal cylinder without disrupting the axon or endoneurium."*
    - Since there is *no structural disruption*, there is **no Wallerian degeneration**
    - It has excellent prognosis, and it recovers within 4–6 weeks.
  - **Axonotmesis:** "tmesis" means "to cut";
    - It is *moderate in severity* and occurs due to traction.
    - Structurally, the *"axons and myelin sheath are disrupted, whereas endoneurium or perineurium intact."*
    - Since there is *structural injury*, there is **Wallerian degeneration and regeneration**
    - Spontaneous recovery is usually good. However, the recovery may take 6–18 months.

Table 41.1: Differences between three types of nerve injury.

	Neuropraxia	Axonotmesis	Neurotmesis
Definition	- Focal conduction block to nerve impulses in the axonal cylinder - No anatomical damage	- Injury to axon cylinder - Intact endoneurial or perineurial sheath	Complete severance of axon along with its epineurial sheath
Injured in	Compression	Traction	Laceration/crush
Severity	Mild	Moderate	Severe
Wallerian D and R	None	Yes	Yes
Tinel's sign	None	Yes	Only if repaired
Motor march	None	Yes	Only if repaired
NCV—distal segment excitability	Maintained	Lost	Lost
EMG—fibrillation and denervation potential in muscles	Absent	Present at 2–3 weeks. Also, polyphasic action potential at recovery.	Present at 2–3 weeks
Recovery	4–6 weeks	6–18 months	None without repair
Prognosis	Excellent	Good	Poor

(D: degeneration; R: regeneration; NCV: nerve conduction velocity; EMG: electromyography)

- **Neurotmesis:**
  - The most severe form of injury occurs as a result of laceration/crush injury.
  - Structurally, there is a *"complete severance of nerve along with its epineurium sheath."*
  - Since there is *structural injury*, nerve undergoes **Wallerian degeneration. However, regeneration in the distal end depends upon whether two ends are in contact or not**.
  - It does not spontaneously recover without surgical intervention.
- **Sunderland classification:** Described by Sir Sydney Sunderland in 1951.
  - *First degree:* Myelin injury; rest intact (akin to neuropraxia)
  - *Second degree:* Axon injury; rest intact
  - *Third degree:* Endoneurium cut; rest intact } (akin to axonotmesis)
  - *Fourth degree:* Perineurium cut; rest intact
  - *Fifth degree:* Entire trunk cut (akin to neurotmesis).

NEURONAL WALLERIAN DEGENERATION-REGENERATION

After the physical injury to the nerve, it undergoes a process of degeneration within 24–36 hours of injury, followed by regeneration, known as Wallerian degeneration and regeneration. Both proximal and distal segments undergo the Wallerian changes known as primary (indirect) and secondary (direct), respectively.
- **Primary retrograde/indirect Wallerian degeneration** occurs *in the proximal segment*, wherein the degeneration proceeds to just the proximal node of Ranvier from the injury site. Also, transient disturbance in the cell body is noted as swelling, chromatolysis, and recovery.

Chapter 41: Approach to Peripheral Nerve Injuries

- **Secondary/direct Wallerian degeneration**: It occurs *in the distal fragment* until the end of the neuron. The changes observed in Wallerian degeneration are:
  - The axon cylinder and myelin sheath break down and get fragmented.
  - After 4–7 days, macrophages enter the area to clear the debris.
  - By 2–4 weeks, the process of debris clearance is over.
  - Neurilemma, endoneurium, and Schwann cells escape the injury and remain intact.
- **Process of regeneration:**
  - The residual Schwann cells release growth factors that stimulate axonal sprouting from the proximal end of the axonal cylinder. Also, Schwann cells form a cell column known as 'Bands of Bungner,' which provides a pathway for axonal growth.
  - Around 50–100 sprouts regrow from the proximal end of the axonal hillock. The growing sprouts enter the endoneurium hollow tube. Only one sprout grows into the endoneurium, and the rest degenerate. The intact endoneurium provides a track to reach the neuromuscular junction.
  - Schwann cells begin the process of remyelination when contacted by axonal sprouts.
  - The rate of nerve regeneration is 1 mm per day.
  - If the axonal sprouts do not manage to migrate into the endoneurial tube or this migration is interrupted, it leads to 'neuroma' formation. It could be end-neuroma or neuroma-in-continuity.

CLINICAL DIAGNOSIS OF A NERVE INJURY

A detailed history and examination of the patient should be performed.

- **Inspection for** attitude, deformity, scars, muscle wasting, skin changes, trophic changes (smooth and shiny skin, ulcerations, and subcutaneous tissue atrophy) and local temperature.
- **Palpation of nerves** include tenderness and thickening of the nerves.
- **Active and passive movements** at the joint must be assessed. **Muscle wasting** should be measured.
- **Sensory examination:** The main objective of the sensory examination is to assess the level of the lesion or the nerve involved. Peripheral nerves carry all types of sensation, which are further distributed to various tracts of the spinal cord [anterior and lateral spinothalamic tract (ASTT, LSTT), posterior column tract (PCT)]. In a peripheral nerve injury, assessing any one sensation (commonly crude touch) in their autonomous zone suffices. However, in case of a nerve root injury (brachial plexus), the sensation assessment is according to the dermatomal pattern as nerve root is part of many nerves.
- **Motor examination** includes: *Bulk* (nutrition) of muscles, *Tone* of muscles; *Power* (MRC grading)—grade 0–5, *Reflexes* (superficial and deep), *Coordination* of movements, and *Abnormal movements*. Coordination and abnormal movements *are essential in CNS examination rather than PNS affections!*
- **Autonomic examination:** For peripheral nerve affection involving the sympathetic nervous system supply to the skin, *sympathetic skin response* (SSR) can be confirmed. SSR test uses an electric current to stimulate sympathetic nerves. The tests measure the change in electrical resistance,

Sensations in various tracts of spinal cord
ASTT: Crude touch, pressure
LSTT: Pain, temperature
PCT: Fine touch, proprioception, vibration, stereognosis, 2-point discrimination, tactile discrimination, tactile localization

which is altered in the presence of sweat. Another test is the starch iodine test. However, in routine clinical practice, autonomic examination is not performed.
- **Signs of nerve recovery:**
  - The *recovery in sensations, motor power, and reflex response* at each follow-up must be noted.
  - The presence of *Tinel's sign and motor march phenomena* are important signs of nerve recovery. They are typically observed in axonotmesis and repaired neurotmesis, while they are absent in neuropraxia.
    - *Tinel's sign (Hoffman sign):*
      - The nerve is gently tapped or percussed along its course in a *'distal to proximal direction.'* A positive Tinel's sign is indicated by a transient tingling/shock-like sensation in the nerve distribution area, persisting for several seconds.
      - Tinel's sign is felt due to hypersensitive regenerating nerves. However, it is suggestive only for sensory recovery, not motor one.
      - Tinel's sign is of prognostic significance only if "distal progression" exists on each follow-up. A static Tinel's sign, i.e., when elicited at the same point on each follow-up, is of a negative value as it is suggestive of neuroma formation.
      - The typical response—tingling/shock of Tinel's sign fades as myelination occurs and is not present after complete myelination of the regenerating nerve.
    - *Motor march:* During the Wallerian regeneration, the muscles nearest to the point of injury recover first due to early innervation, followed by distal ones. This phenomenon is called a motor march. It is observed in axonotmesis and repaired neurotmesis but not in neuropraxia.

INVESTIGATIONS

- **X-ray of the affected part** to rule out fracture and dislocation.
- **Electrodiagnostic studies:** Nerve conduction velocity (NCV) and electromyography (EMG) studies are helpful in diagnosis, location, the extent of the injury, treatment planning prognosis, and recovery pattern of nerves and muscles. *NCV and EMG must be performed after 3 weeks of the primary injury.*
  One can also perform a strength-duration curve (SDC) to assess normal, partially innervated or denervated muscle.
  Note: The description of EMG, SDC, and NCV is discussed after the description of factors affecting nerve recovery.
- **Other relevant investigations** confirm other causes of nerve affection. For example, nerve biopsy in a suspected case of Hansen's disease, serum vitamin B_{12} level.

TREATMENT OF NERVE INJURIES

The treatment of the nerve injury, which could be conservative or operative, depends upon the type (traumatic/other) and severity (neuropraxia/axonotmesis/neurotmesis) of the nerve injury.
- **Traumatic nerve injury:** Most commonly, **closed fractures and dislocations result in neuropraxia/axonotmesis** type of nerve injury, whereas **open injuries may result in neurotmesis**.

- **Nontraumatic nerve injury:** The management (conservative/operative) of non-traumatic nerve affection is based on the etiology and its possible outcome. Furthermore, the treatable cause must also be treated, e.g., Hansen's disease, vitamin B_{12} deficiency.

MANAGEMENT OF TRAUMATIC NERVE INJURY

It can be managed by "conservative or operative means," depending upon the type of nerve injury. The initial basis of managing a nerve injury is based on the fact that ***closed fractures and dislocations generally result in neuropraxia/axonotmesis***, whereas ***open injuries may result in neurotmesis***.

Neuropraxia and axonotmesis respond to the conservative method, while neurotmesis requires operative intervention. A brief outline of the management of all three types of nerve injuries is mentioned in **Flowchart 41.1**.

- **The conservative/wait-n-watch approach** is indicated in: (i) Neuropraxia and (ii) the initial treatment of axonotmesis.
  - Neuropraxia always recovers within 3–6 weeks with conservative treatment.
  - Axonotmesis is initially given a conservative trial for 3–4 months. If the nerve shows progressive and satisfactory clinicofunctional recovery, conservative treatment is continued; otherwise operative option is opted.

The conservative treatment comprises three standard principles:

1. ***Splinting of the affected part in the functional position:*** The splinting in the functional position ensures that even if stiffness persists in the affected part, the part/joint is stiff in the functional position, which enables the patient to perform a specific primary function that needs a functional position.

Flowchart 41.1: Algorithm to treat traumatic nerve injuries.

(Rehab: rehabilitation; ES: electrical stimulation)

2. ***Passive mobilization*** of all the affected joints and encourage the active movement of unaffected joints.
3. ***Electrical stimulation of the paralyzed muscle*** to prevent disuse atrophy.

Green hash line in **Flowchart 41.1** indicates that late cases of axonotmesis cases, which present after 9–12 months of primary injury without any recovery, are directly taken up for tendon transfers/arthrodesis as nerve repair may not yield fruitful result due to degeneration of Schwann cells, endoneurial tubes, neuromuscular junction, and irreversible muscle atrophy.

- **Operative treatment:** *The principle of nerve repair is that nerve repair should be done in a clean vascular field in a tensionless fashion.* The indications of nerve exploration/repair are:
  - Neurotmesis
  - No/poor recovery after conservative treatment of axonotmesis
  - Open nerve injuries
  - No recovery after nerve repair (for tendon transfer).

There are a variety of operative treatments performed after the nerve injury, such as:
A. **Neurolysis**: Release of the intact nerve from scar tissue/callus entrapment.
B. **Coaptation**: Approximating severed nerve ends (fascicle to fascicle).
C. **Primary or secondary nerve repair (neurorrhaphy)** with or without nerve grafting. Nerve repair could be epineurial/perineurial/epi-perineurial.
   - Nerve graft is taken from the sural/saphenous/greater auricular nerve.
D. **Neurotization** implies nerve transfer. It is a common treatment option for brachial plexus injuries.
E. **Tendon transfer** is done in situations like:
   - Nerve is no more amenable to repair
   - Failed nerve repair.

   Box 41.1 lists the principles of tendon transfer.
F. **Arthrodesis** is performed when there is no possibility of tendon transfer. ***However, it should be avoided in insensate limbs*** as arthrodesis may fail and may result in trophic ulcer formation due to a rigid limb.

The specific management of common nerve injuries are briefly mentioned in **Table 41.2**.

> **Box 41.1:** Principles of tendon transfer.
> - Age of the patient should be more than 5 years
> - The joint, which must move after tendon transfer should not be stiff
> - Power of tendon should be grade 4 or more
> - Synergistic muscle transfer preferably
> - The plane of transfer should be scar free
> - It should be of similar strength and excursion
> - Transferred tendon should not affect existing function
> - It should have a straight line of pull

FACTORS INFLUENCING NERVE RECOVERY

- **Type of nerve injury:** Neuropraxia has the best prognosis, followed by axonotmesis. Neurotmesis carries the worst prognosis.
- **Age:** Children have a better prognosis.

Table 41.2: Specific management of common nerve injuries.

Nerve palsy	Conservative (splint)	Common tendon transfer/static procedure
Radial nerve	**Cock up splint:** Prevents wrist and finger drop **(Fig. 41.3)**	***Modified Jones transfer*** For wrist extension: PT to ECRB Finger extension at MCP: FCU/FCR to EDC Thumb extension: PL to EPL
Median nerve	**Splints maintaining** thumb abduction and opposition **(Fig. 41.4)**	• **Low median palsy:** Restore thumb abduction and opposition ***"Bunnell's opponensplasty":*** FDS of ring finger transferred to APB (via FCU pulley) • **High median palsy** – Restore thumb IP flexion: Brachioradialis to FPL – Restore long finger flexion: Side-side suture of FDP of the ring and little finger to FDP of index and middle finger

Ulnar nerve	**Knuckle bender splint:** Keeps MCP flexed and IP extended **(Fig. 41.5)**	• **Restore thumb adduction:** FDS to adductor pollicis
		• **Index finger abduction:** APL/ECRL to 1st dorsal interossei
		• **Reverse clawing effect:** Three common transfers are described wherein the 'selected tendon' is transferred to the extensor hood via the lumbrical canal volar to the transverse metacarpal ligament.
		  1. ***Paul Brand's:*** ECRL/ECRB transfer
		  2. ***Fowler's:*** EI, EDM transfer
		  3. ***Bunnell's:*** FDS of middle or ring finger transfer
		Static procedure
		Zancolli's capsulodesis: Volar capsule of MCP is shortened

Common peroneal nerve (CPN)	**Foot drop splint** also known as ankle foot orthosis **(Fig. 41.6)**	In foot drop due to CPN palsy, the tibialis posterior (TP) tendon is transferred by two methods: 1. **Ober's circumtibial transfer:** The TP tendon is routed around the tibia and transferred over the 3rd metatarsal base/lateral cuneiform 2. **Barr's/Watkins transfer:** The TP tendon is routed through the interosseous membrane and transferred over 3rd metatarsal base/lateral cuneiform

(IP: interphalangeal; PT: pronator teres; ECRL/B: extensor carpi radialis longus/brevis; FCU: flexor carpi ulnaris; APB: abductor pollicis brevis; FPL: flexor pollicis longus; FCR: flexor carpi radialis; EI: extensor indicis; EDM: extensor digiti minimi; MCP: metacarpophalangeal)

- **Level of injury:** More proximal the injury, the more incomplete is the recovery.
- **Type of nerve:** Sensory/motor
    ◆ Pure sensory or gross motor nerves, such as radial nerve: ***Better prognosis***
    ◆ Fine motor (ulnar/median): ***Poor prognosis***
- **Mechanism of injury:**
    ◆ A direct, sharp cut that can be sutured: ***Better prognosis***.
    ◆ A crush of large segment/chemical injury/severe traction injury damaging a significant segment/conditions causing extensive nerve fibrosis: ***Poor prognosis***.

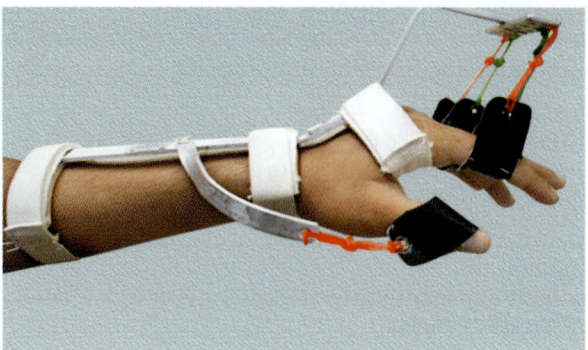

Fig. 41.3: Dynamic cock up splint for radial nerve palsy.

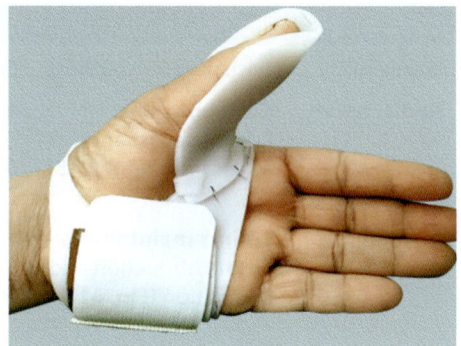

Fig. 41.4: Thumb abduction splint for median nerve injury.

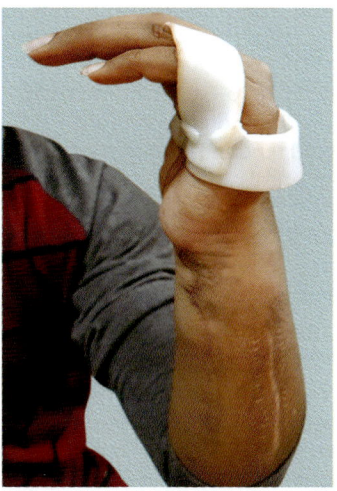

Fig. 41.5: Knuckle bender splint for ulnar nerve injury.

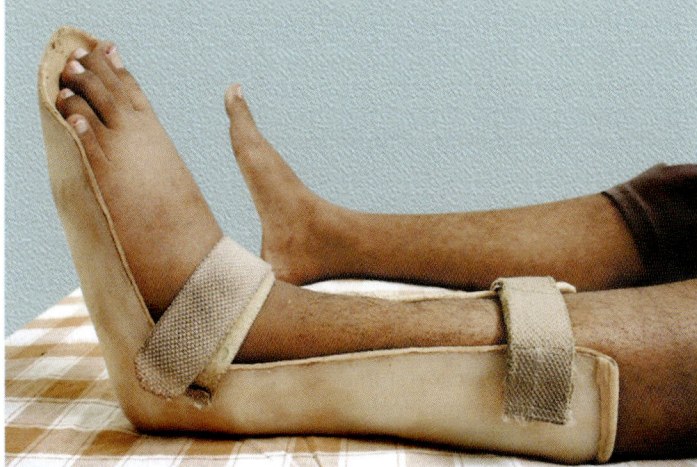

Fig. 41.6: Foot drop splint for common peroneal or sciatic nerve injury.

- **The delay between injury and repair:** Delayed repair can have a poor prognosis as endoneurial tubes and Schwann cells degenerate. The limit is 18–24 months. Further, the target muscle becomes 'irreversibly atrophied' by 12–18 months affecting the outcome even if the nerve regenerates—furthermore, the neuromuscular junction degenerates affecting the function of a recovered nerve.
- **Tension at repair site:** Tensionless repair in the vascular field should be the aim.
- **The gap between nerve ends:** Larger the gap, poor is the recovery.
- **Associated condition:** Local infection and ischemia lead to poor prognosis.

COMPLICATIONS OF NERVE INJURY

- Failed regeneration of nerve
- Muscle atrophy and contractures
- Neuropathic pain

- Ulcers at the insensate areas of the skin
- Economic losses
- Psychological issues.

BASICS OF EMG, SDC, AND NCV

- **Electromyography (EMG):** EMG is the graphic recording of the electrical activity of muscles at rest and voluntary contraction through a needle electrode inserted into the muscle.

    Uses of EMG:
    - To differentiate between complete and incomplete nerve injuries
    - Status of regeneration of nerve
    - To differentiate between neuropathy and myopathy.

    Patterns of EMG: The EMG patterns in normal, denervated, and reinnervated muscles are discussed below:
    - *Normal innervated muscle*: A normal muscle at rest has its muscle action potential (MAP). However, it remains unrecordable as the stronger nerve action potential suppresses it.
    - *Denervated muscle:* When a muscle denervates, the MAP becomes recordable at rest, forming the basis of **denervation potentials**. However, these denervation MAPs are recordable only after 2–3 weeks of the injury to the nerve. Hence, EMG must be performed 2–3 weeks after the nerve injury.
    If there is no denervation potential at the end of three weeks, it indicates an intact nerve.
    - *Post-denervation:* **Reinnervation polyphasic motor unit potentials** indicate recovering nerve. Lack of renervation potentials after 12 weeks of the injury, nerve recovery is unlikely and forms the basis of indication for nerve exploration.
    Note: MAP due to "nerve injury denervation" differs from myopathy 'multiphasic potentials', which helps differentiate neuropathy from myopathy.

- **Strength-duration (SD) curve (Fig. 41.7):**
    - A SD graph relating the varying intensity of an electrical stimulus within the physiological limit (galvanic/faradic) to the length of time it must flow to evoke muscle response effectively.
    - *SD curve plotting determines whether the stimulated muscle is innervated, partially innervated, or denervated*.
    - The physiological limit of stimulation is expressed as rheobase and chronaxie. Rheobase is the minimum stimulus strength that evokes a response. Chronaxie is the stimulus duration required to stimulate a muscle when the stimulus strength is set to exactly at double rheobase.
        - *Faradic current*: Low strength, short duration
        - *Galvanic current*: High strength, long duration.
    - *While plotting the SDC (Fig. 41.7), the curve tends to shift to the right if denervated.*
        - *Normally innervated muscle (a):* The muscle is stimulated by reducing the current from 300 ms to 0.01 ms; the current required proportionately increases.
        - *Denervated muscle (b):* It needs a current of longer duration or higher strength (Galvanic current).
        - *Partially innervated muscle (c):* The SDC of partially innervated muscle lies between the normal and denervated muscle curve with a 'kink' in the SDC.

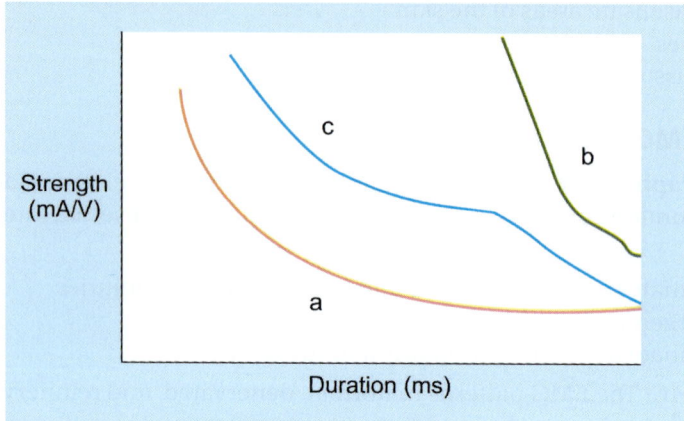

Fig. 41.7: Strength-duration curve of a normal muscle (a), denervated muscle (b), and partially innervated muscle (c).
(ms: millisecond; mA: milliampere; V: volt)

- **Nerve conduction study (NCS):** The study of the speed of conduction of an electrical impulse in a nerve by stimulating it through a surface-based electrode.
  The NCV studies aim for the following parameters of nerve conduction.
  Latency, amplitude, duration, and area under action potential curve.
    - *Latency*: Time between stimulus onset and onset of the peak (milliseconds)
    - *Amplitude*: The size of the response (microvolts)
    - *Duration*: Time from onset of the peak to return to baseline
    - *Area*: Represents several nerve fibers activated
    - Nerve conduction velocity = $\dfrac{\text{Distance traveled between two points}}{\text{Conduction time taken}}$

Timing of Performing NCS in Peripheral Nerve Injuries

If the nerve is in continuity, distal motor axons remain excitable for up to 1 week after injury, and sensory axons remain excitable for up to 2 weeks.
- **0–2 weeks:** Not required
- **2–4 weeks:** Best for baseline study; can distinguish between neuropraxia and axonotmesis
- **3–6 months:** Follow-up study; extent of reinnervation documented
- **6–12 months:** Follow-up study; extent of reinnervation at a greater distance from the injury site is documented.

Interpretations of NCS

- ***Sensory NCS:*** Distal stimulation of sensory nerve with the proximal recording [sensory nerve action potential (SNAP)]; *more sensitive than motor NCS.*
- ***CMAP for motor or mixed nerves:*** It is called compound motor action potential (CMAP). When a motor nerve is stimulated, CMAP represents the summation of all motor potentials recorded due to the recruitment of various motor units. *CMAP reduces in proportion to the volume of nerve injury, i.e., CMAP will reduce by 25%, if 25% of the motor nerve fibers are damaged.*
- ***Decreased amplitude/latency indicate nerve compression/neuropraxia.***

Common Conditions Diagnosed with NCV

Traumatic nerve injuries, mononeuropathy (carpal tunnel syndrome), polyneuropathy (diabetes), radiculopathy, myopathy, and muscular dystrophies.

Notes

CHAPTER 42

Specific Nerve Injuries

COMMON NERVE INJURIES

- Spinal accessory nerve
- Long thoracic nerve
- Thoracodorsal nerve
- Suprascapular nerve
- Axillary nerve
- Musculocutaneous nerve
- Radial nerve
- Median nerve
- Ulnar nerve
- Femoral nerve
- Sciatic nerve-tibial and common peroneal nerve component.

■ SPINAL ACCESSORY NERVE (SAN)

- **Originates from:** Medulla oblongata to upper cervical spinal cord (till C6)
- **Motor supply:** Sternocleidomastoid (SCM) and trapezius
- **Course:** Once it is out of the cranial fossa from the foramen magnum, it runs along the internal carotid artery to reach the sternocleidomastoid. It further pierces the muscle, runs into the posterior triangle, and supplies the trapezius muscle **(Fig. 42.1)**.
    - *Function of sternocleidomastoid:* Turn and tilt neck, neck flexion
    - *Function of trapezius:* There are three parts of trapezius, upper, middle and lower, which elevate, retract and depress scapula, respectively.
- **Injury to SAN** could occur in surgeries involving posterior triangle, such as lymph node biopsy, lymphadenectomy, and radical neck dissection.
- **Clinical features of SAN palsy:** It commonly results in trapezius weakness more than sternocleidomastoid, as injuries to SAN frequently occur distally while supplying trapezius.
    - *SCM weakness:* Difficulty in turning and tilting the neck.
    - *Trapezius weakness:* Lateral winging of scapula and difficulty in mid-arm abduction in the scapular plane.
- **Motor function tests of SAN:**
    - *Sternocleidomastoid*: Turn and tilt the neck, and neck flexion.
    - *Trapezius*: Shoulder shrugs against resistance, mid-arm abduction strength in the scapular plane.

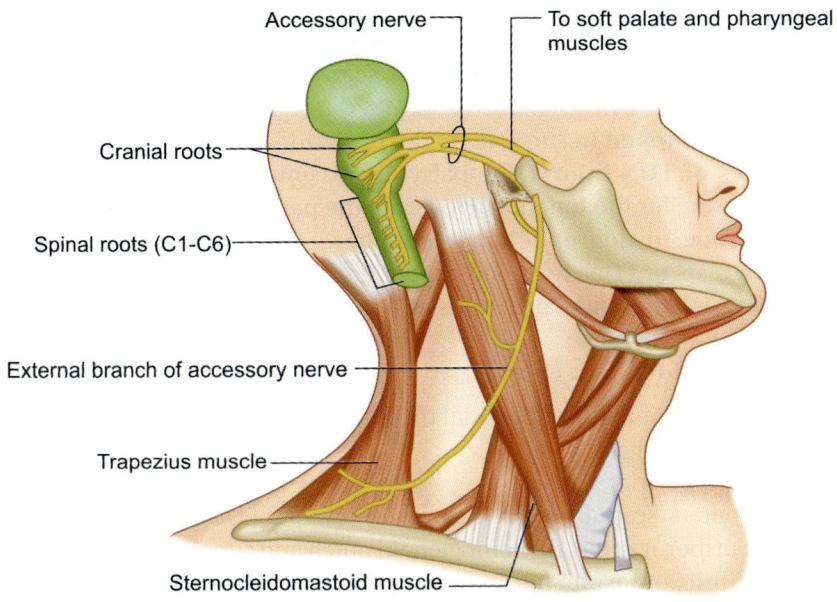

Fig. 42.1: Course and motor supply of spinal accessory nerve.

LONG THORACIC NERVE (LTN) (NERVE OF BELL)

- **Root value:** C5-C7
- **Motor supply:** Serratus anterior (boxer's muscle)
- **Course:** It descends into the cervicoaxillary canal while running behind the brachial plexus and further lies over the outer surface of serratus anterior **(Fig. 42.2)**.
- **The function of serratus anterior:** Protraction of scapula. Hence, it helps arm elevation above 90°. It also helps boxers as it protracts scapula while throwing a punch.
- **Injury to LTN could occur in** sports where there is a major blow to the sides of the ribs, or during radical mastectomies wherein axillary lymph node dissection is done.
- **Clinical features of LTN palsy:** *Medial winging of the scapula,* or trouble in elevating arm.
- **Motor function test of LTN:**
    - *Serratus anterior:* Wall pushing leads to medial winging of the scapula in case of LTN palsy.

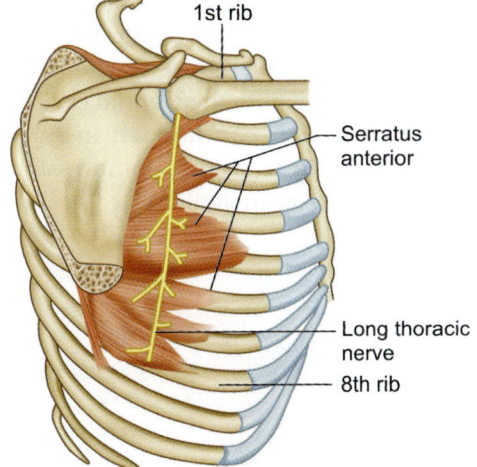

Fig. 42.2: Course and motor supply of long thoracic nerve.

THORACODORSAL NERVE (TDN)

- **Originates from:** Brachial plexus
- **Root value:** C6-C8

- **Motor supply:** Latissimus dorsi (Rower's muscle)
- **Course:** It follows the subscapular artery and runs on the posterior wall of the axilla **(Fig. 42.3)**.
- **Function of latissimus dorsi:** Depression of scapula; adduction, internal rotation, and extension of the arm.
- **Injury to TDN can happen in** surgeries of the posterior axillary wall.
- **Clinical features of TDN injury:** The palsy of latissimus dorsi is well-tolerated as other muscles compensate for the function. However, the patient may find difficulty in climbing while holding a rope, rowing, or holding a crutch.
- **Motor function tests of TDN:** Keep the patient's arm in 90° abduction and then ask him to adduct against resistance and palpate posterior axillary fold.

SUPRASCAPULAR NERVE (SSN)

- **Originates from:** Upper trunk of brachial plexus
- **Root value:** C5-C6
- **Course:** Runs via posterior triangle deep to trapezius and parallel to the inferior belly of omohyoid and enters scapula by passing under the suprascapular notch and innervates supraspinatus. Further, it enters the spinoglenoid notch and supplies infraspinatus **(Fig. 42.4)**.
- **Motor innervation:** Supraspinatus and infraspinatus
    - **Function of the supraspinatus:** Abduction of the arm. Further, along with infraspinatus, it helps to keep the head of the humerus centered in the glenoid for adequate abduction or elevation by the deltoid.
    - **Function of infraspinatus:** External rotation of the arm. Together, supra- and infraspinatus assist in shoulder abduction and keeping the head of the humerus centered onto the glenoid cavity, further helping the deltoid in flexion and abduction.
- **Injury to SSN can happen in** surgeries of the posterior triangle (lymph node biopsy), brachial plexus injury, compression at transverse suprascapular or spinoglenoid notch (usually by a ganglion cyst).

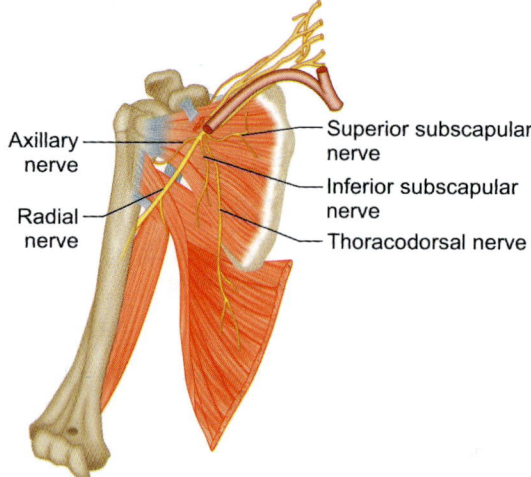

Fig. 42.3: Course and motor supply of thoracodorsal nerve.

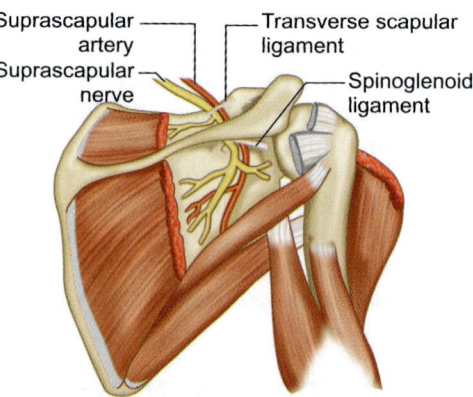

Fig. 42.4: Course and motor supply of suprascapular nerve.

- **Problem after the injury to SSN:** Due to supraspinatus and infraspinatus palsy, patient presents with weakness in abduction and external rotation of the arm.
- **Motor function test of SSN:**
  - *Supraspinatus:* Full can and empty can test
  - *Infraspinatus:* External rotation lag test.

AXILLARY NERVE (AN)

- **Originates from:** Posterior cord of brachial plexus
- **Root value:** C5-C6
- **Course:** It lies in the axilla below and anterior to the subscapularis muscle. It enters quadrangular space and winds around the surgical neck of the humerus, goes posteriorly along with posterior circumflex humeral vessels. It supplies deltoid and teres minor. The axillary nerve forms a "pseudoganglion" before it supplies teres minor **(Fig. 42.5)**. Anatomically, it lies 4–5 cm distal to the lateral acromion margin over lateral aspect of the shoulder. This is important to remember while operating on lateral aspect of shoulder.
- **Sensory innervation:** Lateral aspect of the arm
- **Motor innervation:** Deltoid, teres minor
  - *Function of the deltoid:* Arm flexion, abduction, and extension by the deltoid's anterior, mid- and posterior penna, respectively.
  - *Function of teres minor:* External rotation at the shoulder joint.
- **Injury to AN can happen in** shoulder dislocation, proximal humerus fractures, during surgical approaches—anterior approach to the shoulder around the subscapularis, and the transdeltoid lateral approach to the shoulder, and accidental injection over upper lateral aspect of the arm.

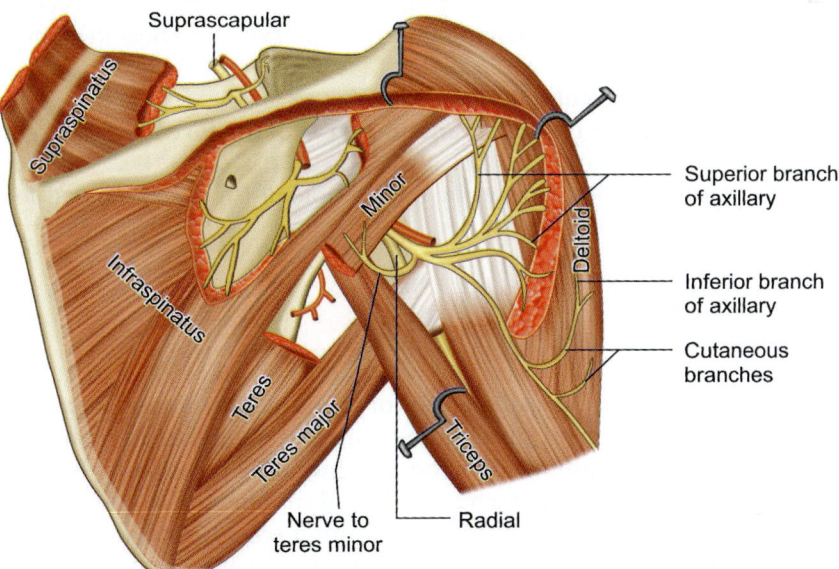

Fig. 42.5: Course and motor supply of axillary nerve.

- **Clinical features of AN palsy:** Due to deltoid palsy, there is wasting of deltoid **(Fig. 42.6)**. Also patient would have weakness in arm flexion, abduction, and extension. Due to teres minor palsy, there will be weakness in external rotation at the shoulder.
- **Clinical assessment of axillary nerve**
  - **Sensory assessment:** Assess sensation over the upper lateral aspect of the arm (regimental badge sign).
  - **Motor assessment**
    - *Deltoid*: Test for arm abduction strength, swallow tail sign for extension strength.
    - *Teres minor*: Assess external rotation strength in 90° abduction of arm. Hornblower sign is positive.

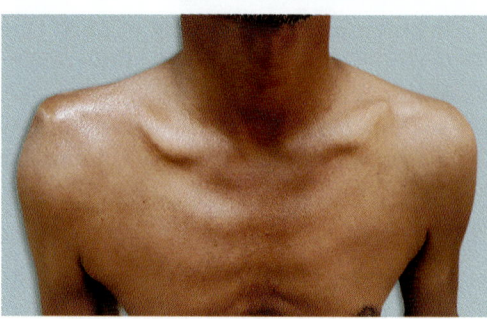

Fig. 42.6: Right deltoid wasting due to axillary nerve palsy.

MUSCULOCUTANEOUS NERVE

- **Originates from:** Lateral cord of brachial plexus
- **Root value:** C5-C7
- **Course:** It penetrates the coracobrachialis to enter the arm between the biceps and brachialis. It further descends and pierces the deep fascia of the elbow and continues downwards as the lateral cutaneous nerve of the forearm **(Fig. 42.7)**.
- **Sensory innervation:** Lateral aspect of the forearm
- **Motor innervation:** Biceps, brachialis, coracobrachialis
  The function of biceps, brachialis: Elbow flexion. The biceps also help in supination.
- **Injury to the musculocutaneous nerve can happen** during the *anterior approach* to the shoulder, or *Latarjet surgery* performed for anterior shoulder recurrent dislocation.
- **Problem after the injury to the musculocutaneous nerve:** Weakness in elbow flexion and forearm supination.
- **Clinical assessment of musculocutaneous nerve**
  - **Sensory assessment (as lateral cutaneous nerve of the forearm):** Sensation over the lateral aspect of the forearm.
  - **Motor assessment:** Elbow flexion by biceps brachii (in the supinated forearm) and brachialis (in the pronated forearm).

RADIAL NERVE (RN)

- **Originates from:** Posterior cord of brachial plexus.
- **Root value:** C5-T1.
- **Course:** Radial nerve lies in the axilla posterior to the axillary artery. It exits the axilla via triangular space posteriorly and supplies the long and medial head of the triceps before it enters the spiral (radial) groove over the mid-humerus posteriorly. It then enters the spiral groove alongside profunda brachii vessels and supplies the lateral head of the triceps and anconeus. After crossing the spiral groove from medial to lateral, radial nerve moves anteriorly by penetrating the lateral intermuscular septum. It then supplies brachioradialis and extensor carpi radialis longus (ECRL). RN further descends and crosses the elbow joint near the radial head, and divides into superficial (sensory) and deep branch (pure motor).

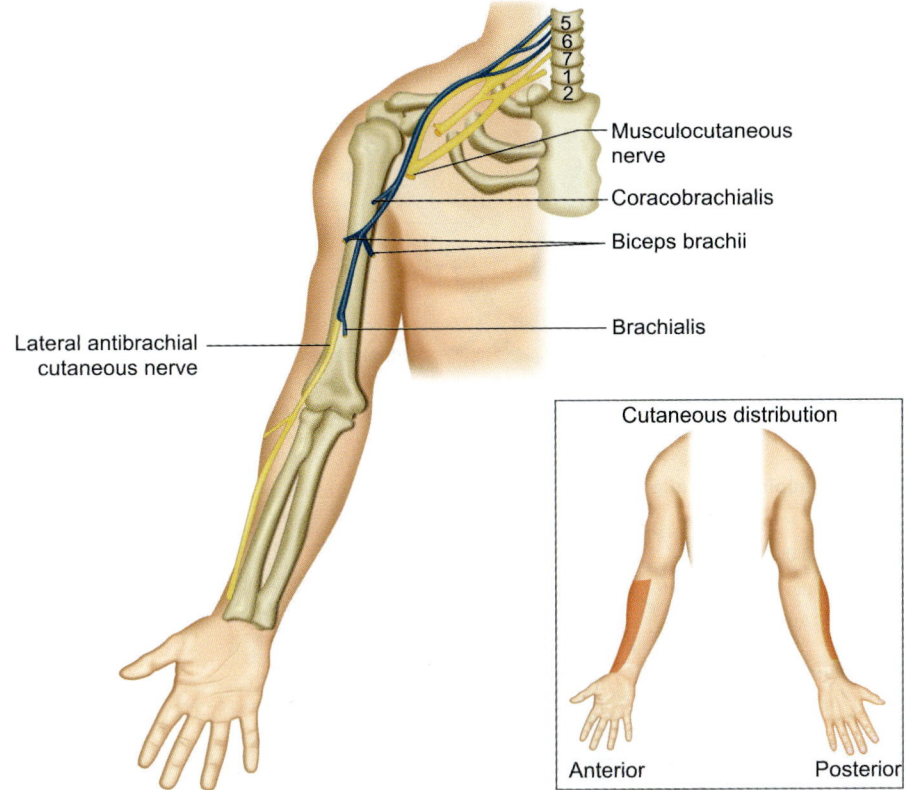

Fig. 42.7: Motor supply and cutaneous innervation of musculocutaneous nerve.

The superficial sensory branch continues distally in the forearm under the brachioradialis muscle and crosses the wrist to supply radial 3½ of the dorsum of the hand and 3½ fingers except for the nailbed (supplied by median nerve). The deep motor branch known as posterior interosseous nerve (PIN) supplies extensor carpi radialis brevis (ECRB), and further penetrates and supplies the supinator and all other extensor compartment muscles. PIN ends as a "pseudoganglion" under the extensor retinaculum and supplies wrist and intercarpal joints **(Fig. 42.8)**.

- **Sensory innervation:** Lower lateral aspect of the arm and posterior arm, proximal 1/3rd lateral forearm, posterior forearm and dorsum of the hand.
- **Motor innervation:** Triceps, anconeus, brachioradialis, and ECRL are innervated by the radial nerve. PIN innervates ECRB, supinator and the rest of the entire extensor compartment of the forearm **(Fig. 42.8)**.
- **The function of muscle supplied by the radial and PIN**
    - *Triceps:* Elbow extension
    - *Brachioradialis*: Elbow flexor and weak forearm supinator
    - *ECRL, ECRB*: Wrist extension and radial deviation
    - *Supinator:* Forearm supination
    - *ECU (extensor carpi ulnaris)*: Extension and ulnar deviation at the wrist
    - *ED (extensor digitorum)*: Extension of fingers at metacarpophalangeal (MCP) joint
    - *EPL (extensor pollicis longus):* Thumb extension at interphalangeal (IP) joint.

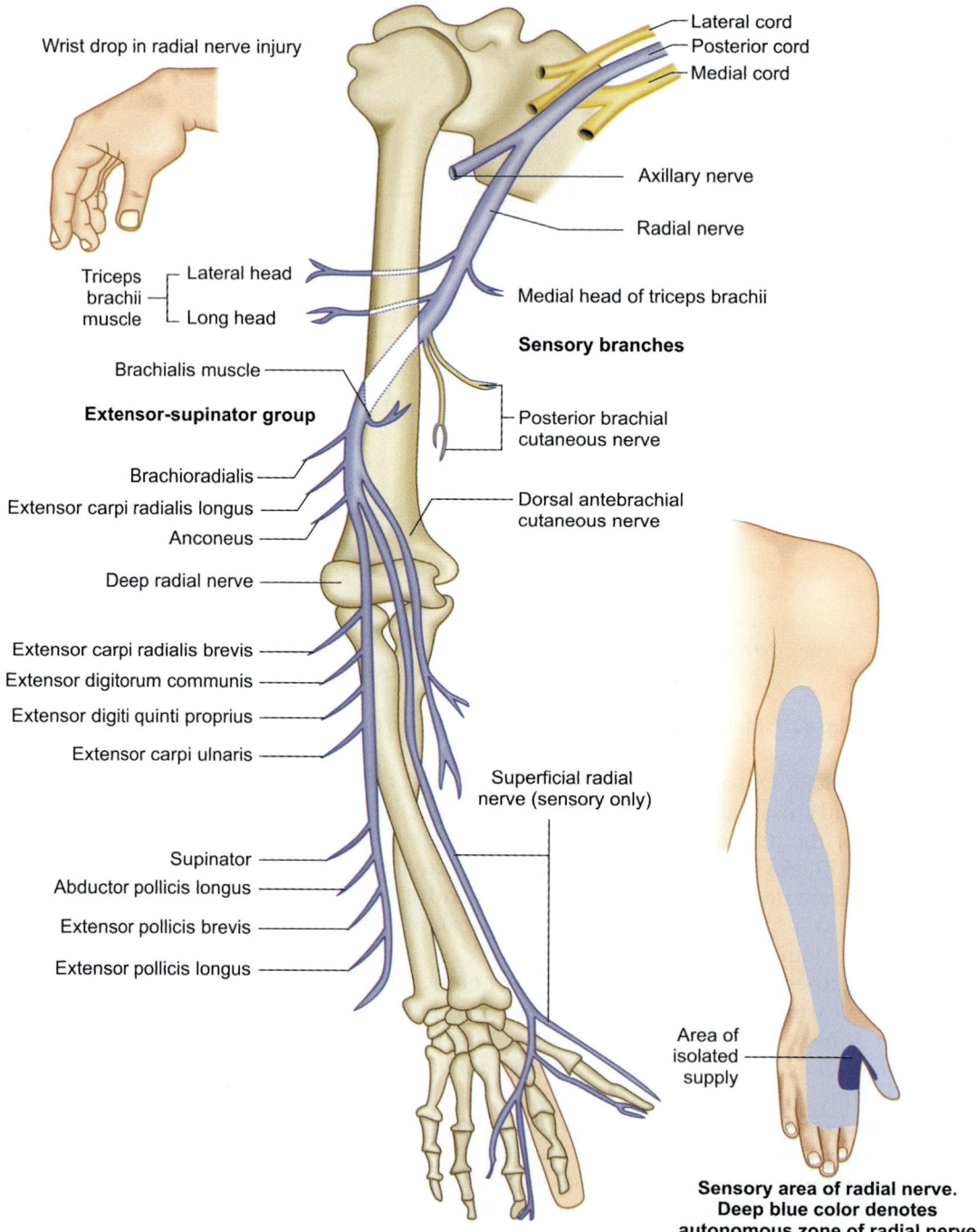

Fig. 42.8: Motor supply (left image) cutaneous innervation (right image) of radial nerve.

- *APL (abductor pollicis longus):* Extension at 1st CMC joint
- *EPB (extensor pollicis brevis):* Extension at MCP joint
- *EDM (extensor digiti minimi):* MCP extension at little finger
- *EI (extensor indicis):* MCP extension at index finger

- **Injury to the radial nerve could happen in** fracture shaft humerus, Holstein-Lewis fracture (lower one-third oblique or spiral # of humerus shaft), whereas PIN palsy is seen in Monteggia fracture-dislocation.
- **Clinical features of radial and posterior interosseous nerve palsy:**
    - High radial nerve injury (in the axilla): Weakness in elbow extension, *wrist, thumb, and finger drop. Loss of sensation over dorsum of 1st webspace.*
    - Low radial nerve palsy (in the spiral groove or just before it supplies ECRL): *Wrist, thumb and finger drop* **(Fig. 42.9)**. *Loss of sensation over dorsum of 1st webspace.*
    - PIN palsy: *Thumb and finger drop* (loss of IP and MCP extension). No sensory loss (as PIN is pure motor nerve)

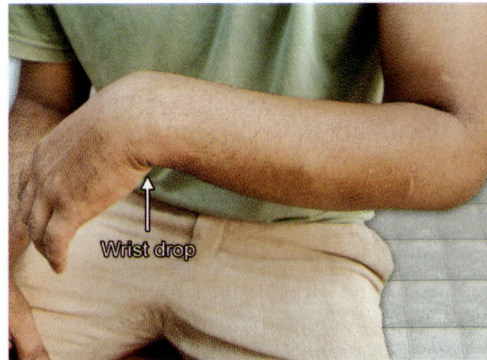

Fig. 42.9: Left side wrist drop due to radial nerve palsy.

- **Clinical assessment of radial and PI nerve**
    - **Sensory assessment:** Check sensation over the dorsum of first web space (autonomous zone for radial nerve).
    - **Motor assessment of major muscles**
        - *Triceps:* Elbow extension
        - *ECRL, ECRB:* Wrist extension and radial deviation
        - *ECU:* Wrist extension in ulnar deviation
        - *Brachioradialis:* Elbow flexion in mid-prone
        - *Supinator:* Forearm supination. However, isolation of various supinators is not possible.
        - *EPL:* Thumb extension at IP joint
        - *ED:* Dorsiflexion at MCP joint.
- **Management of radial and posterior interosseous nerve palsy:** The general management of radial nerve/PIN would be similar to conservative management of a nerve injury *(Refer Chapter 41)*. Specific management of radial nerve injury is discussed below.
    - **Splintage: Dynamic cock-up splint** should be applied during the day, which prevents wrist and finger drop allows active flexion at MCP and IP joints **(Fig. 42.10A)**. *Static cock up splint* should be applied at night **(Fig. 42.10B)**.

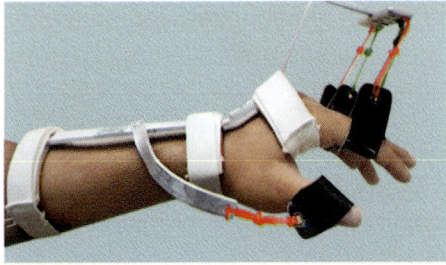
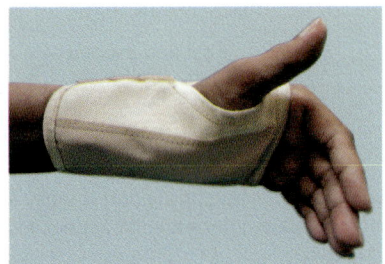

Fig. 42.10A: Dynamic cock up splint for radial nerve palsy.

Fig. 42.10B: Static cock up splint.

- **Modified Jones tendon transfer**
  - **For wrist extension:** Pronator teres to ECRB.
  - **Finger extension at MCP:** Flexor carpi ulnaris/flexor carpi radialis to extensor digitorum communis.
  - **Thumb extension:** Palmaris longus to extensor pollicis longus (EPL).

MEDIAN NERVE (MN)

- **Formed from:** Medial and lateral cord of brachial plexus
- **Root value:** C6-T1
- **Course:** After originating in the axilla, MN stays lateral to the axillary artery as it descends the arm, crosses it halfway down, and goes medial to the axillary artery. *It has no motor supply in the arm.* After crossing the cubital fossa, it enters the forearm and stays between flexor digitorum profundus (FDP) and flexor digitorum superificialis (FDS). There, it gives two branches; the anterior interosseous nerve (AIN) and the palmar cutaneous branch. *AIN supplies flexor pollicis longus, FDP and pronator quadratus.* In the distal third of the forearm, the median nerve emerges beneath FDS to lie medial to flexor carpi radialis (FCR) and lateral to palmaris longus, enters the carpal tunnel and divides into the recurrent motor branch and palmar digital nerves. The former supplies thenar muscles (opponens pollicis, abductor pollicis brevis), superficial head of flexor pollicis brevis, and lateral two lumbricals, whereas digital branches supply sensation over the volar aspect of 3½ digits, including nailbeds **(Fig. 42.11)**.

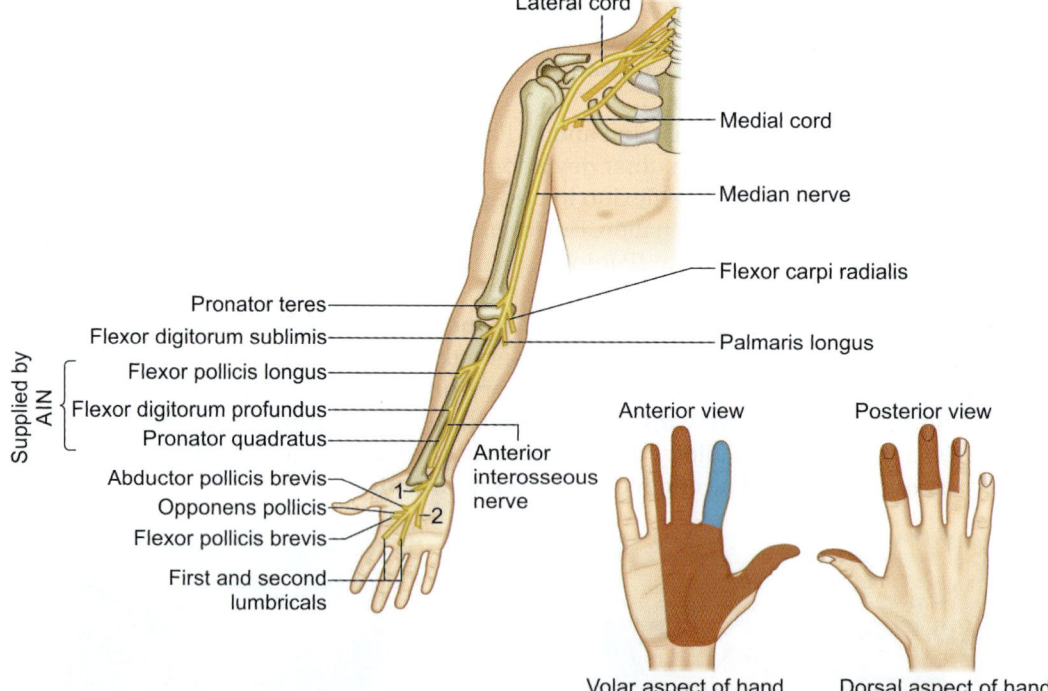

Fig. 42.11: Motor supply (left image) and cutaneous innervation (right image) of median nerve. The deep blue color on volar aspect of index finger indicates autonomous zone of median nerve.
(AIN: anterior interosseous nerve)

- **Sensory innervation:** The digital branches of median nerve supply radial 3½ fingers on volar aspect including nail beds.
- **Motor innervation:** Entire flexor compartment of the forearm except for FCU (flexor carpi ulnaris) and medial two heads of FDP (flexor digitorum profundus). Further, it supplies muscles of thenar eminence [abductor pollicis brevis (APB), opponens pollicis (OP), superficial head of flexor pollicis brevis (FPB)] and lateral two lumbricals.
- **Injury to the median nerve can happen in** supracondylar fracture humerus (extension type), elbow dislocation, compartment syndrome, carpal tunnel syndrome, and lunate dislocation.
- **Clinical features after the median nerve injury:** Patients complain of weakness in wrist, finger and thumb movements result in poor holding of objects, and grip. There may be an *ape thumb deformity* **(Fig. 42.12)**, which is more obvious in combined median and ulnar nerve palsy.
    - **High median nerve injury (above the elbow):** Weakness in wrist flexion, finger flexion, thumb flexion, thumb abduction, and opposition. There will be *ape thumb deformity*.
    - **Low median nerve palsy (after mid-forearm):** Weakness of thumb flexion, opposition, and abduction. Patients will have *ape thumb deformity*.
- **Clinical assessment of median nerve**
    - *Sensory assessment:* Volar tip of the index finger (autonomous zone)
    - *Motor assessment:*
        - *Flexor carpi radialis (FCR)*: Wrist flexion and radial deviation
        - *Pronator teres and quadratus*: Forearm pronation
        - *FDS* for PIP joint flexion and *FDP* for DIP joint flexion (only radial two fingers)
        - *FPL*: Flexion of thumb IP joint
        - *APB*: Pen test for thumb abduction
        - *Opponens pollicis:* Thumb opposition
        - *Ochsner's clasping index/pointing index sign is positive*

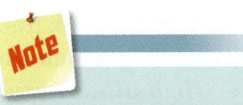

Carpal tunnel syndrome
Compression of median nerve under the flexor retinaculum of the wrist

- **Treatment of the median nerve injury:** The general management would be similar to conservative management of a nerve injury (*Refer Chapter 41*). The specific management of median nerve injury is discussed below.
    - **Splintage:** Thumb abduction splint is used to prevent thumb adduction contracture **(Fig. 42.13)**.
    - **Tendon transfer:** *Bunnell opponensplasty* to restore opposition. *For improving thumb flexion*, brachioradialis to FPL transfer. For further details, *Refer Chapter 41, Table 41.2*.

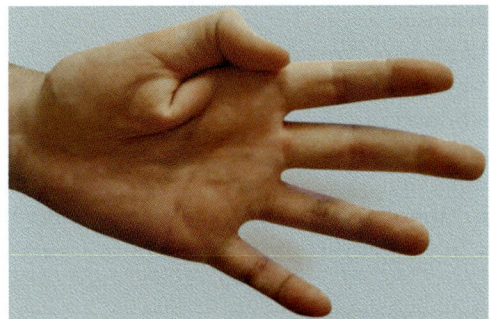

Fig. 42.12: Ape thumb deformity.

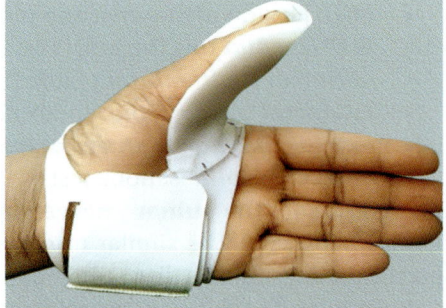

Fig. 42.13: Thumb abduction splint.

ULNAR NERVE (UN)

- **Originates from:** Medial cord of brachial plexus
- **Root value:** C8-T1
- **Course:** After originating in the axilla, it descends on the posteromedial aspect of the arm and crosses the elbow behind the medial epicondyle. It enters the forearm between the humeral and ulnar heads of flexor carpi ulnaris (FCU). It then supplies muscles in the forearm (FCU and medial two tendons of FDP). It descends and enters the hand via Guyon's canal above the flexor retinaculum and supplies muscles in hand-dorsal and palmar interossei, hypothenar muscles [abductor digiti minimi (ADM), flexor digiti minimi (FDM), opponens digiti minimi (ODM), and palmaris brevis], medial two lumbricals, adductor pollicis, and deep head of flexor pollicis brevis **(Fig. 42.14)**.
- **Sensory innervation:** Medial one and half fingers of the hand
- **Motor innervation:** FCU and medial two tendons of FDP in the flexor compartment of the forearm, hypothenar eminence (ADM, FDM, ODM), interossei, adductor pollicis and medial two lumbricals.
- **Injury to an ulnar nerve can happen in** brachial plexus injury, supracondylar humerus fracture (flexion type), elbow dislocation, cubitus valgus due to nonunion of lateral condyle humerus as tardy ulnar nerve palsy, compartment syndrome, and cubital tunnel syndrome, and hamate hook fracture.
- **Features/problems after the injury to the ulnar nerve:**
    - *High ulnar nerve injury (above or around the elbow)*: Weakness in wrist flexion in ulnar deviation (FCU palsy), FDP weakness in medial two fingers, interossei, medial two lumbricals, hypothenar muscles, and adductor pollicis. It presents as an ulnar paradox **(Box 42.1)**. Loss of sensation over ulnar border of the hand.
    - *Low ulnar nerve palsy (after mid-forearm or above the wrist)*: It presents as "classic ulnar claw hand" involving medial two fingers with weakness of hypothenar muscles, interossei, medial two lumbricals, and adductor pollicis **(Fig. 42.15)**. Also, there is loss of sensation over ulnar border of the hand. **Box 42.2** briefly describes the claw hand deformity.

    The combined median and ulnar palsy result in a 'complete claw hand' due to palsy of lateral lumbricals also.
- **Clinical assessment of ulnar nerve**
    - **Sensory assessment:** Sensations over the ulnar border of the little finger.
    - **Motor assessment**
        - *FCU*: Flexion of the wrist and ulnar deviation
        - *FDP (medial two fingers)*: Test for DIP flexion of medial two fingers
        - *Abductor digiti minimi*: Little finger abduction
        - *1st dorsal interosseous*: Index finger abduction
        - *Palmar and dorsal interosseous:* Card test
        - *Adductor pollicis*: Book test or Froment's sign
- **Treatment of the ulnar nerve injury:** The general management would be similar to described in Chapter 41. Specific management is discussed below.
    - *Splintage:* Knuckle bender splint is used to prevent MCP hyperextension **(Fig. 42.16)**

Cubital tunnel syndrome

Compression of ulnar nerve behind medial epicondyle

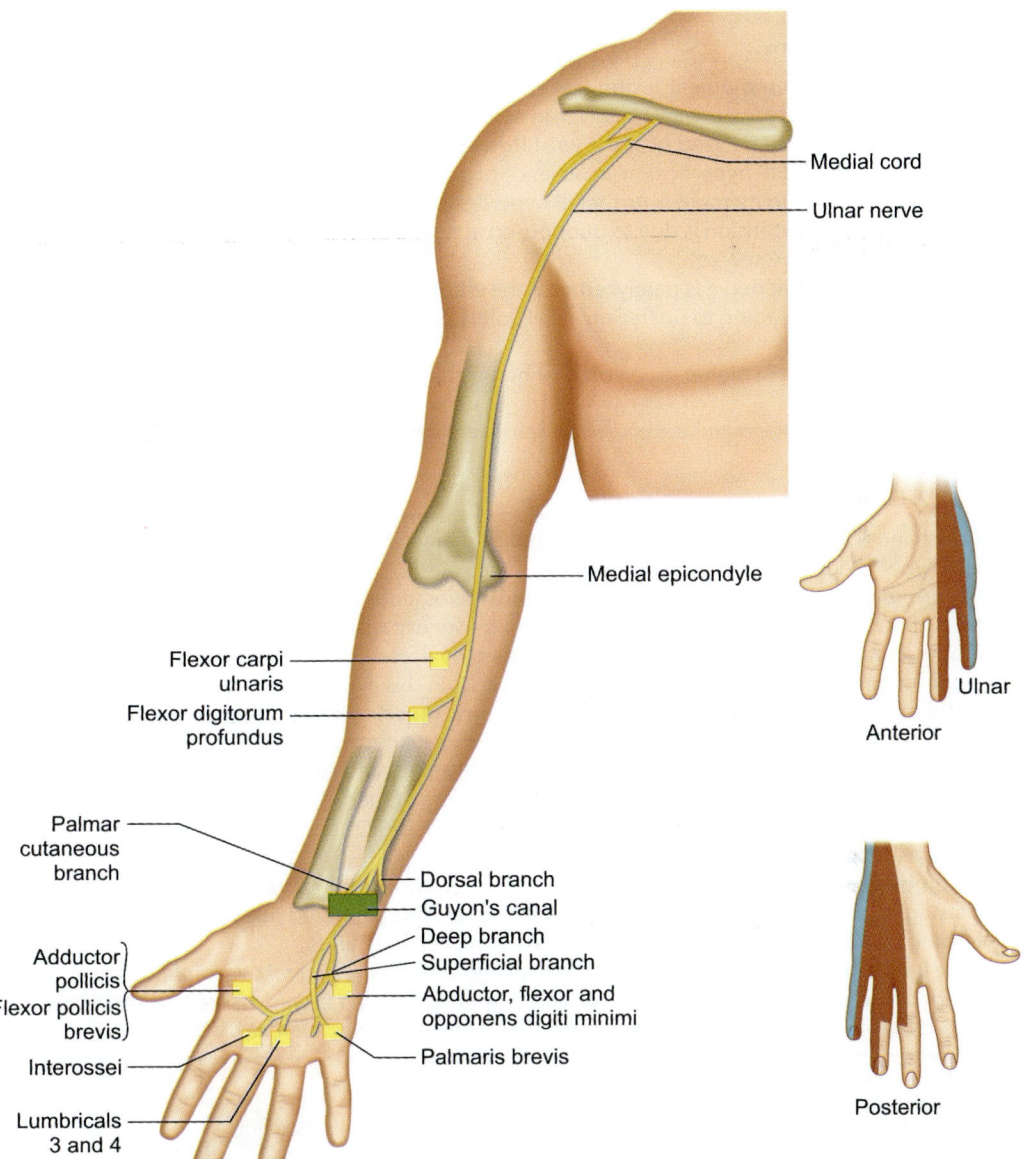

Fig. 42.14: Motor supply (left image) and cutaneous innervation (right images) of ulnar nerve. The deep blue color on ulnar border of little finger indicates autonomous zone of ulnar nerve.

- **Tendon transfer:** *Paul Brand, Bunnell's and Fowler's tendon transfers, Zancolli's capsulodesis.* For details, *Refer Chapter 41, Table 41.2.*

FEMORAL NERVE (FN)
- **Formed by:** Ventral rami of the posterior division of L2-4
- **Root value:** L2-4

Box 42.1: Ulnar paradox.

Usually higher the neurological lesion, severe is the paralysis and consequently **more obvious deformity in extremity** is the rule. However, in case of ulnar nerve injury, there is a paradox!

- When ulnar nerve is paralyzed near the wrist **(lower lesion)**, it leads to classic claw hand with MCP hyperextension and IP hyperflexion. In absence of action of interossei and lumbricals which flex MCP and extend IP joint; there is further IP hyperflexion is due to unopposed FDS and FDP action where MCP hyperextension is due to unopposed action of extensor digitorum. This makes claw deformity "look more severe".
- However, when ulnar nerve is paralyzed near the elbow **(higher lesion)**, it also paralyses FDP to 4th and 5th finger leading to no flexion at DIP joints. So clawing is "not so prominent" as compared to lower lesion.

This is the paradox that in higher lesion of ulnar nerve, the clawing is less prominent vis-à-vis low lesion at the wrist.

Box 42.2: Claw hand.

- Claw hand is also known as "intrinsic minus hand" characterized by hyperextension at MCP joint and hyperflexion at IP joints of fingers.
- **In normal condition:** Along with lumbricals, the interosseous muscle is responsible for flexion at MCP joint and IP joint extension while it joins extensor expansion. (*Note:* The extensor expansion is a structure on dorsum of fingers which is formed by dorsal digital expansion, extensor hood and extensor aponeurosis. The finger extensor tendons join this expansion).
- **Pathoanatomy:** Claw hand is due to **lack of intrinsic muscle power** (interossei and lumbricals) and overacting extrinsic [FDS, FDP (if spared) and finger extensors] at MCP and IP joints.
  When there is paralysis of ulnar nerve, the flexion at MCP and extension at IP action of medial two lumbricals and interossei is lost resulting in clawing of medial two fingers. Also, extension at MCPs by finger extensors and finger flexion at IP joint by FDS and FDP (overacting extrinsic) exaggerates clawing.
- In combined median and ulnar nerve palsy, the lateral two lumbricals are also paralyzed leading to clawing of lateral two fingers also. The thumb also remains paralyzed due to palsied median nerve leading to adducted thumb resembling hand of ape (Simian hand).

Note: In isolated median nerve palsy, there is no clawing even though lateral two lumbricals are paralyzed as major action on MCP flexion and IP extension is by interossei and is only assisted by lumbricals. Since, interossei are normal in isolated median nerve injury, the clawing does not take place.

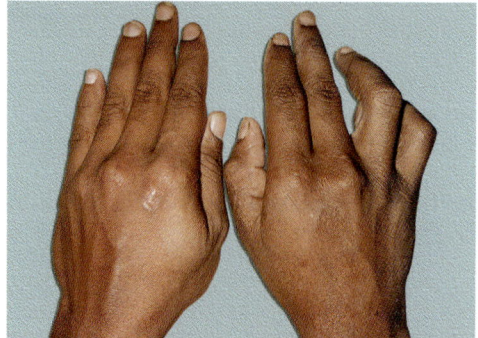

Fig. 42.15: Claw hand (right) showing MCP hyperextension and PIP flexion.

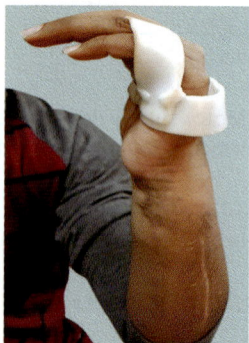

Fig. 42.16: Knuckle bender splint for claw hand.

- **Course:** The nerve descends in the abdomen from the lumbar plexus through psoas major muscle. The nerve further travels down into the thigh behind the mid-inguinal point. It divides into anterior and posterior branches, which supply the hip flexor and knee extensor, respectively **(Fig. 42.17)**.
- **Sensory innervation:** Anteromedial thigh and anteromedial leg and foot (saphenous nerve)
- **Motor innervation:** Hip flexor (iliacus, sartorius, pectineus), knee extensor (quadriceps)
- **Injury to the femoral nerve can happen** in direct trauma, anterior hip dislocation, iatrogenic
- **Problems after the injury to the femoral nerve:**
  - Loss of knee extension
  - Mild loss of hip flexion.
- **Clinical assessment of femoral nerve**
  - Sensory assessment
    - The anteromedial aspect of the thigh
    - The anteromedial aspect of the leg via the saphenous nerve.
  - Motor assessment
    - *Quadriceps*: Knee extension.

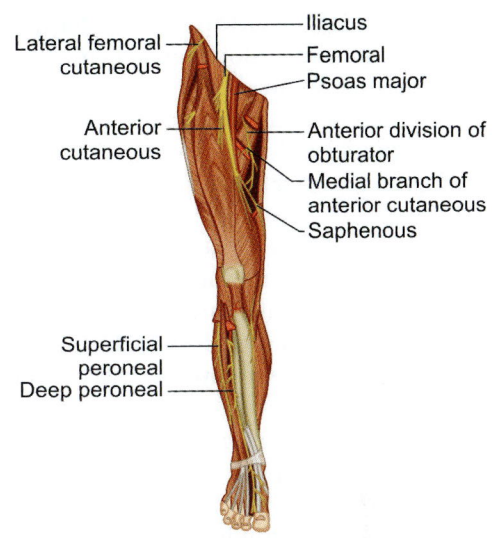

Fig. 42.17: Course and motor supply of femoral nerve.

Meralgia paresthetica
Compression of lateral cutaneous nerve of thigh below the ASIS under the inguinal ligament. It causes paresthesia over lateral aspect of thigh.

SCIATIC NERVE (SN)

- **Formed by:** Anterior and posterior divisions of lumbosacral plexus
- **Root value:** L4-S3
- **Course:** After exiting from the greater sciatic notch, the nerve descends in the gluteal region below the pyriformis behind the hip joint. It lies over the external rotators of the hip and further descends into the thigh under the deep head of the biceps femoris. In the posterior thigh, the 'tibial component' of the sciatic nerve innervates hamstring muscles. At the popliteal fossa apex, it divides into the common peroneal and tibial components **(Fig. 42.18)**.
- **Sensory innervation:** There are no direct sensory innervation of sciatic nerve. However, it innervates skin of lateral aspect of leg, heel and entire foot via its branches (common peroneal and tibial). Note that medial aspect of leg and medial border of foot is supplied by saphenous nerve.
- **Motor innervation:** Sciatic nerve supplies all hamstrings (semitendinosus, semi-membranosus, biceps femoris, and adductor magnus). Later, it supplies muscles of the entire leg and foot through common peroneal and tibial nerves.

- **Injury to the sciatic nerve can happen** in posterior dislocation of the hip, posterior surgical approaches to the hip, direct trauma, and injection into the gluteal region.
- **Problems after the injury to the sciatic nerve:**
  - Loss of knee flexion
  - Loos of all motor activity at ankle and foot (flail foot).
- **Clinical assessment of the sciatic nerve**
  - **Sensory assessment:** Assess the sensory function of the tibial and common peroneal nerve. Tibial nerve supplies plantar aspect of the foot. The deep component of CPN supplies dorsum of the 1st interdigital web space, while superficial component of CPN supplies rest of the dorsum of foot.
  - **Motor assessment:**
    - *Hamstrings*: Knee flexion
    - *Test for all ankle and foot muscles.*

COMMON PERONEAL NERVE (CPN)

- **Root value:** Dorsal component of L4-S2
- **Course:** It descends distally along the lateral wall of the popliteal fossa under the belly of the biceps femoris. Further, it *winds around the neck of the fibula between the peroneus longus and bone* and divides into the superficial and deep peroneal nerve. The superficial peroneal nerve supplies the lateral compartment, while the deep peroneal nerve supplies anterior compartment muscles **(Fig. 42.19)**.
- **Sensory innervation (Fig. 42.20):**
  - *Superficial peroneal nerve*: Dorsum of the foot except for 1st interdigital cleft, medial and lateral borders of the foot
  - *Deep peroneal nerve*: 1st interdigital cleft.
- **Motor innervation:** *Anterior* [tibialis anterior (TA), extensor hallucis longus (EHL), extensor digitorum longus (EDL), and peroneus tertius (PT)] and **lateral compartment** (peroneus longus and brevis) of the leg.

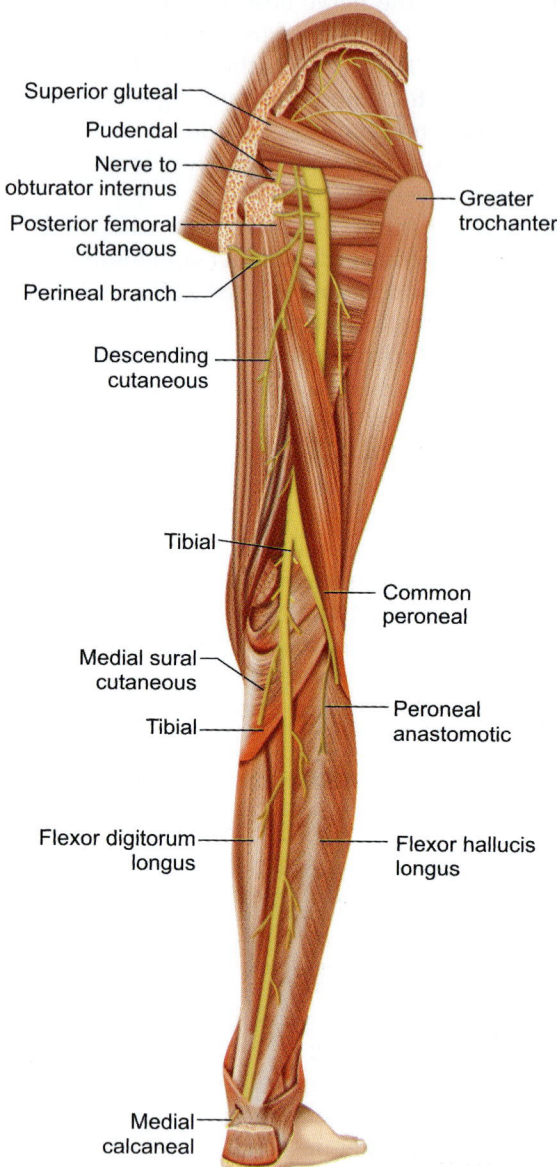

Fig. 42.18: Course and motor supply of sciatic nerve.

- **Injury to the CPN nerve can happen in** fibular neck fracture, knee dislocation.
- **Features/problems after the injury to CPN:** The typical feature of CPN injury is *foot drop and high stepping gait.*
  - Loss of ankle dorsiflexion due to tibialis anterior palsy results in footdrop and there is loss of eversion also due to peroneal longus and brevis palsy.
  - Loss of great and lesser toe extension (EHL and EDL).
- **Clinical assessment of CPN**
  - **Sensory assessment:**
    - ***Dorsum of first web space:*** Deep peroneal nerve
    - ***Rest of the dorsum:*** Superficial peroneal nerve.

  Note: Sensation on the medial border of the foot: Saphenous nerve. Sensation on lateral border: sural nerve **(Fig. 42.20)**.

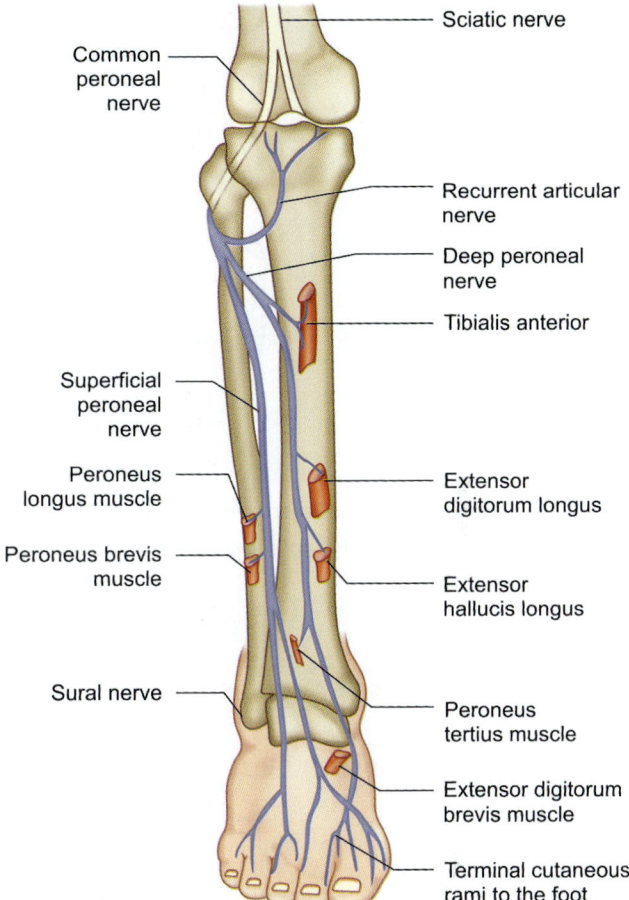

Fig. 42.19: Course and motor supply of common peroneal nerve.

  - **Motor assessment:**
    - ***Tibialis anterior:*** Dorsiflexion at the ankle while the subtalar joint is kept in inversion.
    - ***EHL, EDL:*** Extension of the great toe and smaller toes at MTP and IP joints, respectively.
    - ***Peroneus longus and brevis:*** Eversion at subtalar joint.
- **Treatment of the common peroneal nerve injury:**
  - The general management would be similar to described above.
  - ***Splintage:*** **Footdrop** splint is used to ankle plantar flexion, which may result in equinus deformity **(Fig. 42.21)**
  - ***Tendon transfer:*** To restore ankle dorsiflexion, tibialis posterior tendon is transferred to the dorsum of the foot via Ober's transfer/Barr's transfer. For details, *Refer Chapter 41, Table 41.2.*

TIBIAL NERVE

- **Root value:** Ventral component of L4-S3
- **Course:** It descends distally in the center of popliteal fossa and enters the leg under the arch of the soleus. In the popliteal fossa, it supplies gastrocnemius, popliteus, plantaris, and soleus muscles. Further, it descends and goes behind the medial malleolus under the flexor retinaculum and enters the foot. It divides into medial and lateral plantar nerves

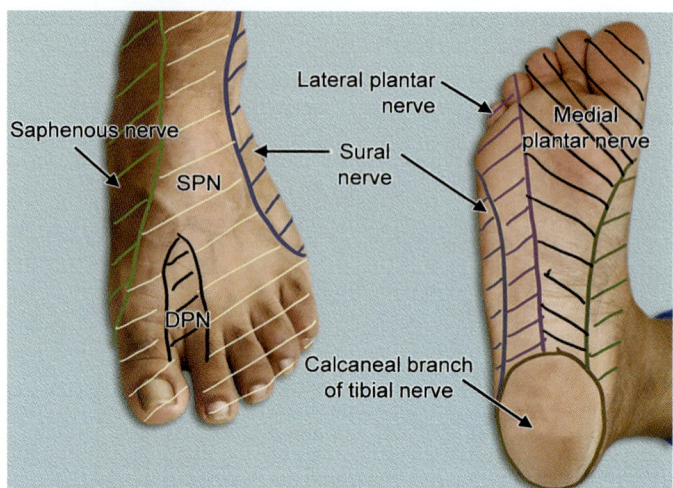

Fig. 42.20: Sensory innervation of the foot (dorsum and plantar side).
(SPN: superficial peroneal nerve; DPN: deep peroneal nerve)

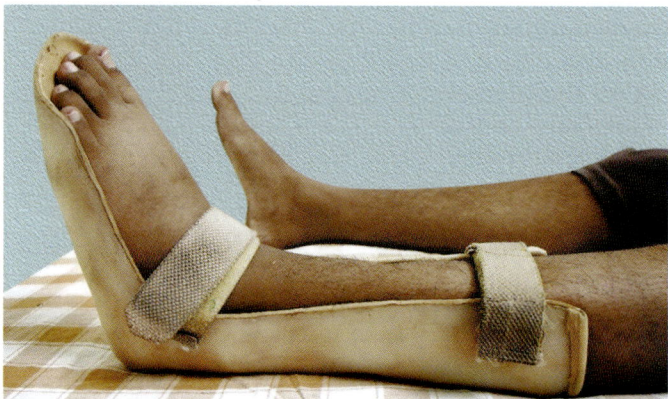

Fig. 42.21: Foot drop splint or ankle foot orthosis.

and supplies the entire four layers of foot muscles along with the skin of the plantar region **(Fig. 42.22)**.
- **Sensory innervation:** Plantar aspect of the foot via medial and lateral plantar nerves.
- **Motor innervation:** All muscles of the posterior compartment of the leg and plantar aspect of the foot **(Fig. 42.22)**.
- **Injury to the tibial nerve can happen in** knee dislocation, proximal tibia fractures, compartment syndrome of leg, and compressive neuropathy under the flexor retinaculum.
- **Problems after the injury to the tibial nerve:**
    - Loss of ankle plantar flexion (Gastrocsoleus)
    - Weak inversion (tibialis posterior)
    - Loss of plantar flexion of toes
    - Claw toes occurs after injury to the posterior tibial nerve near the ankle, leading to palsy of all foot intrinsic muscles

Chapter 42: Specific Nerve Injuries

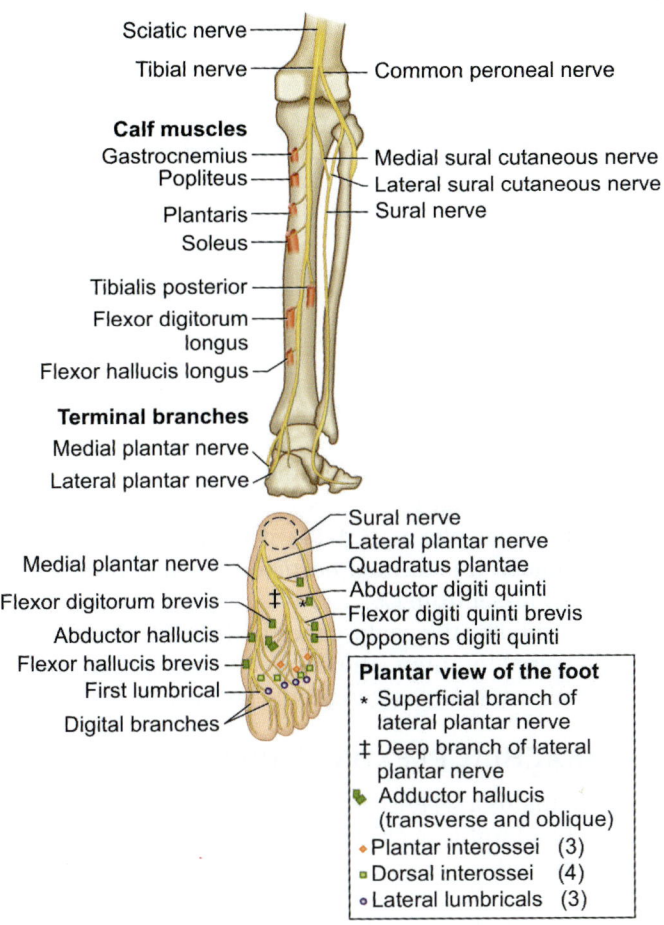

Fig. 42.22: Course and motor supply of tibial nerve.

- Calcaneus deformity
- High stepping gait if there is a common peroneal nerve palsy too.
- **Clinical assessment of tibial nerve**
    - **Sensory assessment:** Assess sensation over plantar aspect of the foot.
    - **Motor assessment:**
        - *Tendo-Achilles:* Ankle plantar flexion while standing on a tiptoe.
        - *Tibialis posterior:* Inversion at the subtalar joint while the ankle is in plantar flexion.
        - *Great toe flexor hallucis longus (FHL) and lesser toe flexor digitorum longus (FDL) plantar flexion:* Plantar flexion at the MTP and IP joints of the toes.

Tarsal Tunnel syndrome
Compression of tibial nerve under the flexor retinaculum behind the ankle.

CHAPTER 43

Brachial Plexus Injury

SURGICAL ANATOMY

- The brachial plexus is a plexus of nerves formed by the *ventral (anterior) rami* of the lower four cervical and the first thoracic (i.e., C5, C6, C7, C8, and T1) spinal nerves **(Fig. 43.1)**.
- The brachial plexus is divided into five anatomic sections—nerve roots, trunks, divisions, cords, and terminal branches **(Fig. 43.1)**.
- It is termed *prefixed* brachial plexus (C4-T1) if C4 has a significant contribution and lesser from T1, and similarly, it is termed *postfixed* brachial plexus if T2 has a significant contribution (C5-T2) and lesser from C5.
- The spinal nerves are formed by the coalescence of the ventral and dorsal nerve rootlets as they pass through the spinal foramen. There can be two types of lesions depending upon the injury site—preganglionic and postganglionic lesions.

MECHANISM OF BRACHIAL PLEXUS INJURY

The primary mechanism remains a *severe traction injury* during.
- **High-velocity injury:** Road traffic accident, fall of a heavy object over the shoulder, or fall with shoulder neck abducted.

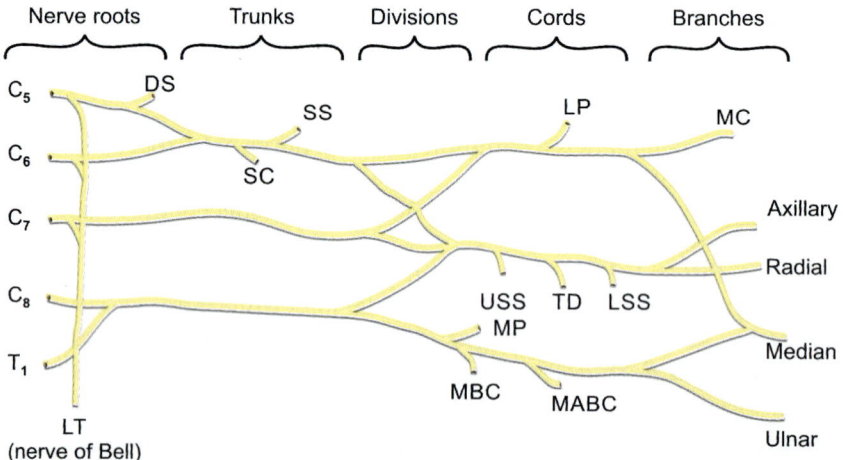

Fig. 43.1: Diagrammatic representation of brachial plexus formation.

(DS: dorsal scapular; LT: long thoracic; SS: suprascapular; SC: subclavius; LP: lateral pectoral; USS: upper subscapular; TD: thoracodorsal; LSS: lower subscapular; MP: medial pectoral; MBC: medial brachial cutaneous; MABC: medial antebrachial cutaneous; MC: musculocutaneous)

- **During birth:** Shoulder dystocia
- Stab or open injury to the neck.

As the plexus passes from the cervical spine between the scalenus anterior and scalenus medius muscles of the neck and beneath the clavicle bone en route to the arm, it is vulnerable to injury.

TYPES OF BRACHIAL PLEXUS INJURIES

Preganglionic and Postganglionic Lesions

- **Preganglionic lesion:** If a nerve root is avulsed from the spinal cord, it is called a preganglionic lesion, i.e., disruption proximal to the dorsal root ganglion **(Fig. 43.2A)**. The characteristics of preganglionic brachial plexus injuries are mentioned in **Box 43.1**.
This type of injury cannot recover, and it is surgically irreparable. Hence, it carries a poor prognosis.

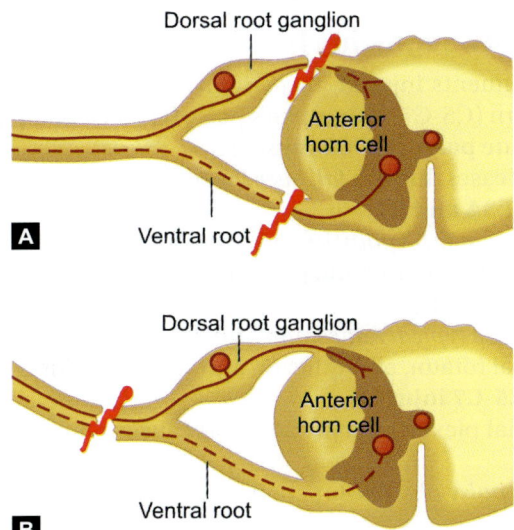

Figs. 43.2A and B: (A) Preganglionic injury; (B) Postganglionic injury. The zig-zag red dashed line shows the area of injury.

Box 43.1: Characteristics of preganglionic brachial plexus injuries.

- Associated spine fractures
- Severe burning sensation in upper limb with insensate limb
- Horner's syndrome
- Normal triple axon reflex (histamine test) due to intact dorsal root ganglion (absent in postganglionic lesions)
- Palsy of rhomboids and serratus anterior leading to medial winging of scapula
- Upper motor neuron signs in lower limb
- Nerve conduction velocity (NCV) detects normal sensory action potentials due to intact dorsal root ganglion
- Electromyography (EMG) reveals denervation potential in posterior paraspinal muscles

- **Postganglionic lesion:** In this type of lesion, there is a rupture of a nerve root distal to the ganglion or of a trunk or at the formation of a peripheral nerve **(Fig. 43.2B)**. It is characterized by abnormal axon triple reflex (only redness and wheal, no flare).
  This type of injury is surgically repairable and carries the potential for recovery, so it has a better prognosis.

Supraclavicular and Infraclavicular Lesions

- **Supraclavicular lesions (65%):** Typically occur in motorcycle accidents; as the rider collides with the ground or another vehicle, his neck and shoulder are wrenched apart. In the most severe injuries, the arm is practically avulsed from the trunk with a rupture of the subclavian artery.
- **Infraclavicular lesions (25%):** Usually associated with fractures or dislocations of the shoulder joint and are associated with axillary artery injury in about ~25% of cases. Clavicle fractures rarely damage the plexus, only if caused by a direct blow.
- **Combined lesions:** Seen in ~10% of cases.

According to the Roots/Segments Involved

Depending upon the segments injured, these injuries are further classified into Erb's palsy (C5-C6), Erb's-plus pattern (C5-C7), Klumpke's palsy (C8-T1), and pan-plexus injury.

- **Erb's or Erb-Duchenne palsy (C5-C6 injury)**
  - It is seen in 15% of cases due to a *fall over the tip of the shoulder or during birth* (shoulder dystocia) **(Figs. 43.3A and B)**.
  - The *injury occurs at an Erb's point* (where six nerves from the upper trunk meet, namely, C5 and C6 nerve roots, anterior and posterior divisions, suprascapular nerve, and nerve to subclavius) **(Fig. 43.3C)**.
  - Erb's palsy results in a *typical Policeman's tip deformity* characterized by loss of shoulder abduction, external rotator, elbow flexor, and wrist extension **(Fig. 43.4)**.
- **Erb's-plus pattern (C5-C7 injury)**
  - A common brachial plexus injury (~20–35%) causes neurological deficits in the upper limbs.
  - It consists of *Erb's palsy plus features of partial or complete C7 or middle trunk injury.*

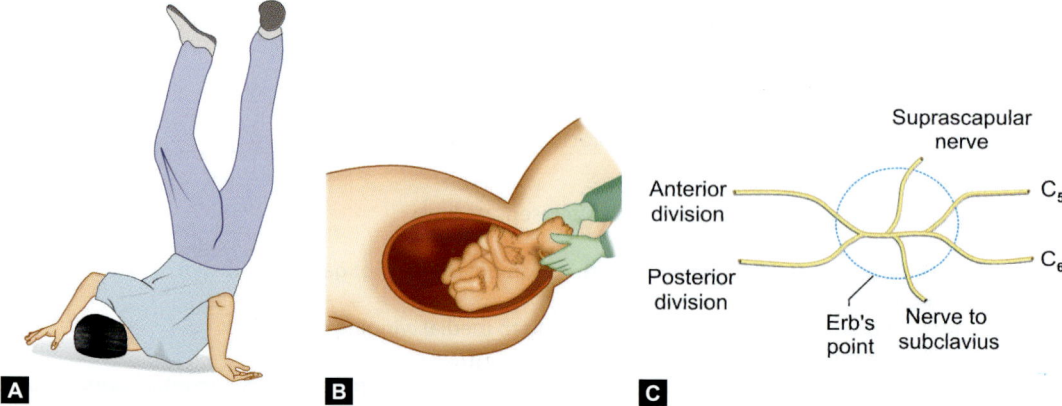

Figs. 43.3A to C: Mechanisms of injury in Erb's: (A) Stretching at Erb's point following a fall on the shoulder; (B) Birth injury at the time of delivery; (C) Erb's point.

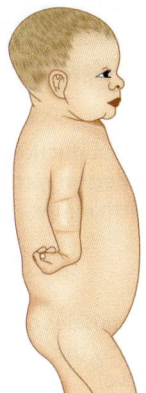

Fig. 43.4: Policeman's tip/porter's tip/waiter's tip position: Adducted, internally rotated arm with extended elbow, pronated forearm in Erb's palsy.

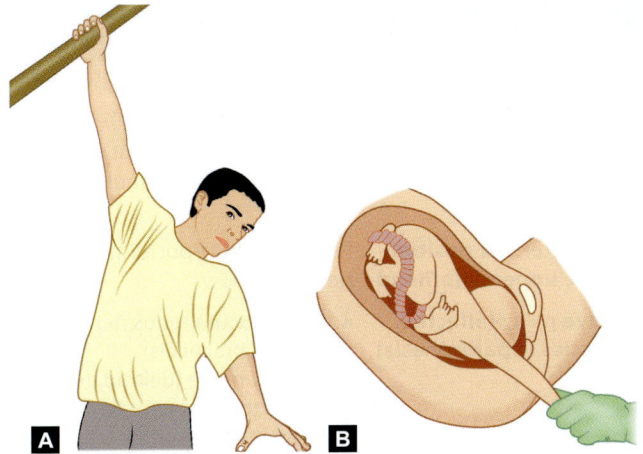

Figs. 43.5A and B: Mechanisms of injury in Klumpke's palsy. (A) Hyperabduction of the arm; (B) Birth injury.

- It results in variable weakness in the elbow, wrist, and sometimes finger extensors.
- The C7 distribution to the wrist and finger extension and even to the flexor digitorum profundus muscles varies between patients and leads to different degrees of weakness.
- Sensory disturbances in the proximal part of the arm, thumb, index, and middle fingers may be present.
- **Klumpke's or Dejerine–Klumpke's palsy (C8-T1 Injury)**
    - It is a *less common* (~10%) but *severe form of* brachial plexus injury.
    - Due to *hyperabduction injury to the shoulder* while a fall or *a birth injury* (**Figs. 43.5A and B**)
    - Associated loss of sympathetic supply to the eye and face
    - Involvement of the lower roots can result in *Horner syndrome,* characterized by
        - *Miosis* (constricted pupil)
        - *Ptosis* of the upper eyelid
        - *Anhydrosis* (loss of hemifacial sweating)
        - *Enophthalmos.*

    Table 43.1 outlines the difference between Erb's and Klumpke's palsy.
- **Pan-Plexus (C5-T1) injury**
    - It is the *most common form* of injury seen in 50–75% of patients with supraclavicular brachial plexus injuries.
    - These patients commonly have a *completely flail arm and insensate hand.*
    - Postganglionic injury (particularly of C5) is often present in these cases, with preganglionic lesions affecting other nerves.

DIAGNOSIS

- **Detailed clinical examination:** Examination of brachial plexus injury patients must be carried out in a standardized and thorough manner. The main objective is to establish the location of the nerve injury (preganglionic, i.e., root, or postganglionic, i.e., nerve, trunk, division, cord, or branches) and the severity of the lesion (i.e., partial or complete for each element of the brachial plexus).

Table 43.1: Differences between Erb's and Klumpke's palsy.

Features	Erb's palsy	Klumpke's palsy
Nerve roots affected	C5 and C6	C8 and T1
Mode of injury	Stretching at Erb's point following a blow or fall on the shoulder, delivery	Forced hyperabduction of arm, e.g., falling person catch a tree/pole and birth injury
Characteristic position of the upper limb/hand	Policeman's tip/porter's tip/waiter's tip position	Claw hand
Nerve palsy (affected muscles in parenthesis)	<ul><li>Musculocutaneous nerve (biceps brachii, brachialis)</li><li>Axillary nerve (deltoid, teres minor)</li><li>Nerve to subclavius (subclavius)</li><li>Suprascapular nerve (supraspinatus, infraspinatus)</li><li>Brachioradialis, supinator, and extensor carpi radialis longus</li></ul>	All intrinsic muscles of the hand (as supplied by the ulnar and median nerve)
Sensory loss (sometimes)	Along the outer aspect of the arm at the lower part of the deltoid, radial side of forearm and thumb	Along the medial border of the forearm and hand (ulnar nerve distribution)
Autonomic signs	Absent	Present (Horner's syndrome)

- **Plain radiographs:** Cervical spine, chest, shoulder girdle, and humerus to be taken in patients with high-energy traumatic brachial plexus palsy to rule out associated upper limb fractures and dislocations.
- **Electrodiagnostic evaluation** of the brachial plexus is performed with electromyography and nerve conduction studies. It is usually *performed after 3-6 weeks* of primary injury.
- **Magnetic resonance imaging (MRI):** MRI of the brachial plexus is performed, especially in traumatic injuries, to locate the level of the lesion. It is usually *performed after 3 weeks* of primary injury.

TREATMENT

- **Conservative/observation**
    - All postganglionic brachial plexus injuries are observed and periodically assessed for several months for gradual sensorimotor recovery. Surgery is preferred if there is no recovery or not-a-functional recovery.
    - Physiotherapy to avoid stiffness and retain mobility at the joints.
    - Appropriate counseling of the patient is a must to understand neurological recovery patterns and time taken for recovery.
- **Surgery:** It is indicated for sensorimotor deficit and pain relief. The indication for surgery are—
    - Preganglionic injuries
    - Open brachial plexus injuries are explored immediately.
    - When there is no hope for spontaneous recovery or further functional recovery after waiting for several months expecting gradual spontaneous recovery.

Various surgical options for brachial plexus injury are:
- ***Exploration and neurotization:*** In neurotization, a functional nerve is transferred (in part/whole) to a more important paralyzed nerve to restore a paralyzed muscle function.
- ***Nerve repair with or without nerve graft***
- ***Tendon transfers***
- ***Arthrodesis***
- ***Free muscle transfer***
- ***Surgery for pain relief:*** Nerve transfer/neurosurgical procedure like DREZotomy.

Counseling of the patients and their family: It is crucial to inform the patient about the possible surgical options, risk-benefit ratio, postoperative rehabilitation program, success rate, prolonged recovery time, and the possibility of additional surgery.

SECTION 12

Congenital and Other Pediatric Disorders

SECTION OUTLINE

44. Congenital and Other Pediatric Disorders
    - Congenital Talipes Equinus Varus
    - Congenital Vertical Talus
    - Developmental Dysplasia of the Hip
    - Multiple Congenital Contractures
    - Coxa Vara
    - Slipped Capital Femoral Epiphysis
    - Perthes' Disease and Other Osteochondrosis
    - Perthes' Disease (Legg-Calve-Perthes Disease)
    - Pes Planus/Flat Foot
    - Pes Cavus
    - Spina Bifida
    - Skeletal Dysplasias—Achondroplasia
    - Osteogenesis Imperfecta/Brittle Bone Disease/Lobstein Vrolik Disease
    - Congenital Pseudoarthrosis of Tibia
    - Congenital Knee Dislocation

12

Congenital and Other Pediatric Disorders

CHAPTER 44

Congenital and Other Pediatric Disorders

CONGENITAL TALIPES EQUINUS VARUS (CTEV)

INTRODUCTION

- It is the *most common congenital musculoskeletal birth defect*. It is also known as club foot as the deformed foot resembles a 'golf club' **(Fig. 44.1)**.
- Its incidence is 0.8–4.4/1,000 living birth.
- It is *bilateral in 50%* of cases. The right side is twice affected more than the left.
- *Boys are twice more likely to get affected* than girls (male:female: 2:1).
- High concordance rate among monozygotic twins.

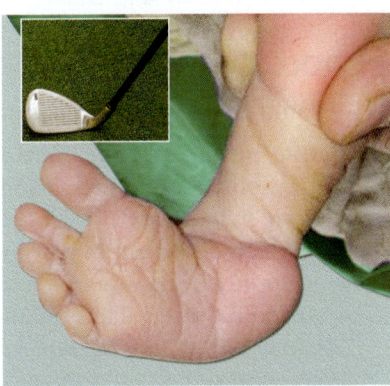

Fig. 44.1: Unilateral right club foot resembling a Golf Club (inset image).

DEFINITION OF CONGENITAL TALIPES EQUINUS VARUS

CTEV is a congenital foot and ankle disorder characterized by equinus (plantar flexion) deformity at the ankle joint, inversion at the subtalar joint, forefoot adduction at the midtarsal joint, and cavus deformity **(Figs. 44.2A to C)**. Cavus implies that the medial arch of the foot is higher than normal.

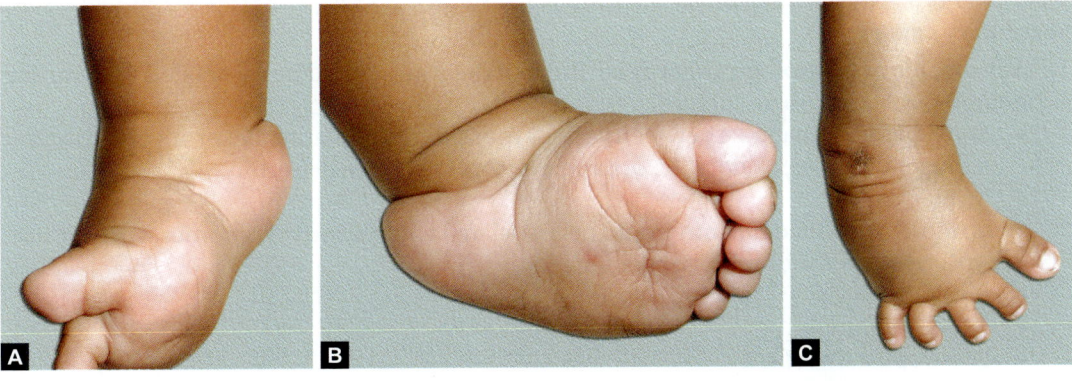

Figs. 44.2A to C: Deformities in CTEV. (A) Equinus (plantar flexion) at the ankle joint and cavus; (B) Inversion (sole facing medially); (C) Forefoot adduction.

The interpretation of each word of 'congenital talipes equinus varus' (CTEV) is mentioned below:
- **Congenital:** Present since birth.
- **Talipes (Talus + Pes):** Deformity around ankle and foot.
- **Equinus:** The heel is elevated like a horse's, leading to plantar flexion at the ankle joint.
- **Varus:** It is the combination of inversion at the subtalar joint and forefoot adduction.

Deformities of a CTEV foot at the various joints are mentioned in **Table 44.1**.

Table 44.1: Site of deformities in CTEV.

Hindfoot	Forefoot-midfoot
Equinus at ankle	Adduction at midtarsals
Inversion at subtalar joint	Supination in forefoot
	Midfoot-Cavus

ETIOLOGY

CTEV could be primary or secondary.

Idiopathic/primary CTEV: There are no known causes, including normal spine and neurological status. However, genetic and various other hypothesis are implicated in CTEV, such as:

1. **Genetic hypothesis:**
   - 1° relatives are more commonly affected
   - It could be *autosomal recessive* or *autosomal dominant with incomplete penetrance*
   - It could be multifactorial inheritance.
2. **Mechanical or positional hypothesis** suggests that *malposition* in the uterus due to *oligohydramnios* could result in a foot deformity. Oligohydramnios results in pressure on foot, resulting in abnormal position of the foot causing the deformity.
3. **Bone/joint hypothesis** postulates that positional bony abnormalities underlie the anomaly.
4. **Connective tissue hypothesis:** A primary abnormality of the connective tissue resulting in muscular, tendinous, and fascial abnormality could be responsible for CTEV.
5. **Vascular hypothesis:** Fibrosis of local tissues probably due to ischemia of calf muscle due to unknown factors could result in muscle contracture resulting in deformity.
6. **Developmental arrest hypothesis:** Several authors suggested that clubfoot may arise due to an arrest of the normal medial rotation of the foot in late fetal development.

Secondary causes:

1. **Neurogenic or teratologic disorders:** The foot deformity could be associated with various neurological conditions, such as
   - *Spina bifida:* Imbalance between various muscle groups plantar flexor, invertor become stronger due to weak dorsiflexors and evertors result in a deformity.
   - Myelodysplasia
2. **Syndromic:** The foot deformity could be associated with various syndromes, such as
   - Arthrogryposis multiplex congenita
   - Myelodysplasia
   - Tibial hemimelia
   - Diastrophic dwarfism
   - Amniotic band syndrome (Streeter's dysplasia).

RELEVANT PATHOANATOMY: STRUCTURES CONTRACTED AND AREAS AFFECTED IN CTEV

The *principal pathology in CTEV is medial talonavicular subluxation*. The talar neck is deviated medially, calcaneum is in varus, navicular and cuboid are displaced medially. Further, most of the medial and posterior soft tissues of the ankle-foot are contracted. Various joints, bones, ligaments, capsules, muscle-tendon of the foot and ankle are involved, which are mentioned in **Table 44.2**.

Table 44.2: Involvement of major structures in CTEV pathology.

Joints involved	Contracted capsule of joints	Ligaments, fascia contracted	Muscle/tendon contracture
Ankle, subtalar, calcaneocuboid, and talonavicular	Ankle, subtalar and talonavicular	Deltoid, talonavicular spring (plantar calcaneonavicular), posterior talofibular, calcaneofibular, interosseous talocalcaneal, and plantar fascia	Tendoachilles, tibialis posterior (TP), flexor digitorum longus (FDL), flexor hallucis longus (FHL), and abductor hallucis

CLASSIFICATION AS PER ETIOLOGY

The CTEV is classified based on the etiology and correctability of the deformity.
- **Idiopathic clubfoot:**
  - *Postural (extrinsic)*: Deformity due to external pressure or faulty posture, which is easily correctable.
  - *Rigid (intrinsic)*: Internal contracture of muscle/tendon/capsule/muscle.
- **Neurogenic, syndromic clubfoot**.

CLASSIFICATION AS PER CORRECTABILITY OF DEFORMITY

- **Mild CTEV** is a passively over-correctable deformity.
- **Moderate CTEV** is passively just correctable deformity or can reach a neutral position.
- **Severe deformity** cannot be corrected up to the neutral position.

CLINICAL FEATURES

The clinical features of CTEV vary in age groups, whether the child is non-walking or walking.
- **Non-walking age group**
  - *The foot and heel size:* The affected foot and heel are smaller.
  - *Deformity:* A typical equinus, varus and cavus deformity is noted in the ankle and foot **(Fig. 44.3A)**.
  - *Creases:* Medial and posterior creases are deep and prominent **(Fig. 44.3B)**.
  - The lateral malleolus and head of the talus are prominent, while the medial malleolus is inconspicuous.
  - Toes appear splayed **(Fig. 44.3C)**.
- **Late cases/children with CTEV in the walking age group:**
  - There are callosities over the lateral border of the foot **(Fig. 44.4)**.
  - Wasting of calf muscles is noted.

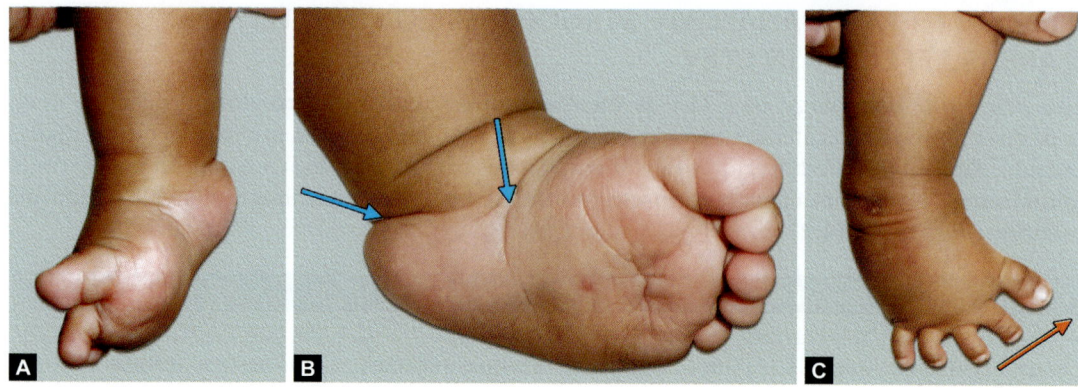

Figs. 44.3A to C: Deformities in CTEV. (A) Equinus at the ankle joint; (B) Inversion at subtalar joint. Medial and posterior deep creases (arrows); (C) Forefoot is adducted with splayed toes (orange arrow).

Further, the examination of CTEV is never complete without the examination of the following triad (CTEV-DDH-spina bifida).

Always rule out other neurological or syndromic causes of CTEV, e.g., spina bifida, arthrogryposis multiplex congenita.

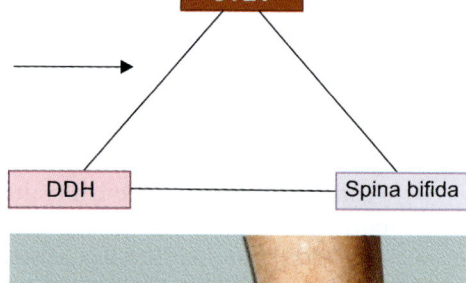

CLINICAL SCORING TO ASSESS THE SEVERITY OF DEFORMITY

Pirani and Dimeglio scores are used to assess the severity of CTEV.

- **Pirani score:** It is a score which uses three variables, each from mid and hind foot, to assess the *severity of the CTEV*. It can also be used to *monitor the progression of correction* with the cast. The Pirani score allocates 0, 0.5, and 1 for each of the six clinical features from midfoot and hindfoot:

    - Medial crease
    - Lateral border of the foot } **Midfoot**
    - Lateral head of talus
    - Posterior crease
    - Empty heel } **Hindfoot**
    - Ankle dorsiflexion

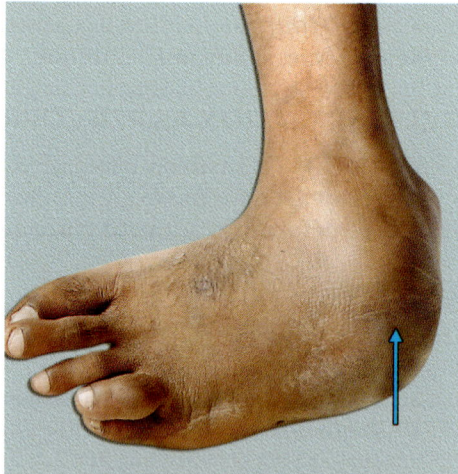

Fig. 44.4: Neglected CTEV. Note callosity below lateral malleolus (blue arrow).

The higher the score, severe is the deformity.

- **Dimeglio score** is based on the degree of reducibility of four deformities: **D**erotation of carpopedal block, **A**dduction of forefoot, **V**arus, and **E**quinus (DAVE). Each factor gets point 1–4. Additional one point is alloted for posterior and medial crease, cavus and hypertonia.

INVESTIGATIONS

- **Plain X-ray of the foot and ankle (Fig. 44.5), including the lower tibia:** Various angles are measured to assess the severity of deformity, such as:
  - Talocalcaneal angle anteroposterior and lateral
  - Tibiocalcaneal angle
  - Talofirst metatarsal angle.

The normal and abnormal angles are mentioned in **Table 44.3**.

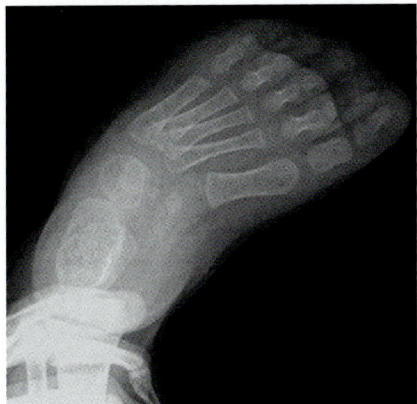

Fig. 44.5: X-ray foot in CTEV.

Table 44.3: Various angles measured in a normal and CTEV foot-ankle. Note that all angles decrease in CTEV (cf. congenital vertical talus where all angles increase).

Angles	Normal (in degrees)	CTEV
Talocalcaneal "Kite" angle (in AP view)	20–40	<20
Talocalcaneal angle (in lateral view)	>35	<35
Tibiocalcaneal angle	60–90	Decreased
Talo-first metatarsal angle (AP)	5–15	Negative

TREATMENT OF CTEV

It is essential to understand that the treatment of primary idiopathic and secondary clubfoot (neurogenic and syndromic) are different. The former can usually be managed by conservative methods, whereas the latter requires operative intervention. The **neurogenic CTEV** foot requires restoration of neurological imbalance at the foot and ankle (by tendon transfers), along with soft tissue correction. Otherwise, the deformity will recur due to persistent neurological imbalance. **Syndromic CTEV** is usually rigid and, therefore, often requires surgical releases.

TREATMENT OF IDIOPATHIC CTEV (FLOWCHART 44.1)

Traditionally, there are two management options for an idiopathic CTEV; typical and more favored **'conservative serial casting'** or **'surgical soft tissue release and/or bony correction.'** The treatment choice depends on the tissue pliability, which in turn may depend upon the chronicity of the deformity. In a newborn or a young child, the soft tissue contractures are less rigid, and bones are not yet deformed. Therefore, CTEV deformity in a younger child often responds to serial casting resulting in deformity correction. In contrast, the CTEV deformity in an older child is rigid or less pliable to stretching during serial casting due to rigid soft tissue contracture and/or deformed bones. Therefore, a rigid CTEV deformity in an older child may require surgical correction. However, as per current recommendations, treatment of CTEV in all ages including adults begins with casting. The aim is to stretch the soft tissues even if surgery is required as magnitude of surgery and soft tissue dissection and stretching is reduced.

Typically, younger children (<2 years) are given a trial of serial manipulation and cast application, whereas older kids (>2 years) may require surgical treatment if the conservative

Flowchart 44.1: Treatment algorithm in managing CTEV.

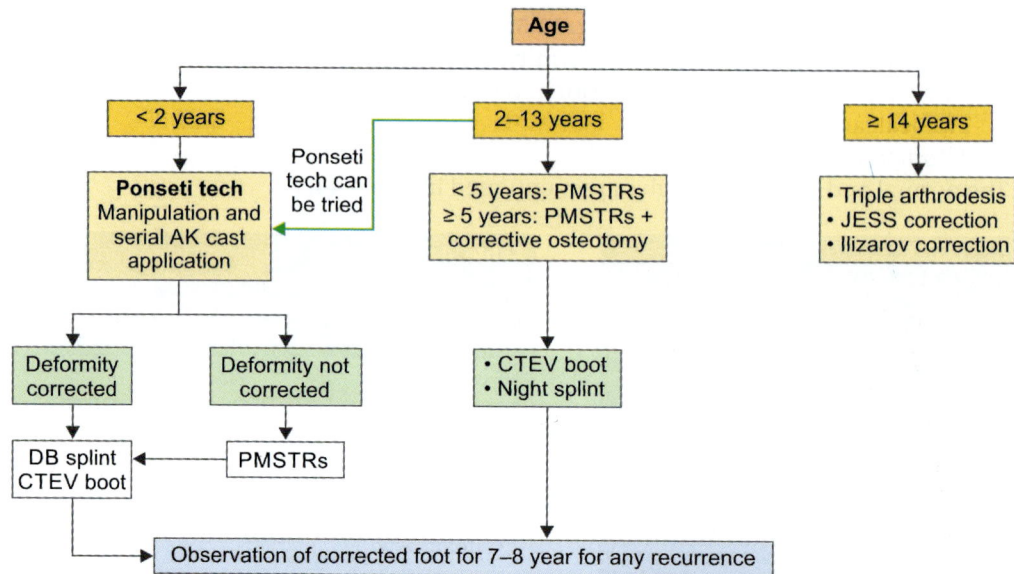

(PMSTRs: posteromedial soft tissue release; JESS: Joshi's external stabilization system)

trial of serial casting fails. The surgical correction involves soft tissue release and/or bony surgery. The bony surgery (corrective osteotomy or fusions) is added if the child is older than 4 years. After 14 years of age, only surgical procedure is recommended. The details of interventions are discussed here.

From Birth till 2 Years of Age

- At birth, *manipulation of the CTEV foot is initiated by the mother* after every feed for several minutes. A flexible deformity responds to manipulation and may get corrected. However, most cases need manipulation and casting followed by bracing.
- **Serial manipulation and POP cast:** Most CTEV foot require serial manipulation and above-knee POP cast application **(Fig. 44.6)**. *The order of correction during serial manipulation is "CAVE": Cavus, adduction, varus, and equinus.* Note that if 'CAVE' order is not followed, it may result in Rocker bottom foot deformity (*See* **Fig. 44.13**).
  The cast is changed every week or two.
- **Methods of serial casting:** *Ponseti and Kite.*
  - **Ponseti's method** is currently the method of choice with >95% success rate in correcting the deformity. It also gives more rapid and constant correction. *In the Ponseti method, the equinus is always corrected by percutaneous tendoachilles tenotomy.*

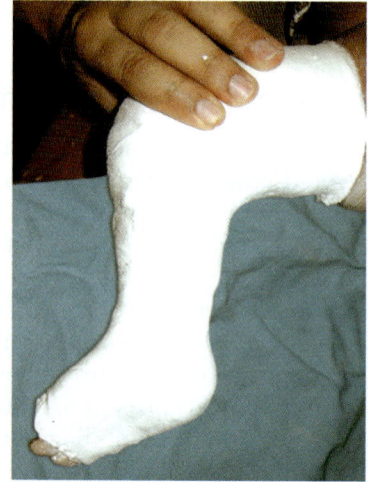

Fig. 44.6: Above knee cast application in CTEV.

- **Kite's method** is an older method of treatment comprising *only serial manipulation for all deformities*. Compared to Ponseti, Kite's method requires longer times to correct deformities.
  Note: The detailed differences between the two methods are mentioned in **Table 44.4**.
- **Post-correction bracing:** Once the deformity is corrected, a non-walking child is given Dennis Brown (DB) splint to be worn for 23 hours/day **(Fig. 44.7)**. Once the child starts walking, the CTEV boot **(Fig. 44.8)** is worn during the daytime, and the DB splint is worn at night. The details of DB splint and CTEV shoes are mentioned on *page 530*.
- **Post-correction follow-up:** The child must be kept under clinical monitoring for 7–8 years to look for any recurrence of deformities.

Surgical correction is performed if the deformities fail to get corrected during serial casting.

Table 44.4: Differences between Ponseti and Kite's methods.		
	Ponseti method	**Kite's method**
Cavus	Corrected first	Not mentioned
Fulcrum for correction: **Correction achieved**	Lateral part of the talar head ■ Forefoot adduction ■ Hindfoot varus	Calcaneocuboid joint ■ Forefoot varus ■ Hindfoot varus corrected by direct calcaneum eversion
Hindfoot equinus correction	Achieved by tendo-Achilles tenotomy	By cast wedging or serial casting
Advantage	Deformity gets corrected within 5–6 manipulations and cast applications	More POPs may be required, but often ends up in soft tissue release

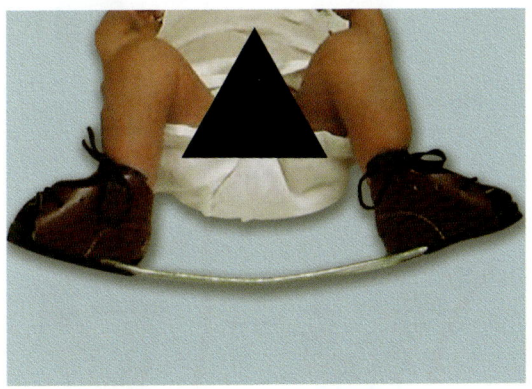

Fig. 44.7: Dennis Brown splint.

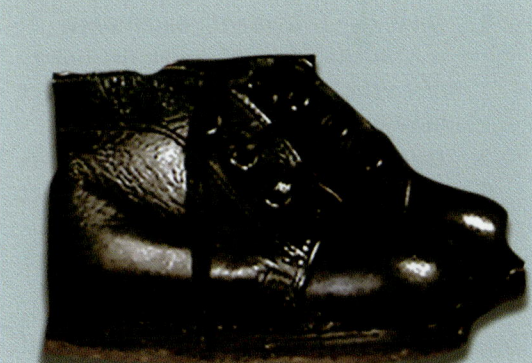

Fig. 44.8: CTEV boot. (*Note:* Boots are always above the malleolus level, while shoes end below the malleolus).

Age: 2–13 Years

Currently, many surgeons try serial casting with the Ponseti technique to correct CTEV deformity, even in kids > 2 years. However, if failed to achieve correction due to rigid deformities, patients may require surgical correction.

Surgical correction involves soft tissue releases and/or bony surgery.

- **Soft tissue surgery:** In CTEV, the soft tissue contractures are on the posterior and medial sides of the ankle-foot. Therefore, typically posteromedial soft tissue release surgery *(PMSTRs)* is performed. *The details of PMSTRs are mentioned in* **Table 44.5.**

Table 44.5: Structures released/lengthened during posteromedial soft tissue releases (PMSTRs).

Side	Tendon lengthening/ tenotomy	Capsule/fascia release	Ligament released
Posterior	TA lengthening by Z plasty	Ankle joint	Post talofibular, calcaneofibular
Medial	Lengthening of TP, FDL, and FHL	Naviculo-cuneiform and cuneiform-first metatarsal in severe cases	Talonavicular, superficial deltoid, and spring *Severe cases*: Interosseous Y ligament between talus and calcaneum
Plantar	FDB and AH released from the calcaneum	Plantar fascia	

(TA: tendoachilles; FDL: flexor digitorum longus; FHL: flexor hallucis longus; TP: tibialis posterior; FDB: flexor digitorum brevis; AH: abductor hallucis)

- **Bony surgery:** The bony correction (corrective osteotomy/arthrodesis) is added only if the child is 5 years or older. Due to the predominant cartilage content in a bone, early bony surgery may result in a small foot or failed fusion. Various corrective osteotomies performed in the foot are as follows:
  1. *Dwyer's calcaneal osteotomy:* It is a *lateral closing wedge osteotomy of calcaneum* performed to correct hindfoot varus **(Fig. 44.9).**
  2. *Dilwyn-Evan's procedure:* It is *calcaneocuboid fusion* to correct forefoot adduction **(Fig. 44.10).**
  3. *Wedge tarsectomy*: Between 8–11 years to correct forefoot adduction.

The details of bony procedures are mentioned in **Table 44.6.**

- **Post-surgical correction:** After the surgical correction, an *above-knee cast* is applied for six weeks.
- **Maintain correction:** After cast removal, the child is given a **CTEV boot during day time** and **a DB splint at night** to maintain the correction.

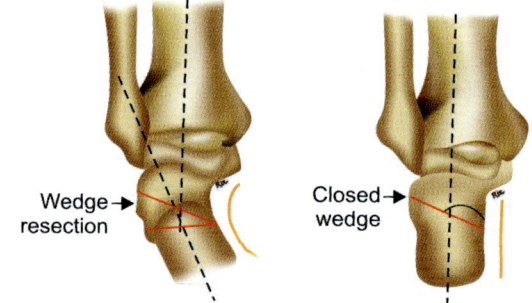

Fig. 44.9: Dwyer's calcaneal closing wedge osteotomy.

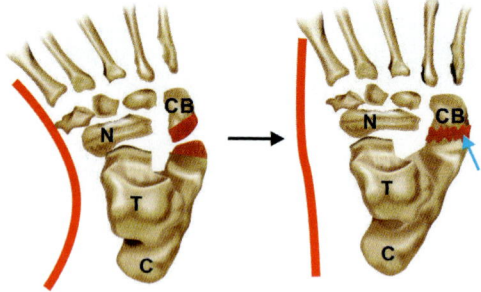

Fig. 44.10: Dilwyn Evans procedure. Shaded red area over calcaneum and cuboid are resected and arthrodesed. Blue arrow shows fused calcaneocuboid joint. Red line represents medial border of foot.
(C: calcaneum; T: talus; N: navicular; CB: cuboid)

Table 44.6: Outline of various bony procedures in CTEV.

Name	Age	Procedure	Corrects
Dwyer's osteotomy (Fig. 44.9)	≥ 5 years	Calcaneal lateral closing wedge osteotomy	Heel varus
Dilwyn Evan's osteotomy (Fig. 44.10)	≥ 5 years	Calcaneocuboid fusion	Forefoot adduction
Wedge tarsectomy	8–11 years	Dorsolateral wedge tarsectomy involving the talonavicular and calcaneocuboid joint	Forefoot varus
Triple arthrodesis (Fig. 44.12)	>14 years	Fusion of three joints: Talonavicular, Talocalcaneal, Calcaneocuboid	All deformities

Age ≥14 Years

Kids who are older than 14 years usually require surgical management of the deformity as the soft tissues are rigid, bones are deformed, and joints are subluxated. Commonly, two procedures are performed to correct the deformity.
1. ***Joshi's external stabilization system (JESS)* (Fig. 44.11) *or Ilizarov method*** can be tried for up to 16 years for the correction of deformity.
2. ***Triple arthrodesis:*** It is a preferred method of treating a neglected CTEV in a child older than 14 years of age **(Fig. 44.12)**. In triple arthrodesis, three joints are fused—talocalcaneal, talonavicular and calcaneocuboid.
   Note: Triple arthrodesis should be avoided in insensate foot.

Why bony procedures are avoided in kids <5 year?
Bony procedures are avoided in patients <5 years of age as it leads to resection of cartilaginous bone. Cartilaginous bone resection would result in: ▪ Lead to small foot due to resection of cartilage and further growth impairment of foot. ▪ Also, two ends of cartilage will fail in fusion, if attempted.

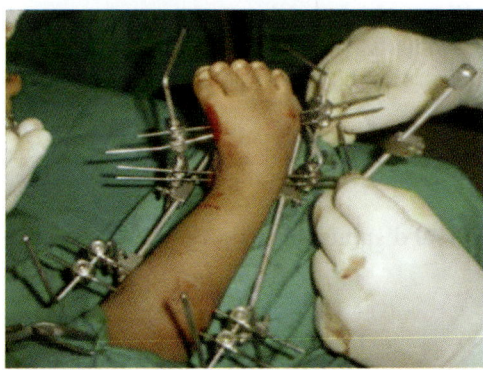

Fig. 44.11: JESS application on a CTEV foot.
(*Courtesy:* Dr Shah Waliullah, KGMC, Lucknow)

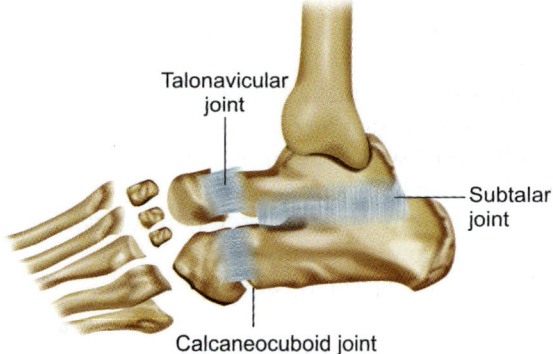

Fig. 44.12: Triple arthrodesis.

ORTHOSIS USED IN CONGENITAL TALIPES EQUINOVARUS

- **Dennis Brown splint (Fig. 44.7):** It is a dynamic splint, not a static one. As the child kicks his one limb, the connecting bar pushes the other foot into eversion and dorsiflexion, helping correct the deformity and making it a dynamic splint.
- **CTEV boot characteristics (Fig. 44.8):** CTEV boots are 'boot and not shoe' as boot extends above the ankle while shoes stay below the ankle. There are three important characteristics of a CTEV boot:
  1. *No heel:* To prevent equinus
  2. *Medial border straight and stiff:* To prevent forefoot adduction
  3. *Lateral border raise:* To prevent inversion.

CONGENITAL VERTICAL TALUS

DEFINITION

A congenital foot condition that presents as a **rigid flat foot with convex contour of the sole**, also known as *"rigid rocker bottom foot"* deformity with a *characteristic radiological picture of irreducible dorsal dislocation of the navicular on the talus.*

It is known as the rocker bottom foot due to the resemblance of the convex sole with the rocker bottom chair whose legs are attached two curved bars allowing rocking back and forth **(Fig. 44.13)**.

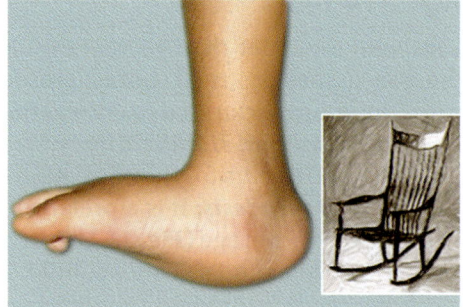

Fig. 44.13: Rocker bottom foot. Inset picture shows rocker bottom chair.

ASSOCIATION

It is uncommon to have congenital vertical talus (CVT) as a standalone deformity. Most cases are associated with:
- Arthrogryposis multiplex congenita (AMC)
- Spina bifida.

PATHOANATOMY

The principal pathology of CVT is **tight tendoachilles, which initiates the equinus and valgus of the calcaneum and further verticality of the talus**. The dorsal tendons [extensor digitorum longus (EDL), extensor hallucis longus (EHL), tibialis anterior] become tight and pull navicular dorsally. Various CVT characteristics are:
- Dorsal dislocation of navicular
- The vertical orientation of the talus
- Calcaneal eversion
- Contracture of anterolateral muscles of the foot, dorsal displacement of peroneal tendons, which now act as dorsiflexors
- Tendoachilles (TA) contracture.

CLINICAL FEATURES

- Rigid flat foot with rocker bottom foot (convex sole) deformity **(Fig. 44.13)**
- *Forefoot*: Valgus, abducted

- *Talus*: Shifted toward sole and medially giving a rocker bottom foot
- *Hindfoot*: Equinovalgus, tight tendoachilles
- *Peg-leg gait*: Forefoot push-off is limited
- *Neurological examination is a must, as many cases are associated with spina bifida.*

INVESTIGATIONS

- **Plain X-ray:** Foot and ankle
  - Vertically oriented talus **(Fig. 44.14)**
  - Forced plantar flexion lateral view of the foot shows persistently dislocated talonavicular joint.
- **Magnetic resonance imaging (MRI) spine:** If there is suspicion of neurological disorder.

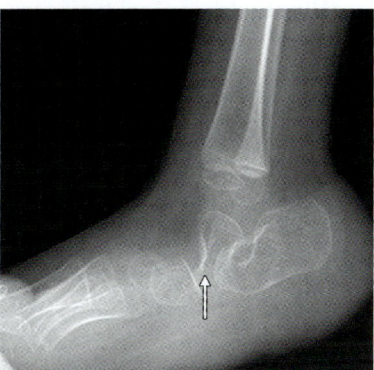

Fig. 44.14: X-ray shows vertical talus (white arrow).

TREATMENT

- **Early cases:** Age less than 12 months
  - Early cases respond to serial manipulation (stretching of TA) and closed reduction of the talonavicular (TN) joint and cast application. Many cases require percutaneous TA tenotomy, TN joint reduction, and k-wire fixation.
- **Late cases:** Age 1–3 years
  - Late cases require open reduction of dislocated TN joint and k-wire fixation and lengthening of contracted tissues (TA, extensor digitorum longus, extensor hallucis longus, peroneal tendons, and tendoachilles).
- **After 3–5 years:** Triple arthrodesis.

DEVELOPMENTAL DYSPLASIA OF HIP

DEFINITION

Developmental dysplasia of hip (DDH) typically refers to patients born with hip dislocation or hip instability.

TERATOLOGIC HIP DISLOCATION

Teratologic dislocation of the hip is defined as a congenital dislocation of hip, which is **irreducible by gentle manipulation at birth**. It is often associated with arthrogryposis, spina bifida, or spasticity.

ETIOLOGY/RISK FACTORS

- **Racial background:** *Native American and Caucasians* have a higher incidence.
- **Positive family history, genetic:** *Ten times higher* chance in a newborn if parents had developmental dysplasia of the hip (DDH).
- **Females:** DDH is more common in females (male:female: 1:6)
- **First child:** More common in the first child

- **Breech delivery:** More common in kids with breech delivery
- **Left side:** It is more prevalent on the left side (L>R: 2–3:1)
- **Ligament laxity**
- **Oligohydramnios:** Intrauterine crowding
- **Associated neuromuscular abnormality:** Cerebral palsy, arthrogryposis multiplex congenita (AMC), and spina bifida.

Risk factors for DDH: *Remember 'Fs', R and S*

Family history, **F**irst child, **F**emale, **F**aulty uterine position, crowding and tissues (Breech, Oligohydramnios, ligament laxity), **R**acial (caucasians) and **S**ide (left)

SURGICAL PATHOANATOMY

The pathoanatomy of DDH varies from mild acetabular dysplasia to minor subluxation to a frank dislocation of the femoral head. There are changes in acetabulum, femoral head, labrum, acetabular fat, ligamentum teres, and surrounding capsule-muscle-tendons **(Fig. 44.15)**. **Table 44.7** briefly mentions the pathoanatomy of a DDH patient.

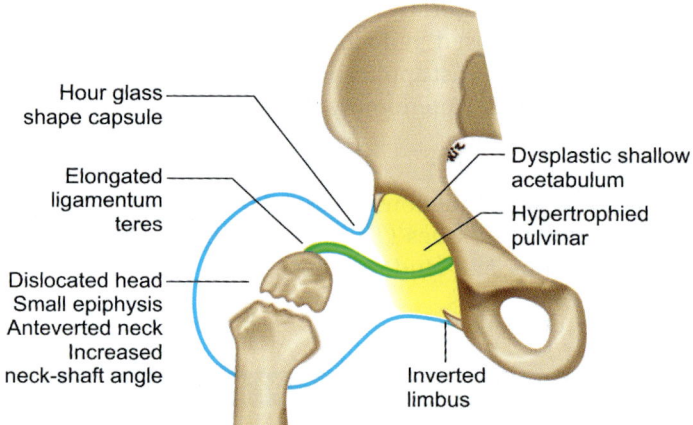

Fig. 44.15: Illustrative image showing pathological changes in developmental dysplasia of hip.

Table 44.7: Pathoanatomy of structures involved in developmental dysplasia of the hip (DDH).

Structure	Alteration
Femur head and neck	Dislocated head, small epiphysis, increased neck shaft angle (coxa valga) and increased anteversion of neck
Acetabulum	Dysplastic, shallow and steep roof
Muscle around hip	Adductor contracture
Capsule of hip joint	Hourglass contracture (as compressed by crossing the iliopsoas tendon)
Acetabular limbus	Inverted (folded inwards) toward the acetabulum
Ligamentum teres	Elongated and hypertrophied

Before the clinical features of DDH are discussed, readers must understand two critical tests to assess DDH—**Barlow's and Ortolani tests**.

Chapter 44: Congenital and Other Pediatric Disorders

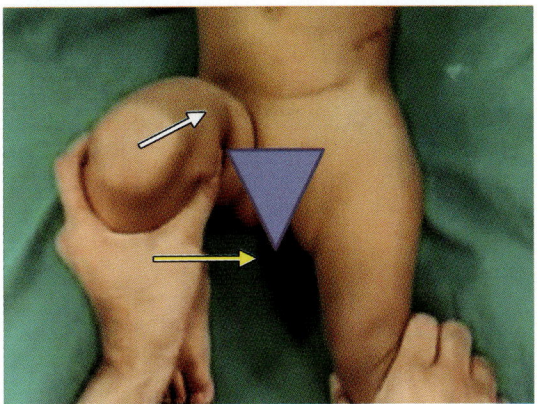

Fig. 44.16: Barlow's test. White and yellow arrows signify posterior push to the femur and adduction of hip, respectively.

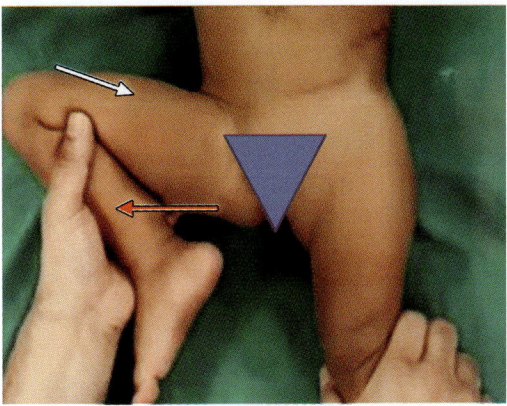

Fig. 44.17: Ortolani test. White and orange arrows signify anterior push to the femur and abduction of hip, respectively.

- **Barlow's test:** With the child in a supine position, the hip and knee are flexed up to 90°. Then, fingers are kept around the greater trochanter and thumb toward the inner aspect of the thigh. Then, the *hip is adducted*, and a gentle posterior push is given, resulting in dislocation of the hip **(Fig. 44.16)**.
- **Ortolani's test:** With the child in a supine position, the hip and knee are flexed up to 90°. Then fingers are kept around the greater trochanter and thumb toward the inner aspect of the thigh. Then *hip is abducted*, and a gentle anterior push is given **(Fig. 44.17)**. If the hip is in a dislocated position, it reduces the hip with a clunk (palpable/audible).

Trivia Pnemonic: How to remember Barlow and Ortolani test?
Barlow: It can be understood with hindi words- 'bahar-lo', which means take it out.
Ortolani: O to I (outside to inside)

The Ortolani test is more significant as it signifies that the hip is relocatable (reducible) by the closed method, whereas the negative Ortolani test suggests that the hip is stable or irreducible.
The positive Barlow test indicates an unstable hip joint.

CLINICAL FEATURES: DEPENDS UPON THE AGE OF PRESENTATION

- **Up to 2–3 months**
  Mother may complain difficulty in applying diaper (due to difficult abduction of thigh) or feeling a clunk during abduction-adduction as hip goes in and out of the acetabulum.
  - Asymmetric thigh folds **(Fig. 44.18)**
  - The hip is dislocatable and relocatable—Barlow's and Ortolani tests are positive **(Figs. 44.16 and 44.17)**.
- **After 3–6 months**
  - Asymmetry of the thigh and gluteal folds
  In unilateral DDH, the affected *greater trochanter is at higher level* than normal side
  - *Shortening of thigh* may be noted
  - **Limited abduction at the hip**

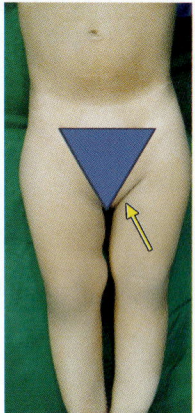

Fig. 44.18: Assymetric thigh fold (yellow arrow).

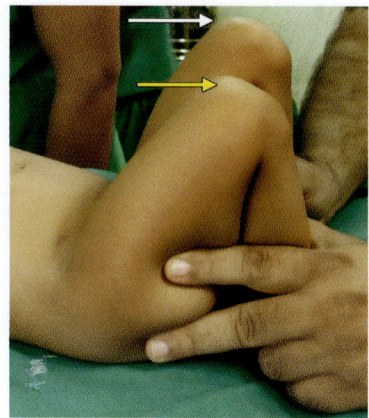

Fig. 44.19: Galeazzi sign (yellow arrow shows lower level of affected thigh, while white arrow shows normal thigh level).

- *Galeazzi sign is positive:* The knee of the affected side is at a lower level than the normal side **(Fig. 44.19)**.
- *Telescopy test positive*
- The *vascular sign of Narath* is positive.
- *Barlow's and Ortolani tests are positive.* However, these tests may become negative with advancing age due to fixed contractures.
- **Children who start walking**
- Superior location of greater trochanter in unilateral cases
    - *Increased lumbar lordosis*
    - *Galeazzi test and vascular sign of Narath positive*
    - *Positive Trendelenburg test*
    - *Trendelenburg gait in unilateral and Waddling gait in bilateral cases.*
    - *Ortolani and Barlow's may be negative due to irreducible hip*

Always look for neurological causes: *Spina bifida.*

INVESTIGATIONS

Most cases of DDH can be diagnosed with the help of a *plain radiograph of both hips*. Another investigation that may help diagnose DDH in *infants younger than six months is USG*, as the hip cartilage is poorly formed.

- **Plain X-ray of the hip:** Several important findings can be observed in a DDH **(Fig. 44.20)**
    - *Dislocated or subluxated hip* indicated by broken Shenton's line and femoral head position in quadrant other than inferomedial **(Fig. 44.20)**.
    - *Dysplastic acetabulum*, which is measured by acetabular index and center-edge angle.
        - *Acetabular index* is an angle between the Hilgenreiner line and the margin of the acetabulum **(Fig. 44.21)**. It is increased in DDH indicative of a dysplastic shallow acetabulum.

> **Important**
> **Shenton's line**
> Shenton's line is formed by superior border of obturator foramen, inferior part of acetabulm, femoral head and neck.

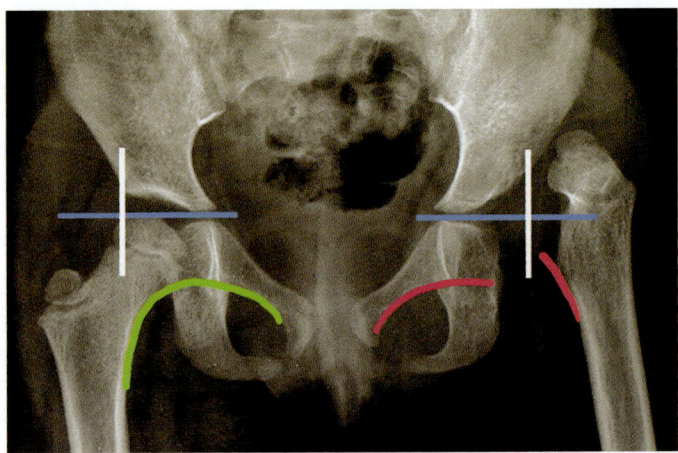

Fig. 44.20: X-ray of DDH showing the dislocated head of the femur on the left side. The green line denotes normal Shenton line, whereas interrupted red line indicates disrupted Shenton's line. The white line denotes the "Perkins line," and the blue line denotes the "Hilgenreiner line" dividing the acetabular area into four quadrants. The femoral head must lie in the inferomedial quadrant. The head position in any other quadrant indicates subluxation/dislocation.

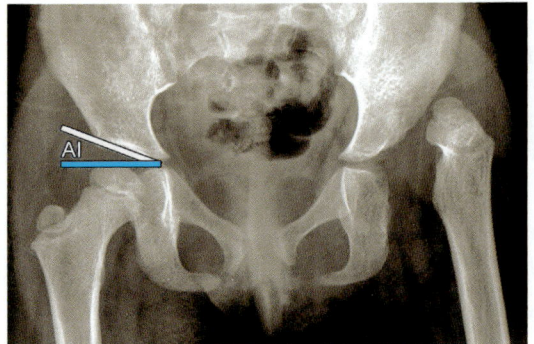

Fig. 44.21: X-ray of the hip showing acetabular index (AI) on normal side of the hip.

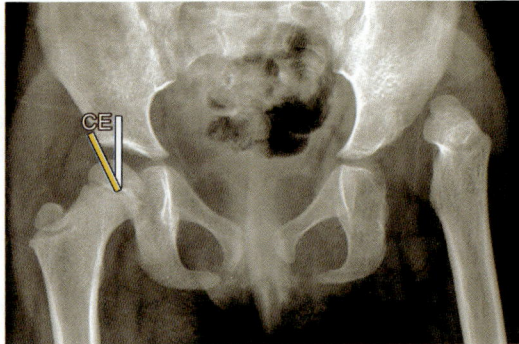

Fig. 44.22: X-ray of the hip showing center-edge (CE) angle on normal side of the hip.

- **Center-edge angle (of Wiberg)** is an angle between Perkin's line and center of the head **(Fig. 44.22)**. It is decreased in DDH. *Note that it is useful in children older than 6 years.*
- **Ultrasonography (USG)** is a *good screening tool for patients with a positive family history but a normal clinical examination.* It can be used in *children younger than six months of age* wherein femoral head is poorly ossified to be visualized on a plain X-ray. Two angles are measured during USG-alpha and beta (Graf angle). Alpha angle is a measure of the angle between ilium and the roof of acetabulum, while the beta angle is a measure of the angle between the labrum and ilium **(Fig. 44.23)**. Normally, the alpha angle should be >60°, and the beta should be less than 55°. *Alpha angle decreases with severity, while beta increases with severity.*

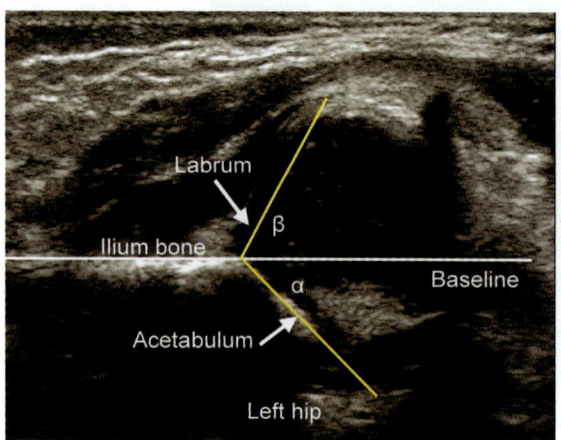

Fig. 44.23: USG of a DDH child showing alpha and beta angles.

> **Box 44.1:** Summary of DDH treatment.
> - **Age <6 months:** CR and Pavlik harness/von Rosen splint
> - **Age 6–18 months:** CR/OR and hip spica application
> - **Age 18 months–6 years:** OR, VDO, femoral shortening, and pelvic osteotomy
> - **Age 7–10 years:**
>   – Unilateral DDH—OR, VDO, femoral shortening, and pelvic osteotomy
>   – Bilateral DDH—no treatment
> - **Age >10 years:** No treatment (uni- or bilateral). Later arthrodesis or THR can be planned as an adult
>
> (CR: closed reduction; OR: open reduction; VDO: varus derotation osteotomy)

TREATMENT

At any age, DDH treatment involves the fulfilment of three major principles.
1. **Concentric reduction of the hip into the acetabulum**
2. **Maintain reduction till the hip is stable in the acetabulum**
3. **Follow-up till skeletal maturity.**

The treatment of DDH is based upon two facts—age of presentation and reducibility of the hip by closed/open methods. **Box 44.1** and **Flowchart 44.2** summarize the treatment protocol of DDH.

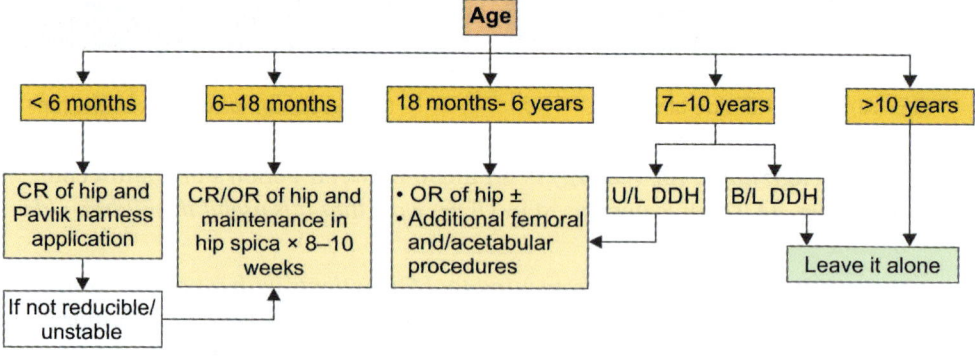

Flowchart 44.2: Treatment algorithm to manage developmental dysplasia of hip (DDH) in various age groups.

- **Age: Newborn to 6 months**
  In this age, most DDH are reducible by closed methods. Therefore, following protocol is used to manage DDH.
  ◆ Closed reduction of the hip
  ◆ Maintain reduction by Pavlik harness/Von Rosen splint **(Fig. 44.24)**.

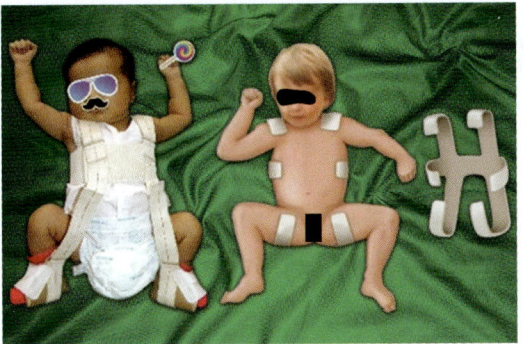
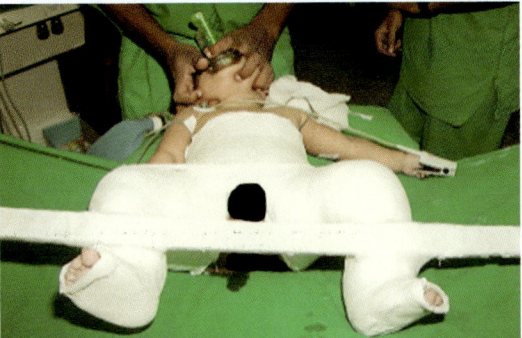

Fig. 44.24: Pavlik harness (left image) and Von Rosen splint (right image).

Fig. 44.25: Hip spica in flexion, abduction.

Note: Pavlik harness is contraindicated in teratological hip dislocations, spasticity and spina bifida.

- **Age: 6–18 months**
  In this age, many of the DDH are reducible by closed methods, whereas some may require open reduction. Therefore, following protocol is used to manage DDH.
   - Closed reduction (CR) should be done under general anesthesia (GA). Once CR is successful, maintain the reduction in hip spica application in 90° flexion and 45° abduction of the hip for a few weeks **(Fig. 44.25)**.
   - If CR under GA fails, open reduction (OR) should be done followed by hip spica application.
   - Later, once the hip is stable without spica, Von Rosen splint/hip abduction orthosis is applied. The splint is continued till the hip is clinically stable.
- **Age: 18 months till 6 years**
  In this age group, *closed reduction is usually unsuccessful due to severely contracted tissues and deformed bones and joints* (see **Table 44.7**) *and hence should not be tried. A forcible CR can cause avascular necrosis of the hip.*
   - The **treatment of choice** is open reduction of the hip followed by maintenance of reduction in hip spica.
     Furthermore, due to severely contracted tissues and deformed bones, often additional procedures are required to achieve a stable and concentrically reduced hip, such as:
     - Adductor tenotomy, femoral shortening
     - Varus derotation osteotomy (VDO) of the femur **(Fig. 44.26)**

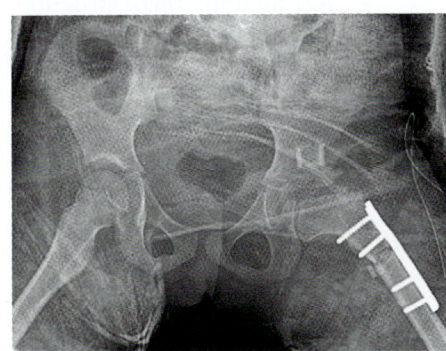

Fig. 44.26: X-ray shows varus derotation osteotomy (VDO) on the left side.

Rationale of VDO in DDH
Since the femoral head neck is in valgus and anteversion, femur shaft is osteotomized below the lesser trochanter and positioned into varus (to decrease valgus) and derotated to reduce anteversion.

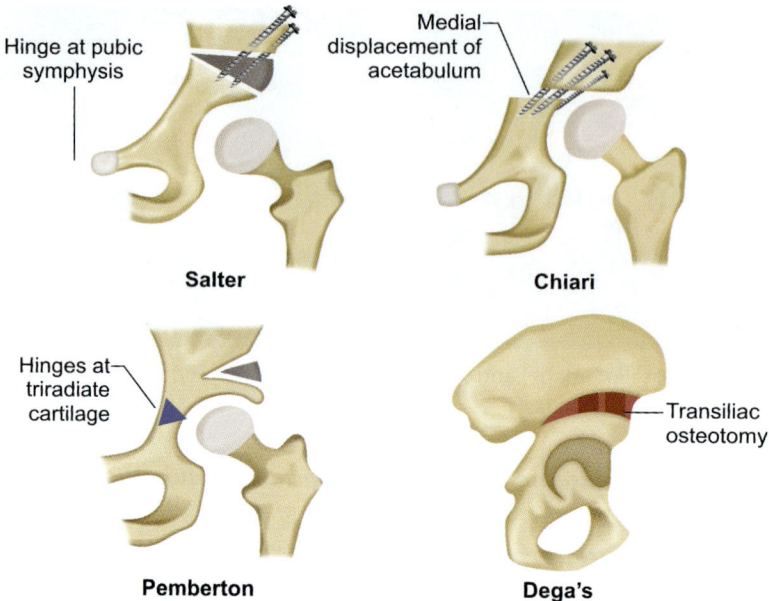

Fig. 44.27: Various pelvic osteotomies performed in DDH to improve acetabular coverage of the femoral head.

- Acetabulum reconstruction is performed to improve femoral head coverage by various osteotomies, such as Salter's, Dega, Chiari, and Pemberton acetabuloplasty **(Fig. 44.27)**. (*Note:* Details of osteotomy aren't needed for undergraduate teaching).
- **Age: 7–10 years**
  In this age group, closed reduction is not possible. However, the treatment depends upon uni- or bi-laterality of the DDH.
  - ***Unilateral DDH:*** Open reduction, VDO, femoral shortening, and pelvic osteotomies can be attempted. However, the rate of complications is high, and outcomes are unpredictable.
  - ***Bilateral DDH:*** Bilateral DDH can be left as mostly:
    - Limp is less noticeable than unilateral DDH
    - May continue to walk with a limp for many years
    - The result of treatment is less predictable, and the chances of avascular necrosis (AVN) are quite high
    - Later, patients may require total hip replacement (THR) in or after the 4th or 5th decade if the patient develops symptomatic secondary osteoarthrosis of the hip.
- **Age: Over 10 years:** Unilateral or bilateral DDH in a child more than 10 years, can be left alone. It may require THR during adulthood if the patient develops secondary osteoarthrosis severe enough affecting the activities of daily living.

COMPLICATIONS AFTER DDH

- 2° osteoarthritis of the hip
- Avascular necrosis due to attempts of reduction (open/closed)
- Shortening of the limb.

MULTIPLE CONGENITAL CONTRACTURES

DEFINITION

A nonprogressive congenital disorder involving multiple stiff joints (>2) causing severe restriction in mobility and activities of daily living **(Fig. 44.28)**.

ETIOPATHOGENESIS: IDIOPATHIC

- It is either *neurogenic* (90%) or *myopathic* (10%).
- Some mothers have shown *antibodies to acetylcholine receptors* leading to the depletion of anterior horn cells.

CLINICAL FEATURES

These patients have *normal intelligence, face, and visceral function*. The musculoskeletal features are:
- Bilateral symmetrical deformities
- Absent skin creases **(Fig. 44.28)**
- Joints are fixed in flexion or extension.

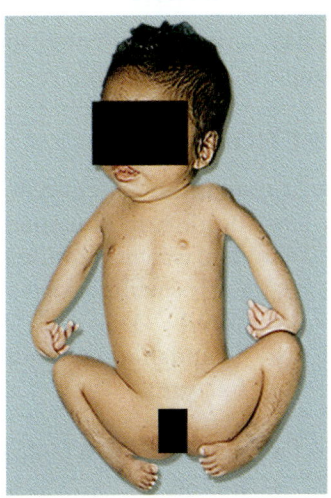

Fig. 44.28: Multiple congenital contracture (MCC) of upper and lower limbs. Note absent elbow crease.

Upper Limb

- **Arm** adducted and internally rotated
- **Elbow** extended
- **Wrist** flexed, and ulnar deviated.

Lower Limbs

- **Hip:** Flexed, abducted, and externally rotated teratologic dislocation or subluxation common
- **Knee:** Hyperextended or flexed
- **Ankle-foot:** Equinovarus, club foot, and vertical talus.

TREATMENT

Treatment of MCC usually requires surgical correction as contractures are very rigid and may be associated with subluxation or dislocation of the joints. Various surgical options are:
- Extensive soft tissue release surgery followed by serial casting and orthotic support
- Open reduction of dislocations
- Epiphysiodesis
- Corrective osteotomies.

PROGNOSIS

The chance of recurrence remains high.

COXA VARA

◼ DEFINITION

Coxa vara is a hip condition wherein the neck shaft angle is less than 120°.

◼ ETIOLOGY

- **Congenital:** There is a defect in endochondral ossification in the medial aspect of the femur. Gradual weight-bearing leads to stress fracture and later varus with retroversion of femoral neck.
- **Acquired**
    - Traumatic—malunion of intertrochanteric fracture
    - Perthes' disease
    - Slipped capital femoral epiphysis
    - Rickets
    - Postinfection squeal—TB.

Femoral neck shaft angle and femoral anteversion

Normal **femoral neck shaft angle** varies between 125°–135° with global mean of 126°.

Femoral anteversion refers to the orientation of the femoral neck in relation to the femoral condyles at the level of the knee. In most cases, the femoral neck is oriented anteriorly as compared to the femoral condyles known as anteversion, whereas posterior orientation of femoral neck with respect to the femoral condyle is known as femoral retroversion. Normally, the femur is 8–15° anteverted.

◼ CLINICAL FEATURES

- **Limp:** Due to pain and shortening
- **Shortening** of limb
- **Gait:** Trendelenburg gait in unilateral and waddling gait in bilateral coxa vara.
- **Hip movements:** Abduction and internal rotation are restricted.

◼ INVESTIGATIONS

Plain X-ray of the hip (Fig. 44.29)
- *Reduced neck shaft angle* ($\beta < \alpha$)
- *Fairbank's triangle* is present in congenital coxa vara
- *Hilgenreiner's epiphyseal (HE) angle* is increased (normal: <25°). Note that HE angle is an angle between a line through the proximal femoral physis and the Hilgenreiner line.

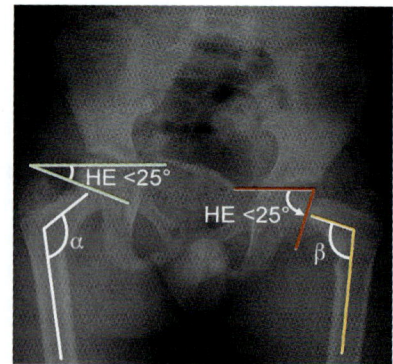

Fig. 44.29: X-ray of hips showing coxa vara of left hip. α and β are neck shaft angle.

(HE: Hilgenreiner epiphyseal angle)

Fairbank triangle

A triangular metaphyseal fragment in the inferior aspect of femoral neck surrounded by radiolucent Y. It represents a zone of abnormal ossification with an interposed triangular segment of dystrophic bone.

TREATMENT

The treatment depends upon Hilgenreiner's epiphyseal angle.
- **Hilgenreiner's epiphyseal angle:** *25–45°*
  - Observe
- **Hilgenreiner's epiphyseal angle:** *45–60°*
  - Observe serially for any increase in angle.
  - Valgus derotation osteotomy is performed, if pain and limp increase with the progression of varus.
- **Hilgenreiner's epiphyseal angle:** *>60°*
  - Corrective valgus derotation osteotomy

SLIPPED CAPITAL FEMORAL EPIPHYSIS (SCFE)

DEFINITION

A disease of proximal femoral physis leading to the slip of the femoral metaphysis anteriorly and proximally with respect to the femoral epiphysis **(Fig. 44.30)**.

Note: The term SCFE is a misnomer as it is the metaphysis which slips and epiphysis remains in its place in the acetabulum due to its attachment with ligamentum teres.

Incidence: It is more common in adolescent males who are between 12–15 years of age. 20–40% of cases are bilateral.

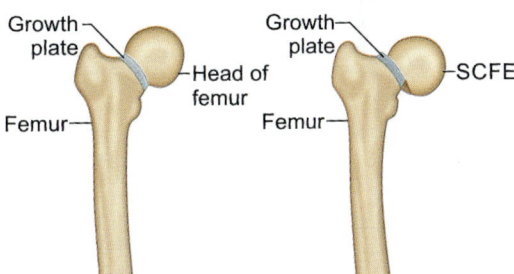

Fig. 44.30: Left image is of a normal hip, while right image shows separated physis from metaphysis.

ETIOPATHOGENESIS

Risk Factors

- Males are more affected than females (male:female—2:1)
- ***Obesity is the most critical risk factor!***
- Occurs at ***adolescence***
- ***Often associated with endocrine disorders***
  - **Hypogonadism:** The growth hormone induces physeal hypertrophy, whereas the gonadal hormone causes physeal maturation. Any imbalance between two hormones can result in SCFE
  - Hypothyroidism
  - Chronic renal osteodystrophy.

Pathogenesis

One must suspect SCFE in an adolescent, an obese male child with or without endocrinal disorders who presents with hip pain and a limp (Fig. 44.31).

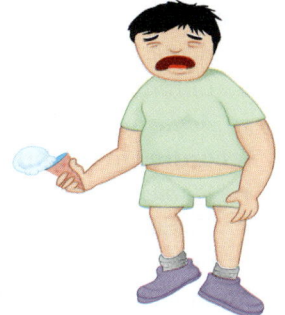

Fig. 44.31: Illustration showing an obese child complains of hip pain. The ice cream slipping from the cone represents SCFE.

(*Courtesy:* Dr Aarthi, MBBS, KMC, Manipal)

SCFE seems to be a mechanical failure of a weak physical plate. The growth plate seems weak due to an imbalance between circulating gonadotrophins, weakness in the perichondrial ring and more oblique orientation during the growth period. Therefore, a weak physeal plate is prone to separation during growth, especially in an obese child. **Flowchart 44.3** summarizes the pathogenesis of SCFE.

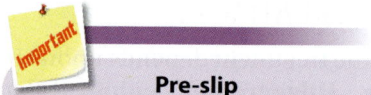

Pre-slip

The SCFE slip happens through the hypertrophic zone of cartilage of physis.

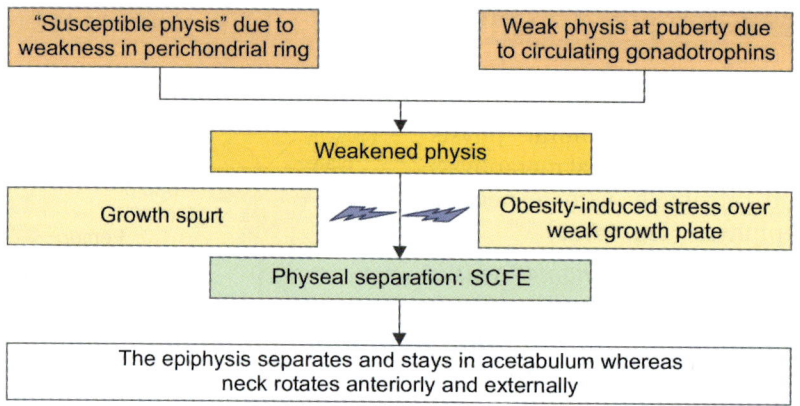

Flowchart 44.3: Pathogenesis of slipped capital femoral epiphysis (SCFE).

CLASSIFICATION

SCFE has been classified according to the *time of presentation (temporal), stability of the hip, and radiological angle measurement*.

- **Temporal**
    - *Acute*: Slip within 3 weeks
    - *Chronic (85%)*: Slip greater than 3 weeks
    - *Acute on chronic*.
- **According to stability (Loder classification)**
    - *Stable slip*: Patient can walk with or without the crutch
    - *Unstable slip*: Unable to ambulate even with a crutch (USG shows effusion, no metaphyseal remodeling)
- **Southwick angle**: It is the angle between the femoral head and the shaft. The degree of slip (mild/moderate/severe) is classified based on difference between the southwick angle of normal and affected side. If both hips are involved, consider 10° as unaffected hip reference on lateral X-ray.
    - *Mild*: Less than 30°
    - *Moderate*: 30–50°
    - *Severe*: Greater than 50°.

Pre-slip

There is a condition known as 'pre-slip' wherein the adolescent child complains of hip pain without any significant obvious X-ray abnormality. The internal rotation is restricted. In such cases, an MRI of the hip is useful.

CLINICAL FEATURES

Symptoms
- **Pain:** The pain around the hip is one of the common symptoms. Often, pain radiates to the thigh and the knee.
- **Limp** is often present.

Signs
- *The affected lower limb is externally rotated.*
- **Gait:** The child may walk with an *out-toeing gait* due to external rotation deformity.
- **ROM assessment:** *There is a loss of internal rotation, flexion, and abduction.*
- **Limb length**: There may be *limb shortening*
- *Trendelenburg sign is positive.*

INVESTIGATIONS
- **Plain X-ray of both hips**: Anteroposterior (AP) and frog leg lateral view.
  Earliest signs are wide and irregular physis with rarefaction in its juxtaphyseal region.
  - *Trethowan sign:* Normally, a line drawn along the superior border of the femoral neck *(Klein line)* must intersect some part of the femoral head. It should be assessed both in AP and frog leg view. A non-intersecting Klein line indicates SCFE **(Figs. 44.32A and B)**.
  - *Southwick angle (slip angle)* is increased **(Fig. 44.33)**.
- **MRI** is rarely performed in radiologically confirmed SCFE. However, it may be useful in a preslip situation.
- **USG:** Absence of effusion and metaphyseal remodeling indicates a stable slip.
- **Investigations for the associated endocrinal disorder, if any**.

TREATMENT
Treatment of SCFE aims to prevent further slip and promote closure of the physis. Since the reduction of the slipped physis is not easy and may result in AVN of the head femur, *commonly, insitu pinning is the preferred treatment.*

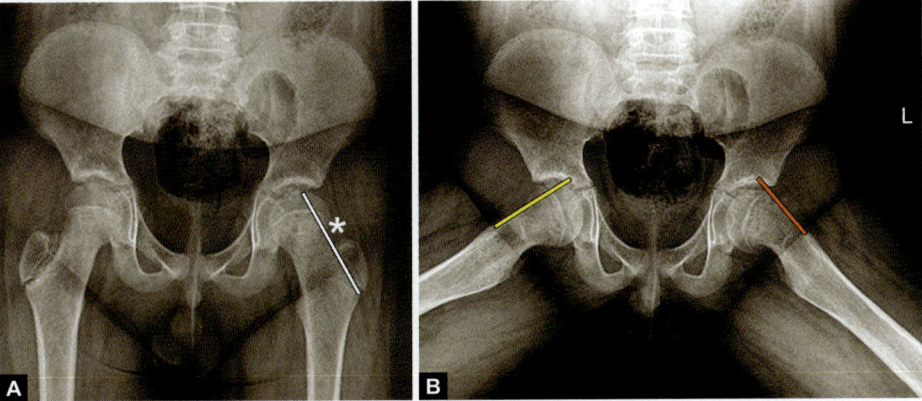

Figs. 44.32A and B: (A) Klein line intersecting the femoral head in AP view of the hip; (B) In the frog leg view, the yellow line intersects, while the orange line does not intersect the femoral epiphysis indicating SCFE on left side.

Section 12: Congenital and Other Pediatric Disorders

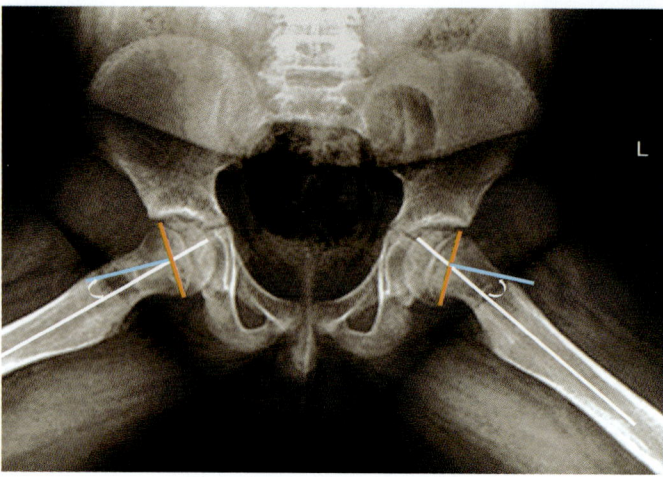

Fig. 44.33: Southwick angle measurement in frog leg view. Right hip SW angle is normal while left hip is increased, implying the possibility of SCFE on the left side. White line represents long axis of femur, whereas orange line joins anterior and posterior edge of physis (physeal line). Blue line is perpendicular to physeal line. Southwick angle is angle between long axis of femur and blue line.

Southwick angle: It is the angle between the perpendicular to the line joining the anterior and posterior tip of physis and the long axis of the femur. The angle is measured bilaterally and the slipped side angle is subtracted from the normal side angle.

Mild slip is when the difference is less than 30°, moderate is 30–50°, and severe is greater than 50°. 10° is the normal control value to be used in the bilateral case.

- **Stable slip:** Closed reduction and percutaneous pinning with cancellous screws **(Fig. 44.34)**.
- **Unstable slip:** Gentle reduction and percutaneous in situ pinning with cancellous screws.
- **Other "normal" hip:** Observe or consider prophylactic pinning.
- *For chronic stable, clinically significant and severe slip* may require certain femoral osteotomies, such as Dunn's, Modified Dunn or Southwick. (Details are out of scope of this chapter).

■ COMPLICATIONS

- **Avascular necrosis of the hip:** Higher chance in unstable hips.
- **Chondrolysis:** Idiopathic necrosis of the articular cartilage of the hip followed by severe pain and stiffness. Often, it occurs due to pin/screw penetration into the hip joint.
- **2° hip osteoarthritis**.

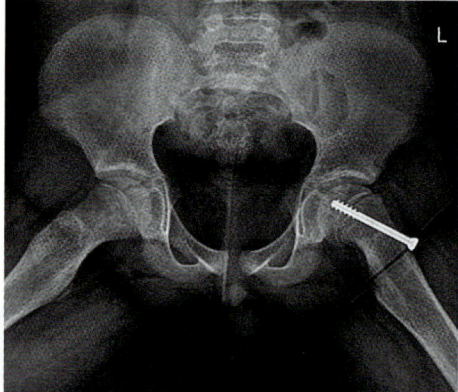

Fig. 44.34: Percutaneous in situ pinning.

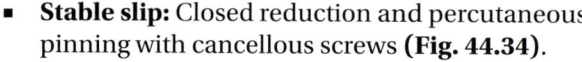

■ DEFINITION OF OSTEOCHONDROSIS

Aseptic avascular necrosis of epiphysis or a small bone (carpals/tarsals).
- It occurs in children and adolescents, often during the period of rapid growth.
- The cause is mostly avascularity, minor trauma, or repetitive stress.

In case of aseptic necrosis of bones in childhood: High chance of spontaneous return of blood supply and recovery.

In case of aseptic necrosis of bones in adults: Poor chance of return of blood supply and recovery.

TYPES

- **Pulling type**: Due to pulling by the tendon
  - *Osgood Schlatter disease*: Tibial tuberosity
  - *Sinding-Larsen-Johansson disease*: Lower pole of patella
  - *Sever's disease*: Calcaneal apophysis
  - *Iselin's disease*: Fifth metatarsal base.
- **Crushing type:** Due to undue compressive stress over the bone
  - *Proximal femur epiphysis*: Perthes disease
  - *Second metatarsal head*: Freiberg disease
  - *Navicular*: Kohler's disease
  - *Lunate*: Kienbock's disease
  - *Scaphoid*: Preiser's disease
  - *Capitellum*: Panner's disease/little leaguer's elbow
  - *Vertebral ring epiphysis*: Scheuermann's disease
  - *Vertebral central epiphysis*: Calve disease
- **Splitting type:** Small fragment of cartilage separates from the subchondral bone. It is known as osteochondritis dessicans (OCD)
  - Osteochondritis dessicans of the medial femoral condyle, the anteromedial dome of the talus, and capitellum.

PERTHES' DISEASE (LEGG-CALVE-PERTHES DISEASE)

Arthur Legg (United States), Jacques Calve (France), and George Clemens Perthes (Germany) described this condition separately. Thus, the eponym Legg-Calve-Perthes originated.

DEFINITION

Perthes' disease is a self-limiting idiopathic avascular necrosis of femoral head epiphysis in children from 5 to 15 years due to temporary ischemia leading to a cycle of avascular necrosis, deformation and subsequent revascularization of the femoral head.

DEMOGRAPHIC DETAILS

- 30/100,000 children (variable in different geographical areas).
- **Age of children affected:** 5–15 years.
- Perthes' disease is more common in the west coast of India.

- **Gender:** It is more common in males (male:female—3:1).
- It is bilateral in 10% of cases.
- Often, these kids are shorter than their siblings and show disproportionate growth of the appendicular skeleton.

ETIOLOGY AND RISK FACTORS

Broadly, the etiology of Perthes' disease remains idiopathic. Many theories are implicated in the avascular necrosis of the femoral head, such as:

Temporary ischemia of the head is the most accepted one. Others are:
- Venous hypertension in the head and neck of the femur.
- The disease of epiphyseal cartilage.
- Genetic.
- Trauma.

PATHOGENESIS

The pathogenesis of Perthes has been described in four stages: Stage of synovitis, stage of avascular necrosis, stage of fragmentation, and residual/healed stage.

First stage: *Stage of synovitis*
- Synovial hypertrophy and joint effusion
- Cartilage hypertrophy
- Head size increases medially
- Lateral displacement of the femoral head.

Second stage: *Stage of avascular necrosis*
- Necrotic trabeculae of infarcted head collapse
- Neovascularization of metaphysis
- New bone laid on dead trabeculae
- Head shape is still normal, and ossific nuclei become dense.

Third stage: *Stage of fragmentation (revascularization)*
- Immature woven bone replaces infarcted trabeculae
- Vulnerable to deformity (biologically plastic)
- The head cannot stand the stress resulting in a flattened, fragmented head.

Fourth stage: *Residual or healed stage*
The necrotic bone is replaced by mature bone.

CLASSIFICATION

Based upon plain X-ray findings, three classifications are used to assess the stage of Perthes':
- **Modified Elizabethtown classification**
    - *Stage I (avascular necrosis of the femoral head):* Dense and sclerotic bone
    - *Stage II (fragmentation):* Fragmented, flat epiphysis
    - *Stage III (regeneration):* More fragmentation with regeneration (new bone over necrotic bone)
    - *Stage IV (healed):* Healed with complete re-ossification and no residual necrotic area.

- **Catterall Classification (Fig. 44.35)**
  - *Group I:* Only anterior epiphysis involved
  - *Group II:* Anterior epiphysis + central sequestrum
  - *Group III:* Only a small part is not involved
  - *Group IV:* Complete head involvement.
- **Herring lateral pillar classification (Figs. 44.36A to C)**
  The epiphysis is divided into three pillars—central, medial, and lateral
  - *Herring A:* Only the central pillar is fragmented, intact lateral pillar
  - *Herring B:* Central and less than 50% of lateral pillar fragmented
  - *Herring C:* Central and greater than 50% of lateral pillar fragmented.

CLINICAL FEATURES

Symptoms

- **A painless limp** is one of the earliest signs of Perthes' disease.
- **Pain in the hip:** Sometimes, there can be pain in the hip, which exacerbates on activity. Often, the pain radiates to the thigh/knee.

Signs

- **Gait:** Many kids may have *Trendelenburg gait*.
- **Tenderness** is present over the hip joint.
- **Trendelenburg test is positive.**

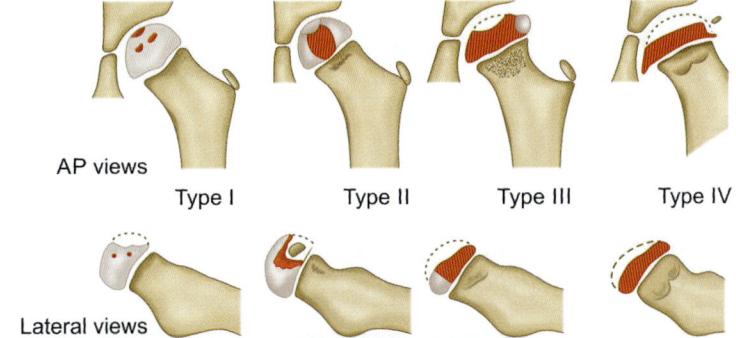

Fig. 44.35: Catterall classification.

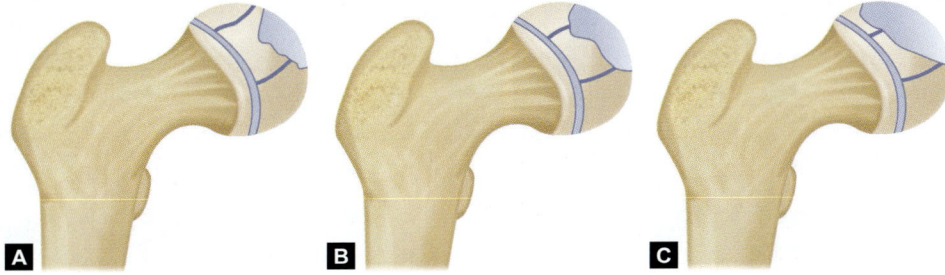

Figs. 44.36A to C: Herring classification.

- **Range of movement** (ROM) at the hip: The ***abduction and internal rotation is limited***. Sometimes, global restriction of ROM is present.
- **Sectoral or Catterall sign:** When the hip is gradually flexed, it moves into an obligatory external rotation.

INVESTIGATIONS

- X-ray of the pelvis with both hips AP (Fig. 44.37A) and frog leg lateral view (Fig. 44.37B): The radiological features depends on the Elizabethtown stage of the disease.

  Early signs
  - Widened medial joint space due to effusion
  - Smaller and horizontal femoral epiphysis
  - Fragmentation of femoral epiphysis with subchondral lucency (Crescent sign)
  - Increased density of epiphysis.
  - **Signs of healing:** Healing is evident by new woven bone formation which is less radiodense and starts from periphery.

  Late signs
  - ***Sagging rope sign:*** A thin sclerotic line crossing the femoral neck
  - ***Coxa magna:*** Enlarged femoral head
  - ***Coxa breva:*** Smaller femoral head
  - ***Coxa plana:*** Flattened femoral head (like a mushroom).
- **Bone scan:** Earliest positive as "cold spot".
- **MRI of both hips:** It can diagnose Perthes at the earliest when plain radiographs are normal.

'Catterall' radiological head at risk sign (indicate poor prognosis).
- Metaphyseal cyst
- Lateral extrusion of femoral head
- Horizontal growth plate
- Ossification lateral to epiphysis
- Gaze sign.

TREATMENT

The principles of treatment are:
- *Achieve and maintain hip ROM,* and *relieve weight bearing*
- *Concentric containment of femoral epiphysis* within the acetabulum
- *Prevent deformity of the femoral head.*

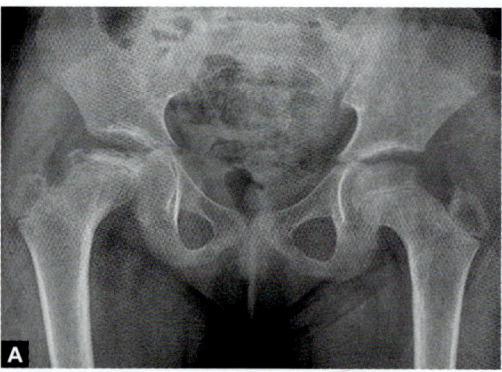
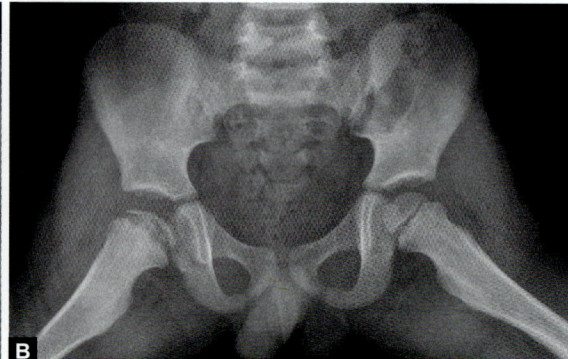

Figs. 44.37A and B: Perthes disease: AP view (A) and frog leg view (B) showing right side Perthes disease.

The decision of treatment are based on certain parameters, such as *age, clinical presentation, hip motion, and radiological findings-extent of epiphyseal involvement, Catterall group, and stage.*

- ***Age of patient:*** Younger patients will have more remodeling potential. So, conservative treatment is advocated in less than 5 years of age.
- ***Clinical presentation:*** Acute disease (with painful stiff hip) vs. chronic Perthes (with mobile hip). Avoid surgery in acute stage
- ***Hip motion:*** If hip ROM is restricted, surgery is not performed.
- ***Radiological parameters:***
  - ***Epiphyseal involvement:*** Less than 20% extrusion of the femoral head does not require surgery.
  - ***Catterall group*** III and IV would require surgery
  - ***Elizabethtown I and II*** require surgery.

A. **Acute Perthes' disease with pain and limited movement:** The goal is to restore painless ROM by:
  - Rest, analgesics
  - Skin traction (below/above knee) to relieve pain, spasm and prevent/correct deformity.
  - Limitation of activity
  - Abduction (Broomstick) cast **(Fig. 44.38)**
    The abduction cast aims to put the extruded head back into the acetabulum for better remodeling.

B. **The treatment of chronic Perthes depends upon the age of the patient and epiphyseal involvement (Flowchart 44.4).**

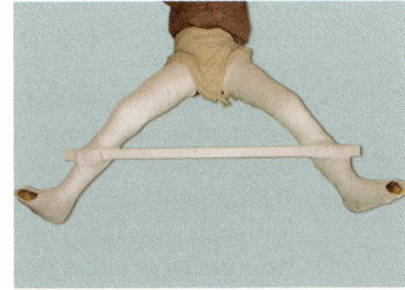

Fig. 44.38: Broomstick cast in Perthes.

Flowchart 44.4: Treatment algorithm of Perthes' disease in various age group and Elizabethtown stage.

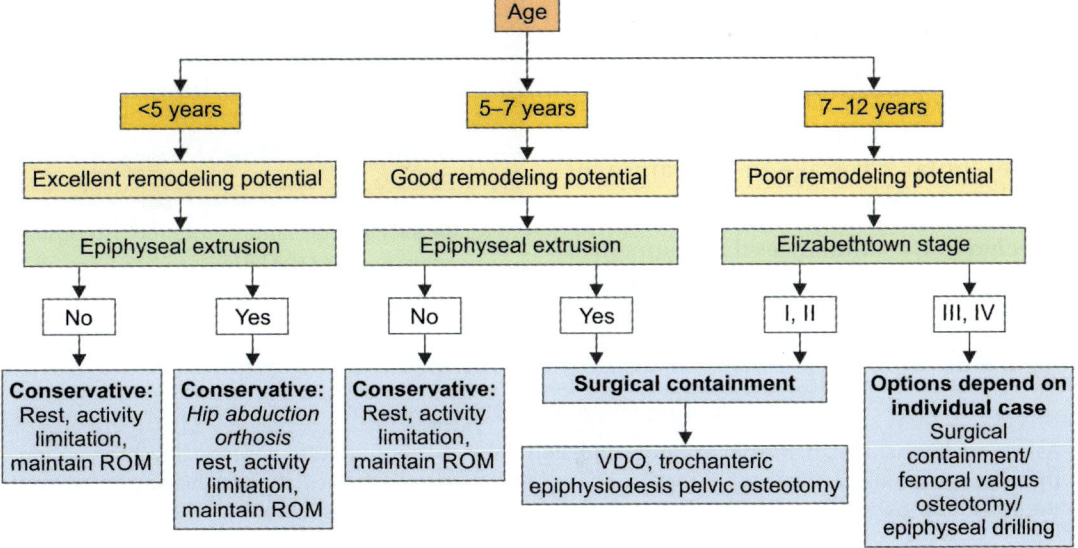

The summary of Chronic Perthes' treatment is as follows:
- **Age less than 5 years:** Usually, conservative treatment is the key in this age group, as the femoral head remodeling is excellent. The conservative treatment comprises limited activity, analgesics. Hip abduction splint is added if there is epiphyseal extrusion. Serial clinical and radiological monitoring of femoral head remodeling must be done.
- **Age 5-7 years:** Usually, remodeling of the femoral head is good in this age group. The decision regarding conservative or operative management depends on femoral epiphyseal extrusion.
    - *Conservative* if there is no epiphyseal extrusion
    - *Operative* if there is epiphyseal extrusion. For femoral head containment, Varus derotation osteotomy of femur, trochanteric epiphysiodesis with/without pelvic osteotomy is performed.
- **Age 7-12 years:** The remodeling potential of the femoral head is poor, especially if a large part of the femoral head is involved. The decision regarding standard containment procedure or salvage/conservative management depends on Elizabethtown classification.
    - If Elizabethtown Stage I, II: Standard femoral head containment surgery (Varus derotation osteotomy of femur, trochanteric epiphysiodesis with/without pelvic osteotomy)
    - If Elizabethtown Stage III, IV: The prognosis is poor in such stages. Therefore, either patient is managed conservatively or sometimes salvage procedures, such as valgus osteotomy, or epiphyseal drilling are performed.

Various commonly performed operative procedures for femoral head containment in Perthes' are:
- *Femoral varus derotation osteotomy* improves femoral head coverage under the acetabulum for better coverage and remodeling **(Fig. 44.39)**.
- *Pelvic osteotomies, such as* Salter, Chiari, Pemberton, Steel, Dega, or Ganz can be performed to improve the femoral head's acetabular coverage or containment (*see* **Fig. 44.27**).

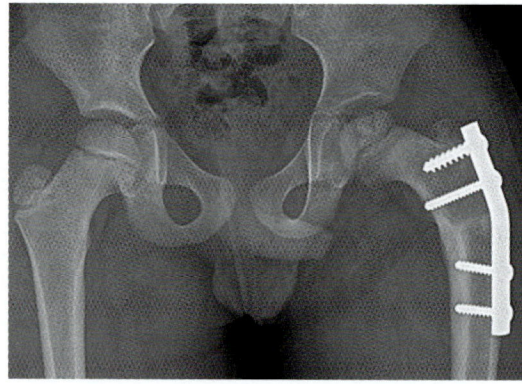

Fig. 44.39: Femoral varus derotation osteotomy of the left hip.

Flowchart 44.4 summarizes the treatment of Perthes' disease according to the age group.

What is femoral head containment?

As per my teacher Prof. Benjamin Joseph, " Containment is the term used to describe any intervention that places the anterolateral part of the femoral epiphysis well into the acetabulum thereby protecting the vulnerable part of the epiphysis from being subjected to deforming stresses."

PROGNOSTIC FACTORS OF PERTHES' DISEASE

- Younger patients have a better prognosis as they have higher remodeling potential.
- Poorer prognosis if there is the presence of Catterall at risk head signs, extensive subchondral fracture lines, aspherical femoral head and Herring C type head.

FLAT FOOT/PES PLANUS

DEFINITION

A condition wherein the medial longitudinal arch (MLA) of the foot is collapsed, leading to the entire sole coming into contact with the ground **(Figs. 44.40A and B)**.

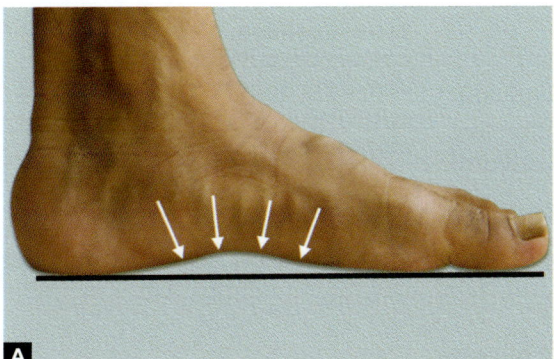
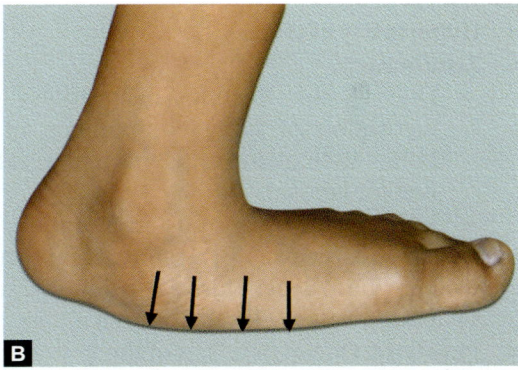

Figs. 44.40A and B: Normal and Pes planus foot: (A) Normal foot, wherein medial longitudinal arch (multiple white arrows) is not in contact with ground; (B) Flat foot, wherein the medial longitudinal arch (multiple black arrows) is in contact with the ground.

SURGICAL ANATOMY OF FOOT ARCHES

There are three arches in a foot—medial, lateral, and transverse **(Fig. 44.41)**. These arches are formed and maintained by foot bones and soft-tissue support.

Bony Component of Arches

- ***Medial longitudinal arch (MLA)*** is formed by calcaneum, talus, cuneiforms, navicular, first to third metatarsals. The "talonavicular" bony wedge is the keystone of the arch.
- ***Lateral longitudinal arch*** is formed by the calcaneum, cuboid, and fourth-to-fifth metatarsals.
- ***Transverse arch:*** Midtarsal joint and tarsometatarsal joints form the transverse arch of foot.

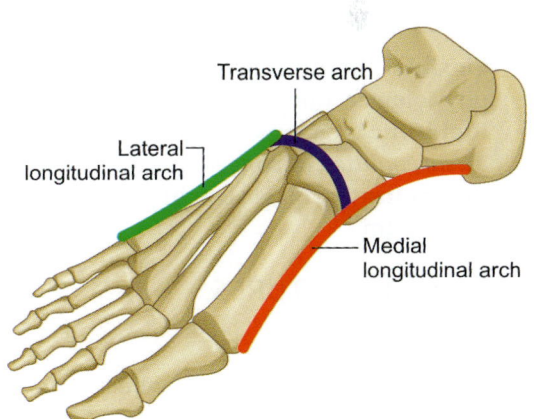

Fig. 44.41: Arches of the foot.

Soft Tissue Support of Arches

- **Tendons:** *Tibialis posterior*
  - It is the most critical dynamic elevator of the medial arch.
  - Other foot muscles (intrinsic and extrinsic) help in maintaining the arch.
- **Ligament:** *Spring ligament* is the most important static support of the medial arch.
- **Fascia:** *Plantaris fascia*
  - Dorsiflexion of the toes tightens the fascia and helps in elevating the arch.

ETIOLOGY

- **Congenital:** Tarsal coalition, vertical talus
- **Physiological:** Flat foot is a common finding up to 7 years of age.
- **Hyperlaxity of tissues**
- **Traumatic:**
  - Due to the fractures/dislocations with the disruption of bony components of the key bones such as the talus, navicular, calcaneum, first metatarsal
  - Injury to the tibialis posterior tendon.
- **Tibialis posterior (TP) dysfunction** is one of the most frequent cause, especially in older women due to degenerative attritional rupture of tendon/chronic tendinitis. A dysfunctional TP tendon fails to elevate the arch.
- **Paralytic:** Due to paralysis of the foot-ankle muscles.
- **Neuropathic arthritis (Charcot's foot):** Common in diabetics
- **Arthritis of the foot.**

Tarsal Coalition: A condition of foot wherein the tarsal bones are fused to each other, such as calcaneotalar, and calcaneocuboid coalition. ***It is one of most common cause of rigid flat foot.***

TYPES OF FLAT FOOT

- **Flexible:** The arch collapses during weight bearing and reappears when offloaded. Mostly physiological due to ligament laxity.
- **Rigid:** The arch remains collapsed during weight bearing/offloaded times It is seen in the *tarsal coalition or congenital vertical talus.*
- **Compensatory:** It is seen in genu valgum, peroneal tendon spasm, or malunited fracture calcaneum.

CLINICAL FEATURES

Symptoms

Patients with flat foot may remain *asymptomatic.* Some of them complain of *foot pain* during prolonged standing.

Signs

- Pes planus deformity is noted with the collapse of the medial longitudinal arch of the foot **(Fig. 44.40B)**.
- Forefoot in pronation and abduction.
- The finger cannot be insinuated beneath the medial longitudinal arch.

- **Too many toe sign:** The patient is made to stand, and the foot is observed from behind. Normally, the heel and tendo-Achilles (TA) mask the visibility of the first-to-fourth toe, and only the fifth toe is visible just lateral to the calf.
  However, in flat feet wherein the forefoot is in pronation, abduction leads to the visibility of many toes laterally from behind.
- **Jack test** is done to check the flexibility of the arch
  During the passive dorsiflexion of the great toe by the clinician, the MLA becomes accentuated in a flexible foot, wheres there is no change in arch concavity in a rigid foot.

INVESTIGATION

X-ray of the foot and ankle: AP and lateral view
- *Meary angle:* Lateral X-ray of the foot can help assess Meary angle, which is a measure of angle between long axis of talus and 1st metatarsal. It is decreased in flat foot **(Fig. 44.42)**.
- In the case of rigid flat feet, X-rays helps rule out **tarsal coalition (Fig. 44.43)**. A CT scan of the foot further helps assessing the tarsal coalition.

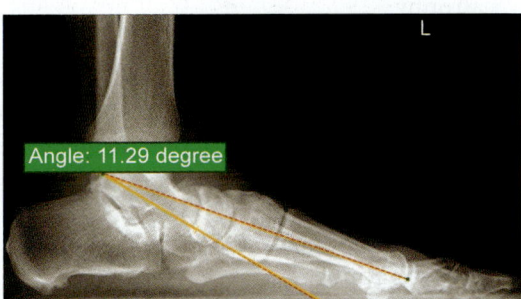

Fig. 44.42: Meary's angle between 1st metatarsal and talus.
(*Courtesy:* Dr Krishna Prasad, KMC, Manipal)

TREATMENT

The treatment of flat foot depends upon the cause, severity of symptoms and type of the flat foot.
- **Treat the cause, if any:** Tibialis posterior rupture (repair/reconstruct), or paralysis (tendon transfer, nerve repair).
- **Physiological flat foot/due to ligament laxity**
  - Serial observation, reassurance
  - Intrinsic foot muscle and tibialis posterior strengthening exercises
  - Tendo-Achilles stretching
- **Flexible foot**
  - Intrinsic foot muscle and tibialis posterior strengthening exercises
  - **Footwear modification:** Medial arch support with elongated and crooked Thomas heel
  - **Surgical:** Rarely, calcaneal lengthening osteotomy can be performed.
- **Rigid foot**
  - Observe, muscle strengthening.
  - Tarsal coalition resection
  - Subtalar or triple arthrodesis.

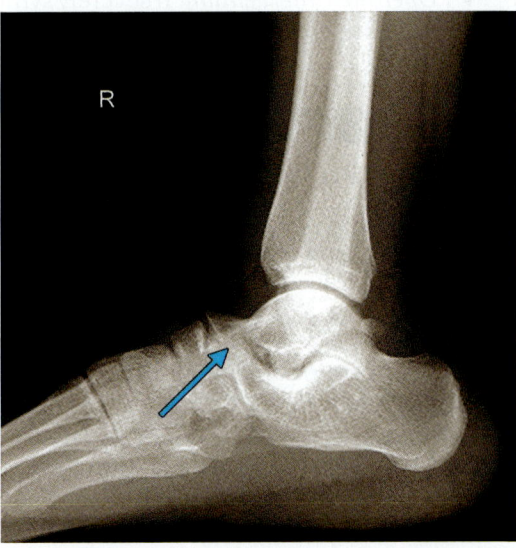

Fig. 44.43: Right foot lateral X-ray shows talocalcaneal tarsal coalition (blue arrow).

PES CAVUS

- **Definition:** Pes cavus is exaggeration of medial longitudinal arch of the foot **(Fig. 44.44)**.
- **Etiology:** *Usually, Pes cavus is a result of neuromuscular conditions* leading to muscle imbalance around the foot and ankle joint, such as post-polio residual paralysis, cerebral palsy, spina bifida, traumatic (foot compartment), hereditary sensory motor neuropathy/charcot Marie tooth disease/peroneal muscular atrophy.

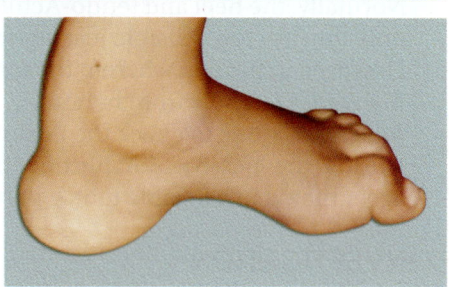

Fig. 44.44: Pes cavus with exaggerated medial longitudinal arch.

- **Clinical feature**
    - *Calcaneocavus deformity,* a hindfoot deformity characterized by dorsiflexed calcaneum, plantar flexed forefoot (equinus of forefoot), and an elevated medial arch.
    - There are *callosities under the metatarsal head.*
    - *Coleman block test* is performed to assess if hindfoot deformity is secondary and correctable.
    - A *detailed neurological evaluation* is a must to rule out any neurological condition.
- **Investigations:**
    - Plain X-ray of the foot-Meary Angle (calcaneal axis-ground) is increased
    - *CT and MRI scan of the foot* can be performed for bony and soft tissue assessment.
- **Treatment:**
    - *Conservative treatment:* Patient with milder deformities with mild-moderate symptoms can be managed with standard nonoperative interventions including activity modification, analgesics, and custom orthoses.
    - *Operative intervention:* If severely symptomatic, surgical correction can be performed—soft tissue release, tendon transfers, calcaneal osteotomy, or talar neck osteotomy.

SPINA BIFIDA

DEFINITION

Spina bifida (SB) is a type of neural tube defect (NTD) characterized by the failure of fusion of vertebral arches.

RISK FACTORS

- **Peri-conceptional lack of folic acid** is considered to be one of the major risk factors for spina bifida
- **Genetic:** Trisomy 18, 13, and 22q deletion
- **Family history:** Women born with SB or had a previous child with SB
- **Antenatal exposure to drugs,** such as valproate, carbamazepine, methotrexate, and isotretinoin
- **Other risk factors:** Maternal obesity, and maternal diabetes. An maternal core body temperature increase due to fever, sauna bath, or hot tub can increase the chance of NTD.

PATHOGENESIS

Usually, the neural tube closure occurs between the 23rd and 26th days after fertilization. As a result of genetic and environmental effects, NT fails to close, leading to NTDs. Typically, the vertebral bodies develop around the notochord. Two projections arise from the vertebral body that grows around the neural canal to form the vertebral arch. The fusion of two halves occurs from front to back, starting from the thoracic region first, then extending cranially and caudally. *Spina bifida results from the failure of fusion of the vertebral neural arch or NT*.

CLASSIFICATION OF SPINA BIFIDA

There are two types of spina bifida—occulta and aperta
- **Spina bifida occulta:** Occulta means "hidden"
  It occurs because of the non-fusion of the posterior arch of the vertebra. However, the unfused arch remains covered by the skin. And therefore, there is no exposure of the cord on the surface. However, clinically, several patients may have tell-tale signs over the region of SB such as dimple, tuft of hair, etc.
- **Spina bifida aperta/cystica (Fig. 44.45):** The layers of the spinal cord and/or its contents herniate over the surface via a defect in posterior arches and skin—subcutaneous tissue. There are three types of spina bifida aperta:
  1. *Meningocele*: A cystic swelling of the dura and arachnoid herniates through the posterior vertebral defect while nerve roots and cord remain inside.
     - *Typically, it is not associated with any neurological deficit.*
  2. *Myelomeningocele*: It is the *most common type of SB cystica.*
     - A cystic swelling of the dura and arachnoid along the nerve roots or cord tissue herniates through the posterior vertebral (arch) defect.
  3. *Myelocele/myeloschisis*: It is *the most severe form of SB.*
     - In this type of SB, the open neural plate is covered by the epithelium, and the neural plate is spread out on the skin surface.

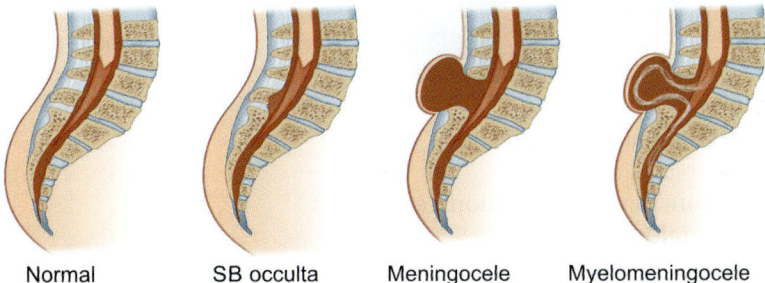

Fig. 44.45: Various types of spina bifida.

CLINICAL FEATURES

Spina Bifida Occulta (SBO)

- SBO mainly occurs in the lumbar or sacral region covered by skin **(Fig. 44.46)**. It is diagnosed accidentally when a radiograph of the spine is taken.
- It is *largely asymptomatic*. However, it can rarely cause low back pain.

- It may have *overlying tell-tale signs* such as:
  - Tuft of hair
  - Pigmented nevus
  - Hemangioma
  - Dimple
  - Palpable gap at the posterior aspect of spine
  - Lipoma.
- In the majority of patients, there is no neurological deficit. However, some patients may have a fibrous cord or lipoma causing subtle neurologic signs resulting in a cavus foot.

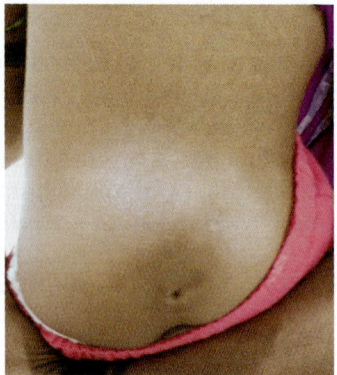

Fig. 44.46: Spina bifida with a dimple in the skin.

Spina Bifida Cystica/Aperta

The clinical features varies according to the type of spina bifida cystica.
- **Meningocele:** Unless the nervous system is involved, there are no symptoms or signs other than meningocele **(Fig. 44.47)**. Sometimes, the patient presents with *tethered cord syndrome*.
- **Myelomeningocele/myelocele:** Typically, it is associated with lower limb sensorimotor features. The sensory deficit results in trophic ulcers and Charcot's arthropathy, while motor deficit results in various musculoskeletal features, such as:

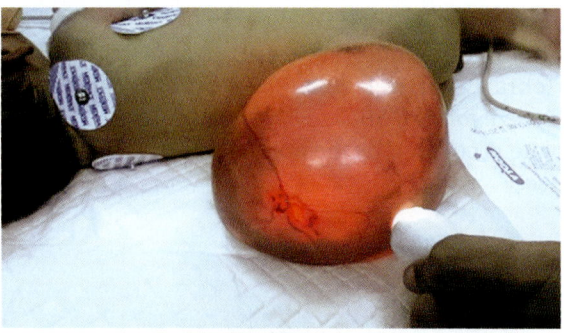

Fig. 44.47: Meningocele.
(*Courtesy:* Dr Saraswathi V, Bengaluru)

Note

What is tethered cord syndrome (TCS)?
Normally, the spinal cord hangs loose in the canal, free to move up and down with growth, and with spine movements. In TCS, abnormal tissues fix the spinal cord to the end of spinal canal or any other point, and hence limit its movement and flexibility. These patients may have back pain, leg pain, or tingling or numbness in lower limbs.

- *Hip:* Dislocation, flexion-abduction deformities
- *Knee:* Flexion deformity
- *Foot:* Club foot, valgus deformities
- *Bladder and bowel control disturbance:* Incontinence, UTI
- Pressure sores.

Other associated problems
- Kyphoscoliosis
- Arnold Chiari II malformation, hydrocephalus
- Absent or underdeveloped corpus callosum
- Higher mental functions and cognitive ability may be affected
- Oculomotor affections.

INVESTIGATIONS

- **Intranatal:** Raised alpha-fetoprotein (AFP)
- **Postnatal**
  - *X-ray:* Spine
  - *MRI of the spine* to rule out tethered cord syndrome or other spinal cord anomalies.

TREATMENT

In Spina Bifida Occulta

No treatment is required unless fibrous cord or lipoma causing any symptoms.

In Spina Bifida Cystica

- The treatment of choice is 'surgical closure of the defect'.
- The orthopaedic aims of the treatment in spina bifida cystica/aperta are:
  - **Obtain the best possible locomotor function in several ways:**
    - *Correct deformities*
      - Tendon lengthening and tendon transfer
      - Contracture release
      - Corrective osteotomy
      - Reduction of dislocations.
    - *Maintain deformity correction:* Restore muscle imbalance by:
      - Denervation of overactive muscle
      - Tendon transfer
      - Bracing.
  - **Care of foot:** Prevent or minimize sensory loss and treatment of pressure sores.

SKELETAL DYSPLASIAS

Skeletal dysplasias are a large heterogeneous group of disorders comprising abnormalities of bone or cartilage growth or texture.

ACHONDROPLASIA

It is the most common skeletal dysplasia and the most common cause of dwarfism.

Genetics: Autosomal dominant.

Clinical features

- These kids have *normal intelligence.* However, the *motor milestones are delayed.*
- **Rhizomelic dwarfism:** The dominant feature is *proximal limb shortening compared to the distal*—the arm is shorter than the forearm, and the femur is shorter than the tibia **(Fig. 44.48)**. However, *trunk size is appropriate for age.*
- Frontal bossing is obvious.
- **Starfish hand:** Short stubby hand with the length of fingers the same.

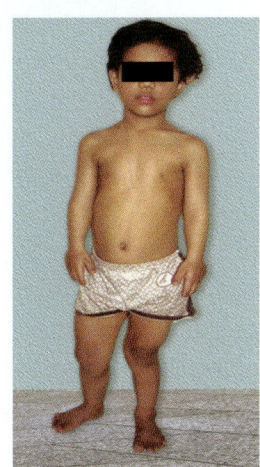

Fig. 44.48: Rhizomelic dwarfism in a patient of achondroplasia.

- ***Trident hand:*** The ring and middle fingers are divergent.
- Thoracolumbar kyphosis.
- Exaggerated lumbar lordosis.
- Protuberant abdomen.
- Low back pain with symptoms of lumbar canal stenosis, neurogenic claudication, and numbness.

Diagnosis
- Prenatal diagnosis can be established by *ultrasound*
- X-rays of skull, spine, hand, pelvis help in establishing key findings.

A. Spine **(Fig. 44.49A)**
   - *Decreased interpedicular distance and anteroposterior diameter*
   - *Posterior vertebral scalloping.*
B. Pelvis **(Fig. 44.49B)**
   - *Champagne glass pelvis*: Iliac blades are flattened, giving rise to a pelvic inlet that resembles a champagne glass. The acetabular angles are horizontal and the sciatic notch is small.
   - *Square shape iliac bone.*
C. Long bones
   - *Short and wide*
   - *Genu varum*
D. Hand
   - *Short phalanges*

Treatment
- Symptomatic treatment for back pain.
- Decompression procedure for lumbar canal stenosis.
- Limb lengthening procedures for shortening.

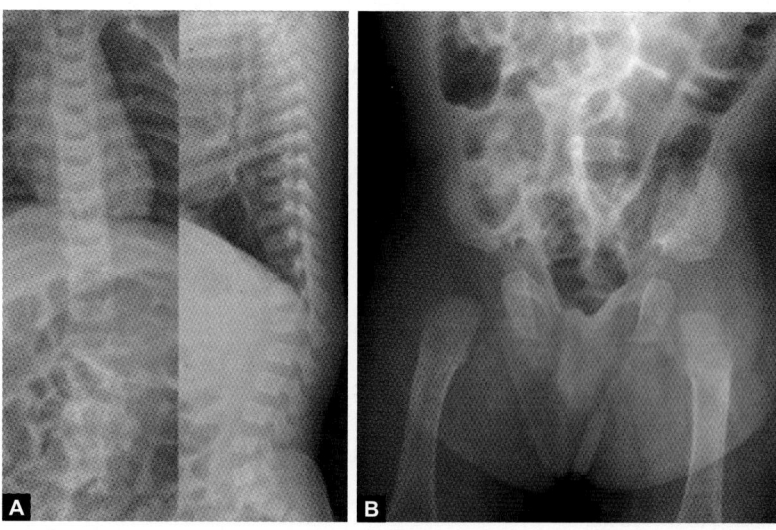

Figs. 44.49A and B: Achondroplasia: (A) Spine X-ray shows decreased interpedicular distance and posterior vertebral border scalloping; (B) Pelvis X-ray shows square shape iliac bone and champaign glass pelvis.

OSTEOGENESIS IMPERFECTA/BRITTLE BONE DISEASE/ LOBSTEIN VROLIK DISEASE

■ DEFINITION

A hereditary condition resulting from a *decrease in normal collagen type I resulting in brittle bones,* which fracture easily.

■ GENETICS

Ninety percent have COL1A1 and COL1A2 genetic mutations responsible for *abnormal collagen cross-linking.*

■ TYPES OF OSTEOGENESIS IMPERFECTA

There are several types of osteogenesis imperfecta (OI). First four types are more common, whereas others are less frequent. The prognosis of OI depends upon the types of OI. ***Type II is the most severe form of OI.***
- **Type I: Autosomal dominant,** mild type blue sclerae, stature is slightly short or normal for family, good prognosis.
- **Type II: Autosomal recessive,** most severe, perinatal mortality due to respiratory compromise. Severely short stature.
- **Type III: Autosomal recessive,** severe, survivable form, numerous fractures, bowed bones normal sclerae, very short stature.
- **Type IV: Autosomal dominant,** moderate severity normal sclerae, survivable, variably short stature.
  Recently, three more type of OI have been described making it a total of seven types.
- **Type V: Autosomal dominant (AD),** moderate severity, multiple fractures with hypertrophic callus, interosseous membrane clacification, variably short.
- **Type VI: Uncertain inheritance/AD**, moderate severity, mild short stature.
- **Type VII: Autosomal recessive**, moderate severity, mild short stature.

■ PATHOPHYSIOLOGY

It is characterized by abnormal collagen, and decreased production of collagen and osteoid. Therefore, bone remodeling is abnormal, resulting in poor-quality bone, causing fractures quickly.

■ CLINICAL FEATURES

Since type I collagen is present in bones, ligaments, skin, teeth, sclera, and the heart, the clinical features of OI are present in many areas.
- **Orthopaedic manifestations**
    - Short stature
    - Fragility fractures with poor remodeling; hence progressive bowing of the bones is observed in long bones-Sabre shin appearance of the tibia **(Fig. 44.50)**.
    - Spine-scoliosis
    - Ligament laxity.
- **Systemic features**
    - *Eye:* Blue sclera is characteristic **(Fig. 44.51)**
    - *Teeth:* Dentinogenesis imperfecta (brownish teeth)

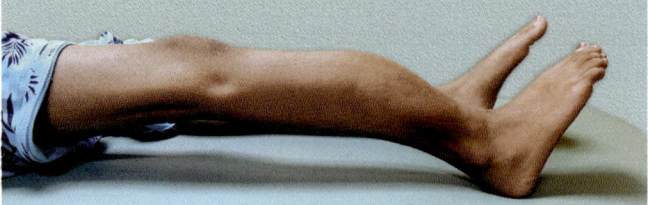

Fig. 44.50: Sabre shin appearance of tibia in osteogenesis imperfecta.

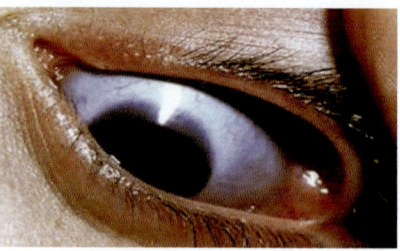

Fig. 44.51: Blue sclera.

- ***Face:*** *Dysmorphic face*
- ***Ear:*** *Hearing loss due to otosclerosis*
- ***Skin:*** *Subcutaneous bleeding tendency*
- ***Heart:*** *Mitral valve (MV) prolapse and aortic regurgitation*

▪ INVESTIGATIONS

Plain X-rays are the preferred initial line of investigations (Fig. 44.52A and B).
- *Long bones:* Diffuse osteopenia, thin cortex, anterior bowing of tibia **(Fig. 44.52B)**, popcorn calcifications, growth arrest lines/zebra stripes. There can be multiple pathological fractures.
- *Hip:* Coxa vara **(Fig. 44.52A)**
- *Spine:* Codfish vertebra
- *Skull:* Wormian bones, thin calvaria.

Laboratory investigation: Mild ALP elevation.
Prenatal investigation: USG can help establishing the diagnosis.

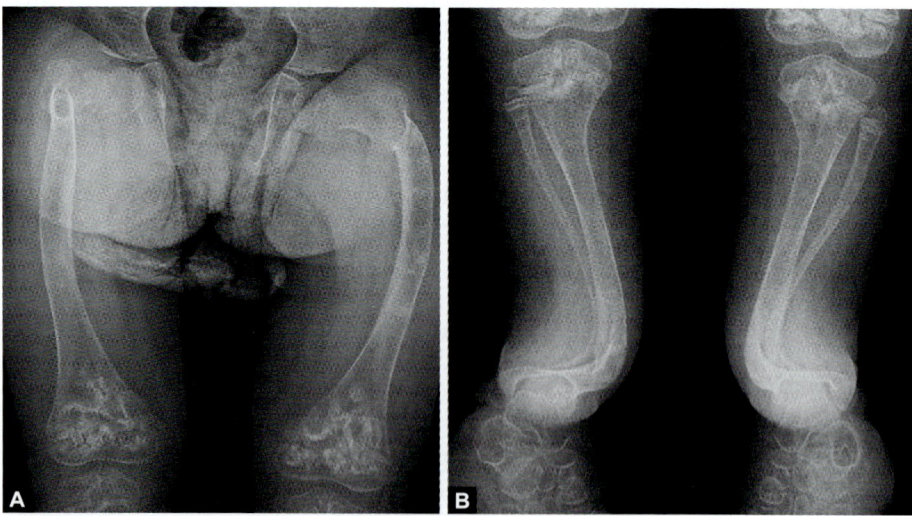

Figs. 44.52A and B: X-ray of hip, femur and tibia of a patient with osteogenesis imperfecta showing marked bowing deformity in the lower limbs, severe osteoporosis, thin bones, and coxa vara. Dense lines in the tibia and femur are compatible with zebra stripe sign due to bisphosphonate therapy. Metaphyseal widening distal femur and proximal tibia with lucent and sclerotic foci (popcorn calcification).
(*Courtesy*: Professor Hitesh Shah, KMC, Manipal)

TREATMENT

The treatment of OI comprises prevention of fracture, treatment of fractures and limb and spine deformities.
- **Fracture prevention**
    - Bracing
    - Bisphosphonates are used to reduce fracture rate and bone pain.
    Note: Chronic use of bisphosphonate causes the radiological appearance of multiple parallel lines in bones known as zebra lines.
- **Fracture treatment:** Internal fixation of long bones with telescopy rods or rush rods.
- **Treatment of deformities:** Corrective osteotomy and internal fixation (intramedullary device).
- **Scoliosis:** Observation/deformity correction.

CONGENITAL PSEUDOARTHROSIS OF TIBIA (CPT)

Definition: It is a congenital *anterolateral bowing of the tibia* with pseudoarthrosis.

Etiopathology: Mainly idiopathic. 40–80% of cases may be associated with neurofibromatosis (NF). There is a *fibrous hamartoma formation at the fracture site,* which prevents osteogenesis, thus making CPT a difficult condition to treat.

Bowing of tibia

Anterolateral bowing: Seen in congenital pseudoarthrosis of tibia.
Anteromedial bowing: Associated with fibular hemimelia, equinovalgus deformity, absence of lateral rays of foot, or tarsal aplasia.
Posteromedial bowing: Congenital anomaly with associated calcaneovalgus deformity of the foot mostly identified after birth. Usually resolves at its own.

Clinical features: Usually, it is a unilateral characterized by:
- Anterolateral bowing of the tibia, which is usually at the middle-lower third tibia **(Fig. 44.53)**.
- The child may be born with bowing, a fractured tibia, or an attenuated tibia which fractures some months later. Fracture fails to unite, leading to pseudoarthrosis with a short and bowed tibia
- Look for café au lait spots/neurofibroma (associated with NF1).

Investigations: Plain X-ray **(Fig. 44.54A)**.

Treatment: It is treated like nonunion, which requires open reduction, internal fixation with a rush rod and bone grafting **(Fig. 44.54B)**. Ilizarov technique is used if there is shortening and deformity.

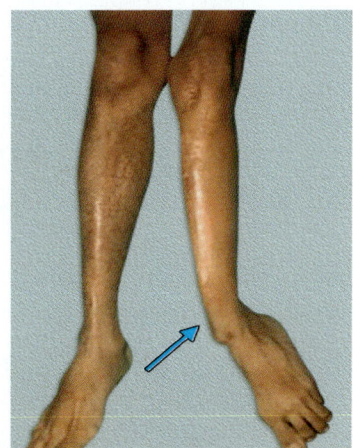

Fig. 44.53: Congenital pseudoarthrosis of tibia with anterolateral bowing of left leg (arrow).

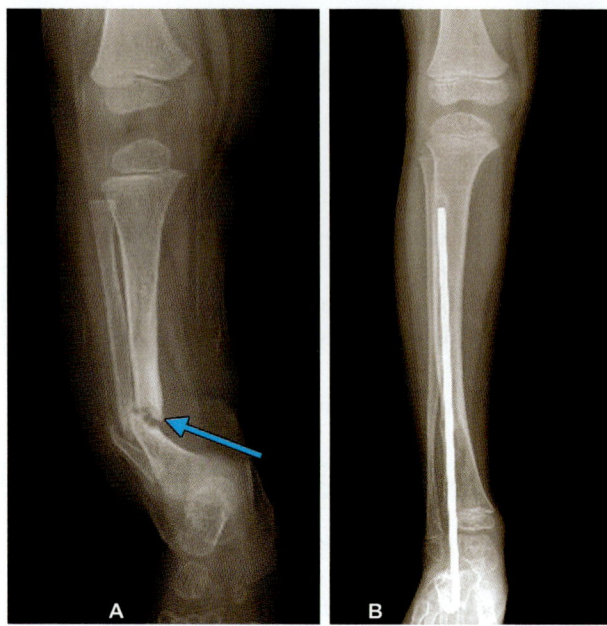

Figs. 44.54A and B: (A) Pseudoarthrosis of tibia (blue arrow); (B) Healed pseudoarthrosis after ORIF, grafting and rush rod application.

(*Courtesy:* Professor Hitesh Shah, KMC, Manipal)

CONGENITAL KNEE DISLOCATION

Definition: Hyperextended knee at birth and cannot be flexed easily **(Fig. 44.55)**.

Associated conditions: It could be an isolated deformity or can be associated with arthrogryposis multiplex congenita (AMC), Larsen's syndrome, CTEV, or DDH.

Pathology: Tight and short quadriceps (contracture), absence of ACL.

Treatment: Surgical correction of the deformity.

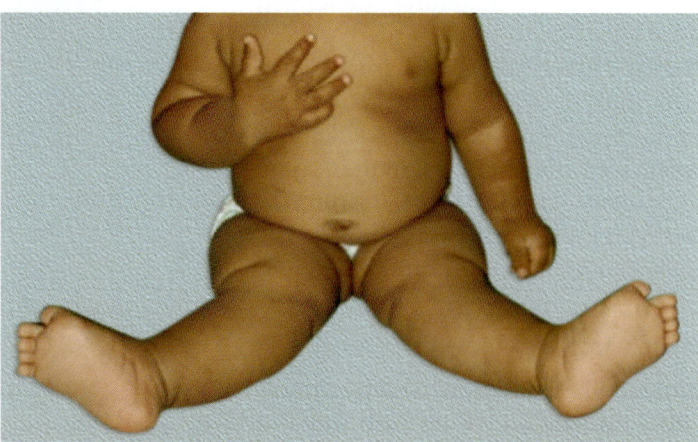

Fig. 44.55: Bilateral congenital dislocation of the knee.

SECTION 13

Regional Conditions

SECTION OUTLINE

45. **Upper Limb Disorders**
    - Frozen Shoulder
    - Rotator Cuff Tendinopathy
    - Acute Calcific Tendinitis
    - Rotator Cuff Tear
    - Painful Arc Syndrome
    - Tennis Elbow
    - Golfer's Elbow
    - Dequervain's Tenosynovitis
    - Carpal Tunnel Syndrome
    - Dupuytren's Contracture
    - Ganglion
    - Compound Palmar Ganglion
    - Trigger Finger

46. **Spine and Lower Limb Disorders**
    - Torticollis
    - Kyphosis
    - Scoliosis
    - Cervical Rib
    - Avascular Necrosis of Femoral Head
    - Femoroacetabular Impingement
    - Baker's Cyst
    - Genu Varum and Genu Valgum
    - Osteochondritis Dessicans of Knee
    - Synovial Chondromatosis
    - Discoid Meniscus
    - Osgood Schlatter Disease
    - Chondromalacia Patella
    - Plantar Fasciitis
    - Morton's Neuroma
    - Retrocalcaneal Bursitis
    - Various Toe Deformities

CHAPTER 45

Upper Limb Disorders

FROZEN SHOULDER

■ DEFINITION

Frozen shoulder is a soft tissue condition of the shoulder **characterized by insidious onset of pain and loss of movement** with no identifiable cause.

Note that frozen shoulder is also known as adhesive capsulitis/periarthritis shoulder. However, currently, frozen shoulder is the most preferred term.

■ CLASSIFICATION

- **Primary/idiopathic frozen shoulder** is the one with no identifiable cause
- **Secondary frozen shoulder:** The stiffness in the shoulder is secondary to an infection, inflammation, trauma or tumor.

■ ASSOCIATED CONDITIONS

Although there is no clarity on causation, certain conditions such as **diabetes mellitus (DM), thyroid dysfunction and dyslipidemia** are strongly associated with frozen shoulder. It is also observed after angioplasty.

■ ETIOPATHOGENESIS

The exact etiology of a frozen shoulder is still **obscure (idiopathic)**. However, there is a strong association between frozen shoulder and **diabetes and thyroid dysfunction**.
- **Pathology:** In frozen shoulder, there is a *contracture of the coracohumeral ligament (CHL), rotator interval and shoulder joint capsule.*
  There are three pathological-clinical stages of frozen shoulder.
  1. **Freezing stage (0–6 months):** Pathologically, it is characterized by *severe inflammation of capsule, rotator interval and CHL*. Clinically, this stage is characterized by *severe pain*. Range of movements (ROM) is decreased, especially abduction and rotations.
  2. **Frozen stage (6–12 months):** Pathologically, it is characterized by *fibrosis and contracture of CHL and capsule* following inflammation. Clinically, this stage is characterized by *decreased pain, but the loss of ROM is profound and global in all three planes*.
  3. **Thawing stage (12–18 months):** Pathologically, it is characterized by gradual fibrosis resolution to normal or near normal. Clinically, this stage is characterized by *minimal pain, whereas ROM gradually starts improving towards the normal range*.

CLINICAL FEATURES

Frozen shoulder commonly affects patients aged between 40–60 years. Many of them have diabetes or thyroid dysfunction. Their *main complaint is insiduous onset pain and loss of movement affecting their sleep and daily activities.*
- **Pain** is moderate to severe in intensity, which is felt more at night. Due to pain, the patient cannot sleep on the affected side. The pain radiates over the deltoid or on the lateral aspect of the arm. The pain starts diminishing later in the frozen or thawing stage.
- **Loss of movements:** The patient cannot reach the overhead object or take the hand to the back of the head, back pockets or back (dorsolumbar spine).

Examination: *The most significant finding in the frozen shoulder is the limitation of both active and passive movements.*
- Tenderness is present over the anterior and posterior aspects of the shoulder, especially joint lines and rotator interval.
- **Range of movement (ROM):** The loss of both *active and passive range of motion is the most classical finding of frozen shoulder.* In most cases, the ROM loss is global, i.e., in all three planes.
- **The strength of rotator cuff** remains nearly normal (though difficult to assess due to pain).

INVESTIGATIONS

Although frozen shoulder is a clinical diagnosis, investigations are performed to rule out secondary causes.
- **X-ray:** To rule out secondary causes of frozen shoulder, such as tumors and infections. It also detects osteoporosis of the humeral head.
- **USG and/or MRI:** In a primary frozen shoulder, *MRI/USG can detect thick capsule, coracohumeral ligament and contracted rotator interval.* However, they are not performed routinely to confirm frozen shoulder, and is performed to rule out 2° causes such as underlying rotator cuff tear, infection, or a tumor.
- **Serum investigations** to rule out DM, hypothyroidism, and dyslipidemia.

TREATMENT

Most frozen shoulder patients respond to conservative treatment in all three clinicopathological stages while a few require surgical treatment. The general plan in three stages is:
1. **Freezing stage:** Always conservative.
2. **Frozen stage:** Mostly conservative; occasionally surgical if there is no response to conservative treatment.
3. **Thawing stage:** Mostly conservative and rarely surgical.

- **Conservative treatment:** The aim is to provide *pain relief, retain and regain ROM of the shoulder and gradually regain shoulder strength.*
    - **Pain relief** can be achieved by:
        - *NSAIDs* or other analgesics, local anti-inflammatory topical application
        - *Intra-articular steroid injection* is of great help to reduce pain and inflammation, especially in freezing or early frozen stage. By reduction in inflammation, pain decreases considerably, which helps the patient perform physiotherapy.
        - *Pain relieving physiotherapy*, such as moist heat, shortwave diathermy, transcutaneous electrical nerve stimulation (TENS), and local ultrasound massage, help relieve pain.

- ♦ **Physiotherapy for retaining and regaining ROM:** Once the pain starts decreasing, active and passive mobilization of shoulder movement is initiated, along with cuff and scapular muscle strengthening.
- ♦ **Treatment of underlying associated condition,** such as DM, hypothyroid, and dyslipidemia.
- **Surgical option are** *arthroscopic capsular release* or *manipulation of shoulder under general anesthesia (MUGA)*, which are explored if conservative treatment fails to relieve pain and stiffness even after 8–10 months of conservative treatment.
  - ♦ *Arthroscopic capsular release* is preferred over MUGA as the tight capsule, and coracohumeral ligament release is performed in a controlled fashion, which is visualized during arthroscopy.
  - ♦ *Manipulation under general anesthesia (MUGA)* is a technique wherein the tight shoulder is mobilized under anesthesia to break the tight capsule forcibly. However, MUGA is contraindicated if there is osteoporosis of humeral head, as it can lead to fracture during manipulation. Furthermore, manipulation could cause rotator cuff or labral tear. Hence in modern orthopaedics, it is mostly avoided, or it should be performed with extreme caution.

ROTATOR CUFF TENDINOPATHY/TENDINITIS

Tendinopathy of rotator cuff commonly involves supraspinatus. Sometimes biceps tendon, infraspinatus and subscapularis are also involved.

ETIOPATHOGENESIS

Risk factors: Apart from aging, repetitive overhead activities (occupational or sports related) can predispose rotator cuff for tendinopathy followed by appearance of small tear in the cuff.

There are intrinsic and extrinsic factor involved in pathology of RC tendinopathy.
- **Intrinsic factor:** *Aging and hypovascularity of the tendon*, which renders rotator cuff tendon weak
- **Extrinsic factor:** *Acromial spurs* can damage the supraspinatus tendon while arm is repeatedly taken in forward flexion or abduction.

CLINICAL FEATURES

Rotator cuff tendinopathy occurs in patients who are in their 30s–50s. Their typical complaints are:

Symptoms
- Pain during overhead activities, which radiates towards the deltoid insertion.
- Often, shoulder pain is felt more at night while lying on the affected side disturbing the sleep.

Signs
- Tenderness present over the supraspinatus insertion
- Neer's impingement sign +
- Hawkin's sign ± (for subacromial bursitis)
- ROM is nearly full. However, it may be terminally painful.
- Strength of supraspinatus (full can and empty can test): Normal or slightly weak.

INVESTIGATIONS

- **X-ray of the shoulder (AP, outlet view):** Mostly, it is normal. Sometimes, it may show acromial spur, sourcil sign in acromion, and calcification in rotator cuff.
- **MRI:** Diagnostic investigation, which can detect tendinopathy and associated tears.
- **USG:** Less sensitive and specific than MRI. However, it is cheaper, no claustrophobia, and dynamic assessment of tendons is possible.
- **Serum investigations:** Rule out DM, hypothyroidism.

TREATMENT

Most cases respond to conservative treatment, while a few may require surgical debridement.

- **Conservative:** Mostly nonoperative treatment is sufficient.
  - *Rest*
    - Activity reduction and modification
    - Avoid provocative movements.
  - *Pain relief*
    - NSAIDs/other analgesics
    - Local anti-inflammatory topical applicants
    - Hot/cold pack
    - Subacromial injection of corticosteroid: If subacromial bursitis inflammation not responding to NSAIDs and other conservative options.
    - Subacromial platelet-rich plasma (PRP) injection: It might help in tendon healing and pain relief. However, the outcomes reported in various studies are inconsistent.
  - *Physiotherapy*
    - Pain relief: Hot/cold pack, interferential therapy, shortwave diathermy
    - Achieving full ROM
    - Muscle strengthening exercises of rotator cuff and scapular muscles.
  - *Treatment of underlying metabolic pathologies*, such as DM, thyroid dysfunction.
- **Surgery:** Only if conservative treatment fails >6 months
  Arthroscopic subacromial decompression: In this surgery—
  - Inflamed subacromial bursa is excised
  - Acromial spur is removed
  - Frayed tendon surface is debrided
  - If there is a concomitant rotator cuff tear, it is repaired.

ACUTE CALCIFIC ROTATOR CUFF TENDINITIS

Among all degenerative conditions of the shoulder, it is only condition which has an *"acute onset and is very painful."*

PATHOGENESIS

There is *gradual dystrophic calcification* in the degenerated part of the cuff over months and years. Occasionally, there is sudden rupture of this calcific deposit into the subacromial space leading to severe acute inflammation in the subacromial space, resulting in severe pain and restriction of movement of shoulder. Often, there is pseudopalsy of the shoulder.

CLINICAL FEATURES

- *Moderate-severe, acute shoulder pain* (nontraumatic) usually with a short history of a few days.
- Generalized tenderness over the greater tuberosity
- *Severe restriction of motion* (active and passive), which appears as pseudopalsy.
- Generally, no special tests can be performed due to severe pain.

DIAGNOSIS

- **Plain X-ray is diagnostic:** "Calcification" can be seen in the rotator cuff **(Fig. 45.1)**
- **MRI or USG** is usually not required. However, it can confirm the diagnosis.
- Rule out underlying metabolic pathology, such as DM, thyroid dysfunction.

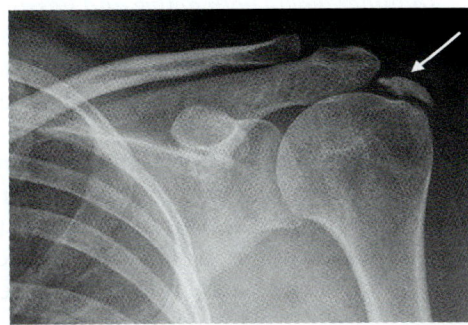

Fig. 45.1: Calcification in supraspinatus (arrow).

TREATMENT

Most patients respond to conservative treatment while a few may need surgery.

Conservative treatment

- **Pain relief:** NSAID or other analgesics for 2–3 weeks, local ice pack. Sometimes, a local steroid injection is helpful to reduce inflammation and pain.
- **Rest** by arm sling.
- **Barbotage:** Those who do not respond to NSAIDs, rest or steroid injection may require Barbotage. Barbotage is Ultrasound-guided needling of the calcific deposit followed by subacromial injection of steroid.

Surgical treatment: *Arthroscopic removal of calcific deposit* can be performed in case of failed conservative treatment including barbotage or if there is recurrent calcification.

ROTATOR CUFF TEAR

Rotator cuff tear is common in patients older than 50–55 years. However, traumatic rotator cuff tears can also occur in younger populations, especially between 40–50 years. It results in pain and limited shoulder movement, affecting the shoulder's function.

ETIOPATHOLOGY

There are **two major causes of rotator cuff tear—degenerative and traumatic.** Rotator cuff tendon degeneration results from aging, overuse, hypovascularity or impingement from the acromial spur causing gradual fraying and tear of the tendon. A frayed or torn tendon results in pain and difficulty in moving the shoulder. The traumatic injury commonly happens after a fall over the shoulder.

Most commonly, tears in the cuff involve the supraspinatus tendon.

CLINICAL FEATURES

Symptoms: The patients with rotator cuff tear present with pain and/or difficulty elevating their shoulders. There may/may not be a history of trauma.

- **Pain:** The patients with rotator cuff tear have pain while moving the shoulder. Pain radiates towards the arm, especially towards the deltoid tip. Often, pain is more at night while sleeping on the affected side.
- **Difficulty or inability to elevate the arm:** A patient with torn tendon(s) may find difficulty in elevating the arm due to loss of power.

Signs
- **Muscle wasting** of the supraspinatus and/or infraspinatus is almost always present.
- **Loss of active movements** but **passive ROM is usually preserved** (*cf. from the frozen shoulder where both active and passive ROM is limited*).
- **Drop arm test** *may be positive:* Passively elevate the shoulder till 180° and ask the patient to 'gradually lower the arm' till their hand reaches waist area. This test is positive if there is pain while lowering the arm, sudden dropping of the arm, or weakness in maintaining arm position during lowering.
- **Assess individual muscles strength by performing specific tests**
    - Full can test for supraspinatus tear
    - External rotation lag test for infraspinatus tear
    - Belly press test for subscapularis tears
    - Hornblower sign for teres minor tear.

INVESTIGATIONS

- **X-ray:** Plain radiograph must be done to rule out arthritis and osteopenia. A massively torn rotator cuff (two or more tendons) may show proximal migration of the humeral head and narrow acromiohumeral space **(Fig. 45.3A)**.
- **MRI** of the shoulder *is diagnostic*. It helps assess the number of tendons torn, tear size, retraction, muscle atrophy and fatty infiltration, which helps decision-making.
- **USG** can be performed to detect RC tear. However, it is operator-dependent, resulting in lower sensitivity and specificity than MRI. Furthermore, assessment of muscle atrophy and fatty infiltration is difficult.

TREATMENT

The rotator cuff tear treatment depends upon the patient's age, prevailing symptoms, difficulties in daily living activities, and tendon's reparability. Smaller or minimally symptomatic tears can be managed conservatively with analgesics and physiotherapy. Larger tears or those failing to respond to conservative treatment, require rotator cuff repair (open/arthroscopic) **(Fig. 45.2A to C)**.

Irreparable tears resulting in pain and dysfunction can be managed with tendon transfer, superior capsule reconstruction (SCR) or reverse shoulder replacement (RSR), depending upon age, torn tendon and joint arthritis **(Figs. 45.3A and B)**. While tendon transfer and SCR are preferred in younger patients (<60 years), RSR is a better choice in patients older than 60–65 years, especially with arthritis.

COMPLICATION

A neglected large or massive size rotator cuff tear could further progress over the years and result in **rotator cuff arthropathy,** wherein there is arthritis of the glenohumeral joint with a defunct degenerated rotator cuff **(Fig. 45.3A)**. Such patients require **reverse shoulder replacement** for pain relief and restoration of forward elevation **(Fig. 45.3B)**.

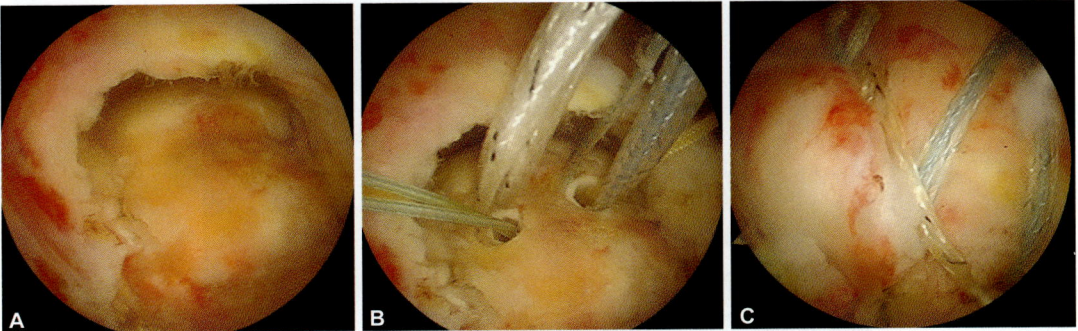

Figs. 45.2A to C: (A) Arthroscopic image of supraspinatus tear; (B) Suture anchors in place; (C) Repair of the supraspinatus.

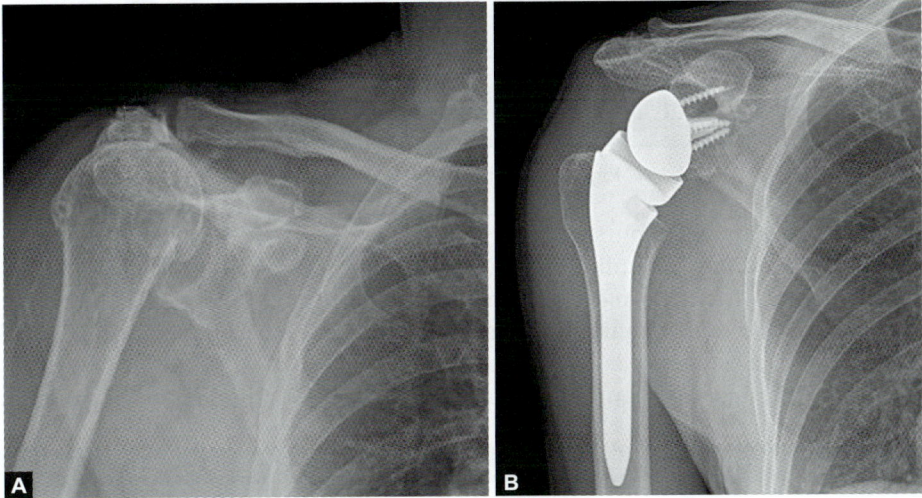

Figs. 45.3A and B: (A) Proximal migration of humeral head with arthritis of joint; (B) Reverse shoulder replacement.

PAINFUL ARC SYNDROME

Painful arc syndrome is *not* an isolated diagnosis but a syndrome of the shoulder, as many pathological conditions can cause painful arc syndrome.

Clinically, it is characterized by an arc of painful abduction, typically between 60°–120°, during abduction from 0–180° wherein the initial (<60°) and later part of abduction (>120°) is painless **(Fig. 45.4)**. It happens because, during the arc of 60–120°, the subacromial space is quite tight. Normally, *during shoulder abduction*, the subacromial structures (bursa, cuff, greater tuberosity, undersurface of acromion) easily navigate in space between the greater tuberosity and the undersurface of the acromion without getting impinged. In contrast, pathological conditions do not allow easy subacromial clearance of these structures, causing pain.

The following conditions could result in PAS as it makes the subacromial space quite tight, and structures get impinged between the greater tuberosity and undersurface of the acromion.

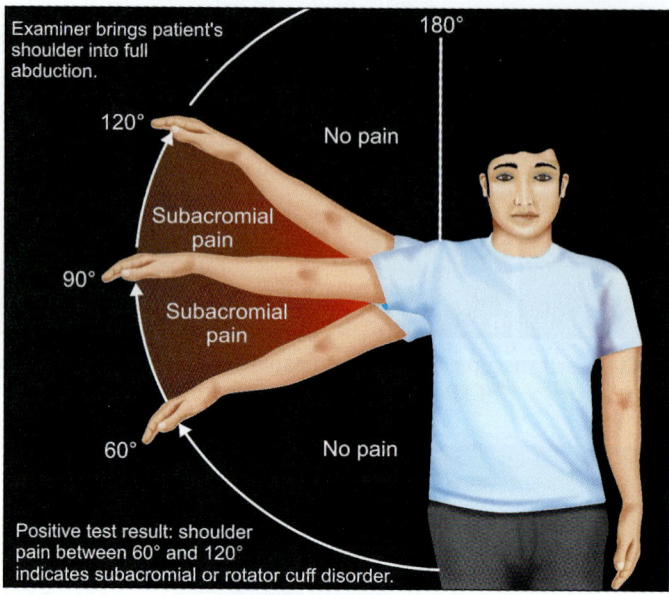

Fig. 45.4: Painful arc syndrome.

- *Subacromial bursitis* (thick bursa)
- *Rotator cuff tendinopathy* results in thick, frayed tendon occupying larger space
- *Rotator cuff tears*—frayed torn edge impinge with acromion
- *Greater tuberosity avulsion* malunion or nonunion causes narrow subacromial space
- *Acromial spur* causes narrow subacromial space.

The clinical features, diagnosis, and treatment of PAS depend on the underlying condition.

TENNIS ELBOW (LATERAL EPICONDYLITIS)

■ DEFINITION

A painful condition of the elbow caused by *"tendinosis of the common extensor tendons on the lateral epicondyle of the elbow.* **It chiefly involves tendon of extensor carpi radialis brevis (ECRB)**".

■ ETIOPATHOGENESIS

- *Repetitive use or overuse of the extensor muscles of the forearm*
- *Commonly seen* in certain racquet sports like tennis, squash and badminton which involve hitting a backhand or occupation that requires repetitive motions of the wrist and forearm include plumbers, painters, carpenters, butchers, musicians (pianists, drummers) or any laborer who swings a tool with their forearm.

■ CLINICAL FEATURES

Tennis elbow is common in age group of 30s–50s.

Symptoms
- Pain over outer aspect of elbow which may radiate down the forearm. It worsens with activity such as playing racquet sports, turning a wrench or tool, lifting a coffee cup or even shaking hands
- Weakened grip strength while holding objects.

Signs
- *Tenderness over the lateral epicondyle* **(Fig. 45.5)**.
- **Cozen's test is positive:** With elbow fully extended and wrist radially deviated, pain is increased when the wrist is subjected to resisted extension.
- Pain with passive wrist flexion as this stretches the extensor tendon.
- Weak grip strength.

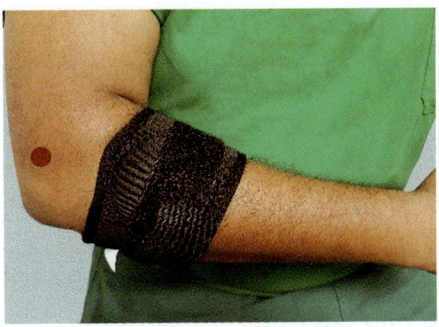

Fig. 45.5: Tennis elbow tenderness over lateral epicondyle (brown dot). Tennis elbow splint over the proximal forearm.

INVESTIGATIONS

Tennis elbow is a clinical diagnosis. Radiological investigations are not routinely performed.
- **X-ray:** Findings are usually normal. Sometimes, calcifications may be seen along the lateral epicondyle.
- **USG:** It helps to detect common extensor tendon tendinosis, partial tears, and calcifications.
- **MRI:** Though it is diagnostic, it is not routinely performed as most findings can be assessed with USG.
- **Serum investigations:** It should be done to rule out DM, or thyroid dysfunction.

TREATMENT

Treatment of tennis elbow is largely conservative. Surgery is rarely needed.
- **Conservative:**
  - *Activity modification, equipment check:* Repetitive wrist work that overstresses the tendon should be avoided. Players should ensure that their techniques are corrected and faulty equipment should be replaced.
  - *Pain relief:* Analgesics, local anti-inflammatory gel, cold pack or hot fomentation.
  - *Physiotherapy:* Muscle stretching and strengthening exercises, ultrasound therapy.
  - *Orthosis:* Tennis elbow splint helps by limiting amount of stress on the injured area, allow healing while patient could still gently use the elbow **(Fig. 45.5)**.
  - *Local corticosteroid injections:* It helps in pain relief by decreasing inflammation.
  - *PRP injection:* It helps pain relief by promoting tendon healing.
  - *Extracorporeal shockwave therapy (ESWT).*
  - *Treatment of metabolic conditions,* such as DM, thyroid disorder.
- **Surgery:** Only if conservative treatment fails for 8–12 months.
  - Debridement and repair of the frayed ECRB tendon attachment over the lateral epicondyle.

DIFFERENTIAL DIAGNOSIS

Radial tunnel syndrome: In this condition, the posterior interosseous nerve is entrapped under the supinator muscle arch over the proximal radius. Clinically, patient experiences pain around the lateral aspect of elbow, which may radiate towards the forearm. However, there is no tenderness over the lateral epicondyle but is just below the radial head above the supinator arch. Pressure over this point leads to a radiating pain along the forearm up to the thumb.

GOLFER'S ELBOW (MEDIAL EPICONDYLITIS)

DEFINITION

Golfer's elbow or medial epicondylitis, is tendinosis of the common flexor muscle origin at the medial epicondyle of the elbow chiefly, **pronator teres (PT) and flexor carpi radialis (FCR)**.

ETIOPATHOGENESIS

- Any activity that requires repetitive wrist flexing, gripping or swinging can cause tendinosis of common flexors origin
- Commonly seen in golfers, bowlers, baseball players, archery, javelin throwing, improper weight training, painting or even while using a computer for too many hours daily.

CLINICAL FEATURES

Golfer's elbow is common in age group of 30s–50s.

Symptoms
- Pain over inner aspect of elbow which runs along the medial aspect of forearm and worsens with wrist and forearm motion. There may be pain while shaking hands.
- Weakness of grip
- There may be tingling and numbness of medial aspect of forearm.

Signs
- Tenderness over the medial epicondyle
- **Reverse Cozen's test is positive:** Pain is reproduced over medial epicondyle with resisted forearm pronation and wrist flexion.
  Always palpate ulnar nerve behind the medial epicondyle to rule out its involvement. It can also cause medial side elbow pain and tingling in forearm.

INVESTIGATIONS

- **Plain radiographs:** Usually normal; sometimes may show calcification.
- **USG or MRI** shows tendinosis of common flexors at medial epicondyle.
- **Serum investigations:** Rule out DM, thyroid dysfunction.

TREATMENT

Treatment of Golfer's elbow is largely conservative. Surgery is rarely needed.
- **Nonoperative/conservative:**
  - *Activity reduction and modification:* Repetitive wrist work that overstresses the tendon should be avoided

- ♦ *Pain relief:* Analgesics, local anti-inflammatory gel, cold packs or hot fomentation
- ♦ *Physiotherapy:* Muscle stretching and strengthening exercises, local ultrasound therapy
- ♦ *Orthosis:* Tennis elbow splint
- ♦ *Local corticosteroid injection:* Care should be taken that ulnar nerve should not be damaged accidentally in the process of injecting a golfer's elbow which is just behind the medial epicondyle.
- ♦ *Platelet-rich plasma (PRP)* injection to promote healing.
- ♦ *Treatment of metabolic conditions,* such as DM, thyroid disorder.
- **Operative/surgery:** Indicated when 8–12 months of conservative treatment fails.
  - ♦ Open debridement of PT and FCR, reattachment of flexor-pronator group.

DE QUERVAIN'S TENOSYNOVITIS

(Syn: BlackBerry Thumb, Texting Thumb, Gamer's Thumb, Washerwoman's Sprain, Mother's Wrist or Mommy Thumb)

■ DEFINITION

De Quervain's disease is **Tenosynovitis of abductor pollicis longus (APL) and the extensor pollicis brevis (EPB) tendons** and the sheath around it, due to chronic overuse of the wrist joint.

■ ETIOPATHOGENESIS

- **Occupations and activities that require repetitive hand and wrist movements** such as playing music, sewing and knitting, frequent texting or typing on mobile devices with thumbs may increase the risk of developing this condition. This may irritate these tendons causing thickening and swelling, which restrains smooth gliding of the tendons through the sheath. Subsequent movements of the thumb cause pain due to friction and perpetuate the cycle of irritation and swelling.
- **Associated conditions:** Diabetes, alcoholism, liver cirrhosis, pregnancy (due to hormonal changes, fluid retention, and debatably, repetitive lifting of the baby as it grows heavier) and rheumatoid disease.

■ CLINICAL FEATURES

De Quervain's tenosynovitis is common in age group of 30s–50s.

Symptoms
- Pain at radial side of the wrist joint—may radiate to forearm and thumb, aggravated by lifting the thumb or when forcefully grasping objects
- Swelling over radial border of wrist
- Difficulty in moving the thumb due to pain.

Signs
- *Tenderness just proximal to the radial styloid* (Fig. 45.6)

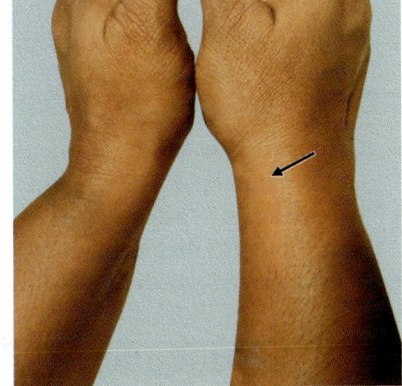

Fig. 45.6: De Quervain's tenderness area (black arrow).

- Sometimes, swelling is observed over the radial styloid area due to inflamed thickened tendons.
- **Finkelstein test positive:** The thumb is just drawn into ulnar deviation without closing the fist/drawing wrist into ulnar deviation. A positive test is indicated by sharp pain along the radial border of the wrist.
- **Eichoff test positive:** The thumb is flexed, drawn into ulnar deviation, held inside the fist, and the patient either actively ulnar deviates the wrist or it is passively deviated by the clinician. A positive test is indicated by sharp pain along the radial border of the wrist.

INVESTIGATIONS

Mostly, De Quervain's is a clinical diagnosis. Radiological investigations are not routinely performed.
- **X-ray of wrist:** Mostly normal. Done to rule out any bone or joint disorder.
- **USG** can confirm tendinopathy of APL and EPB.
- **Serum investigations** to rule out DM, thyroid dysfunction.

TREATMENT

Treatment of De Quervain's disease is largely conservative. Surgery is rarely needed.
- **Conservative:**
    - *Activity modification:* Avoiding repetitive motion of the thumb
    - *Orthosis:* Bracing of the thumb in extension (Fig. 45.7)
    - *Pain relief:* Analgesics, local anti-inflammatory gel, ice pack/hot fomentation
    - *Treatment of metabolic conditions,* such as DM, thyroid disorder.
    - *Local corticosteroid injection:* Injection of corticosteroids into the sheath of the first.
- **Surgery:** Only if conservative treatment fails for 6–8 months. Surgical release of the first dorsal compartment relieves the entrapped tendons.

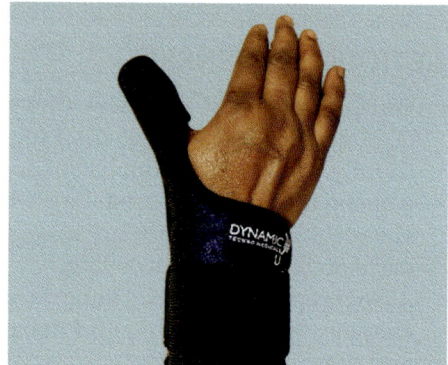

Fig. 45.7: Thumb splint.

DIFFERENTIAL DIAGNOSIS

- **Osteoarthritis of the first carpometacarpal joint:** Pain and tenderness over the 1st carpometacarpal (CMC) joint.
- **Intersection syndrome:** Pain will be more towards the middle of the back of the forearm and about 2–3 inches below the wrist.
- **Wartenberg's syndrome:** Mononeuropathy of superficial branch of radial nerve.

CARPAL TUNNEL SYNDROME

Carpal tunnel syndrome is a painful condition of the wrist and hand caused by compression of the median nerve while it passes through the carpal tunnel (CT).

SURGICAL ANATOMY

The boundaries and contents of carpal tunnel are mentioned below:
- **Radially:** Scaphoid tubercle, trapezium
- **Ulnarly:** Pisiform, the hook of hamate
- **The roof of the carpal tunnel:** Flexor retinaculum
- **The floor of the carpal tunnel:** Proximal carpal row
- **Contents of the carpal tunnel:** 9 *flexor tendons* (four flexor digitorum superficialis, four flexor digitorum profundus and one flexor pollicis longus tendons) and the *median nerve.*

ETIOLOGY

Any condition which decreases the volume of carpal tunnel or space available for the median nerve can cause carpal tunnel syndrome.
- **Conditions compromising space in carpal tunnel:** Malunited Colles' or Smith's fracture, intratunnel tumors, or compound palmar ganglion.
- **Condition causing tenosynovitis, such as** rheumatoid arthritis results in swollen, inflamed tendon reduce CT space.
- **Conditions causing fluid or substance retention:** Hypothyroidism, pregnancy, Cushing syndrome, chronic renal failure, and mucopolysaccharidosis could increase fluid in CT space, causing pressure over the median nerve.
- **Others:** Smoking, alcoholism, repetitive wrist movements, cycling, and throwing.

PATHOLOGICALLY

The compression of the median nerve in the carpal tunnel results in sensory-motor symptoms in hand **(Fig. 45.8)**.

CLINICAL FEATURES

- Carpal tunnel (CT) syndrome is *more common in women.*
- These patients complain of *pain and tingling in their hands, especially in radial 3½ fingers* (in the median nerve distribution area). Pain is severe at night and often awakens the patient, who then shakes their hand vigorously to relieve symptoms.

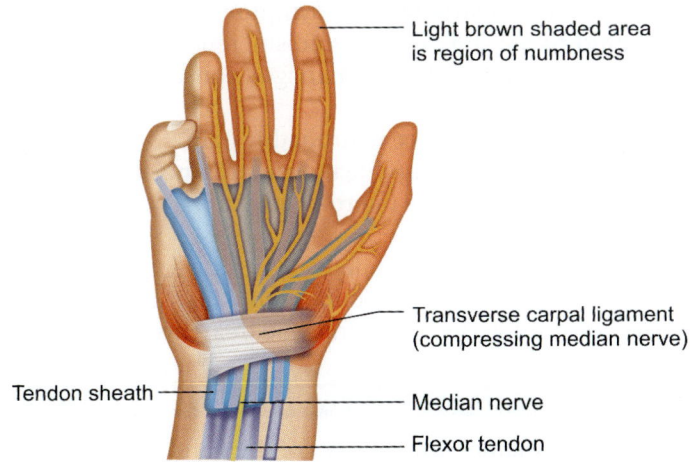

Fig. 45.8: Carpal tunnel entrapment.

- There may be a history of the underlying cause, such as DM, rheumatoid arthritis, trauma, or pregnancy.

Clinical Examination

- Inspection may reveal thenar muscle wasting if the median nerve is severely affected.
- Special tests to diagnose CT syndrome are:
    - ***Phalen's test:*** Folding both hands in extreme palmar flexion >60 seconds produces pain and numbness in the median nerve distribution area.
    - ***Reverse Phalen's test:*** Folding hands in complete dorsiflexion together causes pain and numbness in the median nerve distribution area.
    - ***Durkan's test:*** *It is the most sensitive test for CTS.* Pressure is applied over the median nerve over the carpal tunnel. A positive test is suggested by reproducing pain and numbness in the median nerve distribution area within 30–60 seconds.
    - ***Semmes Weinstein testing:*** Most sensitive sensory test for detecting early CTS.
- A thorough sensorimotor examination of the median nerve is essential to assess the degree of involvement of the median nerve.

INVESTIGATION

Investigations to assess CTS are bifold, one to confirm the median nerve involvement and the other to assess the causation.
- **Plain X-ray of the wrist:** To look for bony causes of CTS.
- **USG/MRI** of the carpal tunnel can detect the size of carpal tunnel and compression of the median nerve. It is also helpful to assess any intratunnel causes of compression, such as a tumor or thickened tendon sheaths.
- **Nerve conduction velocity (NCV) test** can establish the median nerve compression.
- **EMG of muscles supplied by median nerve in hand**. It is rarely performed.
- **Serum investigation:** Rule out systemic conditions predisposing to CTS, such as DM, thyroid function tests, rheumatoid arthritis (RA).

TREATMENT

Treating CT syndrome involves treatment of the symptoms and underlying conditions.
- **Treat associated conditions:** DM, hypothyroidism, renal failure.
- **Conservative:** Mild to moderate cases are managed conservatively with:
    - Analgesics
    - Pregabalin or gabapentin to reduce neuropathic pain
    - A carpal tunnel splint to prevent undue movements/positions of the wrist.
    - Occasionally, intracarpal tunnel steroid injections are helpful in inflammatory conditions.
- **Surgical treatment** is opted in case of failed conservative treatment for >8–12 weeks. The *flexor retinaculum is released* by open/endoscopic method to relieve pressure over the median nerve. Any bony/soft tissue cause must be treated accordingly.

DUPUYTREN'S CONTRACTURE

It is a condition affecting the palmar aponeurosis of the hand resulting in flexion contracture of the fingers.

ASSOCIATED CONDITION

Many conditions would predispose a patient to Dupuytren's contracture, such as *chronic alcoholism, diabetes, HIV, smoking, and antiepileptic medications.*

PATHOLOGY

There is contracture of palmar aponeurosis with preponderance of 'myofibroblast'. The adjacent myofibroblasts connect via extracellular fibronectin to create contracted tissue.

CLINICAL FEATURES

- It affects *middle age-elderly patients*, and is more *common in males* than females.
- Clinically, patients present with *progressive flexion contracture of the finger*. The *ring finger is most commonly involved, followed by the little finger. The flexion deformity occurs at metacarpophalangeal (MCP) and proximal interphalangeal (PIP) joints.*
- Inspection reveals visible and prominent cords over the palm **(Fig. 45.9)**. These cords are also palpable and thickened. Finger extension at MCP joint is not possible.

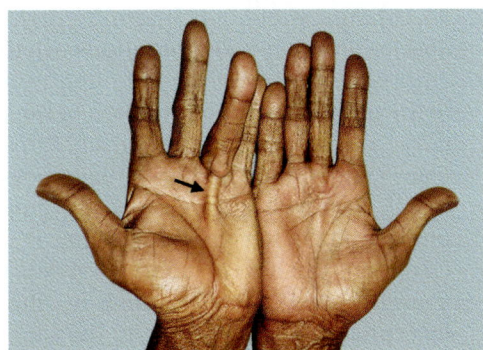

Fig. 45.9: Dupuytren's contracture. Prominent cords in palm (arrow).

INVESTIGATIONS

It is always a clinical diagnosis. Investigations are performed to rule out an underlying condition, such as diabetes.

TREATMENT

One must treat the underlying condition and treat milder deformities conservatively. Surgical treatment is opted for in case of failed conservative treatment or severe deformities.
- **Conservative treatment**
    - Mobilization of contracture, splinting in early cases
    - Local injection of histolyticum collagenase: For cases with less than 5° contracture at MCP and PIP joint.
- **Surgical treatment**
    - *Needle aponeurotomy*: For milder cases
    - *Palmar aponeurectomy with/without skin graft*: For moderate-severe cases.

GANGLION

Ganglion is a small cystic swelling filled with mucin.

ETIOPATHOLOGY

It is *not* a *true* cyst as there is no epithelial lining. There are many theories of its formation, such as synovial herniation/mucous cyst formation/degeneration of connective tissue and cyst formation. Often, it is connected to the underlying joint, such as wrist joint via a stalk. Most are multiloculated.

■ CLINICAL FEATURES

Ganglions are one of the **most common swellings around the wrist** and are *more common in females*.

- It presents as a small pea-size swelling or occasionally larger, on the **dorsum of the wrist** and sometimes on the **volar aspect (Fig. 45.10)**. The swelling is intermittently painful, and the size may show variation with time.
- The volar wrist ganglion are often quite close to the palmar cutaneous branch of the median nerve and the median nerve itself. Proximity of volar ganglion to the nerve may occasionally result in tingling-numbness in hand, and rarely, median nerve compression.
- Ganglions can also occur in the **flexor tendon sheaths**, and when located at the **distal interphalangeal (DIP)** joints, they are termed mucous cysts. Flexor tendon sheath ganglion cause painful movement of fingers. Ganglion cysts within bone, termed **interosseous cysts**, most often affect the scaphoid and lunate and require open surgery for removal.

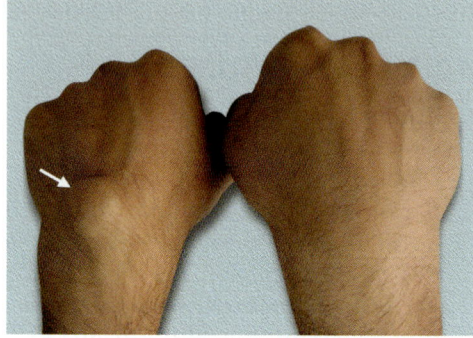

Fig. 45.10: Ganglion over dorsum of left wrist (arrow).

Examination:
- On palpation: It is firm or bony hard.
- Joint ROM is normal. Sometimes, extremes of movement are painful.

■ INVESTIGATIONS

Usually, it is a clinical diagnosis. Plain X-rays are normal. In case of mucous cyst over DIP joint, there may be underlying arthritis of DIP. The USG or MRI confirms the diagnosis.

■ TREATMENT

Smaller swellings which are occasionally painful, can be managed conservatively, while larger ones frequently interfering with the function must be excised.
- **Conservative treatment:** Observation, analgesics, aspiration and intracystic steroid injection.
- **Surgical excision** (open/arthroscopic) is opted if it is *painful, large, interfering with function, nerve compression,* or *recurrence after aspiration*.

Trivia: Histortical treatment of ganglion

In the past, closed rupture of ganglion cyst was one of the treatment option, either by firm massage or the traditional sharp blow with the family Bible. The reported cure rate varies from 22% to 66%.

During our medical school training, our professors jokingly used to say that hit a ganglion with 'Gray's Anatomy' book, which was heaviest of all, to rupture it for healing! Note that *these options are not practiced*!

COMPOUND PALMAR GANGLION

DEFINITION

Compound palmar ganglion is a condition wherein a swelling in the distal part of the forearm communicates with another one in hand across the flexor retinaculum.

PATHOLOGY

A compound palmar ganglion is commonly seen in patients with tuberculosis or rheumatoid arthritis. Typically, it results from **flexor tendon synovitis due to tuberculosis (TB)/ rheumatoid arthritis** (RA) under the flexor retinaculum.

CLINICALLY

The compound palmar ganglion appears as an '**hourglass shape swelling**' extending above and below the flexor retinaculum **(Fig. 45.11)**. Cross fluctuation is positive. There may be associated features of carpal tunnel syndrome.

DIAGNOSIS

Plain X-ray is performed to assess bones and joints. USG or MRI can confirm the diagnosis.

TREATMENT

Treat the underlying condition and the ganglion may subside. In case of no relief, the synovectomy of the affected tendons and bursa can be performed.

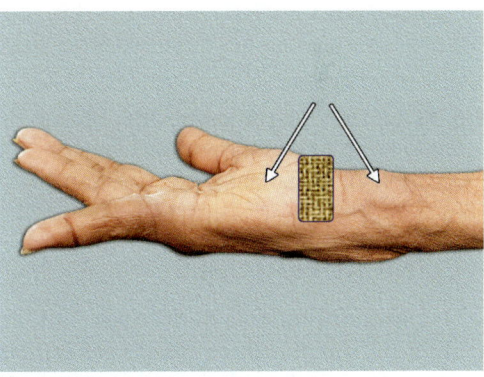

Fig. 45.11: Compound palmar ganglion indicated by two white arrows while brown hashed area indicates flexor retinaculum.
(*Courtesy:* Dr Darshan Jain, Bengaluru)

TRIGGER FINGER

A trigger finger is a condition wherein the finger gets locked in flexion and extends with a sudden click after effort.

PATHOLOGY

Trigger finger occurs due to **stenosing tenosynovitis of flexor tendons**, which results in nodular thickening in the flexor tendon. The nodular thickening hinders back-and-forth movement of the flexor tendon under the A1 flexor pulley, causing locking of the finger **(Fig. 45.12)**.

COMMON ASSOCIATION

Trigger finger is common in patients with diabetes, hypothyroid, rheumatoid arthritis, and amyloidosis. Therefore, always consider taking history regarding these conditions.

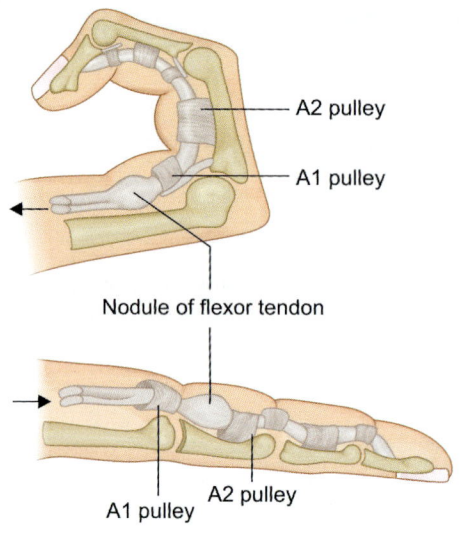

Fig. 45.12: Stenosing tenosynovitis of flexor tendon with a nodule in a trigger finger.
(*Courtesy:* Dr Aarthi, MBBS, KMC, Manipal)

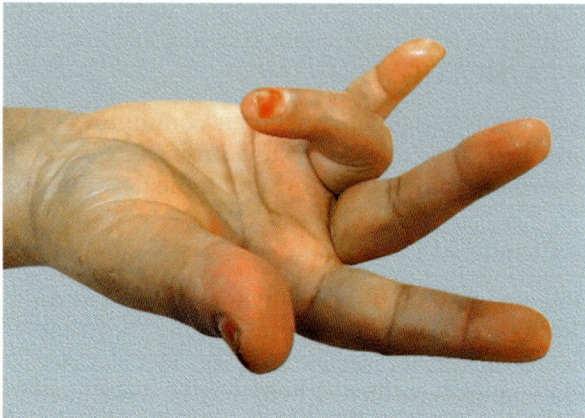

Fig. 45.13: Ring finger stuck in flexion.

CLINICAL FEATURES

- It commonly affects middle age patients.
- Mainly, the *middle or ring finger is involved.* The patient is unable to extend his finger with ease. It extends with a sudden release **(Fig. 45.13)**.
- A *nodule* is often palpable along the finger's flexor sheath.

DIAGNOSIS

The trigger finger is essentially a clinical diagnosis. Plain radiographs of the hand are usually normal.
- **USG** of the involved finger can confirm the flexor sheath tenosynovitis and the presence of the nodule.
- **Blood tests** are required to confirm the presence of DM, RA or hypothyroid.

TREATMENT

Early cases are managed conservatively and treatment of the underlying condition (DM). In case conservative management fails, the release of the A1 pulley is required.
- **Conservative treatment:** Observation, night splint, and NSAIDs
  - Treat underlying condition, if any
  - If the pain does not alleviate with the above, USG-guided local steroid injection into the involved flexor sheath can be tried to reduce inflammation.
- **Surgical management:** If there is no response to conservative treatment, surgical debridement and release of the A1 pulley is performed.

CHAPTER 46

Spine and Lower Limb Disorders

TORTICOLLIS

DEFINITION
Torticollis or wry neck is characterized by a rotational and tilt deformity of the neck, wherein the head tilts to the affected side, and the chin rotates to the other side.

The term torticollis is derived from Latin words *'tortum' means twisted* and *'collum' means neck*.

TYPES OF TORTICOLLIS
- **Congenital/infantile:** It presents within 1–4 weeks of birth.
- **Secondary torticollis:** It could be due to retropharyngeal space infection, cervical lymphadenitis, cervical spine tumor/tuberculosis, posterior fossa tumor, or Grisel syndrome. (Note: Grisel syndrome is a nontraumatic atlantoaxial subluxation which is usually secondary to an infection or an inflammation at the head and neck region. The spine ligament are damaged due to inflammation. It is seen in children).
- **Trochlear torticollis:** Due to fourth cranial nerve palsy resulting in superior oblique muscle (of eye) palsy.
- **Spasmodic:** It is due to recurrent spasm in sternocleidomastoid.

In this section, we will discuss congenital torticollis.

CONGENITAL TORTICOLLIS

DEFINITION
A deformity involving the shortening of the sternocleidomastoid (SCM) resulting in limited rotation and lateral flexion **(Fig. 46.1)**.

COMMON ASSOCIATION
About 5–20% of cases may have developmental dysplasia of hip (DDH). Others are metatarsus adductus and calcaneovalgus feet.

ETIOPATHOLOGY
- **Theory of intrauterine crowding:** A distorted position in-utero could result in ischemia in sternocleidomastoid

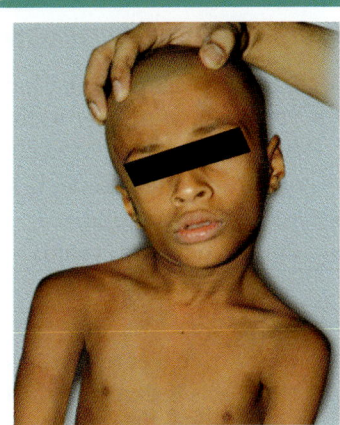

Fig. 46.1: Torticollis.

muscle (SCM) or venous occlusion causing a "compartment-like situation" in SCM. This theory is supported by fact the congenital torticollis in common in breech delivery (13–17%) or cesarean section (16–20%).
- **Repetitive microtrauma in the womb**
- **Birth trauma theory:** Trauma to SCM due to use of forceps/vacuum followed by bleeding in the SCM, leading to hematoma formation (*sternomastoid tumor*). A lump is observed over the SCM at birth. Later, the lump resolves, but the SCM becomes fibrotic and fails to elongate.
- **Sudden changes in calcium levels (in utero)** may result in prolonged SCM spasm followed by contraction.

CLINICAL FEATURES

The patient presents with torticollis.

Clinical examination reveals
- Ipsilateral shoulder elevation
- Asymmetric development of skull and face in infants (plagiocephaly or brachycephaly)
- A mass (8 mm–3 cm) is felt in SCM in 60% of cases
- Neglected torticollis can result in impaired cognitive development due to limited ability to turn, see and hear.
- Assess cervical spine movements.
- *Also assess visual functions*—eye alignment, presence of red reflex, and pupillary reaction to light, to determine whether it fixes and follows objects. Often, there may be a weakness of the oculomotor muscles (superior oblique or lateral rectus); the torticollis results from a compensatory mechanism to improve vision.

INVESTIGATIONS

- **Cervical spine X-ray:** To assess any associated vertebral anomaly
- **MRI neck and brain:** To assess any neurological causes
- **Ophthalmic evaluation:** To rule out gaze (macula) fixing in th eye. If the gaze is fixed in the torticollis, surgical correction of the torticollis is not advisable.

DIFFERENTIAL DIAGNOSIS

- Superior oblique palsy/ocular diseases
- Vertebral anomaly: Hemivertebra, Klippel–Feil syndrome, which is characterized by congenital fusion of two or more cervical vertebra. Klippel–Feil has a classic clinical triad of—short, webbed neck, low hairline, and reduced neck movement.
- Vestibular diseases
- Central nervous system (CNS) and peripheral nervous system (PNS) lesions.

TREATMENT

Nonoperative treatment is recommended if:
- Torticollis is detected during infancy (<1 year) or
- Limitation of neck rotations less than 30°

Nonoperative treatment consist of:
- *Passive stretching of the SCM*
- *Botulinum toxin type—a injection into the SCM*

Operative treatment is recommended if:
- If there is no improvement after 6 months of stretching
- Rotation limitation greater than 30°

Surgery: *Unipolar release/bipolar release/Z-plasty lengthening of the sternocleidomastoid.*

Postoperatively, the correction is maintained in POP or extended cervical brace **(Fig. 46.2)**.

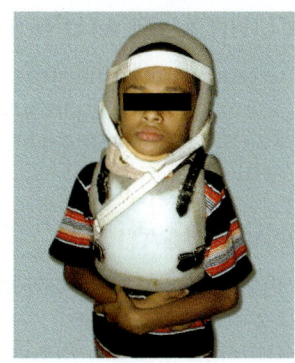

Fig. 46.2: Extended cervical brace.

KYPHOSIS

DEFINITION

Kyphosis is defined as excess dorsal curvature of the spine, especially in the thoracic spine. *Note: Normal thoracic kyphosis from T1–T12 vertebra is 20–40° of Cobb's angle.* Angle more than 45° is called kyphosis.

TYPES

Postural: It is common in prepubertal girls, obese women.

Structural: Structural kyphosis is also known as gibbus. There are three types of structural kyphosis.
1. ***Knuckle:*** Single-level vertebral collapse—tuberculosis (TB), traumatic
2. ***Angular:*** Two to three vertebral collapse—TB spine, osteoporosis
3. ***Round back:*** Four or more vertebral collapse result in round back kyphosis, which is also known as Dowager's hump. Round back kyphosis is seen in:
    - Osteoporosis
    - Ankylosing spondylitis **(Fig. 46.3)**
    - Scheuermann's disease **(Box 46.1)**.

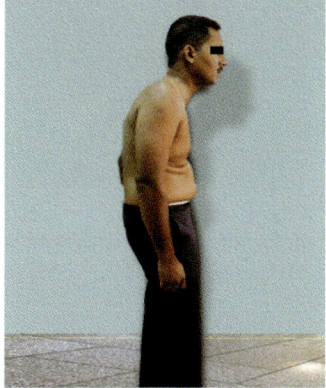

Fig. 46.3: Exaggerated kyphosis of dorsal spine.

> **Box 46.1:** Scheuermann's disease.
>
> - Developmental thoracic kyphosis of adolescence
> - Characterized by anterior wedging of greater than or equal to 5° in 3 or more adjacent vertebral bodies resulting in thoracic kyphosis (curve is usually 45–75°)
> - More common in males
> - Most patients asymptomatic, kyphosis or hunchback noticed by parents. Sometimes, mild back pain
> - X-ray shows wedging of three adjacent vertebra
> - Extension brace (Boston, Milwaukee) is used in curves <75°
> - Rarely, surgery is performed is curve >75°.

CLINICAL FEATURES
- Often, asymptomatic if the lesion is old and healed.
- There may be pain in structural kyphosis.
- The rest of the clinical features depend upon the etiology (e.g., ankylosing spondylitis, Pott's spine).

INVESTIGATIONS
- **Plain X-ray of the dorsal spine:** Anteroposterior (AP) and lateral view
- **CT scan, MRI scan**
- **Other investigations** as per etiology.

TREATMENT
- **Treatment of the etiology:** Tuberculosis, ankylosing spondylitis, osteoporosis as per standard guidelines.
- **Conservative:** Physiotherapy, braces
- **Surgery:** For severe deformity, "corrective osteotomy" can be performed.

SCOLIOSIS

DEFINITION
It is defined as lateral bending of the spine **(Fig. 46.4)**. However, it should be noted that scoliosis is not a uniplaner deformity of the spine.
- The bodies of the vertebra are rotated towards the convexity of the curve
- The spinous processes are rotated towards the concavity of the curve

CLASSIFICATION OR TYPES OF SCOLIOSIS (FLOWCHART 46.1)

The scoliosis could be *postural* and *structural*.
- **Postural scoliosis:** It is a compensatory scoliosis due to:
  - *Muscle spasm:* Acute painful conditions of the spine, such as acute lumbar disc prolapse.
  - *Pelvic tilt:* Due to deformities and contractures around the pelvis and the hip
  - *Limb-length discrepancy*

  Note that postural scoliosis disappears when patient bends forwards or sits, whereas structural scoliosis persists.
- **Structural scoliosis** is a scoliotic deformity due to permanent structural changes in the spine.

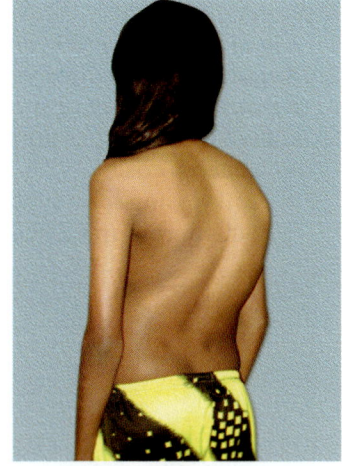

Fig. 46.4: Dorsolumbar scoliotic deformity of spine with right side rib hump.

Flowchart 46.1: Classification of scoliosis.

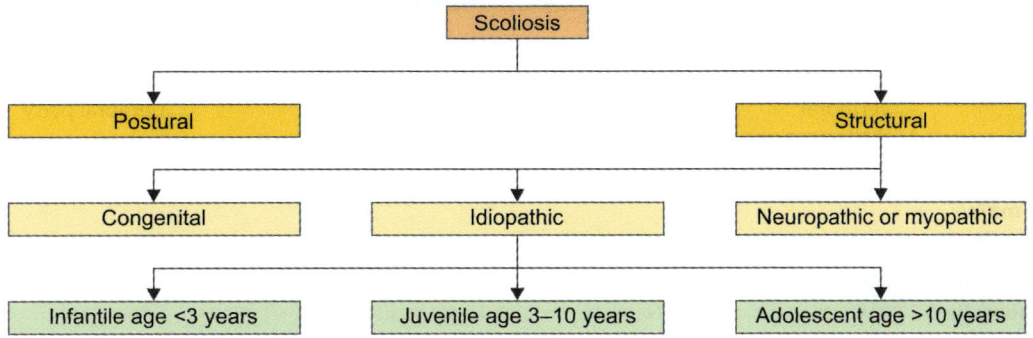

It is of three major types—(i) congenital, (ii) idiopathic and (iii) neuromuscular.
1. ***Congenital:*** It is due to *"congenital bony abnormality of the vertebra,"* wherein either vertebra did not form or failed to segment. Various causes are:
   - *Failed to form*: Hemivertebra
   - *Failed to segment*: Block vertebra/unsegmented bar
   - Mixed type.
2. ***Idiopathic:*** *Unknown cause of scoliosis* possible due to the *"primary contractile disorder of the muscle"*. It is possibly due to:
   - Platelet calmodulin defects
   - Abnormal fibrillin metabolism
   - Disorganized skeletal growth
   - Hormonal (melatonin).
3. ***Neuromuscular disorders:***
   - Cerebral palsy
   - Spinal muscular atrophy
   - Poliomyelitis
   - Spina bifida.

Table 46.1 outlines the difference between postural and structural scoliosis and **Table 46.2** outlines the difference between various structural scoliosis.

Table 46.1: Differences between postural and structural scoliosis.

	Postural scoliosis	Structural scoliosis
Structural changes in the spine	No	Yes
Rotatory deformity	No	Yes
Rib hump	No	Yes
Progression	No	Yes
Postural correction possible	Yes, when the patient • Sits • Bends forwards • When primary pathology is corrected	No

Table 46.2: Differences between various types of structural scoliosis.

	Congenital	Infantile	Juvenile	Adolescent	Neuromuscular
Cause	Congenital vertebral malformations				Poliomyelitis Cerebral palsy
Common in male/female		Male	Female	Female	
Associated anomalies	60% chance • Cardiac, genitourinary • VACTERL syndrome • Klippel–Feil syndrome	• Plagiocephaly • Neural axis abnormality	Neural axis abnormality		
Progression of curve	• Rapid in first three years of life • Block vertebra: Slow progression	• Most resolve spontaneously • If progresses after 5 years, 50% will have a curve of >70°	High risk of progression	High risk of progression if • Curves >25° • Remaining skeletal growth	Rapidly progressive

CLINICAL FEATURES

Symptoms
- Scoliotic deformity of the spine **(Fig. 46.4)**. Always ask about the progression of the curve.
- There may be associated back pain.
- Ask for family and birth history.

Signs
- The scoliotic deformity is noted **(Fig. 46.5)**
- Note the region and direction of the curve
- A rib hump can be noted while the patient bends forward **(Fig. 46.6)**
- ***Adam's forward bending test:*** The patient is asked to stand and bend forward till the back becomes horizontal with the floor. The curve becomes "more obvious."
- Prominent hip and pelvic tilt
- Look for skin signs, such as:
  - *Café-au-lait spots, axillary freckles*
  - *Neurofibromatosis*
  - *Sacral dimples, tuft of hairs, nevus*: In spina bifida
- Complete neurological examination is must to rule out any neurological deficit.
- Systemic examination: 'Head to toe' and the entire systemic examination must be done to rule out associated anomalies **(Box 46.2)**.

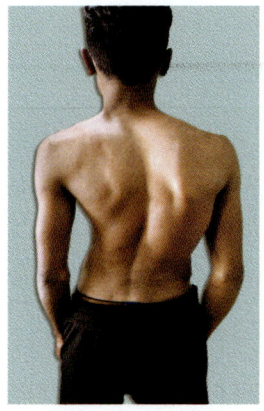 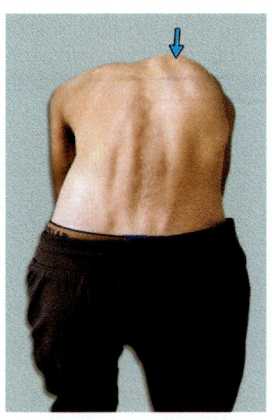

> **Box 46.2:** Associated conditions especially in congenital scoliosis.
>
> - **Cardiac malformations:** 10%
> - **Genitourinary malformations:** 25%
> - **Spinal cord malformation**
> - **VACTERL syndrome:** Vertebral, anal atresia, cardiac, tracheoesophageal fistula, renal and limb defects
> - **Klippel–Feil syndrome**

Fig. 46.5: Scoliotic deformity of dorsolumabr spine.

Fig. 46.6: Adam's test with rib hump on right side (arrow).

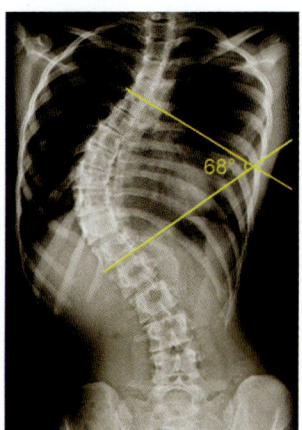 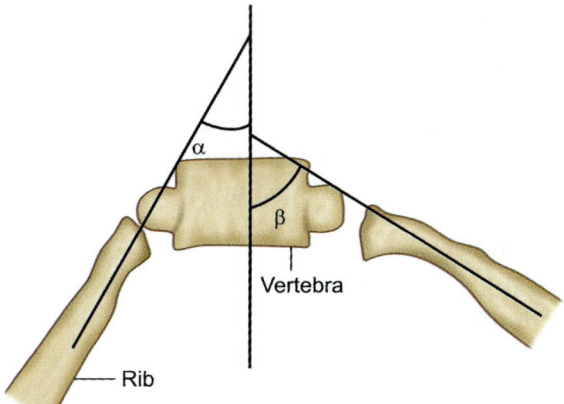

Fig. 46.7: Cobb's angle (left image) and rib-vertebral angle difference (RVAD) measurement (right image) in scoliosis.

INVESTIGATIONS

- **X-rays of the spine:** Full length in posteroanterior (PA) and lateral view:
  - In erect, supine and traction views
  - Lateral bending views to assess the correctability of the curve
  - The angle of curvature can be measured as Cobb's angle and rib-vertebral angle difference (RVAD) **(Fig. 46.7)**.

> - **Cobb's angle:** It is defined as the angle formed between a line drawn parallel to the superior endplate of superior terminal vertebra of the curve and a line drawn parallel to the inferior endplate of the inferior terminal vertebra of curve. A Cobb angle of 10° is regarded as a minimum angulation to define scoliosis.
> - **Rib-vertebral angle difference (RVAD = A–B):** Rib vertebral angle between concave and convex side of curve.

- **X-ray of the pelvis:** It should be done to look for the *"Risser sign."*

> **Risser's sign**
>
> The Risser sign is an indirect measure of skeletal maturity, whereby the degree of ossification of the iliac apophysis by X-ray evaluation is used to judge overall skeletal development. Risser's sign is used to assess skeletal maturity for the treatment of scoliosis as a near mature skeleton carries lesser risk of curve progression and vice versa.
>
> There is the gradual mineralisation of the iliac crest apophysis from anterolateral aspect, which progresses medially towards the spine. It is graded as 0–5. Risser 0 means no apophysis has appeared and indicates years of remaining growth. Risser 4–5 indicates little or no growth remaining.

- **CT scan of the spine with 3D reconstruction:** It helps assess curvature and vertebral anomalies.
- **MRI of the spine:** It is a *must* in congenital scoliosis, which is often associated with:
    - Diastematomyelia: Spinal cord is split vertically
    - Chiari malformation
    - Syringomyelia
    - Tethered cord.
- **Pulmonary function test:** Lung function is often compromised in scoliosis due to impaired thoracic growth and decreased lung volume.
- **Other appropriate investigations** to look for other associated congenital defects—Echo, abdomen–pelvis ultrasonography (USG).

TREATMENT

- **Postural:** Treatment of the cause, such as acute back pain.
- **Structural:** *"The overall goal is to prevent the curve from progressing over time"*, especially during the child's growth period. *Depending on Cobb's angle*, the treatment options vary from observation, bracing or surgical correction.
    - **Observation is advised** *for milder Cobb's angle (<25°) or nonprogressive curves. These patients must be periodically followed up to look for any curve progression.*
      Many infantile curves spontaneously resolve. However, it will progress if Cobb's angle or RVAD is greater than 25°. A high risk of progression is observed in juvenile scoliosis.
    - **Bracing:** Bracing is indicated for curves with Cobb's angle between 25°–45°. Note that the brace is not indicated in congenital scoliosis.
      There are several types of braces—**Milwaukee, Boston, and Charlston**. Currently, many institutions prefer a custom made brace for every patient, which is a modified version of Boston brace.
        - *Milwaukee brace, which is a cervico-thoraco-lumbo-sacral orthosis (CTLSO)*, must be worn 23 hours a day. And, therefore, it has a poor compliance. Also, the mandibular pad could result in mandibular hypoplasia **(Fig. 46.8A)**.
        - *Modified Boston brace, which is a thoraco-lumbo-sacral orthosis (TLSO), works well for thoracic curves*. It has better compliance and does not lead to mandibular hypoplasia unlike Milwaukee **(Fig. 46.8B)**.
        - *Charlston brace, which is a TLSO, works well for lumbar and thoracolumbar curves. It is worn only during night, and therefore has better compliance* **(Fig. 46.8C)**. However, it is not frequently used as correction of curve is poor than Modified Boston brace. *Providence, a TLSO*, is another type of night brace.

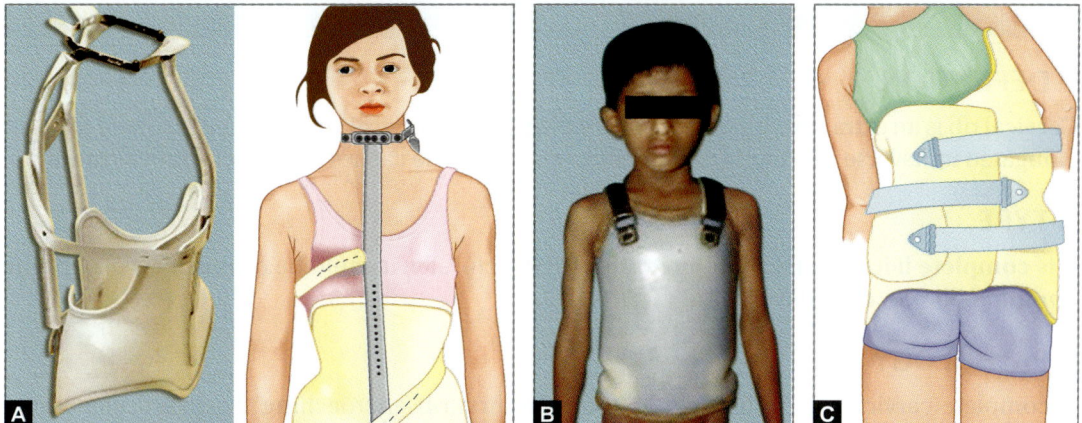

Figs. 46.8A to C: Braces in scoliosis: (A) Milwaukee brace; (B) Modified Boston brace; (C) Charlston brace.

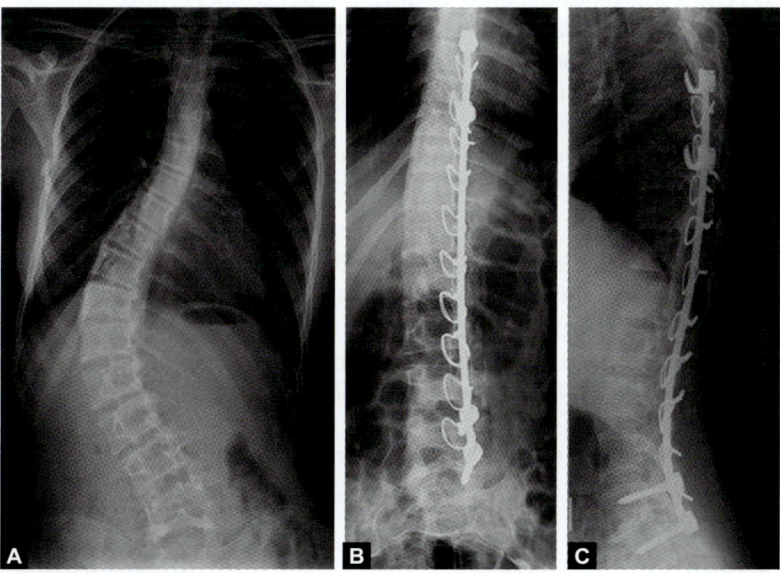

Figs. 46.9A to C: (A) Scoliosis, preoperative; (B and C) Postoperative X-rays showing corrected deformity.

- Other braces are *Lyon, Cheneau*, and *Spincor*. (Details are out of purview of this chapter).

  Note: In past, Minerva POP jacket was used to correct curves with casting. It is no more preferred.

- **Surgical correction of scoliosis (instrumentation and spinal fusion)** is performed when progressive curves with Cobb's angle/RVAD greater than 45° **(Figs. 46.9A to C)**. In kids younger than 5 years where fusion of spine could result in compromised cardiopulmonary function, newer techniques, such as growing rod and vertical expandable prosthetic titanium rib (VEPTR) are used which avoid fusion of spine. (*Details of these surgeries are out of scope of this chapter. Students are encouraged to read about it by themselves*).

CERVICAL RIB

■ DEFINITION

Cervical rib is an extra rib which arises out of the seventh cervical vertebra. It is also said to be an elongated transverse process of C7 vertebra. It is one of the causes of thoracic outlet syndrome.

■ TYPE

It is **complete** if it joins 1st rib or **incomplete**. Structurally, it could be *completely bony, partly bony and fibrous, or totally fibrous*.

■ PATHOLOGY

A complete cervical rib is directed towards the first rib encroaching the interscalene area where the brachial plexus and subclavian vessels lie. As the cervical rib moves forward and attaches over the first rib, it elevates the brachial plexus compressing the lower trunk of the brachial plexus **(Fig. 46.10)**. Rarely, there could be upper trunk compression. Also, there could be compression upon subclavian vessels. This could result in stenosis of subclavian artery followed by 'post-stenotic dilation' of the artery. The blood flow in post-stenosis dilated area turns turbulent resulting in a thrombus formation, which can embolize into the arteries of the upper limb leading to gangrene of the upper limb. Further, compression over the subclavian vein could result in thrombosis causing upper limb edema.

■ CLINICAL FEATURES

- Most cases are asymptomatic and are diagnosed on plain radiograph of the neck.
- **Neck pain** which often radiates towards the medial side of the arm, forearm and hand due to pressure over lower trunk (C8-T1) of brachial plexus. [*cf. intervertebral disc prolapse (IVDP) of the cervical spine where the radiation of the pain is common over the radial aspect of forearm and hand as the IVDP of the cervical spine predominantly occurs in C5-6, C6-7 region*].
  Neck pain may also radiate towards the anterior aspect of chest, shoulder, etc.
- Occasionally, the cervical rib can be palpated at the root of the neck on the anterior aspect.

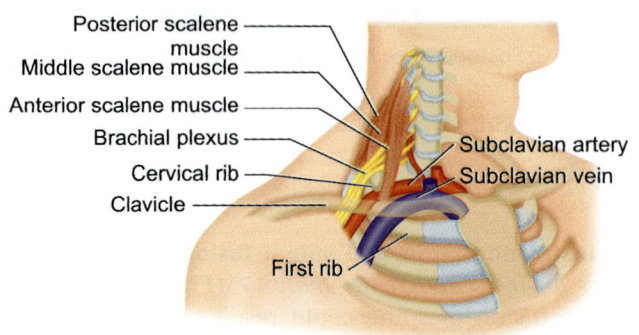

Fig. 46.10: Cervical rib compressing brachial plexus and subclavian artery.

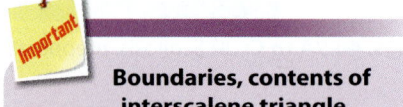

Boundaries, contents of interscalene triangle

- **Borders**
  Anterior: Anterior scalene muscle
  Posterior: Middle scalene muscle
  Inferior: First rib
- **Contents:** Brachial plexus trunk, subclavian artery
  Note: Subclavian vein does not pass through interscalene triangle. It runs beneath scalenus anterior muscle prior to entering the costoclavicular space

- **Neurological features:** Weakness may be noted in the muscles supplied by affected nerve roots. There may be sensory loss in the dermatomes of the compressed roots.
- **Vascular features:** Swelling (venous congestion) in the upper limb, Raynaud's-like features in the hand, cold intolerance, rarely gangrene of fingers.
- **Provocative test:** *Adson's* and *Wright tests* are positive for vascular insufficiency. *Roos test* can assess arterial, venous and neurological compression.

DIAGNOSIS

- **X-ray of cervical spine:** AP view, can diagnose a bony cervical rib **(Fig. 46.11)**
- **MRI scan of the neck** can be performed to detect cervical rib if it is not seen on X-ray. Angiography can be added to MRI if subclavian vascular occlusion is suspected.
- **Nerve conduction velocity** can be performed for nerve conduction study of brachial plexus.

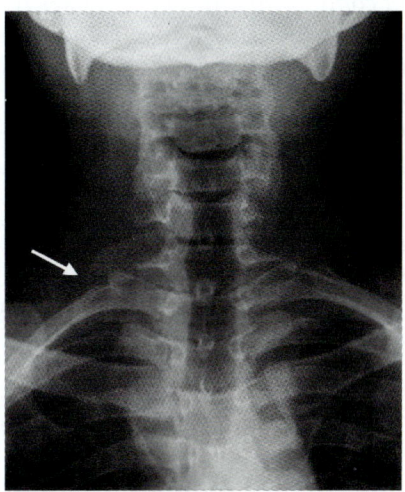

Fig. 46.11: Cervical rib (arrow).

TREATMENT

- **Conservative treatment** should be advised in case of neck pain with/without minor neurovascular symptoms in form of shoulder shrugging exercises, pectoral muscle stretching, analgesics, and pregabalin.
- **Surgical option** is advocated when conservative treatment fails or in case of disabling neurovascular symptoms, *"cervical rib excision along with a sleeve of periosteum"* can be performed.

AVASCULAR NECROSIS OF THE FEMORAL HEAD

Avascular necrosis of femoral is a result of loss of blood supply to the femoral head causing necrosis and collapse of the subchondral bone, followed by hip osteoarthritis.

ETIOLOGY

- **Direct/traumatic**
  Post-traumatic: It is common after a fracture neck femur and dislocation of the hip.
- **Indirect causes**
    - Idiopathic
    - Alcoholism
    - Systemic steroid therapy
    - Irradiation
    - Sickle cell anaemia
    - Caisson's disease
    - Gaucher's disease
    - Hematologic disease: Leukemia, lymphoma
    - Systemic lupus erythematosus (SLE)
    - Hypercoagulable states: Polycythemia vera.

PATHOGENESIS

The blood supply to the femoral head is precarious with end arteries supplying the femoral head **(Fig. 46.12A)**. A normal supply maintains the nutrition of subchondral bone and overlying hyaline cartilage **(Fig. 46.12B)**.

Various direct and indirect causes can damage the blood supply to the femoral head. The **direct 'traumatic' causes** *violate blood supply primarily by damaging the arteries due to tear or compression*. **Indirect causes** *result in arterial or venous thrombosis, raised intramedullary osseous hypertension* causing sinusoidal compression and venous thrombosis, resulting in decreased blood flow to the femoral head causing subchondral bone necrosis and collapse. As a result of subchondral bone death, there is a 'loss of support and nutrition' of hyaline articular cartilage, as the latter is supported by subchondral bone. *The damage to the hyaline cartilage results in hip arthritis* **(Fig. 46.12C)**.

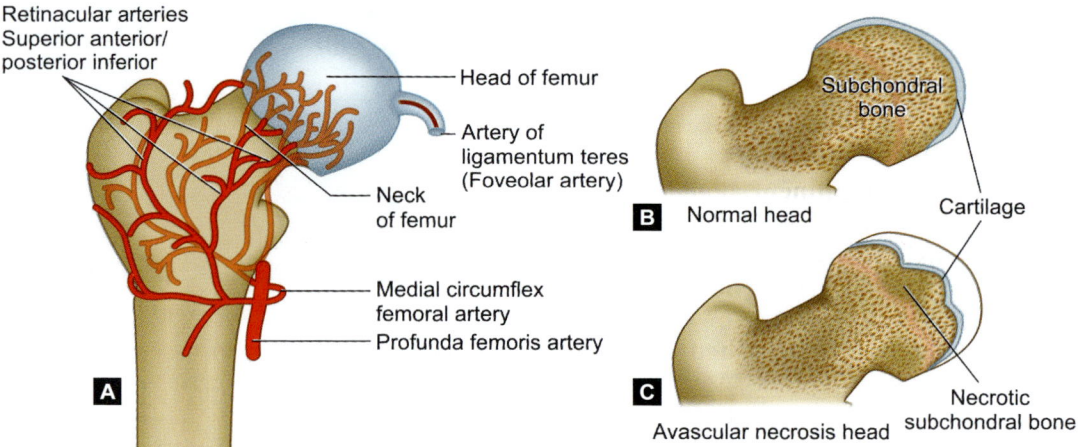

Figs. 46.12A to C: (A) Normal blood supply to femoral head; (B) Normal cartilage and subchondral bone; (C) Avascular necrosis of the femoral head with necrotic collapsed subchondral bone and cartilage damage.

CLINICAL FEATURES

Symptoms: Vague *pain* of mild to moderate intensity around the hip during activities for several weeks to months is the most common symptom of avascular necrosis (AVN) hip. It is followed by *limp*.

Signs
- The hip joint line is tender.
- **ROM:** The *movement at the hip are restricted*, especially abduction and internal rotation.
- **Axis deviation** is characteristic: During hip flexion, there is an obligatory external rotation of the hip.
- Other features of underlying etiology may be present.

INVESTIGATIONS

- **Plain X-ray of the hip:** AP and lateral view **(Fig. 46.13)**. Early cases may show normal hip X-ray. Late cases show sclerosis of femoral head and collapse of subchondral bone. Later, arthritis of hip.

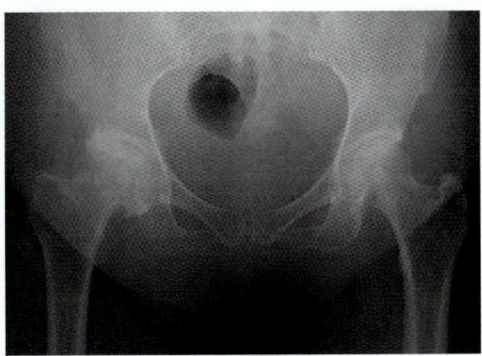

Fig. 46.13: Avascular necrosis (AVN) of right hip.

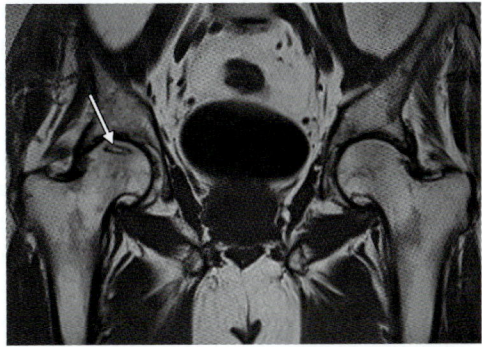

Fig. 46.14: MRI of both hips reveals early AVN of right hip (white arrow) whereas left is normal.

- **Magnetic resonance imaging (MRI)** *is the investigation of choice* **(Fig. 46.14)**. It helps in staging the disease using *Ficat and Arlet classification*. Stages 0–IV [Stage 0: Normal MRI; Stage I: Bone edema; Stage II: Subchondral cyst; Stage III: Subchondral collapse (Crescent sign); Stage IV: Arthritis].

TREATMENT (BASED UPON STAGE OF DISEASE)

The treatment of AVN is based on *disease staging according to the MRI of the hip.*
- **Early stages (I, II) of AVN**
  - ***Bisphosphonates:*** *Bisphosphonates are the drug of choice* in pre-collapse and early cases (Ficat and Arlet 0–II). Bisphosphonates act by inhibiting osteoclasts and thereby preventing subchondral collapse. Hence, it provides pain relief, better mobility and delays further disease progression.
  - ***Core decompression ± fibular grafting (vascularized/nonvascularized):*** Core decompression helps decrease intramedullary venous hypertension of the head of the femur. This helps reduce pain and may help slow down the AVN progression. Further, cortical fibular graft acts as a 'strut' to prevent subchondral collapse. *Note: Core decompression is a procedure wherein an 8–10 mm wide tunnel is bored into the femur starting from the lateral cortex of the femur just below the intertrochanteric ridge to the subchondral area of head femur via the neck femur* **(Fig. 46.15)**
  - ***Autologous cultured osteoblast injection OR bone marrow aspirate concentrate (BMAC)*** into the necrotic area: After core decompression and curettage of necrotic area, autologous cultured osteoblasts or BMAC can be injected into the necrotic area to

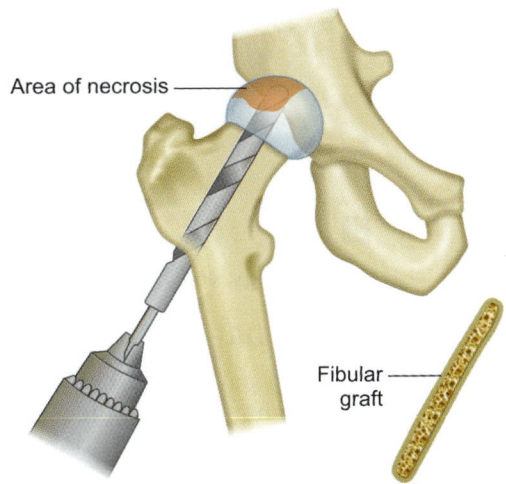

Fig. 46.15: Core decompression with or without fibular grafting for AVN femoral head.

regenerate new bone and restore microcirculation. However, these therapies report variable success and long-term results are awaited.

- **Late stages (III, IV) of AVN:** Hip arthritis
  - ***Total hip replacement is the treatment of choice*** in an arthritic hip to restore a painless, mobile and functional hip joint **(Fig. 46.16)**.
  - ***Arthrodesis (fusion of the hip joint)*** is an option in a young patient wherein THR is not feasible.

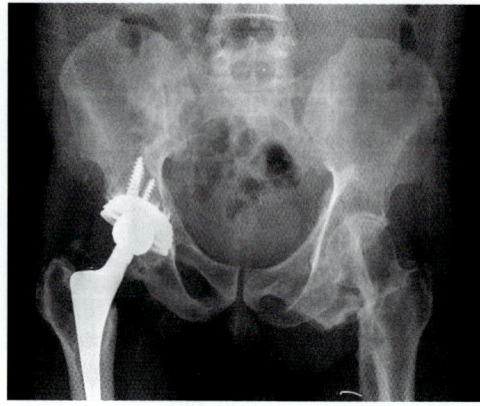

Fig. 46.16: Total hip replacement of right hip.

FEMOROACETABULAR IMPINGEMENT (FAI)

Femoroacetabular impingement is a condition of the hip joint common in young people wherein the femoral head pinches against the acetabulum, especially in flexion-rotation causing cartilage and labrum injury.

ETIOPATHOLOGY

High impact athletic activities or sports (hockey, soccer, basketball) during adolescence can increase chance of FAI. There are **two types of FAI**—*pincer* and *cam-type* **(Figs. 46.17A to C)**. In the pincer type, excessive coverage of the femoral head by the large acetabular rim results in damage to the labrum and femoral head cartilage **(Fig. 46.17A)**. The cam type is characterized by excess aspherical bone near the femoral head-neck junction, resulting in damage to the labrum and cartilage **(Fig. 46.17B)**. Occasionally, there are combined pincer and cam lesions **(Fig. 46.17C)**.

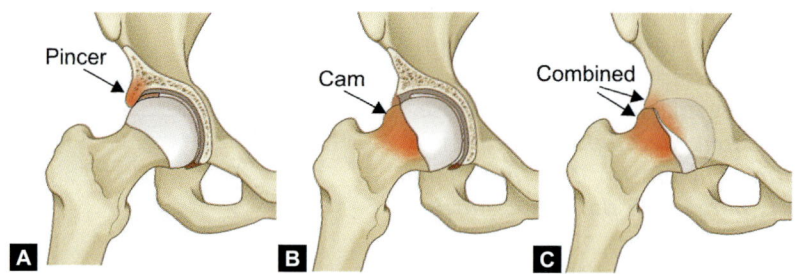

Figs. 46.17A to C: Types of femoroacetabular impingement.

CLINICAL FEATURES

Patients complain of pain in the hip during walking, prolonged sitting, or sporting activity. They may keep their hand around the hip (C-sign). The pain may radiate to the anterior thigh. Activities such as driving, sitting for long can aggravate the pain. Occasionally, there can be catching or clicks.

On examination, the hip *flexion and internal rotation are painful and limited.*

DIAGNOSIS

It can be confirmed by X-ray and MRI of the hip. In cam type, X-ray shows a pistol grip deformity, whereas cross over sign is observed in pincer type.

TREATMENT

Conservative treatment encompasses analgesics, physiotherapy, and activity modification. Surgical options for failed conservative treatment are debridement of cam lesion, labral debridement and repair, and chondroplasty.

BAKER'S CYST

It is also known as *Morrant-Baker's cyst*. The patient presents with pain and swelling in the popliteal fossa with coexisting arthritis/synovitis of the knee.

PATHOLOGY

It is *not* a true cyst. It is located in popliteal fossa *between the medial head of the gastrocnemius and the capsular reflection of the semimembranosus (oblique popliteal ligament)*. Whenever there is a chronic synovial irritation due to underlying intra-articular pathology (synovitis, arthritis, meniscal tear), there is excess synovial fluid formation, which cannot be accommodated in the knee. Therefore, the knee synovium herniates posteriorly in the popliteal fossa through the naturally-occurring rent in the posterior capsule of the knee with a unidirectional valve adjacent to the medial femoral condyle. The excess joint fluid keeps collecting in the cyst due to the unidirectional valve, which allows fluid to flow into the cyst from the joint but not in reverse direction.

Important fact about Baker's cyst

The fact that must be remembered is that "Baker's cyst is almost always secondary to a primary intra-articular pathology in the knee, e.g., osteoarthritis (OA), rheumatoid arthritis." And therefore, the primary pathology must be treated first, which may result in spontaneous resolution of the Baker's cyst.

CLINICAL FEATURES

- Patients complain of pain in the knee along with a *swelling in the popliteal fossa* **(Fig. 46.18)**. The pain increases during full extension, and deep flexion.
- **Foucher's sign positive:** The swelling in popliteal fossa is firm and prominent in an extended knee, whereas it becomes less prominent in a flexed knee.
- The knee may have features of other pathology like osteoarthritis/rheumatoid arthritis.

INVESTIGATIONS

- **X-ray of the knee:** To look for associated knee pathology.
- **MRI of the knee is confirmatory**. It also provides information about the associated knee joint pathology.

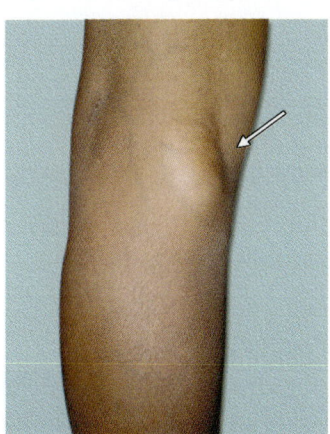

Fig. 46.18: Baker's cyst.

- **USG** can also confirm the diagnosis but does not provide information about the intra-articular pathology.

TREATMENT

Primarily, treat the intra-articular knee pathology, the Baker's cyst may subside. However, if it remains symptomatic even after primary treatment, it may need excision (open or arthroscopic).

COMPLICATION

A Baker cyst can rupture, resulting in cystic fluid leakage into the calf's musculofascial planes causing an intense inflammatory reaction leading to acute onset pain and swelling in the calf. *These features mimic acute onset deep vein thrombosis of the calf veins*, which can be ruled out with venous doppler.

DIFFERENTIAL DIAGNOSIS

Ganglion cyst, semimembranosus bursa, popliteal artery aneurysm. *Note that baker's cyst is usually located below the joint line, whereas semimembranosus bursa lies above the joint line.* Popliteal artery aneurysm is pulsatile in nature.

GENU VARUM AND VALGUM

INTRODUCTION

- In an adult, the *normal lower limb alignment* is 5°–7° of valgus. The kids are born with 10°–15° of genu varus. The varus reverses to neutral alignment and further to 10°–20° of *"physiologic valgus"* by the age of 3–4 years of age and gradually corrects to normal adult valgus of 5°–7° by the age of 8–10 years **(Fig. 46.19)**.
- Average intermalleolar distance (IMD) (for genu valgum assessment) should be less than 8 cm.
- The average intercondylar distance (for genu varum assessment) should be less than 5 cm.

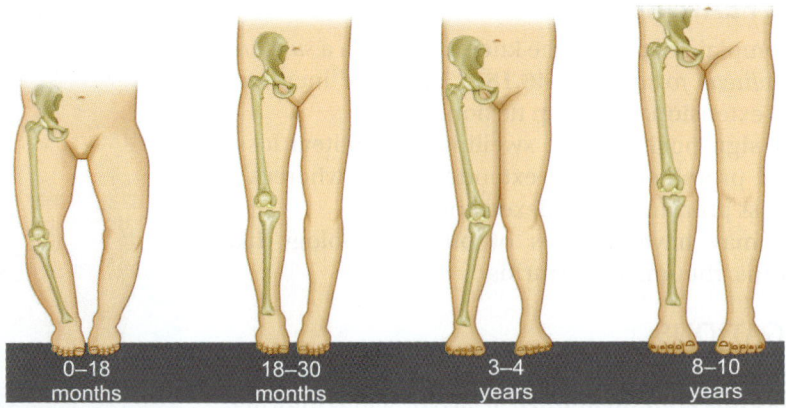

Fig. 46.19: Progression of Infanthood varus to adult valgus alignement of lower limb.

GENU VALGUM (KNOCK KNEE)

DEFINITION

The lateral or outward deviation of the tibia with respect to the knee is called genu valgum **(Fig. 46.20)**.

ETIOLOGY

The normal alignment of the lower limb is mild valgus. Pathologic genu valgum can happen in the distal femur (most common) or the proximal tibia.

The causes of genu valgum vary in children and adults.

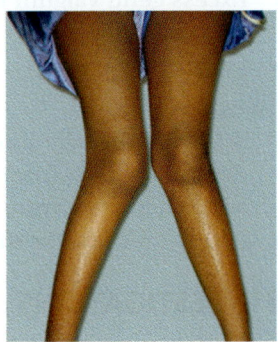

Fig. 46.20: Bilateral genu valgum.

Children

Any condition which partially/completely damages the lateral half of the distal femoral or the upper tibial growth plate results in more growth from the medial side/less growth from the lateral side of the growth plate, resulting in genu valgum. The uni- and bilateral causes vary as mentioned below.
- **Bilateral:**
    - Physiological
    - Metabolic: Rickets. Note that renal rickets is most common cause of pathologic genu valgum in kids
    - Skeletal dysplasia: Spondyloepiphyseal dysplasia
    - Neuromuscular: Cerebral palsy.
- **Unilateral:** It is always pathological
    - Trauma to the growth plate—*Cozen's phenomena*
    - Infections: Osteomyelitis
    - Tumor: Affecting growth plate.

Adults
- *Inflammatory:* Rheumatoid arthritis or other inflammatory arthritis.
- *Traumatic*: Malunited fractures around the knee, chronic medial collateral ligament injuries.

CLASSIFICATION FOR SEVERITY OF BILATERAL GENU VALGUM BY MEASURING INTERMALLEOLAR DISTANCE (IMD)

With patient supine, both knees are brought close to each other and measure IMD. The IMD can be used to classify the severity of genu valgum.
- **Mild:** IMD 8–10 cm
- **Moderate:** IMD 10–15 cm
- **Severe:** IMD greater than 15 cm.

CLINICAL FEATURES
- **Genu valgum deformity (knock knee)** is noted wherein knees touch each other and ankles are apart. The deformity could be progressive/static.

- *Difficulty in running* due to knocking knees
- Excess genu valgum can predispose the knee to *recurrent patella dislocation due to an increased Q angle.*
- Late cases in adults may present as osteoarthritis of the lateral compartment of the knee.

On examination
- *Site of deformity must be assessed by completely flexing the knee:* If the genu valgum deformity arises from the distal femur, it gets masked with knee flexion, whereas it remains as it is if it arises from the proximal tibia.
- Assess the *"intermalleolar distance" and "Q angle."*

INVESTIGATIONS

- **Plain X-ray of the knee:** Anteroposterior (AP) and lateral
- Plain AP X-ray of the entire lower limb from the hip to the ankle **(long leg view)**.
    - To measure the degree of valgus.
- **Other investigations:** As per the etiology.

TREATMENT (FLOWCHART 46.2)

The treatment of the genu valgum depends upon the following:
- Etiology, which must be treated as per standard guidelines, e.g., rickets.
- Age of the patient
- Unilateral/bilateral deformity
- The severity of the deformity, which is calculated according to IMD

1. **Bilateral genu valgum in those less than 6 years of age** should be serially observed. If it further progresses or in case of residual moderate–severe deformity, it can be corrected with temporary hemiepiphysiodesis after 7 years of age.
2. **Unilateral genu valgum deformity is usually pathological.**
    - Investigate and treat local pathology
    - Still can be observed till 7 years

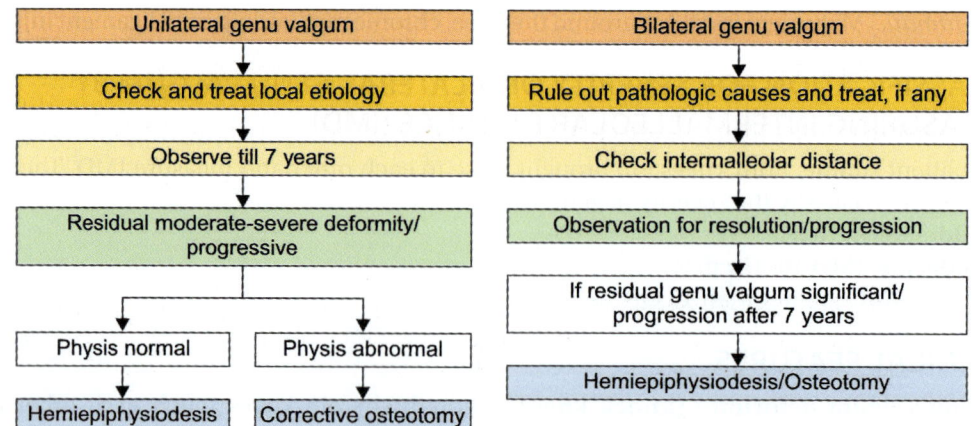

Flowchart 46.2: Treatment algorithm of the genu valgum.

- Leftover moderate–severe deformities/progressive deformity should be corrected with temporary hemiepiphysiodesis/distal femoral osteotomy **(Fig. 46.21)**.

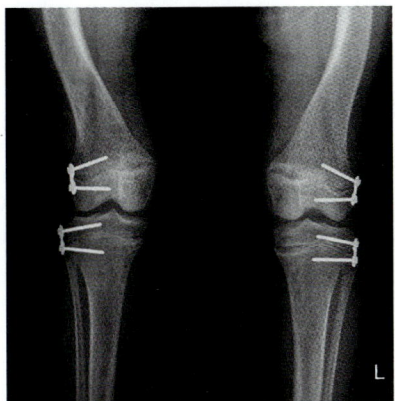

Fig. 46.21: Hemiepiphysiodesis of lateral side of growth plate to correct genu varum.

Hemiepiphysiodesis

Hemiepiphysiodesis is a 'guided growth or growth modulation' procedure in which the longitudinal growth from the physis can be altered, temporarily or permanently.

To temporarily alter/stop the growth from one side of the growth plate, a staple or a plate is placed across the growth plate on one side, stopping the growth from the plate placement. As the other side of the physeal growth continues, this results in correcting the deformity. Later, the plates/staples are removed.

GENU VARUM/BOW LEGS

DEFINITION

Inward/medial bending of the leg is known as genu varum **(Fig. 46.22)**.

ETIOLOGY

The etiology may vary in unilateral or bilateral genu varum.

Bilateral

- Physiologic: Upto 2 years
- Infantile Blount's disease or tibia vara **(Box 46.3)**. It is the most common cause of pathologic genu varum in kids.
- Metabolic: Rickets
- Skeletal dysplasia: Achondroplasia
- Degenerative: Osteoarthritis is the most common cause of bilateral genu varum in adults.

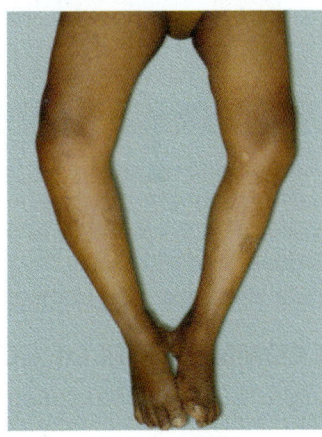

Fig. 46.22: Bilateral genu varum.

Box 46.3: Blount's disease.

A condition wherein abnormal growth of proximal tibial metaphysis results in pathological varus. Infantile variant is bilateral, progressive and associated with internal tibial torsion. Adolescent variant is unilateral and torsion is uncommon. X-ray shows flat medial tibial epiphysis and beak shape adjacent metaphysis. If progressive, it require corrective osteotomy.

Unilateral
- Traumatic: Malunited fracture around the knee, chronic lateral collateral ligament injuries
- Infection
- Tumor
- Adolescent Blount's disease.

CLINICAL FEATURES
- Genu varum deformity is present **(Fig. 46.22)**.
- *Site of deformity must be confirmed by flexing the knee:* If the deformity obliterates with knee flexed, it indicates femoral origin of deformity, whereas a persistent genu varus with knee flexed indicates a tibial origin deformity.
- Late cases in adults may have OA of the medial compartment of the knee.
- Other clinical features pertaining to specific etiology (rickets, etc.)

INVESTIGATIONS
- Plain X-ray of the lower limb (long leg view)
- Relevant investigations to rule out etiology.

TREATMENT
- Treatment of cause, if possible
- *Mild varum:* Conservative, bracing
- *Moderate–severe:* Lateral hemiepiphysiodesis in growing children (*see* **Fig. 46.21**)
- High tibial osteotomy is performed once the growth plate/tibial tuberosity is fused.

OSTEOCHONDRITIS DESSICANS (OCD) KNEE

Osteochondritis dessicans is an idiopathic, focal, subchondral-bone abnormality that can cause instability or detachment of a bone fragment and overlying articular cartilage, with subsequent progression to osteoarthritis. Note that OCD can occur in other joints, too, such as the elbow and ankle.

It is common in young people, and affects boys more than girls.

COMMON SITE OF OCD IN THE KNEE
Lateral surface of the medial femoral condyle (MFC) is the most common site.

ETIOPATHOLOGY
Repeated microtrauma or idiopathic avascularity to the subchondral bone are the proposed causes. Avascular necrosis of subchondral bone is followed by osteochondral fragment separation.

CLINICAL PRESENTATION
Patients complain of knee pain, intermittent swelling, and locking.

EXAMINATION
The findings are non-specific, such as joint line tenderness, effusion, and limited movement.

DIAGNOSIS

X-ray—AP and lateral view may show an OCD fragment **(Fig. 46.23A)**. A *tunnel view of the knee* (knee in 60° flexion) may be helpful. MRI is diagnostic **(Fig. 46.23B)**. Arthroscopy reveals the size and stability of the lesion and the status of overlying cartilage **(Fig. 46.23C)**.

TREATMENT

Conservative treatment is tried in stable lesions, which involves analgesics, rehabilitation and limiting sporting activity. The lesion may heal in 8–12 months. Unstable fragments or those not responding to conservative treatment require surgical treatment. Depending upon the size and stability of the fragment, surgical options include drilling (ante/retrograde) with/without fixation of the lesion **(Figs. 46.24A and B)**, debridement with microfracture/osteoarticular

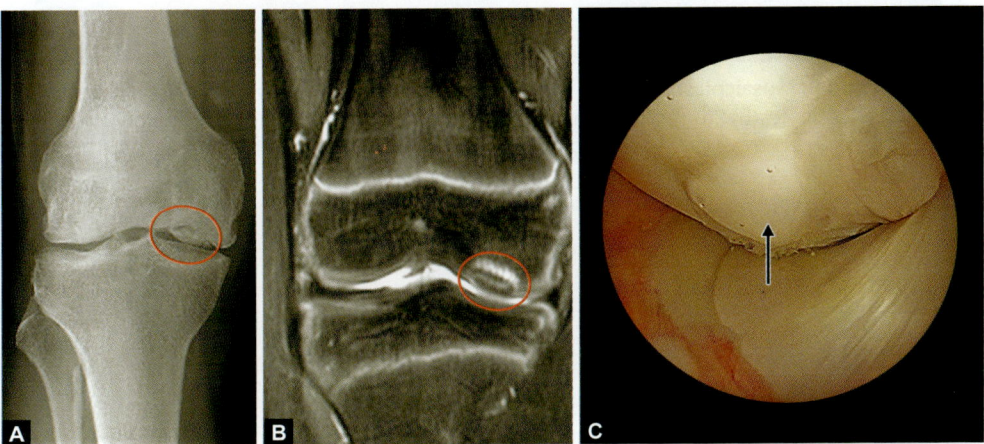

Figs. 46.23A to C: (A) Plain radiograph showing OCD of the right medial femoral condyle; (B) MRI of right knee shows OCD of the medial femoral condyle; (C) Arthroscopic view of OCD of the medial femoral condyle.

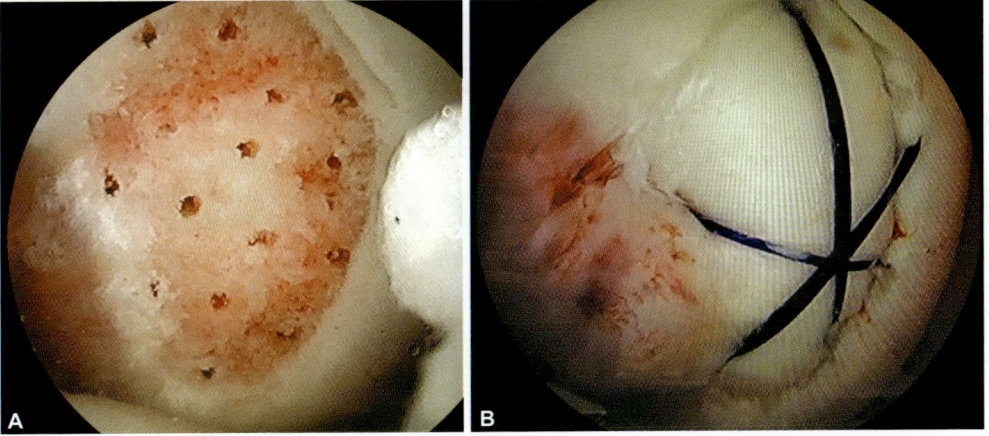

Figs. 46.24A and B: (A) Microfracture of OCD crater; (B) Fixation of OCD with PDS suture.
(OCD: osteochondritis dissecans; PDS: polydioxanone)
(Courtesy: Dr Sujit Jose, Kerala)

articular cartilage transplant surgery (OATS) **(Figs. 46.25A and B)**, and autologous cartilage implantation **(Figs. 46.26A and B)**.

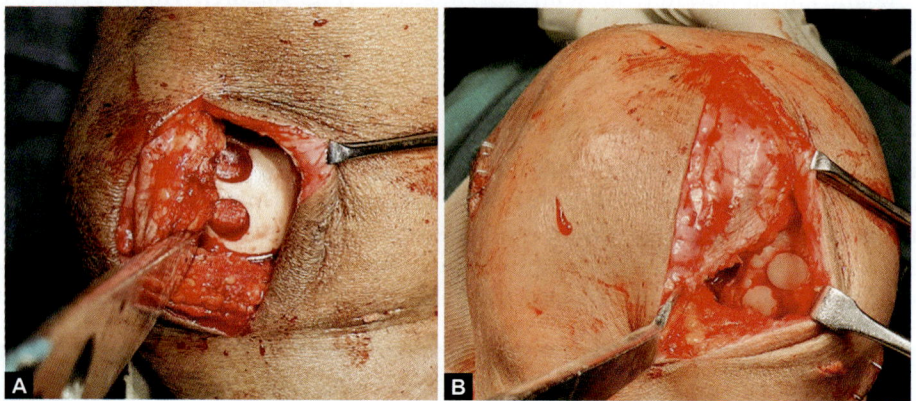

Figs. 46.25A and B: Mosaicplasty or OATS plug. (A) Osteoarticular plugs obtained from lateral femoral condyle; (B) Plugs placed in the OCD defect on medial femoral condyle.
(OCD: osteochondritis dissecans)

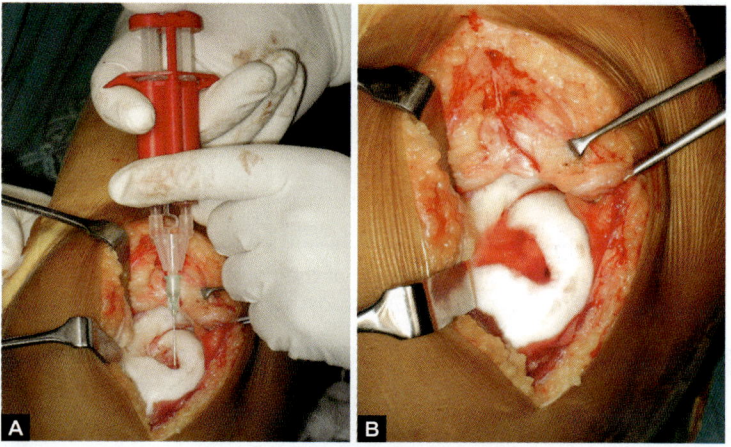

Figs. 46.26A and B: (A) Autologous cartilage implantation (ACI) in the defect; (B) The ACI forms a stable gel in the defect area of cartilage.

SYNOVIAL CHONDROMATOSIS

It is a *synovial proliferative disease associated with cartilage metaplasia resulting in multiple intra-articular loose bodies*. It is observed in patients between 30–50 years of age.

■ CLINICAL PRESENTATION

Pain, locking, and swelling of the joint.

■ EXAMINATION

Single or multiple loose bodies can be felt during palpation. Other palpatory findings are crepitus and synovial hypertrophy.

INVESTIGATIONS
X-ray—multiple loose bodies **(Fig. 46.27)**.

TREATMENT
Open or arthroscopic synovectomy and loose body removal **(Fig. 46.28)**.

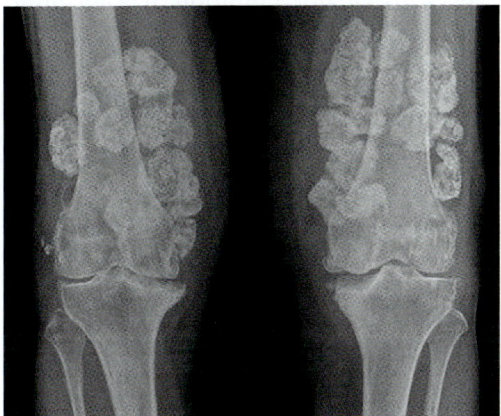
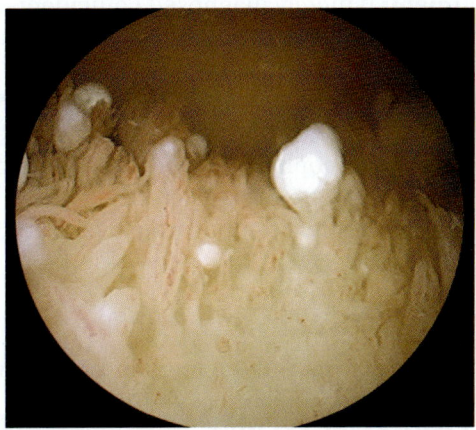

Fig. 46.27: Synovial chondromatosis. X-ray knee shows multiple ossified loose bodies in both knees.

Fig. 46.28: Arthroscopy of knee shows synovial hypertrophy and pedunculated chondromatosis bodies.

DISCOID MENISCUS

It is congenital anomaly of meniscus, wherein the meniscus is thicker and like a disc or saucer shape rather than normal 'C' shape **(Figs. 46.29A and B)**. *Lateral discoid is more common than medial and often, it is bilateral.* Due to abnormal structure, discoid meniscus is more prone for tears, especially horizontal.

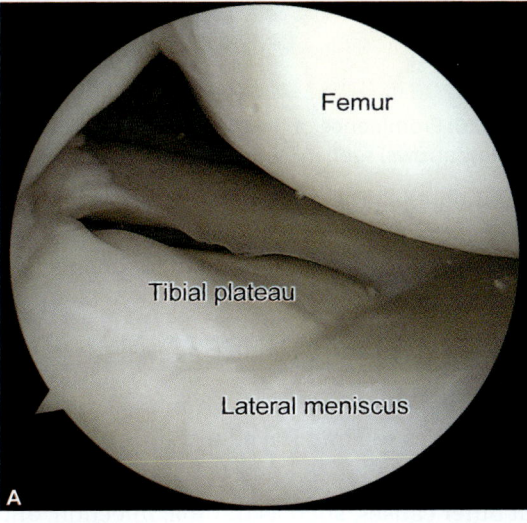
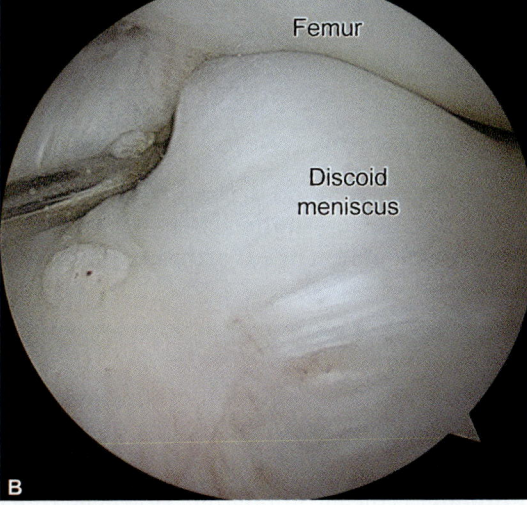

Figs. 46.29A and B: (A) Arthroscopic image of a normal C shape lateral meniscus; (B) Arthroscopic image of a discoid lateral meniscus covering entire tibial plateau.

Clinical features: Often, patients are asymptomatic or may complain of pain. One of the *classic presentation is presence of thud over the joint line, which is palpable and often audible.* It is also known as snapping knee syndrome.

There may be locking or catching. Meniscal tests, such as McMurray's is positive.

Investigation: MRI is diagnostic.

Treatment: If merely diagnosed coincidentally on MRI without any symptoms, it is left alone. Symptomatic ones require arthroscopic partial meniscectomy.

OSGOOD–SCHLATTER DISEASE

It is a traction apophysitis of the tibial tuberosity apophysis in *young adolescent kids who are active in sports.* Often, it is bilateral.

It is one of the common cause of anterior knee pain in young adolescent kids who are active in sports.

■ PATHOLOGY

Avascular necrosis and fragmentation of tibial tuberosity (TT) apophysis.

■ CLINICAL FEATURES

These patients present with anterior knee pain, especially while running, climbing stairs, and squatting. Often patients point their finger over the tibial tuberosity as the point of pain. Pain relieves with rest.

Examination reveals a tender and prominent TT **(Fig. 46.30).**

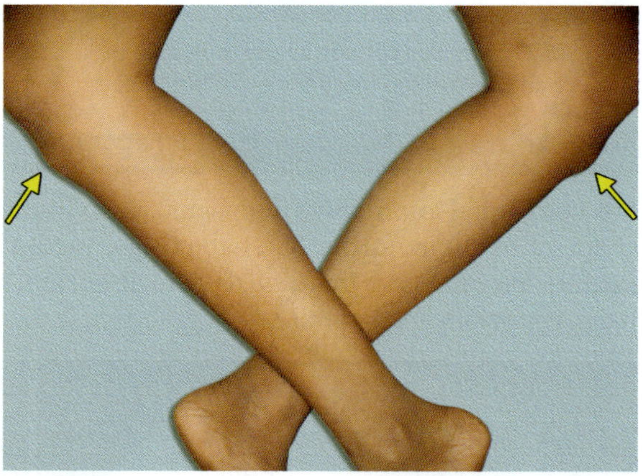

■ DIAGNOSIS

Lateral X-ray of the knee shows fragmented TT.

■ TREATMENT

Fig. 46.30: Prominence of the bilateral tibial tuberosity (yellow arrows) seen in Osgood–Schlatter disease.

Most patients respond to conservative treatment, which includes NSAIDs, physiotherapy, and limit/modify/stop sports activity for several months. Usually self-limiting by six months to a few years. Rarely, it needs arthroscopic/open debridement of frayed separated fragments.

CHONDROMALACIA PATELLA

It is an idiopathic condition of the *young population, especially females from the 2nd to the fourth decade,* wherein the retropatellar cartilage becomes soft and frayed resulting in anterior knee pain. Often, it is bilateral.

Etiology: Typically idiopathic. However, rule out other causes, such as trauma, infection, and inflammation.

Pathology: Softening, fraying and fibrillation of patellar cartilage.

Clinical presentation: These patients present with knee pain, especially while keeping the knee bent for a long time (in the classroom, watching a movie—cinema theater sign), climbing stairs, squatting or sitting cross-legged.

Examination reveals
- Tenderness over the patellar facet.
- Crepitus may be present, and deep flexion is painful.
- *Clarke's test is positive:* In a supine patient, the clinician presses the patella in the trochlear groove, while patient is asked to contract their quadriceps. A painful test indicates chondromalacia.

Diagnosis: X-rays are normal. MRI may show cartilage fibrillation, while arthroscopy is diagnostic **(Figs. 46.31A and B)**.

Treatment: Most patients are managed conservatively by activity modification, physiotherapy, and analgesics. Usually, it is a self-limiting condition of six months to a few years. Rarely, arthroscopic debridement of frayed cartilage is required.

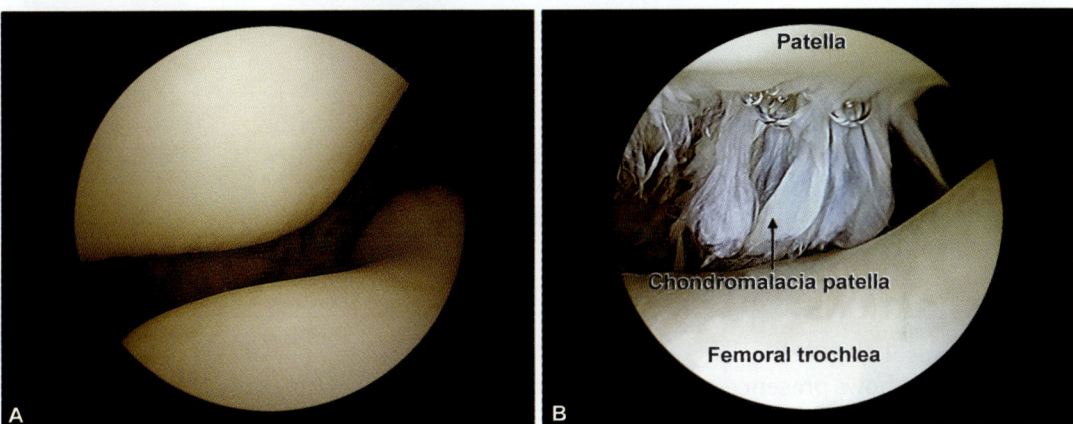

Figs. 46.31A and B: (A) Arthroscopic view of normal patella cartilage (from superolateral portal); (B) Arthroscopic view of cartilage fibrillation in chondromalacia.

PLANTAR FASCIITIS

DEFINITION

It is a painful condition of foot due to chronic degeneration of plantar fascia over the insertion of medial calcaneal tuberosity.

ETIOPATHOGENESIS

- **Training errors** in athletes, *shoes with inadequate support*.
- **Occupations with prolonged standing:** Factory workers, teachers, soldiers, etc.
- **Certain types of activities that place a lot of *stress on heel*:** Long-distance running, ballistic jumping activities, ballet, and aerobics.
- **Obesity:** Extra stress.

- **Structural risk factors:** Pes planus, pes cavus, leg-length discrepancy.
- **Functional risk factors:** Tightness of Hamstring, gastrocnemius—soleus, weakness of the intrinsic foot muscles.
- **Aging and heel fat pad atrophy**.

CLINICAL FEATURES

It is common in people who are in age group of 40s to 60s.

Symptoms

Pain: *Typically sharp, stabbing pain starts over the bottom of the heel when patient takes initial few steps after a period of rest*, e.g., right after getting up in morning or after a period of sitting. It worsens by bearing weight on the heel. Further, the pain improves after taking few steps!

Signs

- Tender medial tuberosity of calcaneus and the medial arch of the foot **(Fig. 46.32)**
- Windlass test: Passive dorsiflexion of toes might reproduce the pain
- Limited ankle dorsiflexion due to tightness of calf muscles or Achilles tendon.
- Look for deformities such as flat-foot, pes cavus, leg-length discrepancy, excessive external tibial torsion, and excessive femoral anteversion.

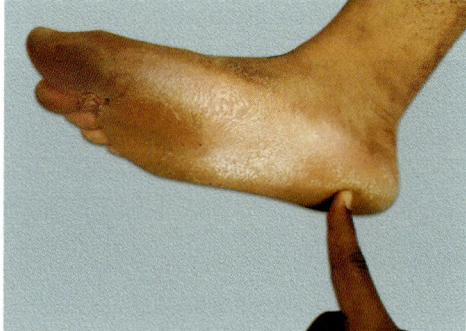

Fig. 46.32: Plantar fasciitis tenderness spot over medial calcaneal tuberosity.

INVESTIGATIONS

Mostly, a clinical diagnosis.
- **X-ray** often shows presence of a spur at undersurface of calcaneum. However, it may not be responsible for symptoms.
- **MRI of the heel and foot:** Mostly performed to rule out other pathologies.
- **Serum investigations:** Rule out diabetes mellitus, hyperuricemia, hypothyroidism.

TREATMENT

Almost all cases respond to conservative treatment, while a very few.
- **Conservative treatment:**
  - Weight reduction.
  - ***Contrast foot bath:*** Heel is subjected to alternate hot and cold therapy by immersing the heel alternatively in hot and cold water.
  - ***Physiotherapy:*** Calf and toe muscle strengthening and stretching exercises.
  - ***Pain relief:*** Analgesics, local anti-inflammatory gel.
  - ***Orthotics:*** Arch supports with excavated heel. Heel inserts/cups may also be tried.
  - ***Night splints*** that passively stretch the calf muscles and the plantar fascia while sleeping.
  - ***Local corticosteroid/platelet-rich plasma injections***
  - ***Extracorporeal shockwave therapy***.

- **Correction of metabolic factors**, such as high uric acid, diabetes mellitus, and hypothyroid.
- **Operative:** If conservative treatment fails >8–12 months
  - Open plantar fascial debridement and release at medial calcaneal tuberosity
  - Percutaneous radiofrequency (coblation) microdebridement of plantar fascia at attachment over medial calcaneal tuberosity.

MORTON'S NEUROMA

It is an *interdigital neuroma commonly found between the 3rd and 4th metatarsal heads*, causing pain in the forefoot. It is common in adults, especially females (female:male 9:1), who prefer to wear shoes with a narrow toebox.

Pathology: Neuroma results from constant compression or repeated microtrauma over the interdigital nerve, resulting in perineural fibrosis **(Fig. 46.33)**.

Clinical presentation: Patients present with pain in the plantar aspect of the forefoot, which worsens during weight-bearing and wearing narrow toebox shoes.

Examination: There is tenderness over the 3rd interdigital space over the plantar aspect. Webspace squeeze test is positive, and causes pain and tingling. *Mulder's click* may be felt while squeezing metatarsals.

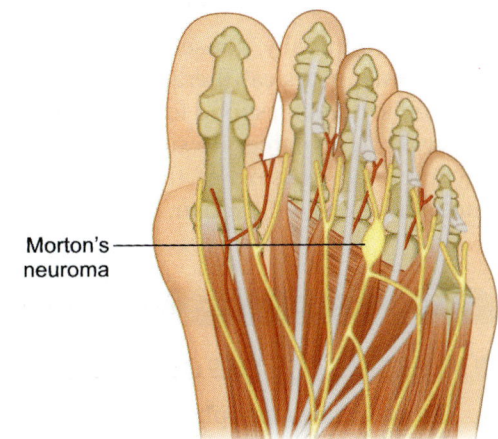

Fig. 46.33: Morton's neuroma.

Diagnosis: It is essentially a clinical diagnosis. The presence of neuroma can be confirmed with USG or MRI of the foot.

Treatment: Conservative treatment involves a wider toebox shoe, avoiding heels, and local steroid injection. If still symptomatic—surgical excision of the neuroma is warranted.

RETROCALCANEAL BURSITIS (HUMP-BUMP/HAGLUND'S DEFORMITY)

It is a condition in adults that presents with heel pain wherein there is inflammation and swelling of the retrocalcaneal bursa resulting in a painful swelling at the back of the heel **(Fig. 46.34)**.

Etiopathology: It may be idiopathic or secondary to an inflammatory condition. There is inflammation of the retrocalcaneal bursa (bursitis), located between the Achilles tendon and the calcaneus. Further, a calcaneal spur grows into the substance of the tendoachilles (TA). In severe cases, there can be a partial or total tear of TA.

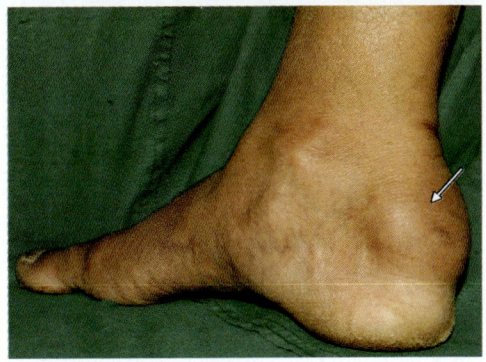

Fig. 46.34: Haglund's bump (arrow).

Clinical presentation: The patient complains of a prominent swelling at the back of the heel and "back of the heel" pain when taking a few steps or walking after rest.

Note: *The pain in plantar fasciitis subsides after taking a few steps, whereas the pain of retrocalcaneal bursitis usually does not subside while walking. Moreover, plantar fasciitis pain is felt under the heel, whereas retrocalcaneal bursitis pain is over the back of the heel.*

Examination: There is a swelling over the posterior aspect of the calcaneum, which is tender on palpation.

Investigations: X-ray of the heel shows a bump at the back of the calcaneum and a spur **(Fig. 46.35)**. USG or MRI of the heel is performed to assess tendinopathy and tears of the tendoachilles.

Treatment: Initially, conservative treatment is tried with NSAID, physical therapy and shoe heel raise. Those who do not respond to conservative therapy or one with TA tears require surgical treatment, which encompasses excision of the retrocalcaneal bursa and bony spur +/– TA repair.

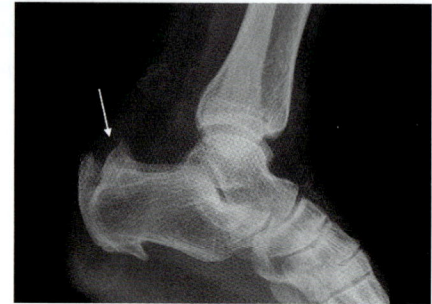

Fig. 46.35: Retrocalcaneal spur growing in tendoachilles tendon (arrow).

VARIOUS TOE DEFORMITIES

TYPES OF TOE DEFORMITIES

- **Claw toe:** Metatarsophalangeal (MTP) hyperextension and proximal interphalangeal (PIP), distal interphalangeal (DIP) flexion
- **Hammer toe:** Proximal interphalangeal flexion, DIP extension, MTP (neutral/extended)
- **Mallet toe:** Hyperflexion of DIP
- **Hallux valgus:** Great toe deviates in valgus
- **Hallux rigidus:** The great toe MTP cannot be extended/dorsiflexed
- **Turf toe:** Hyperextension injury to plantar plate and sesamoid complex of the hallux MTP joint.

VARIOUS BURSITIS

Name	Bursa involved
Shoulder	Subacromial (most common site)
Student's elbow	Olecranon
Weaver's bottom	Ischial tuberosity
Housemaid's knee	Prepatellar
Clergyman's knee	Infrapatellar
Pes anserinus	Medial side of the knee
Retrocalcaneal	Achilles tendon

SECTION 14

Miscellaneous Topics

SECTION OUTLINE

47. Common Procedural Skills
48. Overview of Common Orthopaedic Procedures
49. Overview of Physiotherapy
50. Basics of Imaging in Orthopaedics

14

Miscellaneous Topics

CHAPTER 47

Common Procedural Skills

CASTS IN ORTHOPAEDICS

■ PLASTER OF PARIS CAST

No object is as strongly associated with orthopaedic surgeons as plaster of Paris. It is more colloquially known as POP. *It is made from gypsum*, a naturally occurring material. The name POP is said to stem from an accident involving a house in Paris built over the deposit of gypsum. Accidentally, the place got burnt down. Many people walked over the charred remains of the house and floors with gypsum powder. When rain fell over the floor, footprints in the mud set rock-hard. This led to the discovery of gypsum hardening properties. Chemically, POP is calcium sulphate hemihydrate ($CaSO_4$, $½H_2O$). POP is prepared by heating gypsum ($CaSO_4$, $2H_2O$).

$$CaSO; 2H_1O + heat \rightarrow CaSO, 1/2H_1O + 3/2H_1O \text{ (released as steam)}$$

When water is added, the original material (gypsum: $CaSO_4$, $2H_2O$) is reformed, and heat is released. The idea of incorporating POP in bandages was incepted by Mathijesen and Nikolai Ivanovich Pirogov in 1852, and ever since, it has been an orthopaedic staple **(Fig. 47.1)**. The pros and cons of POP are mentioned in **Table 47.1**.

■ SYNTHETIC CAST

Currently, synthetic cast is also available, which is made up of *fiberglass impregnated with polyurethane polymer*. This substance undergoes polymerization and becomes rigid after

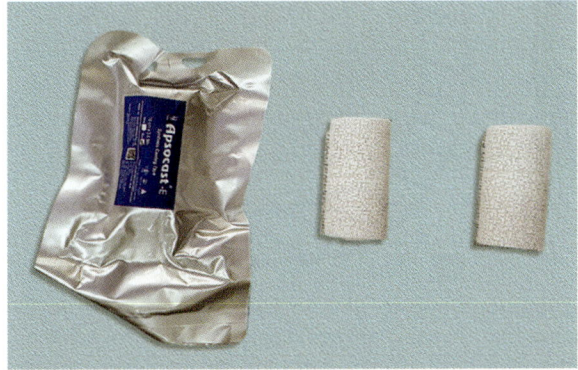

Fig. 47.1: Plaster of Paris bandage and synthetic plaster (wrapped).

Table 47.1: Advantages and disadvantages of POP material.

Advantages	Disadvantages
▪ Cheap ▪ Easily available ▪ Easily moldable and excellent contour of limb can be obtained ▪ Easy to cut with a sharp knife or hand held saw	▪ Heavy ▪ Not very strong, it can be broken ▪ Not waterproof—disintegrates if in contact with water

Table 47.2: Advantages and disadvantages of synthetic cast.

Advantages of synthetic cast	Disadvantages of synthetic cast
Light	Costly
Strong, cannot be broken easily	Not moldable easily, and therefore not used as reduction material
Surface of cast is waterproof	Not easy to cut—need an electric saw

exposure to air/the addition of water. The synthetic cast is lighter and stronger than POP, more expensive and not easily moldable **(Fig. 47.1)**. The pros and cons of the synthetic cast are mentioned in **Table 47.2**.

POP or its analogous materials are used as a **slab (or splint)** or a **cast**. A slab is a non-circumferential construct of the plaster, which *supports the limb on 2/3rd of the limb circumference* and is secured to the limb with wet gauze bandages **(Figs. 47.2A and 47.3A)**, whereas a *cast circumferentially encases the affected part* with POP or synthetic bandages **(Figs. 47.2B and 47.3B)**.

A slab is applied when the limb is swollen, or it is anticipated in due course of treatment as it allows the expansion of the swelling as 1/3rd circumference is covered with mere bandages. And therefore, the chance of developing a compartment syndrome is less in a slab. Slab is also applied if there are blisters on the skin, which need repeated removal of slab to observe the condition of skin and blisters. *(Note: Blisters indicate poor circulation to skin and precompartment like situation)*. In contrast, cast is applied when the swelling has subsided and there is no risk of compartment syndrome and skin does not require repeated observation. Therefore, while considering whether to apply a splint or a cast, one must assess:
- The stage and severity of the injury
- Swelling of the affected limb
- The risk of complications and
- The patient's functional requirements.

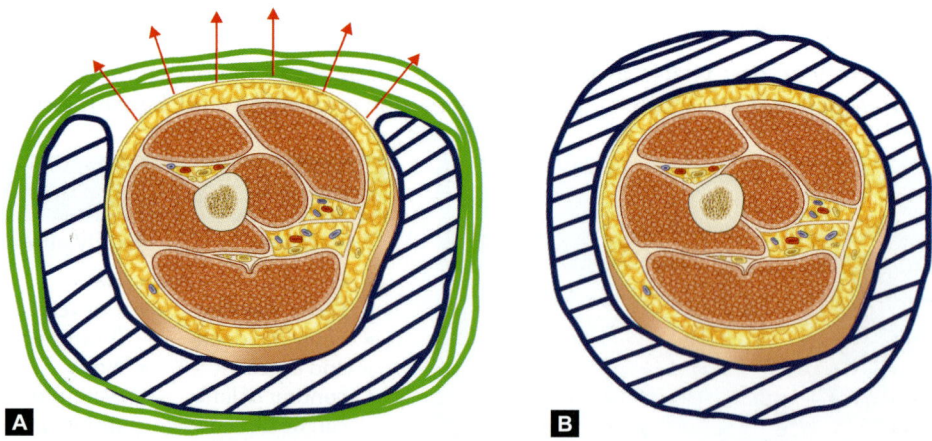

Figs. 47.2A and B: SLAB and cast on the limb: (A) SLAB on the limb. Blue hashed area represents SLAB, whereas green encircling lines represent gauge bandages. The red arrows represent room for swelling expansion through the bandage; (B) CAST on the limb. Blue hashed lines all around the limb depict a cast. *Note*—there is no room for swelling expansion, if any, in the cast.

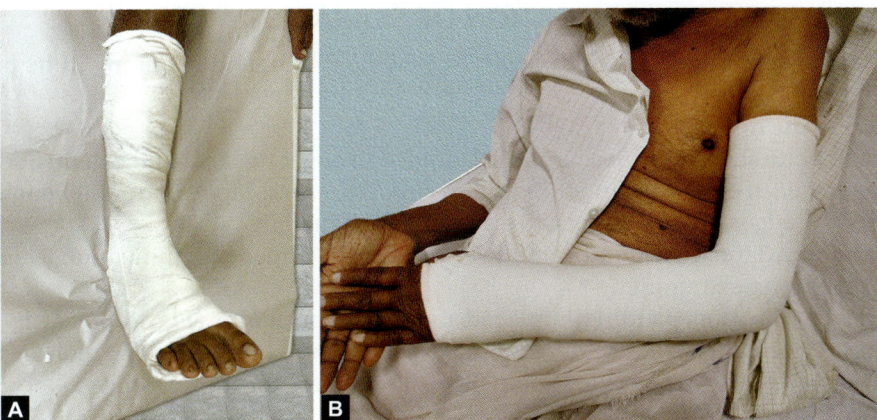

Figs. 47.3A and B: (A) Below knee slab; (B) Above elbow cast.

In general, slab is more widely used in primary care for acute injuries, whereas cast is usually reserved for definitive management of injuries.

Table 47.3 enumerates the difference between the slab and cast.

Table 47.3: Differences between the slab and cast.		
	Slab	**Cast**
Circumference of the limb encircled	2/3rd of the limb	Completely encircles the limb
Strength	Not strong, can break due to limb weight and joint movement	Stronger than slab, and possibility of breakage is less
Fracture retention	It cannot be used to retain a reduced fracture, as reduction can slip due to slab loosening or breakage or poor hold on the limb	It is used to retain fracture reduction
Chance of compartment syndrome	Nearly nil as it allows expansion over 1/3rd area, which is merely covered with cotton and bandage (Fig. 47.2A)	High, especially if it is tight. It does not allow any room of expansion due to circumferential plaster of Paris bandage (Fig. 47.2B)

■ RULES OF APPLICATION OF PLASTER

- Choose the correct size—generally, 4-inch padding and plaster roll are used for the upper and 6-inch for the lower extremities.
- A joint above and below should ideally be included to eliminate movements of the joints on either side of the fractures to avoid fracture displacement.
- No wrinkles should be present over cotton padding.
- Plaster should be moulded with the palm, not fingers, to avoid pressure points.
- The incorporated joints should be immobilized in a functional position.
- The plaster should be snugly fit and not too tight or loose.
- Maintain uniform thickness of the plaster.
- Avoid movement till the plaster sets/dries.

GENERAL STEPS OF APPLICATION OF SLAB/CAST

- Casting and splinting (slab) both begin by placing the injured extremity in its functional position.
- **Preparing the limb:**
    - Stockinette should be measured and applied to cover the area and extend about 10 cm beyond each end of the intended splint site. The excess stockinette will be folded back over the edges of the slab/cast to form a padded margin.
    - Generally, 3 inches wide stockinette is used for the upper extremities and 5 inches wide for the lower extremities.
    - A layer of cotton padding is placed over the stockinette **(Fig. 47.4)**. It is wrapped circumferentially around the extremity; each new layer should overlap the previous layer by 50%. Extra padding should be ensured over bony prominences.
- **Preparing the plaster:**
    - *For slab:* After measurement of desired length, sheets of plaster are layered over each other (8–10 layers for the upper limb, 12–16 layers for the lower limb), creating a slab **(Fig. 47.5)**.
    - *For cast:* The required size and number of plaster rolls should be kept handy before initiating the procedure.
- The prepared plasters should be dipped in cool to tepid water. Cold water will slow the setting process, whereas hot water can hasten the setting of POP.
- **Slab:** After wetting the prepared POP slab, place it over the desired surface of prepared limb, and gently mould it to conform it correctly and smoothen it out. Do not press or pinch it, as this could create a pressure area. Secure the wet slab with gauze bandages, ensuring no constrictions.
- **Cast:** Appropriate-sized plaster rolls should be applied circumferentially over the affected limb; each new layer should overlap half of the previous layer. The cast should be moulded layer by layer.
- Turn back the stockinette if used, catching it in the last layer of bandage. Be careful not to pull the casting bandage back with the stockinette, as this will create a crease at the edge.
- Maintain the limb in the desired functional position until it sets.
- Finally, assess the pulse and the capillary refill time of the extremity. Clean the POP stains from the body.
- The drying time is between 24–48 hours, depending on thickness.

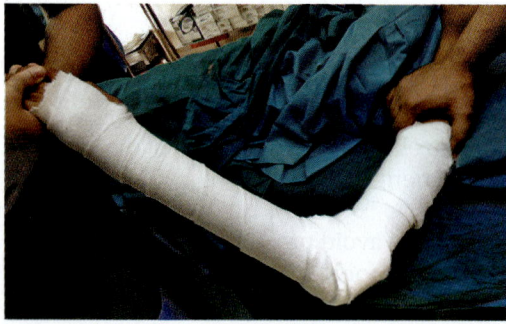

Fig. 47.4: Stockinette followed by compressed cotton over the upper limb.

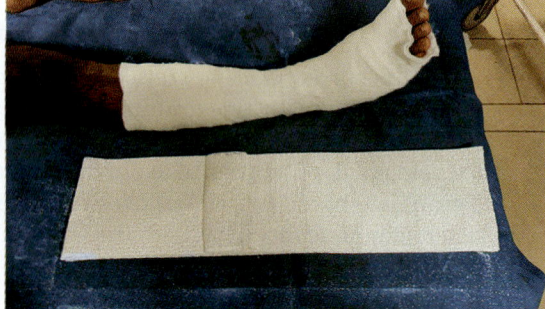

Fig. 47.5: Layers of POP kept ready for slab.

ORTHOPAEDIC USE OF CAST

- To support reduced fracture and dislocation till the fracture and soft tissues heal.
- To correct a deformity, such as CTEV.
- To retain a reduced joint, such as developmental dysplasia of hip.
- To stabilize and rest joints in case of soft tissue injury (ankle sprain, ligament injury, etc.)
- For postoperative immobilization to rest tissues.

INSTRUCTIONS AFTER CAST APPLICATION

- Limb must be kept elevated to avoid swelling.
- Active mobilization of fingers/toes and other free joints must be done to avoid swelling and improve circulation.
- Watch for any bluish discoloration of finger/toes.
- Excessive tightness at any point/area should be informed to the healthcare worker. It may require a release of plaster to avoid necrosis of underlying tissues. Further, increasing pain or painful passive stretch of finger/toes must be reported immediately, as it may indicate pre-compartment syndrome. In such a case, the plaster must be released/opened immediately up to the skin.
- Treat inability to pass stool or vomiting after hip spica as an emergency. Persistent vomiting after hip spica application could be due to spica syndrome.

COMPLICATIONS OF CAST APPLICATION

- **Compartment syndrome** is a disastrous complication, especially if a tight cast is applied. If compartment syndrome is suspected, the cast should be immediately split till the skin and should be removed. Immediate pain relief is a sign that the compartment pressures are normalizing. *Note that a tight cast is the most common cause of compartment syndrome.*
- **Nerve compression** at tight bony points could result in nerve palsy.
- **Skin ulceration:** Usually due to inadequate padding or dent in the plaster **(Figs. 47.6A and B)**.
- **Thermal injury:** Due to the heat release at the time of casting. However, it is rare.

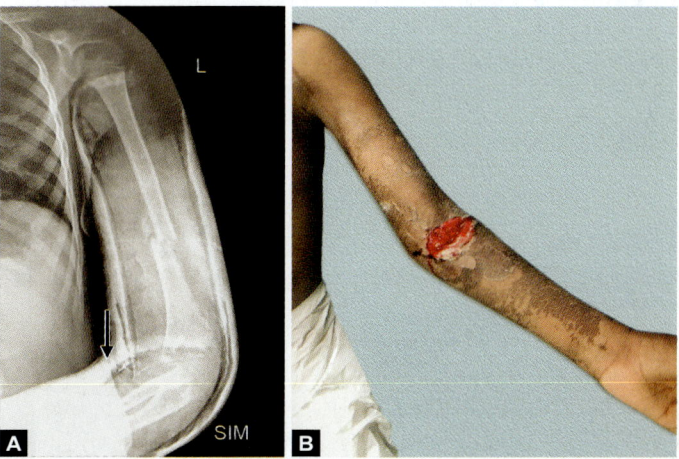

Figs. 47.6A and B: (A) POP ridge or a tight point/dent in cubital fossa (black arrow); (B) POP ridge in cubital fossa causing pressure ulcer.

COMMON CASTS/SLAB

- **Above elbow cast/slab** (*Refer* **Fig. 47.3B**):
  Proximal and distal extent:
  - *Proximal:* Upper one-third of arm
  - *Distal:* Just proximal to the metacarpophalangeal joint or proximal to the distal palmar crease.

  Indications: After the closed reduction in:
  - Both bone forearm fracture
  - Elbow dislocation.
- **Below elbow cast/slab (Fig. 47.7):**
  Proximal and distal extent:
  - *Proximal:* Upper one-third of the forearm
  - *Distal:* Just proximal to the metacarpophalangeal joint or just proximal to the distal palmar crease.

  Indications:
  - Colles' fracture
  - Smith's fracture.
- **Above knee cast/slab (Fig. 47.8A):**
  Proximal and distal extent:
  - *Proximal:* Upper one-third thigh
  - *Distal:* Just proximal to the metatarsophalangeal (MTP) joint.

  Indications: After a closed reduction in:
  - Both bone leg fracture
  - Undisplaced patella fracture.
- **Above knee cylindrical cast/slab (Fig. 47.8B):**
  Proximal and distal extent:
  - *Proximal:* Upper one-third thigh
  - *Distal:* Just above the two malleoli.

  Indication: Undisplaced patella fracture.

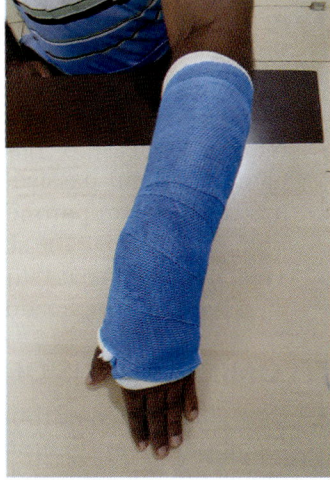

Fig. 47.7: Below elbow cast.

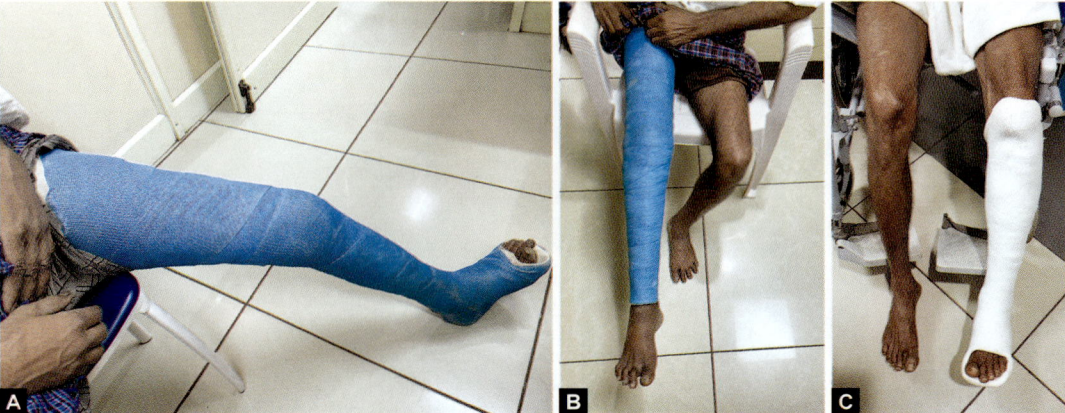

Figs. 47.8A to C: (A) Above knee cast; (B) Above knee cylindrical cast; (C) Patellar tendon bearing (PTB) cast.

Note: In patella fracture, the distal extent of the above knee cast is just above the two malleoli, also known as above knee cylindrical cast.

- **Patellar tendon bearing cast/slab (Fig. 47.8C):**
  It is a functional cast applied in fractures of the tibia after 3–4 weeks of injury to accelerate the healing. Initial 3–4 weeks, the limb remains in standard above knee cast following the closed reduction, which allows soft callus formation in a well-reduced position of the fracture. A functional cast is based on principles that 'controlled limited movements at the fracture site are good for osteogenesis.'
  The proximal and distal extent are:
  - *Proximal:* 2 inches above the tibial tuberosity
  - *Distal:* Just proximal to the metatarsophalangeal (MTP) joint.

  Indications: After a closed reduction in:
  - Both bone leg fracture.

  > **Note**
  > Functional cast can be applied in fractures of tibia-fibula, humerus and radius-ulna.

- **Below knee cast/slab (Fig. 47.9):**
  Proximal and distal extent:
  - *Proximal:* Upper one-third of the leg, four fingers below the tip of the fibula.
  - *Distal:* Just proximal to the metatarsophalangeal joint of the dorsal aspect. In some cases, the POP is extended to the tip of all toes on the plantar aspect, but the dorsum is spared till the MTP joint.

  Indications: After the closed reduction in:
  - Ankle dislocation
  - Undisplaced malleolar fracture
  - Ankle sprain
  - Soft tissue injuries of foot and ankle.

- **Hip spica (Fig. 47.10)**
  Proximal and distal extent of plaster:
  - *Proximal:* Up to nipples.
  - *Distal:* Up to the metatarsophalangeal joint on the affected side and above the knee on the unaffected side.

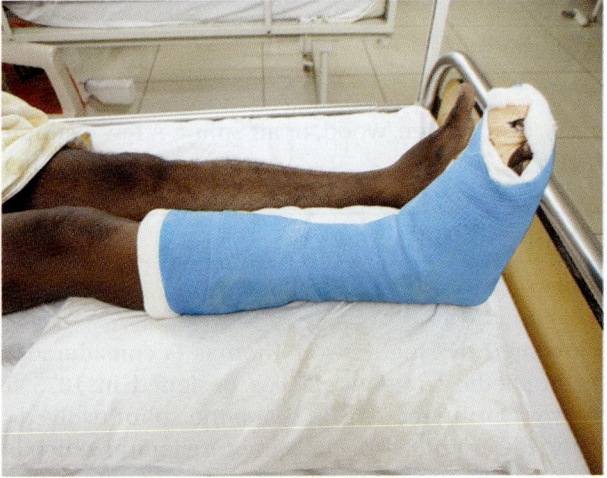

Fig. 47.9: Below knee cast.

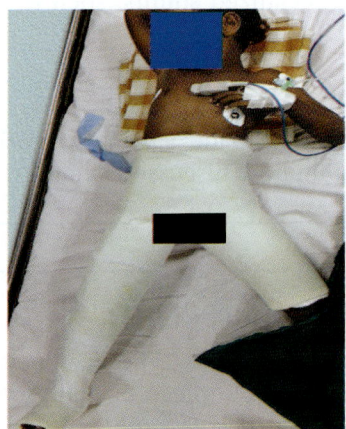

Fig. 47.10: Hip spica cast (in this image, the upper limit of the cast is only up to the lower costal margin).

The two thighs could be connected with a wooden bar to reinforce the strength of the plaster.
- Occasionally, the cast is extended just above the knee on the opposite normal side known as one and half hip spica.

Indications: After the closed reduction in:
- Pediatric femur shaft fracture
- Pediatric undisplaced fracture neck of femur
- Developmental dysplasia of the hip.

SPLINTS IN ORTHOPAEDICS

A splint is a device made of rigid material, which is used to support or immobilize an injured or painful part of the body. A splint can be:
- **Conventional**
- **Non-conventional:** Any rigid object, such as a wooden piece, umbrella, stick, etc.

FUNCTIONS OF SPLINTS

- They are used for *temporary immobilization* of injured body parts facilitating patient transport from the site of injury to the hospital and in the trauma triage. In some cases, they are used as the *definitive method* of managing a fracture/dislocation/soft tissue injuries, such as Thomas knee splint in fracture shaft femur of children or mallet splint (for mallet finger).
- It *helps control pain and prevent injury* to the soft tissues and neurovascular bundle by preventing undue movements.
- It also decreases the risk of converting a minor injury into a major injury, e.g., a closed fracture can become open due to the spike of fracture piercing through the soft tissue due to excessive movement.
- Several splints, such as the Thomas knee and Bohler Braun can also help in traction to the injured limb.
- Specialized splints, such as Dennis Brown splint, cock splint, etc., are used in special cases.

SPLINT MATERIAL

It could be made of plaster of Paris, fiberglass, iron, plastic, wood, or air splint. A few examples of splints are discussed below.

LOWER LIMB SPLINT

THOMAS SPLINT

Thomas splint or "Thomas knee splint" invented by Hugh Owen Thomas is considered an indispensable piece of equipment for orthopaedic surgeons. It was designed in 1875 for *immobilizing knees inflicted with tuberculosis*. During the World Wars, the splint evolved to immobilize and treat trauma sustained to the lower limb, especially fracture femur, which led to a dramatic decrease in mortality due to hemorrhagic shock and fat embolism. Since then, Thomas splint has been an invaluable splint in the management of the fractures shaft femur.

Parts of Thomas Splint (Fig. 47.11A)
- Padded oval metal ring
- Inner and outer sidebars, which are attached proximally to the ring
- The ring is set at an angle of 120° to the inner bar
- A slight convex bulge on the outer sidebar a few inches below the ring accommodates the convexity of the greater trochanter.
- The two sidebars distally join to form a 'W'. The 'W' can have a pulley for traction, or the traction cord is tied to the 'W'.

Measuring the Correct Size of Thomas Splint
Two components of the Thomas splint must be measured—*ring diameter* and *length*.
1. **Ring diameter:** Measure the oblique thigh circumference immediately below the gluteal fold and ischial tuberosity, equal to the padded ring's internal circumference.
   In cases where measurement from the affected side is difficult due to pain, one should measure the diameter of the thigh at maximum girth and add 5 cm to accommodate for swelling.
2. **Length of the splint:** Measure the distance from the crotch to the heel, which should equal the inner bar and add 15–23 cm/6–9". This additional 6–9" is to accommodate the traction cord and spreader.

Thomas knee splint is NOT side specific. It can be used for either side.

Indication
All femur shaft fractures (adult and pediatric population).

How to Apply Thomas Knee Splint
Padding of the TK splint: Multiple 6-inch cotton gauze bandages are spread between the two arms of the TK splint as fashion slings to create a base where the limb can be supported. Over the base of bandages, cotton is kept to make it adequately padded **(Fig. 47.11B)**.

Application of traction to the limb: Apply traction (skin or skeletal) to the leg. The TK splint is applied to the injured limb by passing the limb through the ring space. The limb is gently pulled down, so the ring snugly fits over the groin, below anterior superior iliac spine (ASIS) and ischial tuberosity. While maintaining the traction, the traction cord is either tied to the 'W' (fixed traction) or passed over a pulley on 'W' and weights are tied to the end of the cord (balanced traction). While applying the traction, *the inner traction cord must come from under the bar, whereas the outer traction cord must come above the bar to control traction and rotation of the limb* **(Fig. 47.11C)**. Once the TK splint is applied on the limb, it must be placed over the bed in slight flexion and abduction at the hip.

Complications
- *Pressure sores:* The common areas at risk are the perineum, groin, ischial tuberosity, Achilles tendon (from the edge of gauge bandage), and over the lateral malleolus.
- *Common peroneal nerve palsy*, especially if the leg remains externally rotated and the fibular neck comes too close to the outer bar of the TK splint.
- *Difficult perineal care, bed sore.*

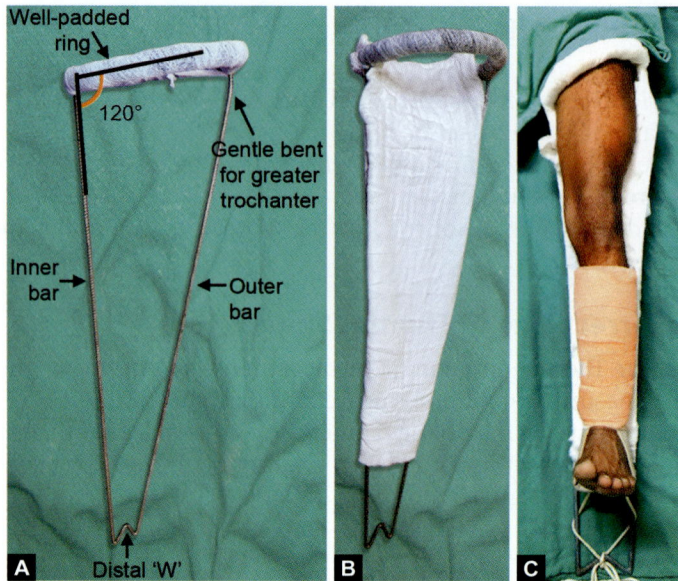

Figs. 47.11A to C: Thomas knee splint. (A) Parts of Thomas splint; (B) Well-padded splint; (C) Thomas splint applied on limb.
(*Courtesy:* Dr Abhishek Agarwal, KGMC, Lucknow)

LISTON'S LONG LEG SPLINT

Liston's long (LL) leg splint is a prefabricated radiolucent splint **(Fig. 47.12A)**. This splint is applied to the lower limb from the pelvis up to the ankle joint **(Fig. 47.12B)**. It can be either flexible or rigid. In the case of a rigid wooden splint, it must be well-padded with cotton and a bandage before applying on to the limb.

Indications

It is used for femur fracture or fracture around the knee joint.

POSTERIOR LEG SPLINT

It is a prefabricated radiolucent splint, either flexible or rigid. It is applied to the posterior aspect of the thigh spanning the knee and the ankle joint **(Figs. 47.13A and B)**.

Indications

- Fractures of the tibia or around the knee joint.
- Soft tissue injuries to the leg, ankle and foot.

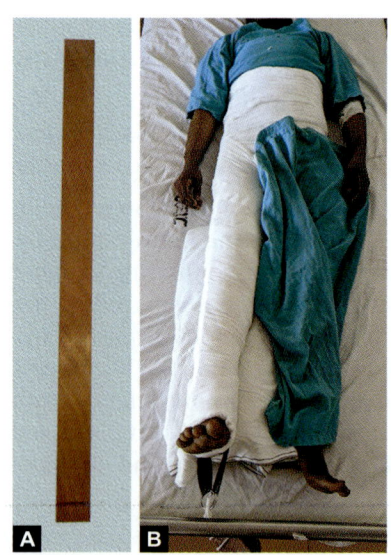

Figs. 47.12A and B: (A) Liston's long splint; (B) LL splint applied from hip to the ankle.
(*Courtesy:* Dr Abhishek Agarwal, KGMC, Lucknow)

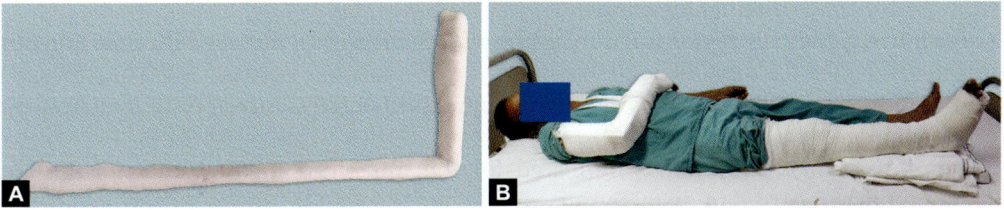

Figs. 47.13A and B: (A) Posterior leg (PL) splint; (B) PL splint applied on the right lower limb.
(*Courtesy:* Dr Abhishek Agarwal, KGMC, Lucknow)

CRAMER WIRE

It comprises two thick parallel wires, with ladder-like thinner wires arranged between them **(Fig. 47.14)**. It is malleable and can be contoured to the limb. The disadvantage of Cramer wire is that it does not sustain a rigid immobilization and casts a radio-opaque shadow in radiographs.

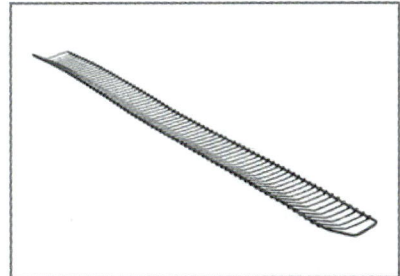

Fig. 47.14: Cramer wire splint.

BOHLER BRAUN SPLINT

It is a common splint used for immobilization in the ward, especially for the fractures around the knee (distal femur and proximal tibia fractures), femur and tibia shaft fractures **(Fig. 47.15A)**.

It is used in conjunction with skeletal traction **(Fig. 47.15B)** and sometimes skin traction. It consists of an iron frame, a bent for the knee and three or four pulleys. The bent for the knee aims to relax gastrocnemius and hamstring muscles, which tend to pull distal femur and proximal tibia # fragments posteriorly, causing injury to the neurovascular bundle. Furthermore, a relaxed muscle helps align the proximal and distal fragments of the fracture. The bent also allows correct direction for the femoral traction via pulleys, and also acts as counter for traction in tibia or calcaneum.

Three pulleys are for traction, and the fourth is to prevent foot drop. Some Bohler frames have only three pulleys.

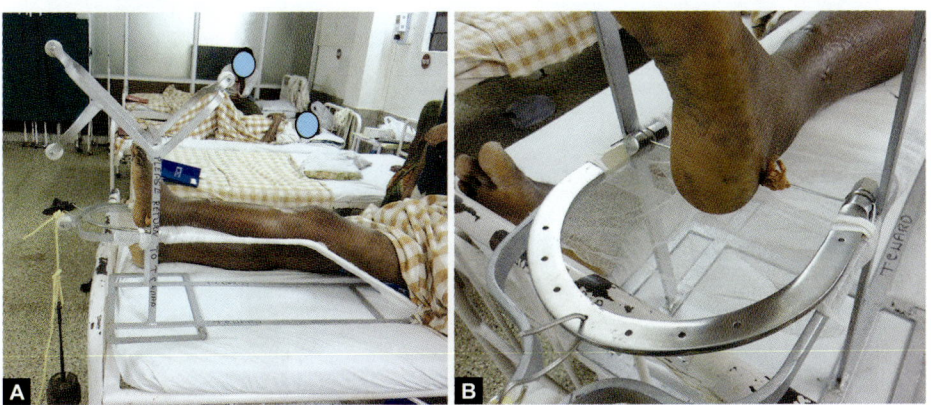

Figs. 47.15A and B: (A) Bohler Braun splint showing bent for the knee, four pulleys and calcaneal traction; (B) Skeletal traction (through calcaneum).

The four pulleys have distinct functions:
1. **Lowermost pulley:** Provides traction in line with the leg. They are used for tibia and fibular injuries.
2. **2nd pulley from bottom:** It is used for supracondylar fracture femur. Traction pin is inserted in proximal tibia.
3. **3rd pulley from bottom:** It is indicated for the mid-third fracture shaft of the femur. Traction pin is inserted in distal femur.
4. **Proximal pulley (directed towards the patient):** It is used to prevent foot drop.

UPPER LIMB SPLINT

LONG ARM POSTERIOR SPLINT

It is applied from the back of the arm up to the wrist and hand.

Indication

Fractures of the humerus shaft, both bones, forearm fracture, and distal radius fracture.

LATERAL ELBOW SPLINT

It is applied on the side of the arm up to the wrist and hand **(Figs. 47.16A and B)**.

Indication

Fractures of the distal humerus, both bones, forearm fracture, and distal radius fracture.

THUMB SPICA SPLINT

It is used to immobilize the thumb. It extends from the nail bed of the thumb to the distal forearm **(Fig. 47.17)**.

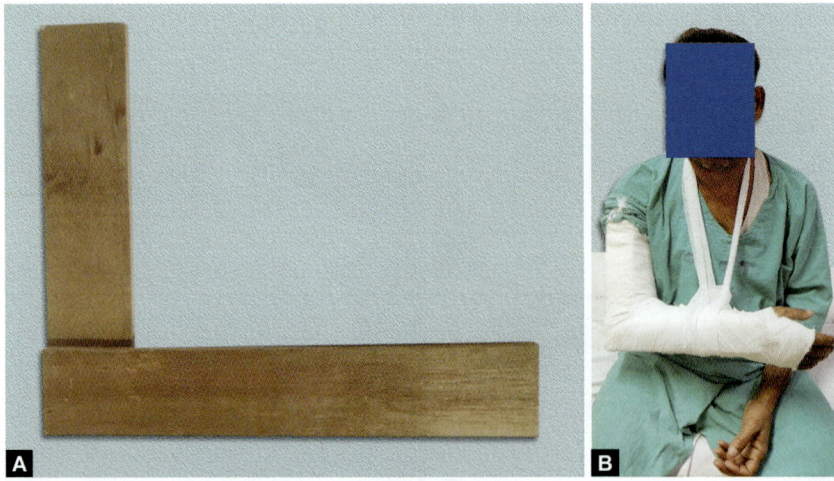

Figs. 47.16A and B: (A) Lateral elbow splint; (B) Lateral elbow splint applied from arm to the wrist.
(*Courtesy:* Dr Abhishek Agarwal, KGMC, Lucknow)

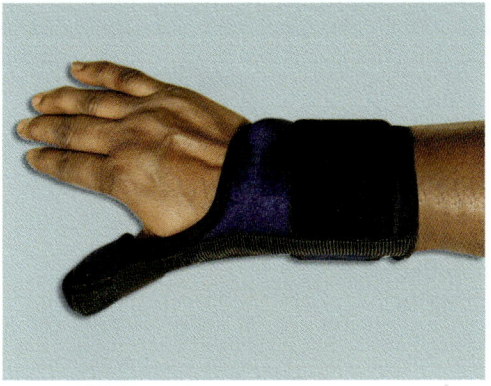
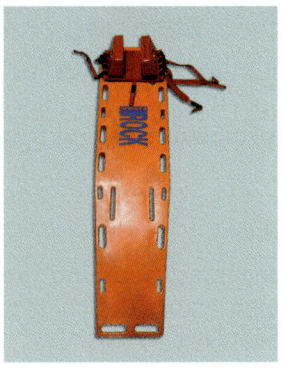
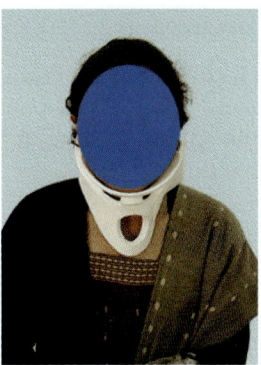

Fig. 47.17: Thumb spica splint.

Fig. 47.18: Spine board with neck support.

Fig. 47.19: Philadelphia collar.

Indications

- Scaphoid fracture
- Gamekeepers's thumb
- First metacarpal fractures.

SPINE

■ SPINE BOARD

It is a rigid board used as a "splint" for suspected or confirmed spine injury **(Fig. 47.18)**. The spine board is always used with head supports, straps, and a hard cervical collar to secure the patient.

■ PHILADELPHIA COLLAR

It is used in cervical spine injury, which encircles the neck and encompasses the chin and posterior head **(Fig. 47.19)**. It prevents movement by supporting the mandible and the occiput. It is made up of two parts—anterior and posterior shell. The anterior part had a hole which aids in tracheostomy (if indicated).

Care of a Patient on a Splint

- Always ensure adequate padding for bony points.
- Regularly check the neurovascular status of the limb once the splint is applied—*color, temperature, capillary filling, sensation and movements.*
- Regularly check the firmness of bandages on the limb to ensure that the splint adequately supports the limb.
- Mobilization of the free joints must be encouraged.
- Adequate perineal care in case of lower limb splints.
- Watch out for deep vein thrombosis, bed sore.

STRAPPINGS

Historically, several common strappings or styles of bandaging have been applied to various injuries around the shoulder, such as Velpeau bandage and figure of eight bandage.

■ VELPEAU BANDAGE

It is a bandage applied for injuries around the shoulder, wherein the arm is strapped across the chest resulting in minimal shoulder movement **(Fig. 47.20)**.

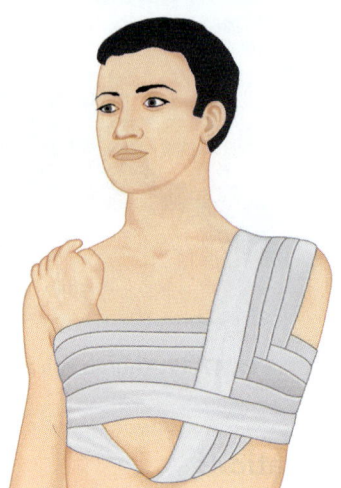

Fig. 47.20: Velpeau bandage.

Technique

A 4–6" broad and 20–30 feet length bandage is required to apply a Velpeau strapping.
- The injured arm-forearm is placed across the chest, and the hand is placed over the normal shoulder's acromion. The turn of the bandage starts from the normal opposite axilla, over the shoulder, in front of the injured arm, and beneath the elbow to pass again to the normal axilla **(Fig. 47.21A)**.
- This step is repeated several times to have multiple diagonal turns, which overlap the injured side clavicle and the arm **(Fig. 47.21B)**.
- It is completed by numerous transverse turns wrist encircling the chest and covering the forearm **(Fig. 47.21C)**.

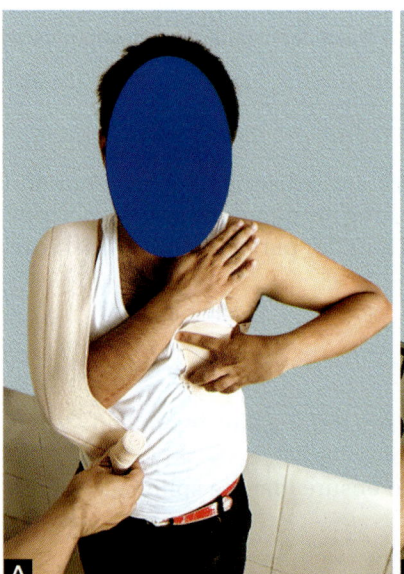 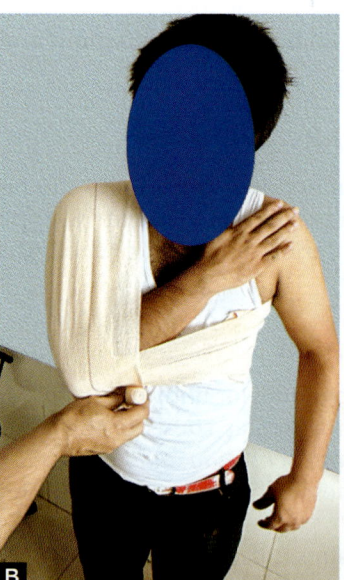 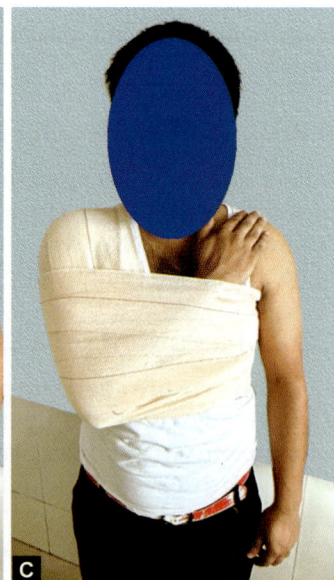

Figs. 47.21A to C: Velpeau bandage application.

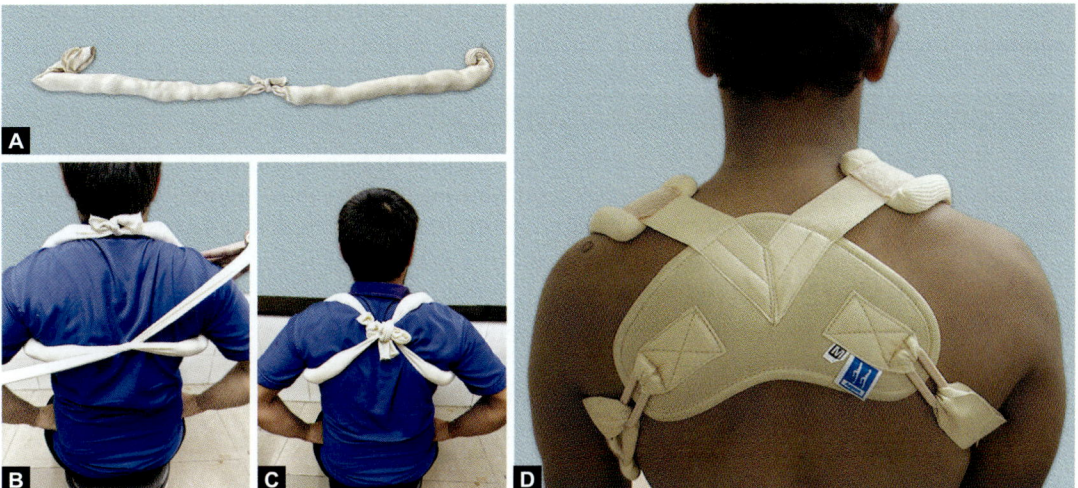

Figs. 47.22A to D: (A to C) show figure of '8' bandage application; (D) Commercially available clavicular brace in situ.

FIGURE OF EIGHT BANDAGE

It is described for the conservative management of the midshaft clavicle fracture. Currently, commercial designs of the figure of '8' bandage are also available.

Technique

The patient should be made to sit on a stool chair with both hands over the waist, and both shoulders must be pushed down and backwards (shoulders retracted) with the spine in extension.
- Examine both shoulders and axilla for any open wounds or bruises. Rule out any neurovascular injury of the upper limbs.
- A 4-6" broad tubigrip or stockinette is taken, which should be long enough to be encircled around both shoulders to be tied at the back between the two scapulae. The stockinette and stuffed with cotton **(Fig. 47.22A)**.
- The center of the stuffed stockinette or tubigrip is placed behind the neck, and both free ends are pulled under the respective axilla to be brought between the two scapulae and tied together **(Fig. 47.22B)**.
- One can also pad the axilla with cotton to avoid the loop getting soggy with sweat. Then, the tied end and loop behind the neck are also connected, giving a figure of '8' appearance **(Fig. 47.22C)**. **Figure 47.22D** shows a commercial clavicle brace in place.

Aftercare

Always check the neurovascular status of both upper limbs by palpating pulses and sensorimotor examination.

Problems after Figure of '8' Bandage

The bandage keeps becoming loose and needs frequent tightening or reapplication, which may defeat the 'immobilization.' The loop part of the bandage in the axilla can cause chafing, discomfort and rarely axillary vein thrombosis. It also gets soiled due to axillary sweat, which can invite infection.

TRACTION

Traction is a pulling method, which is exerted on the part of bones and joints. It is applied to the limb/part distal to the fracture to exert a continuous pull in the long axis of the bone to restore alignment of a fracture through gradual neutralization of muscular forces.

OBJECTIVE OF TRACTION

- Maintenance of fracture reduction or a reduced joint
- Immobilize painful and swollen joint
- Reduce or relieve pain as gradual traction reduces muscle spasm
- Prevent or correct joint deformity.

PRINCIPLES OF TRACTION

- Traction must produce a pulling effect on the affected part
- Traction must be balanced with an opposite counter traction
- The cord/rope for traction must freely move over the pulleys
- The weights used for traction must hang freely.
- The traction (weight) must be gradually increased in increments.

TYPES OF TRACTION

- Skin traction **(Fig. 47.23A)**
- Skeletal traction **(Fig. 47.23B)**
- Manual traction (and countertraction). It is applied over limbs during the fracture or dislocation reduction.

METHODS OF TRACTION

- **Fixed traction:** The traction is applied by pulling the cords which is tied on to the splint, while the counter traction applied by the splint hitching against a part of the body. For example, the Thomas splint hitches against ASIS and ischial tuberosity **(Fig. 47.24)**.

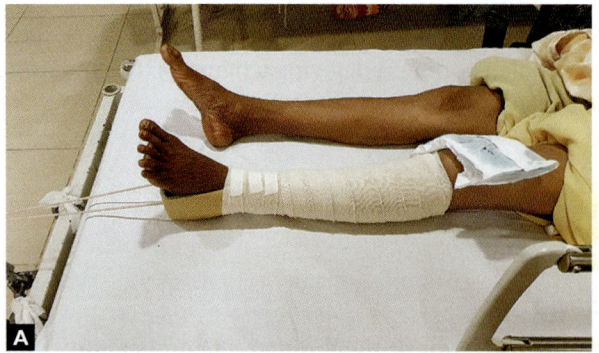 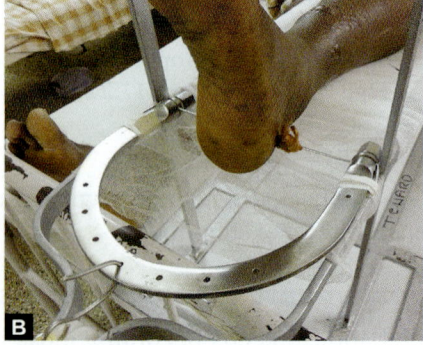

Figs. 47.23A and B: (A) Below knee skin traction; (B) Skeletal traction (through calcaneum).

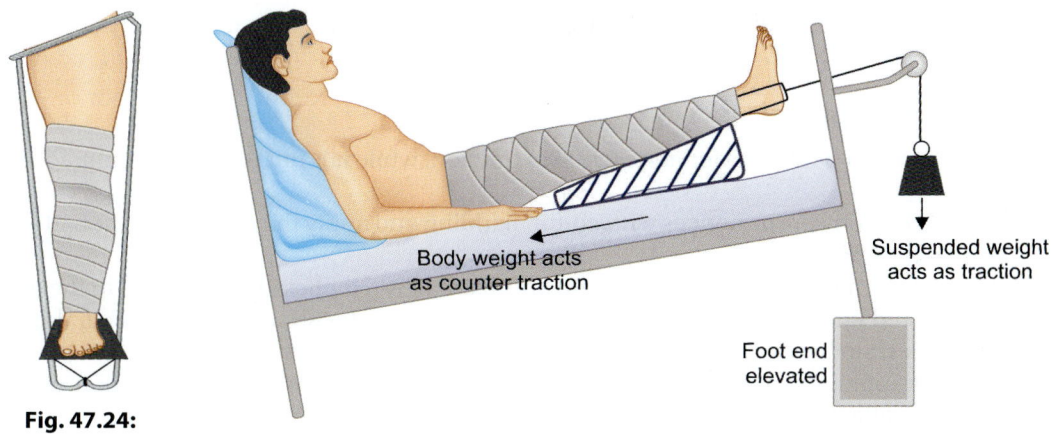

Fig. 47.24: Fixed traction.

Fig. 47.25: Sliding traction.

- **Sliding traction:** The traction is applied by weights hanging freely while counter traction is applied by the weight of the body when the foot end of the bed is elevated **(Fig. 47.25)**.

SKIN TRACTION

In a skin traction, the traction force is applied over a large area of skin, which spreads the load uniformly over the applied area. The biggest advantage is that it is non-invasive and can be easily applied even by paramedics or nurses. Generally, the weight used is 5 lb. The maximum traction weight that can be tolerated by skin traction is **15 lb (6.7 kg)**, or less than 10% of the body weight.

Methods of Applying Skin Traction

There are two types of skin tractions—adhesive and nonadhesive. While the side pads of the former get adhered to the skin as the pad surface has a coat of adhesive materials, the latter is secured to the skin with crepe bandages.
1. **Adhesive skin traction:** In this system, the side pads applied over the side of the limb are made of zinc oxide tapes or other, which directly adhere to the skin. Over the zinc oxide tapes, cotton and bandage are applied to further secure it over the limbs. It does not slip easily and can tolerate more weight. However, the adhesive material can be allergenic and cause itching or skin peeling.
2. **Nonadhesive skin traction:** In this system, the nonadhesive traction pads are applied over the side of the limb **(Fig. 47.26)** and secured with a crepe bandage. Nonadhesive tractions

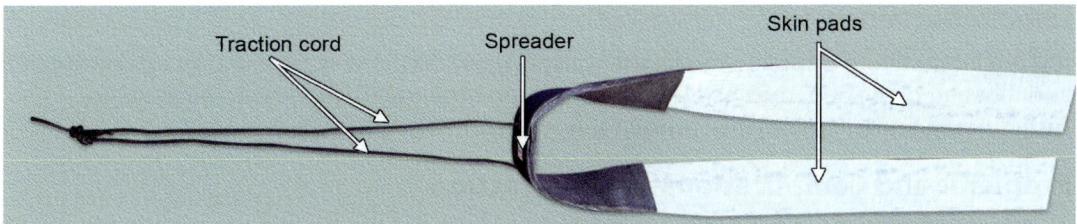

Fig. 47.26: Nonadhesive skin traction.

are easy to apply, and there is no risk of skin allergy. However, it can slip easily and cannot tolerate more weight.

Method of Application
- The limb must be shaved for adhesive skin traction, while it is not required for nonadhesive ones.
- Protect the bony prominences with cotton padding and apply the adhesive or nonadhesive strip to the affected limb.
- Ensure that the spreader should extend approximately 6 inches (15 cm) distal to the end of the affected limb. It is essential to ensure that the spreader should be parallel to the heel. The extra strap beyond the foot should appear like a loose stirrup.
- Apply strapping (generally crepe bandage) over the skin pads to secure traction over the limb, and attach the required weight. Elevate the foot end for counter traction.

Examples of Skin Traction

Above-Knee Skin Traction
The above-knee skin traction is applied mid-thigh up to the ankle using a commercial above-knee traction kit/custom-made materials **(Fig. 47.27)**.

The above-knee skin traction is applied from mid-thigh up to the ankle using a commercial above-knee traction kit/custom-made materials. The maximum skin traction, which can be applied, is 6.7 kg (approximately 8–10% of body weight).

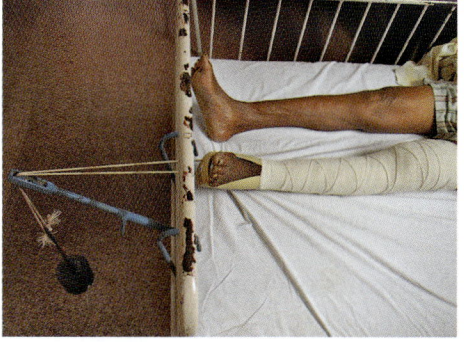

Fig. 47.27: Above-knee skin traction.

Indications
- To relieve pain and spasm from hip pain arising out of synovitis, arthritis of the hip or fracture neck femur/intertrochanteric femur.
- To prevent or correct hip deformity (tuberculosis).

Cervical Traction
It is a "skin traction" applied around the neck, also known as Glisson's or Halter traction **(Fig. 47.28)**. A maximum weight of 1.4 to 2.3 kg is applied and the head end of the bed should be raised to provide counter traction.
Indication: Cervical spondylitis, cervical intervertebral disc prolapse.

Lumbar Traction
It is a "skin traction" applied around the waist **(Fig. 47.29)**. A weight of 4–6 kg can be applied and foot end of the bed must be elevated for counter traction (by the body weight).
Indication: Lumbar spondylitis, lumbar intervertebral disc prolapse.

Problems and Complications of Skin Traction
- A large traction force cannot be applied over the skin. A limited force can be applied and therefore, major deformities are difficult to correct.

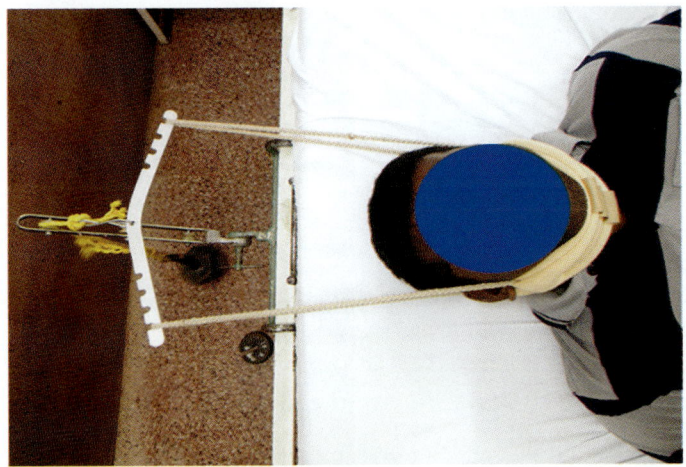

Fig. 47.28: Cervical or Glisson's traction.

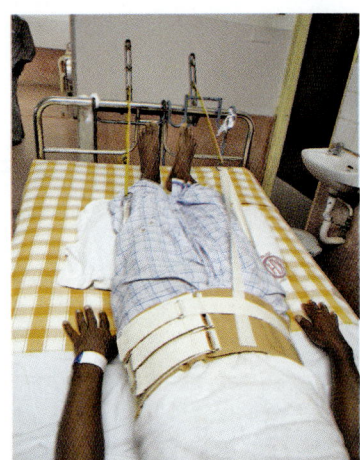

Fig. 47.29: Lumbar traction.

- It cannot be tolerated for long time. It keeps on slipping, which can lead to loss of fracture reduction and therefore, it needs regular reapplication.
- Damage to the skin either due to traction material or force, resulting in blisters or skin peel off.
- Deep vein thrombosis.
- Distal part edema due to compression bandage.

Contraindication of Skin Traction
- Presence of wounds, skin disease
- Vascular injury to the limb, which is under observation.

SKELETAL TRACTION
Traction force is applied directly to the skeleton by a metal pin or a wire inserted through a bone. It is used in cases where *heavy traction is required up to 20% of the body weight* (for example, fractures of the lower limb), or in cases where skin traction is contraindicated.

Advantages of Skeletal Traction
- It can tolerate large loads up to 20% of the body weight. Therefore, large traction can be applied which is essential for maintenance of reduction of long bone fracture in adults.
- It can be applied for long duration and in the limbs with soft tissue injury or skin lesion.

Pins and Wires Used in Skeletal Traction
Commonly used pins or wires for skeletal traction in the limb are the Steinmann pin, Denham pin, and Kirschner (K) wire **(Figs. 47.30A to C)**.
- ***Steinmann pin*** is rigid stainless-steel pin of varying lengths and diameters. It is pointed at one end while the other end is blunt **(Fig. 47.30A)**. After insertion of the Steinmann pin, Bohler stirrup is attached to the pin **(Fig. 47.30D)**. Bohler stirrup allows the direction of the traction to be varied without turning the pin in the bone.

Section 14: Miscellaneous Topics

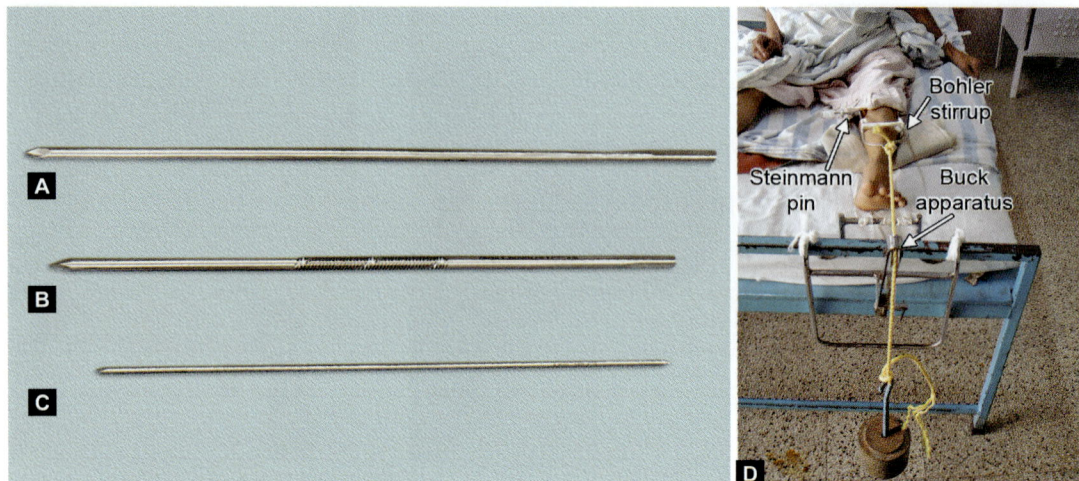

Figs. 47.30A to D: (A) Steinmann pin; (B) Denham pin; (C) K-wire; (D) Upper tibial skeletal traction with Bohler stirrup on Bucks apparatus.

- ***Denham pin*** is similar to the Steinmann pin but has a short raised threaded portion in the middle **(Fig. 47.30B)**, which engages the bony cortex and reduces the risk of pin sliding. It is useful in cancellous bones or osteoporotic bones.
- ***Kirschner (K) wire*** is a flexible stainless steel wire with a small diameter **(Fig. 47.30C)** and is pointed at both ends. They are insufficiently rigid until pulled taut in a special stirrup. The wire may easily cut out through bone if a heavy weight is applied. Therefore, to avoid bending and cutout of a K-wire, it needs to be tensioned for traction.

Site of Skeletal Traction

- ***Lower limb sites:*** Proximal femur (in trochanter), distal femur, proximal tibia and calcaneum
- ***Upper limb sites:*** 2nd, 3rd metacarpal and olecranon
- ***Skull.***

Examples of Skeletal Traction

Upper Tibial Skeletal Traction

- **Indications:** Femur fracture, reduced hip dislocation for maintenance of reduction.
- **Implants** used for upper tibial traction are the Steinmann pin and Denham pin.
- **Site for upper tibial traction:** The pin is inserted 2 cm below and 2 cm posterior to the highest point of the tibial tuberosity **(Fig. 47.31)**. The pin is inserted from the lateral cortex of the tibia to the medial side to avoid injury to the common peroneal nerve.

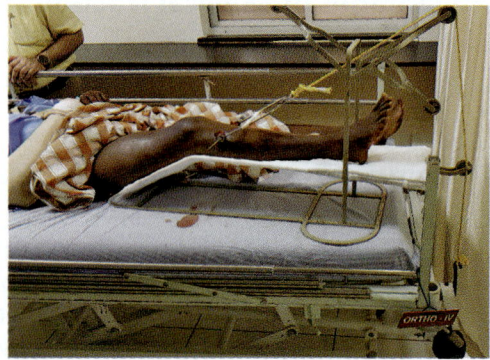

Fig. 47.31: Upper tibial skeletal traction.

- **Risk of upper tibial traction:** Injury to the common peroneal nerve during insertion of Steinmann pin.

Calcaneal Traction

- **Indications:** Tibia fracture
- **Implants** used for calcaneal traction is either Denham pin or K-wire tensioned traction **(Fig. 47.32)**.
- **Site for calcaneum traction:** The pin is inserted 1 cm below and 1 cm posterior to the medial malleolus. The pin is inserted from the medial side of the calcaneum.
- **Risk of calcaneum traction:** Injury to medial neurovascular bundle (tibial nerve, posterior tibial artery).

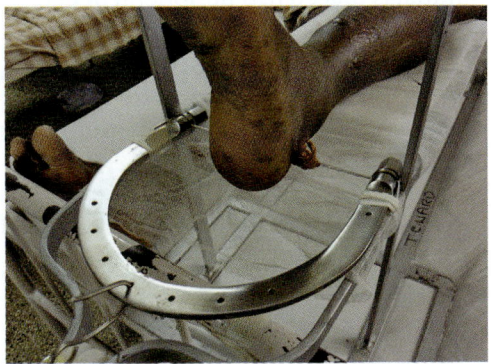

Fig. 47.32: Calcaneal K-wire tensioned skeletal traction.

Skull Traction

- **Indication:** Conservative management of cervical spine fracture/reduced dislocation of the cervical spine for maintenance of reduction
- **Devices used:** Crutchfields tongs **(Fig. 47.33)**, Gardner-Wells tongs **(Fig. 47.34)**.

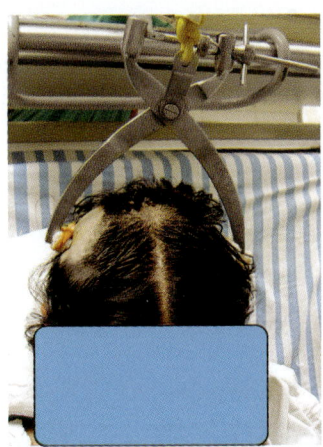

Fig. 47.33: Crutchfield skull traction.

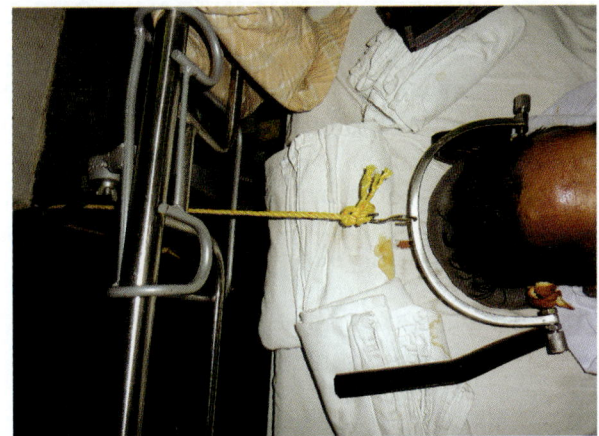

Fig. 47.34: Gardner-Wells skull traction.

Care of Skeletal Traction

The pin insertion site into the bone must be cleaned with saline every day to avoid pin tract infection.

Complications of Skeletal Traction

- Injury to the neurovascular bundle while inserting the pin
- Fracture as pin creates a point of stress riser.
- Pin tract infection. *Osteomyelitis is the most serious complication.*

INTRAVENOUS CANNULATION

Intravenous (IV) cannulation is a procedure performed by a medical specialist where a plastic cannula is placed in a peripheral or central vein.

PERIPHERAL VENOUS IV CANNULATION

Peripheral IV cannulation is performed using IV cannula in one of the peripheral veins of hand, forearm or foot.

INDICATIONS OF CANNULATION

- Fluid resuscitation of patients in trauma
- Maintenance fluids if a patient is fasting
- Administration of antibiotics
- Infusion of blood, blood products
- Before induction of anesthesia.

COMMON SITES OF INSERTION

The common sites of cannula insertion are the dorsum of the hand, ventral side of the forearm, cubital fossa, neck and foot.

PARTS AND SIZE OF THE INTRAVENOUS CANNULA

An intravenous cannula has several parts, depicted in **Figure 47.35**. The size of commercially available cannulas ranges from 24G to 14G. Smaller the number (gauge), the more the diameter of the cannula, allowing more fluid to be infused per minute.

The flow of fluid (mL/min) varies with different sizes:
- 24G cannula: 20 mL/min
- 22G cannula: 36 mL/min
- 20G cannula: 60 mL/min
- 18G cannula: 90 mL/min
- 16G cannula: 180 mL/min
- 14G cannula: 240 mL/min.

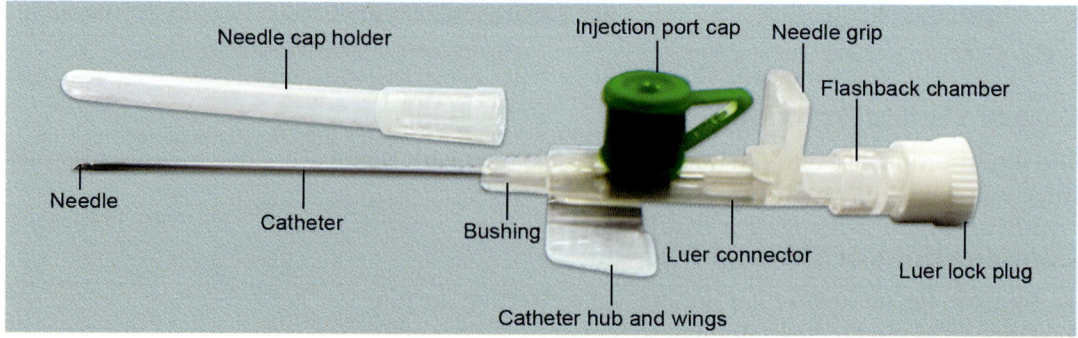

Fig. 47.35: Intravenous cannula.

CONTRAINDICATIONS OF IV CANNULATION

There are no specific contraindications per se. Peripheral lines are better avoided in places with infections, burns or any injury to that part. Irritant solutions with a high osmolarity (>600 mOsm/L), fluids with pH <5 and pH >9, chemotherapeutic agents and vasopressors are better avoided peripherally.

EQUIPMENT REQUIRED FOR IV CANNULA INSERTION

- Intravenous cannula
- Gloves
- Antiseptic solutions like 2% chlorhexidine
- Local anesthetic solution—2% lignocaine
- Intravenous fluids with tubing's attached
- Medical tapes like Durapore™.

PROCEDURE

- Peripheral intravenous cannulation is usually done in the dorsal aspect of the hand, where veins are easily accessible.
- Explain the procedure to the patient and "what and how" you will do it.
- Extend the arm you want to cannulate and support it with an arm board.
- Pronate the arm and look for any visible vein in hand with overhead light, if available.
- Place a tourniquet proximally to the site of cannulation so that there is stasis of blood peripherally and veins become easily visible.
- Clean the area of interest with 2% chlorhexidine and allow it to air dry, and tell the patient that they might feel a slight prick while you are inserting the cannula.
- Infiltrate the skin intradermally with a local anesthetic agent (0.5–1 mL of 2% lignocaine), stabilize the skin with your nondominant hand and then prick the patient with a cannula at 15–20 degrees from the skin **(Fig. 47.36A)**.
- After the skin prick, as soon as you see the backflow of blood in the flashback chamber of the cannula, take the needle (stylet) out by 1 cm.
- At this point, your cannula has just entered the lumen of the vein, decrease the angulation of the cannula and push the cannula further.

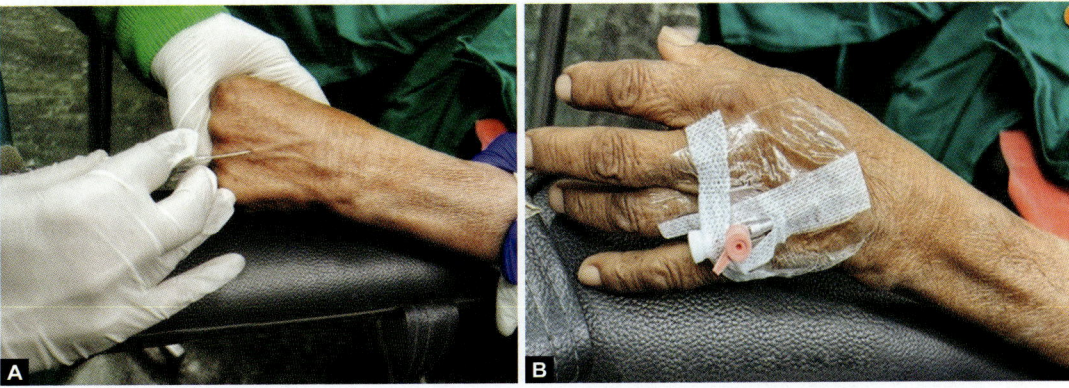

Figs. 47.36A and B: The procedure of intravenous cannulation and intravenous line in situ.

- Follow the path of the vein, holding the stylet in place.
- As soon as the entire length of the intravenous cannula is inside the vein, the stylet is removed completely, and intravenous fluid tubing can be connected to the Luer lock of the cannula.
- The cannula should be taped to the skin with a plaster to prevent dislodgment of the cannula **(Fig. 47.36B)**.

COMPLICATIONS

- Pain
- Arterial puncture
- Thrombophlebitis
- Skin and soft tissue necrosis
- Compartment syndrome.

CENTRAL LINE CANNULATION

Central line cannulation is a procedure in which a larger, centrally placed vein is cannulated using a wide-bore catheter.

The central line catheter has several advantages over peripheral IV cannulations. One, it can stay in the body longer (days to months) than a peripheral IV cannula without much risk of thrombophlebitis compared to a peripheral vein cannula. Two, the wider bore of the central line allows the transfusion of multiple fluids at the same time, including ones which are highly thrombogenic.

INDICATIONS

- When an IV infusion of antibiotics, drugs (chemotherapy) or various other fluids is required for a longer is required.
- In critically ill patients, many parenteral therapies, such as fluids, drugs and other nutrient mixtures, might need simultaneous infusion for a longer period.
- When no peripheral vein is accessible, or there is difficulty in peripheral vein cannulation (e.g., cancer patients, obese).
- For infusions of high osmolarity solutions like potassium chloride, total parenteral nutrition (TPN), which are highly thrombogenic.

SITES

- Internal jugular vein (most common site), right side is more preferred than the left side.
- Subclavian vein, right side preferred.
- Femoral vein.

Commercially, they are available as single-lumen, double-lumen and triple-lumen catheters **(Fig. 47.37)**.

PROCEDURE

- The ***most important precaution while inserting a central catheter is to maintain asepsis.***

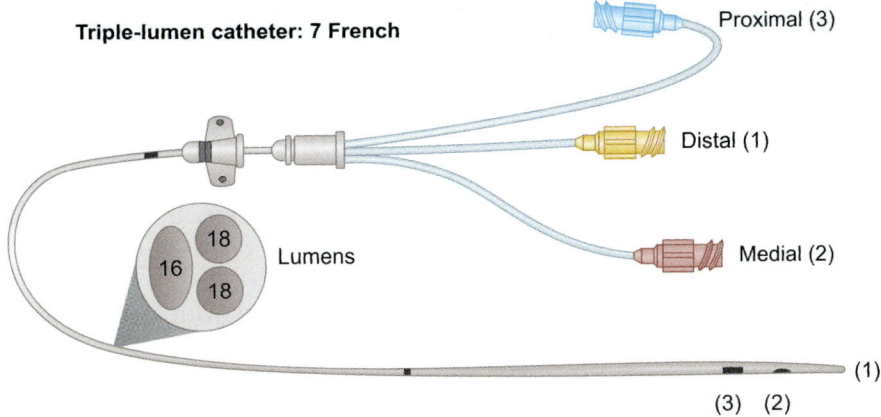

Fig. 47.37: A triple-lumen catheter, with the three infusion ports at the proximal end and their respective openings at the distal end.

- Central vein cannulation can be inserted by landmark or ultrasonography-guided technique (most safe and preferred).
- The modified Seldinger technique is used for the cannulation of central veins.
- USG probe is placed in the site of interest, such as the right side of the neck, with the patient's head turned to the opposite side.
- A 20 g needle is used to probe the vessel of interest (USG guided).
- After the needle enters the vessels, a long, thin guidewire with a flexible tip is inserted through the needle into the vessel lumen.
- The needle is removed and a catheter is advanced over the guidewire and into the blood vessel.
- Check the backflow of blood through each catheter before suturing the catheter to the skin **(Fig. 47.38)**.

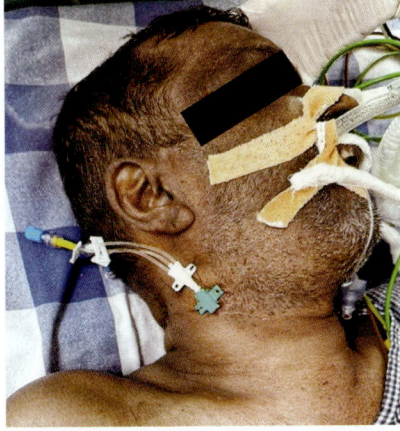

Fig. 47.38: A critically ill patient with triple lumen in-situ in the right internal jugular vein.

COMPLICATIONS

- Malposition of catheter
- Arrhythmias
- Pneumothorax
- Hemothorax
- Injury to major arteries such as carotid artery and femoral artery
- Infections
- Hematoma
- Injury to the neurovascular bundle
- Air embolism.

URINARY CATHETERIZATION

A urinary catheter is a small flexible tube that can be inserted into the bladder through the urethra, allowing urine to drain out.

INDICATIONS FOR CATHETERIZATION

It is performed when patients cannot void urine by themselves, incontinent patients, in situations where hourly urine output monitoring is a must, or when urine should not be allowed to pass via the urethra for surgical/procedure reasons.
- *Cannot void by themselves:* Unconscious patients, patients with a spine or spinal cord injury, prolonged surgery, acute urinary retention
- *Incontinent patients*
- *Urinary input-output monitoring required:* Patients with shock, renal failure
- *Injury/post-procedure:* Post-prostatectomy, urethral repairs/reconstruction, urethral injury.

CONTRAINDICATIONS FOR CATHETERIZATION

- Patients who can pass urine on their own.
- In case of injury around the pelvis (pelvis fracture), there may be blood at the tip of the urethral meatus indicating urethral injury. In such a case, catheterization should not performed and suprapubic cystostomy is preferred.

TYPES OF URINARY CATHETERS

- *Foley catheter:* For extended indwelling catheterization
- *Red rubber catheter:* For intermittent catheterization.

ITEMS REQUIRED FOR FOLEY URINARY CATHETERIZATION (FIGS. 47.39A TO C)

- *Foley catheter:* It comes in various sizes measured in French (Fr). One French equals to 0.33 mm.
- Sterile urine drainage bag—to collect and measure the output.
- 2% xylocaine jelly—water-soluble lubricant jelly
- 10 cc syringe with sterile water for the balloon
- Sterile drapes and gloves
- Sterile saline and betadine—for cleaning and sterilizing the area.

At some centers, the healthcare worker checks the balloon inflation before inserting the catheter.

CATHETERIZATION PROCEDURE

Informed consent is a must and maintain privacy during the procedure of catheterization. Explain the reason and steps of the procedure to the patient (if the patient is conscious and can understand the process and indication) or family. Always enquire about any allergies to latex.
- Catheterization is performed while the patient is supine. Put on sterile gloves
- Clean the penis or the vagina with saline first, then sterilize with betadine
- Drape the area with sterile sheets ensuring only the required area is exposed

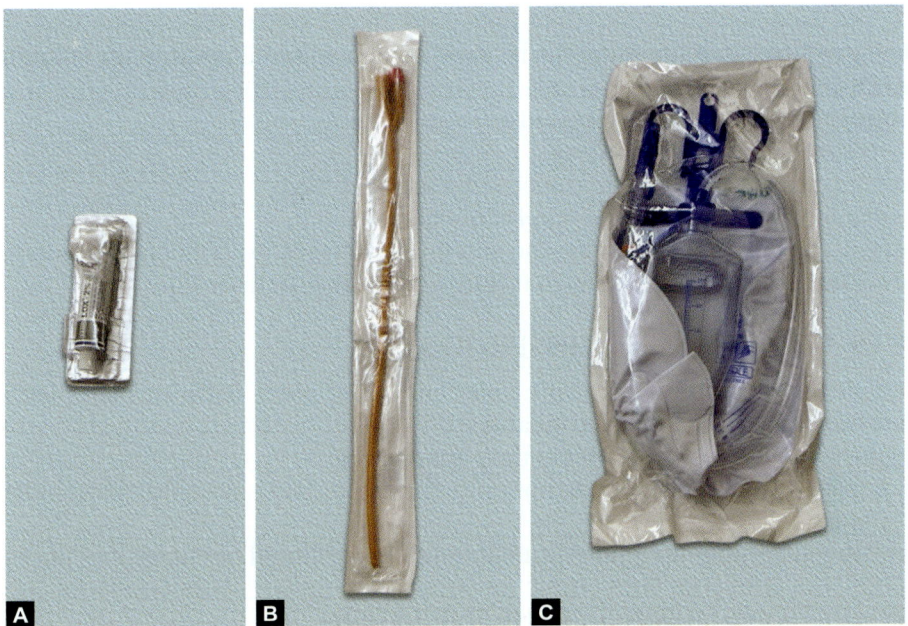

Figs. 47.39A to C: Materials required for indwelling urinary catheterization: (A) Xylocaine jelly; (B) Foley catheter; (C) Urobag.

- ***In male patients:***
    - First step is to anesthetize the urethral tract with xylocaine jelly. Gently straighten and stretch the penis to create slight traction; retract the foreskin and lift the penis at an angle of 90° to the body to straighten the urethral canal. Inject 2% xylocaine jelly into the urethra to anesthetize the tract. The process can cause a stingy sensation in the urethral tract, which must be informed to the patient. Wait for a few minutes for the urethral tract to get anesthetized.
    - Now, lubricate Foley catheter tip to atleast 6–8 cm proximal part with the 2% xylocaine jelly for easy passage of the catheter. Gently straighten and stretch the penis to create slight traction; retract the foreskin and lift the penis at an angle of 90° to the body to straighten the urethral canal. Hold the catheter and gently advance the catheter until urine begins to flow. Keep passing it till the 'Y or bifurcation' of the Foley catheter. Resistance may be encountered while passing the prostatic sphincter—utmost care should be taken not to rupture the urethra.
- ***In female patients:*** Ask the patient to breathe deeply and slowly to relax the sphincter. Slightly flex and abduct the hip and hold the labia apart to expose the urethral tip. Advance the catheter slowly until urine flows out. Keep passing it till the 'Y or bifurcation' of the Foley catheter.

▪ AFTER INSERTION OF THE CATHETER

Always ensure that urine flows out of the catheter before the balloon is inflated. An important point to note is that if the bladder is fully distended, the urine must be allowed to pass slowly into the bag to avoid sudden decompression of the bladder, which in turn may result in hematuria.

- Inflate the balloon with sterile water (generally 10 cc). Inflate the balloon while the Y of the Foley catheter is at the tip of the urethral meatus to avoid inadvertent inflation in the urethra itself
- Gently tug the catheter to see if seated securely
- Connect to the urine collection bag
- Secure the catheter to the inner aspect of the patient's thigh
- Place the drainage bag below the level of the bladder
- Document the size of the catheter, the amount of water in the balloon, the assessment of urine (clear, concentrated, bloody or turbid) and the date of insertion.

CARE OF CATHETER AFTER INSERTION

- Always clean the perineal area with soap and water twice daily and after each bowel movement, especially around the meatus.
- Avoid the use of lotions or powder in the perineal area.
- The catheter should be clamped temporarily if the urine bag is placed at a higher level than the bladder.
- For prolonged indwelling catheterization, the catheter should be changed as necessary.

COMPLICATIONS DURING CATHETERIZATION

- **Injury to the urethra** can occur due to urethral-catheter diameter mismatch or inadvertent balloon inflation resulting in urethral injury while the catheter balloon area is still in the urethral tract. *Therefore, inflate the balloon only after the bifurcation of the Foley is at the tip of the meatus.*
- **Introduction to infection:** It can occur due to unsterile techniques.

COMPLICATIONS AFTER URINARY CATHETERIZATION

- **Urinary tract infection** is quite common, especially in an indwelling catheter (Foley)
- Balloon rupture inside the bladder
- Blockage of catheter: It needs removal and insertion of a new one.

ENDOTRACHEAL INTUBATION

Endotracheal intubation is a highly skilled procedure performed by a medical specialist to secure a patient's airway. Endotracheal intubation aims to provide oxygenation and ventilation to the patient. Generally, a PVC (portex) endotracheal tube is introduced into the trachea through the mouth or nose.

INDICATIONS

- Patient ventilation during general anesthesia.
- Cardiac arrest.
- Low GCS score—if GCS is equal to or less than 8.
- Patients having a high-risk of aspiration.
- Poor respiratory drive—hypoxia, hypercarbia.
- ICU patients with critical illnesses such as pneumonia, emphysema, heart failure or coma.

CONTRAINDICATIONS

There are no absolute contraindications for tracheal intubation, but every patient should be clinically assessed before tracheal intubation. Various conditions can lead to challenging intubation scenarios, which must be kept in mind. Some of the conditions are enlisted below:
- Difficult airway—with reduced or no mouth opening.
- Laryngeal malignancy.
- Large oral malignancy, which may impede insertion of endotracheal tube.
- Trauma to the neck or orofacial bones—fracture of the maxilla and mandible.
- Co-morbidities like obesity.

EQUIPMENTS REQUIRED (FIGS. 47.40 AND 47.41)

- **Laryngoscope:** Macintosh and Miller blade for adults and children, respectively or video laryngoscopes.
- **Endotracheal tubes:**
    - *Male:* 8.0–8.5 cm ID (internal diameter)
    - *Female:* 7.0–7.5 cm ID (internal diameter)

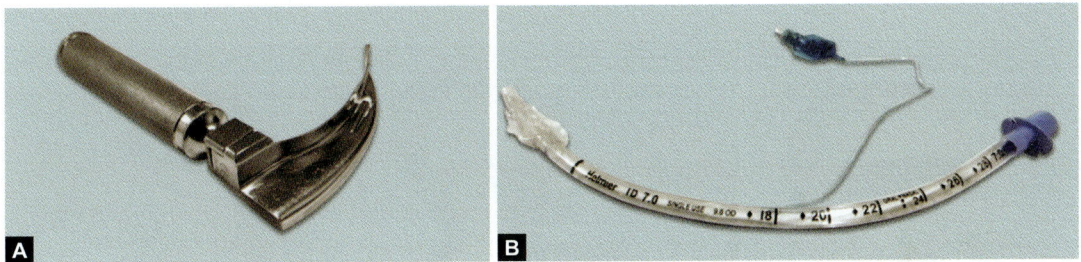

Figs. 47.40A and B: Laryngoscope with a Macintosh curved blade (A) and endotracheal tube (B).

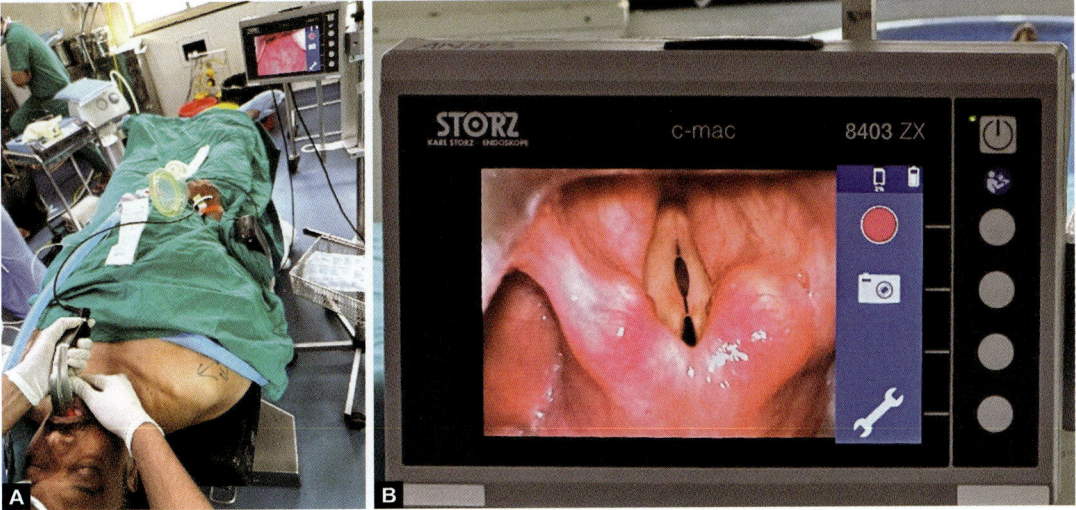

Figs. 47.41A and B: Videolaryngoscope insertion (A) to visualize the oropharyngeal structures (B).

- Intravenous cannula
- Anesthetic drugs.
- Rigid or malleable stylet and bougie.

PREREQUISITES

- Accessing the airway
  - **Rule of 1-2-3:** When a person opens his mouth, you should be able to insinuate **1-finger** in the temporomandibular joint, a **2-finger** distance should prevail between upper and lower incisors, and a **3-finger** distance should be available between the mentum and the thyroid cartilage **(Fig. 47.42)**.
  - **The modified Mallampati test** has four classes **(Fig. 47.43)**. Class I is present when the soft palate, uvula, and pillars are visible; Class II when the soft palate and the whole uvula are visible; Class III when only the soft palate and base of the uvula are visible and Class IV soft palate not seen, only the hard palate is visible. In Mallampati Classes III and IV, a difficult airway might be anticipated.
  - **Neck movement:** Flexion and **extension** (most important) of the neck should be examined. Lack of extension (in cervical spondylitis, ankylosing spondylitis) could result in difficulties during intubation as neck extension is required for intubation.

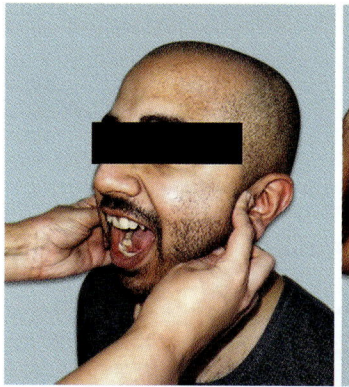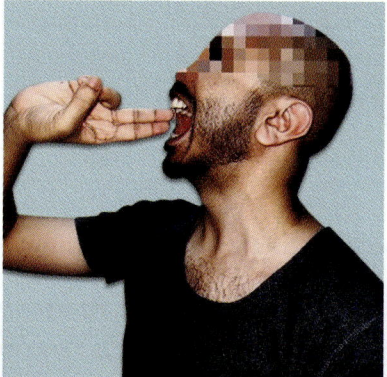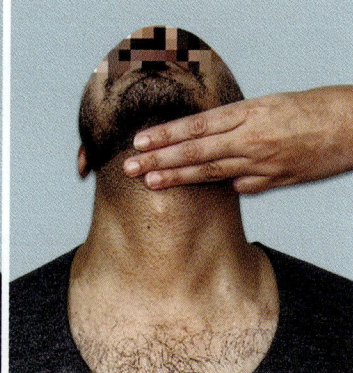

Fig 47.42: Rule of 1-2-3.

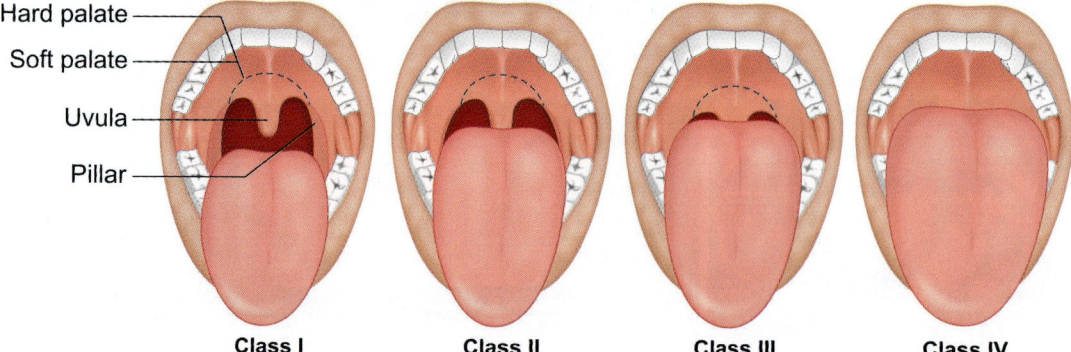

Fig. 47.43: Modified Mallampati test for adequacy of airway.

- There should be a working intravenous cannula on a peripheral or central vein.
- Monitors for continuous hemodynamics monitoring—5 lead ECG, pulse-oximeter, non-invasive blood pressure monitor, and $ETCO_2$.
- Working suction catheter.
- **Defibrillator:** In case of cardiac arrest scenarios.

PROCEDURE

- The patient should be supine with a pillow under the head. Oxygen should be provided continuously to the patient via a resuscitation bag or a bag and mask circuit. Every patient should be induced with anesthetic drugs (e.g., propofol, midazolam) and paralyzed with muscle relaxants (e.g., succinylcholine, vecuronium).
- Place the patient's head-neck in the "sniffing position", which is the most optimal position for endotracheal intubation, where there is an extension at the atlanto-occipital joint and flexion at the rest of the lower cervical spine. Sniffing position aligns oral-pharangeal-tracheal axis to visualize structures and facilitate intubation **(Fig. 47.44)**. To achieve the sniffing position, the head is elevated by placing it on a thick pad, which flexes the lower cervical spine followed by extension of the head (at the atlanto-occipital joint).
- The route of entry is usually through the oral or nasal route. After opening the mouth, the laryngoscope blade is introduced from the right angle of the mouth and passed along the tongue towards the epiglottis.
- After reaching the epiglottis, the tip of the blade is pressed over the vallecula, and the epiglottis is uplifted, revealing the glottic opening and the vocal cords. Once the vocal cords are seen, the endotracheal tube is passed into the trachea.
- After intubation, the pilot balloon of the endotracheal tube is inflated. Confirmation is done by bilateral (B/L) chest rise with ventilation and the 5-point chest auscultation (B/L infraclavicular and B/L mid-axillary and epigastric region).

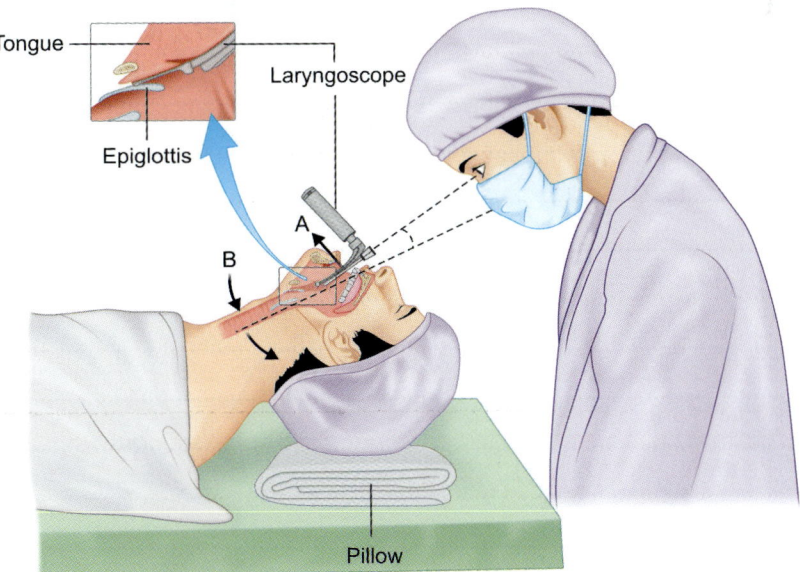

Fig. 47.44: Sniffing position during orotracheal intubation.

COMPLICATIONS

- Injury to tongue, teeth, lips, epiglottis, and arytenoids.
- Hemodynamic instability—tachycardia, hypertension, myocardial ischemia and cardiac arrest.
- Tracheal or subglottic stenosis—late complication.
- Inadvertent insertion of the tube into the esophagus.

CHAPTER 48

Overview of Common Orthopaedic Procedures

CLOSED REDUCTION, OPEN REDUCTION, INTERNAL FIXATION, EXTERNAL FIXATION

■ CLOSED AND OPEN REDUCTION, INTERNAL FIXATION

Closed and open reduction and internal fixation indicates the *technique* employed to reduce a fracture.
- **Closed reduction** means the *fracture site is not exposed* to achieve the reduction. This is similar to the basis of fracture classification—open or closed fractures—'fracture site' exposed or not to the external environment **(Fig. 48.1)**.
- **Open reduction** means the *fracture site is surgically exposed* (or opened) to achieve anatomical reduction of the fracture **(Fig. 48.2)**.
- **Internal fixation** means implants, which are used to maintain fracture reduction, are inside the body (compared to external fixators).

■ ADVANTAGES AND DISADVANTAGES OF CLOSED REDUCTION

- *Advantages:* Preserves the healing biology (fracture hematoma), smaller/no incision, less chance of infection, no or minimal scar and less pain.
- *Disadvantages:* Sometimes, it is difficult to anatomically reduce the fractures, often unsuitable for displaced intra-articular fractures, the requirement of specific traction maneuvers/distraction devices, and the use of a traction table.

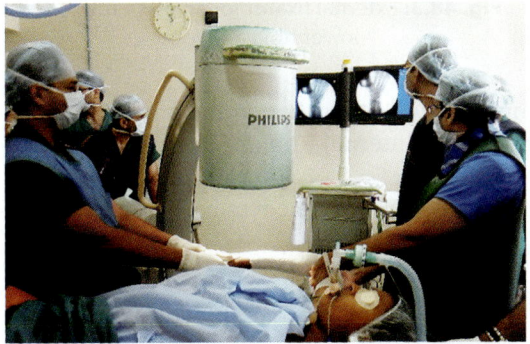

Fig. 48.1: Closed reduction of distal radius fracture by traction—countertraction and assessing the reduction using an image intensifier.

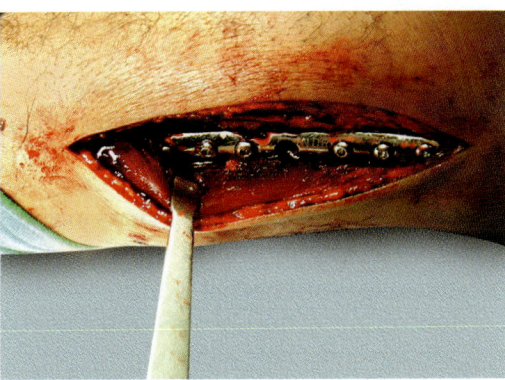

Fig. 48.2: Open reduction of fracture and plate application (internal fixation).

ADVANTAGES AND DISADVANTAGES OF OPEN REDUCTION

- ***Advantages:*** Anatomical fracture reduction is the single most important advantage of open reduction, especially in intra-articular fractures.
- ***Disadvantages:*** Loss of fracture hematoma, risk of introducing infection into the fracture site, bleeding, increased chance of adhesions between site and implant, presence of scar, and more pain is experienced in the postoperative period.

INTERNAL FIXATION

When a fracture is fixed using **'internal implants'**, which are beneath the skin and not seen from outside, it is known as internal fixation **(Fig. 48.2)**. Several examples of internal implants are intramedullary nails, plates, and screws.

Advantages of internal fixation: It provides stable fixation of the fracture.

Disadvantages of internal fixation: An internal implant can increase the possibility of osteomyelitis in the event of deep infection. Such osteomyelitis/deep infections are difficult to eradicate as biofilm can form over the plate/nail creating resistance to antibiotic therapy. In such a case, the implant needs removal, debridement and local antibiotic bead application. The fracture should then be stabilized with an external fixator.

EXTERNAL FIXATION

When a fracture is fixed using an external implant (stays above the skin), it is known as external fixation, e.g., external fixators for open fractures **(Fig. 48.3)**. Note that the reduction of fracture can be achieved either by the closed or open method. A threaded pin (Schanz pin) is passed into the bone. Generally, two pins above and below the fracture site are passed into the bone and connected by single/multiple rods to stabilize the construct, thereby providing stability to the fracture site.

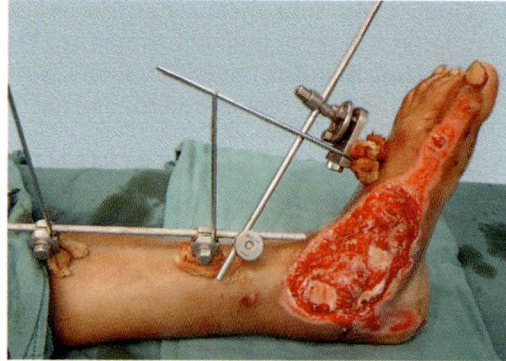

Fig. 48.3: External fixator for an open fracture of lower tibia and foot.

Advantages of external fixator:
- Quick stabilization of a fracture in open fractures.
- Ease of daily dressing of the wound.
- There is a lower chance of intramedullary bone infection other than at the fracture site, as there is no internal implant. Furthermore, absence of internal implant such as nail/plate prevents a biofilm formation.
- Later, plastic surgical procedures to cover the wound, such as flap coverage or skin grafting can be performed easily.

Disadvantages of external fixator:
- The dressing of the pin tracts must be regularly done to avoid pin tract infection.
- Cumbersome to the patient.
- Pin tract infection remains one of the key problems of the external fixator. A major pin tract infection could result in osteomyelitis.

Chapter 48: Overview of Common Orthopaedic Procedures

METHODS OF JOINT RECONSTRUCTION

If the joint surface (cartilage) is damaged due to aging, trauma, infection, or inflammation, it results in arthritis causing pain and deformity, which in turn results in difficulty in daily activities. Therefore, various procedures can be performed to provide pain relief, such as:
- **Replacement arthroplasty** is the partial or total replacement of the joint surface by a prosthesis.
- **Excision arthroplasty** is where one or both joint surfaces are excised.
- **Arthrodesis** is defined as surgical fusion of joint.
  The best form of joint reconstruction is where the surgical method achieves "painless, stable and mobile joint with the adequate power of muscles around the joint". It is possible only with joint replacement. However, in all cases of arthritis, joint replacement is not possible. **Table 48.1** outlines the difference between various methods of joint reconstruction.

Table 48.1: Differences between three methods of joint reconstruction.

	Replacement arthroplasty	Excision arthroplasty	Arthrodesis
Movement	Yes	Excess movement	No movement
Painless	Yes	Yes	Yes
Stable	Yes	Results in unstable joint	Yes
Restoration of power	Yes	Loss of power (as the lever arm is not functional)	Yes

ARTHROPLASTY

TYPES OF ARTHROPLASTY

- ***Partial replacement (Hemi Replacement):*** Only one articulating surface is replaced by a prosthesis **(Fig. 48.4)**.
- ***Complete (Total Joint Replacement):*** Both articulating surfaces are replaced by a prosthesis/implant **(Fig. 48.5)**.
- ***Excision arthroplasty:*** One or both articular surfaces are removed.

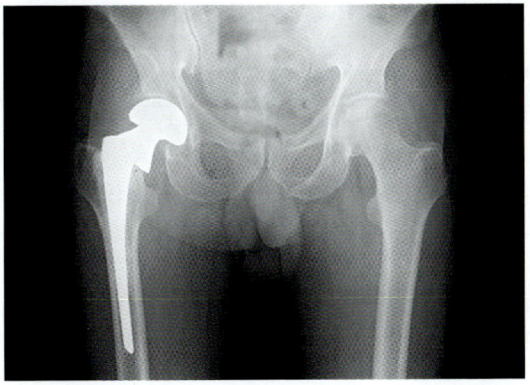

Fig. 48.4: Hemi replacement of the right hip.

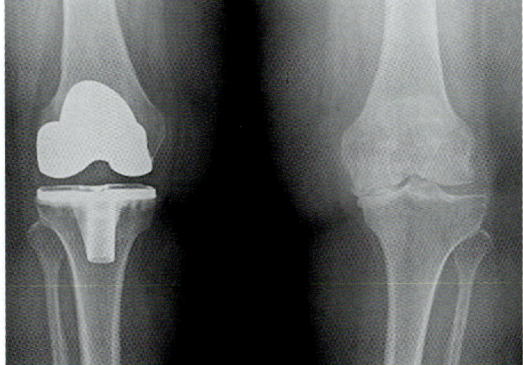

Fig. 48.5: Total knee replacement of the right knee.

Note: Classic excision arthroplasty is described for tuberculosis of the hip wherein the diseased femoral head and neck are surgically excised, known as *"Girdlestone arthroplasty."*

INDICATIONS OF REPLACEMENT ARTHROPLASTY

- **Degenerative or inflammatory arthritis** is the *most common indication for joint replacement wherein* severe cartilage destruction leads to arthritis, causing severe pain, deformity and loss of movement. A total replacement restores the patient's functional status by providing a painless, stable, and mobile joint.
- **Fracture:** Where one/both articular component is not salvageable or fixable, the joint can be replaced, e.g., fracture neck femur in the elderly (>60 years).
- **Massive rotator cuff tear with arthropathy in the shoulder:** Reverse shoulder replacement is performed wherein the convex surface (humeral head) is replaced by a cup component, whereas a ball component replaces the concave surface (glenoid).
- **Tumor prosthesis:** If one or both joint surface has to be excised during tumor resection, it can be replaced by a specialized tumor prosthesis.

CONTRAINDICATIONS OF REPLACEMENT ARTHROPLASTY

- **Infection:** The presence of active local infection or a recent history of infection in the joint is a contraindication for joint replacement. One must wait till there is no clinical or serological evidence of joint infection.
- **Charcot's arthropathy:** A joint replacement would fail due to a lack of pain and proprioceptive sensations from the joint.
- Very young age group as replacement implants in the body can last only up to 15–25 years. However, it is not an absolute contraindication. Following the failure of primary replacement, revision replacement is quite a morbid, challenging and expensive procedure.

COMPLICATIONS OF REPLACEMENT ARTHROPLASTY

- **Infection:** Most serious complication. It requires the removal of the prosthesis, debridement, antibiotic spacer application and antibiotic therapy. Once the infection is cured, joint replacement is performed as a second stage.
- **Periprosthetic fractures**
- **Dislocation of the prosthetic joint**
- **Premature prosthesis wear and loosening.**

ARTHRODESIS

DEFINITION

Permanent surgical fusion of a joint **(Fig. 48.6)**. (*c.f. Ankylosis—Pathological fusion of a joint*).

INDICATIONS

- It is an **alternative to joint replacements** for those painful joints where a replacement cannot be performed due to a lack of prosthesis/failed joint replacement where a replacement cannot be performed due to technical reasons.
- **Infected joints** when replacement is not an option.

- **Instability after muscle paralysis**. The joint involved is fused in a functional position.
- **Deformity correction**, such as Mallet toe.

ADVANTAGE
Arthrodesis results in a painless and stable joint.

DISADVANTAGES
- Arthrodesis results in loss of motion; therefore, movements cannot be performed in the said area.
- Following arthrodesis, there is excess load transfer over other neighboring and distant joints, which gradually undergo arthritic changes over the next several years. For example, an arthrodesed knee can result in arthritis of the hip and spine over the next several years.

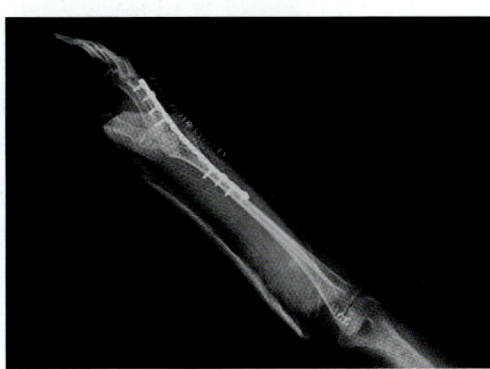

Fig. 48.6: Arthrodesis of the wrist joint using a plate.

PROCEDURE
The cartilage cover of the affected joint is denuded to expose the underlying spongy cancellous bones on either end of a joint. The two raw surfaces are fused together with the help of implants with/without additional bone grafting. **Figure 48.6** shows arthrodesis of the wrist with the plate.

POSITION OF ARTHRODESIS
Each joint is usually permanently fused in a functional position. The functional position of a joint implies that it is the most functional position of the joint, and it remains useful to perform essential functions. **Box 48.1** summarizes the functional position of various joints of the body.

> **Box 48.1:** Functional position of various joints of the body.
>
> **Shoulder:** 20° forward flexion, 20° abduction, 40° internal rotation
> **Elbow:** 90° flexion on right side to facilitate eating; 40–50° flexion on left side to facilitate perineal hygiene
> **Wrist:** 10° dorsiflexion to facilitate grip function of the hand
> **MCP joints of hand:** 90° flexion. **IP joints:** mild flexion
> **Hip:** 10–15° flexion, no adduction/abduction for easier ground clearance during walking
> **Knee:** 5–10° flexion for easier ground clearance of the limb during walking
> **Ankle:** Neutral position to facilitate plantigrade walking.

OSTEOTOMY

DEFINITION
Osteotomy implies surgically cutting a bone (creating a surgical fracture) to correct the alignment, which is required to improve function and/or cosmesis **(Fig. 48.7)**.

INDICATIONS
Varus/valgus, flexion/extension, rotational deformities of a limb or spinal deformities.

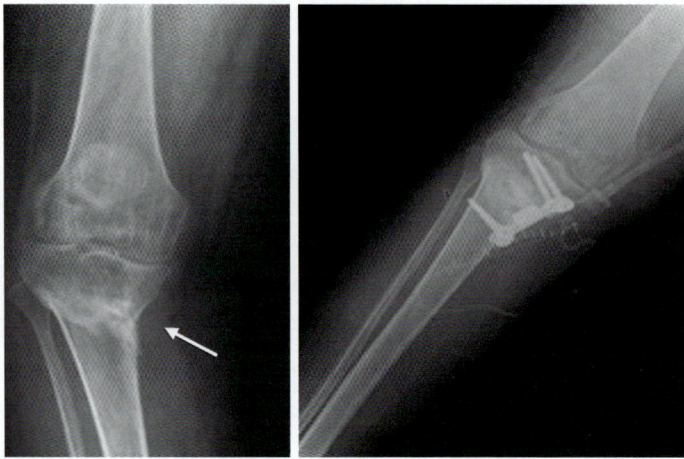

Fig. 48.7: Varus malunion of tibia corrected by high tibial osteotomy.

COMMON EXAMPLES OF OSTEOTOMY IN LIMBS

- **Upper limb:** Malunited Colles' fracture, cubitus varus after supracondylar humerus fractures.
- **Lower limb:** High tibial osteotomy in OA knee, containment varus derotation osteotomy in DDH and Perthes' disease, and corrective osteotomy for Hallux valgus deformity.

SPECIAL OSTEOTOMIES

- **French osteotomy:** Malunited supracondylar humerus (cubitus varus).
- **Pauwell's osteotomy:** Fracture of neck femur.
- **Spinal osteotomy:** Ankylosing spondylitis to correct extreme flexion of the spine.

BONE GRAFTING

Bone grafting is a procedure wherein pieces of bone are obtained (autograft/allograft) for specific indications, such as enhancing healing at the nonunion site, compensating for bone loss, or filling a tumor cavity.

INDICATIONS

- To facilitate **fracture healing**: Used in nonunion or delayed unions of fracture.
- **Void fillers**: Fill defects in bone tumors cavity after curettage or gap nonunion in fractures.
- For arthrodesis.

TYPES OF BONE GRAFT

- **Based on donor types:** Autograft, allograft, xenograft, graft substitutes (synthetic/artificial bone—hydroxyapatite, calcium sulphate), and growth factors [recombinant bone morphogenetic protein (BMPs)].
- **Based on the type of bone:** Cortical/cancellous grafts.
- **Based on vascularity:** Vascularized (with vascular pedicle)/nonvascularized.

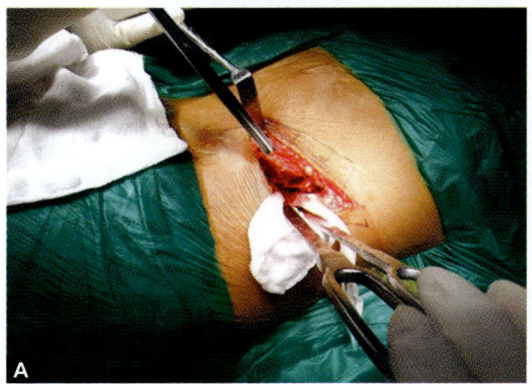 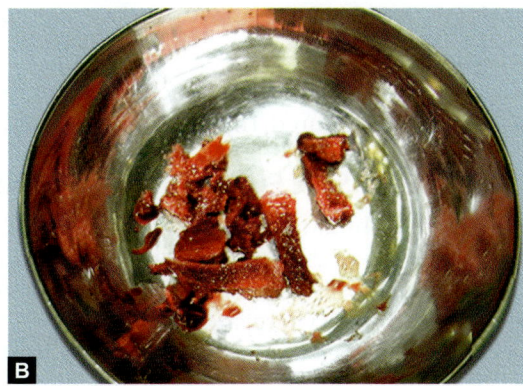

Figs. 48.8A and B: (A) Bone graft harvest from the left iliac crest; (B) The bowl shows harvested cancellous graft.

COMMON DONOR SITES

Iliac Crest, Ribs, Fibula

- **Iliac crest, ribs:** Iliac crest remains the *most common source of cancellous graft* (Figs. 48.8A and B). It is mainly needed to stimulate union at the nonunion site or fill up a defect.
- **Fibula:** It is the *most common source of cortical graft*. It is needed to strengthen or fill larger defects in gap nonunions/tumor cavities.

MECHANISM OF ACTION OF BONE GRAFT

There are three major actions of a bone graft: Three 'O's
1. **Osteoconduction:** The exo- and endoskeleton of the graft act as a scaffold/bridge over which new bone is laid upon.
2. **Osteoinduction:** Recruitment and stimulation of local cells to convert into osteoblast via bone morphogenic protein (BMP), which is present in the bone marrow (of fresh autograft). Recombinant BMPs induce the differentiation of osteoprogenitor cells into osteogenic cells and have the potential to act as autogenous bone graft substitutes.
3. **Osteogenesis:** Transplanted 'live osteoblasts' from fresh bone graft help new bone formation.

Box 48.2 summarizes the function of three types of graft—autograft, allograft, and synthetic graft.

Box 48.2: Function of three types of graft.

Fresh autograft: All three functions—osteoconduction, induction and genesis
Allograft, synthetic graft: Only osteoconduction. No osteoinduction as there is no fresh marrow. No osteogenesis as there are no live osteoblasts
Recombinant BMPs: Provide osteoinduction.

TENDON TRANSFER PROCEDURE

DEFINITION

A tendon transfer is a procedure wherein a healthy tendon with normal and intact neurovascular status is detached from its primary insertion and transferred to a new location to perform a new function.

INDICATIONS
- Muscle paralysis.
- To restore muscle balance across a joint in case of deformity due to muscle imbalance.
- Irreparable injured/ruptured tendon.

PREREQUISITE FOR TENDON TRANSFER
- The joint should be supple and mobile.
- The power of the tendon transferred should be a minimum grade IV, as after the tendon transfer, it loses power by one grade. And to function, the tendon must have grade III power.
- It should be a synergistic transfer.
- The transferred tendon should have a straight line of pull.
- The transferred/donor tendon must be expendable with a similar excursion.
- The patient's age should be a minimum of five years, as the post-tendon transfer requires re-education regarding usage for a newer function.

ARTHROSCOPY

PROCEDURE
Through a keyhole (stab wound) around the joint, a telescope with the camera system is introduced into the joint and intra-articular structures are visualized over a monitor screen **(Figs. 48.9A to C)**. By making several similar keyholes around the joint, instruments are introduced into the joint to perform a procedure. Normal saline is required to distend the joint while performing the various procedure.

Advantages: Smaller incisions result in less bleeding, less postoperative pain, easier rehabilitation, and cosmetic scars. Technically, arthroscopy provides easier access to intra-articular structures and tight corners of the joint.

Disadvantages: Steep learning curve, costly instrumentations, constrained space to operate, and risk of neurovascular injury.

COMMON PROCEDURES WITH ARTHROSCOPE ACROSS THE JOINTS
- *Diagnostic arthroscopy*: If the clinical and radiological diagnosis remains doubtful
- Synovectomy
- Adhesiolysis for a stiff joint
- Loose body removal

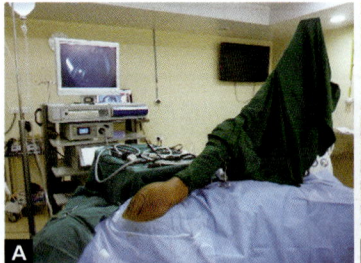 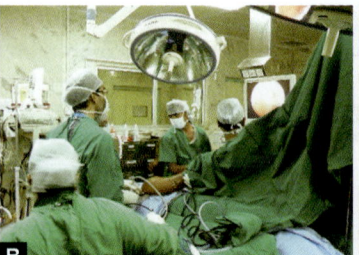 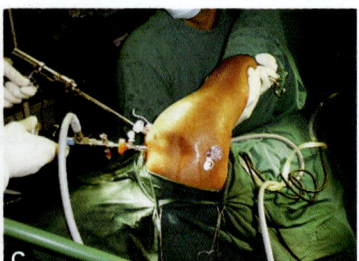

Figs. 48.9A to C: Setup of arthroscopy, small portals, and instruments through it.

- Septic arthritis debridement
- Cartilage surgery.

SPECIFIC JOINT AND PROCEDURES

- ***Knee:*** ACL/PCL surgery, meniscus surgery.
- ***Shoulder:*** Shoulder dislocation—Bankart (Labral) repair, rotator cuff repair, frozen shoulder capsular release.
- ***Elbow:*** Tennis elbow release.
- ***Wrist:*** Carpal ligament repair surgery, scaphoid/distal radius fracture fixation, carpal tunnel release.
- ***Hip:*** Labral surgery, femoral acetabular impingement treatment.
- ***Ankle:*** Ligament surgery.

AMPUTATIONS

DEFINITION

Amputation is the intentional surgical removal of the limb by cutting through the bone or by disarticulating the joint.

Indications of amputation

Alan Apley highlighted the indications as "four Ds."

- **Dead (or Dying):** Includes dry gangrene due to peripheral vascular disease and this is the commonest indication. Other examples of a dead limb include severe trauma, burns and frostbite.
- **Deadly:** Includes conditions which if not eradicated by amputation immediately might prove fatal. Example include gas gangrene and severe sepsis.
- **Dangerous:** Includes conditions such as malignant tumors and crush injuries.
- **Damned nuisance:** Retaining the limb may be worse than having no limb at all, because of:
  - Pain
  - Gross malformation
  - Recurrent sepsis such as chronic osteomyelitis
  - Severe loss of function

PRINCIPLES OF AMPUTATION

The following principles should be considered while performing an amputation to create an ideal stump.
- The scar should be healed and mobile, away from the subcutaneous bony edges.
- The skin should be as sensate as possible.
- The stump should have a cylindrical or conical shape at closure.
- Traumatized tissue must not be retained.
- Myoplastic techniques may be attempted in non-ischemic limbs.

Ideal stump characteristics

- Ideal length
- Conical shape
- Free of scars (except appropriately placed and healed surgical scars)
- No prominent/sharp bone ends
- No sinuses/ulcers
- No neuroma
- Full range of movement at the proximal joint
- Normal sensation at the stump
- Good muscle power

- Nerves should be gently sectioned and allowed to retract into proximal soft tissues to prevent neuroma formation in inappropriate places.
- The bone should be bevelled.

TYPES OF AMPUTATION

- **Provisional amputation** is performed when primary healing is unlikely. The limb is amputated as distal as the caudal condition will allow. Re-amputation and closure of the stump are performed when the local conditions are favorable.
  For example, Guillotine amputation is a type of provisional amputation.
- **Definitive end-bearing** is performed when pressure or weight is to be borne through the stump end. Hence, the scar must not be terminal, and the bone end must not be hollow, which means it must be cut through or near the joint.
  For example, Syme's amputation.
- **Definitive non-end bearing amputation** is performed when the weight is not to be borne at the stump end. This is the most common variety.
  For example, Below knee amputation.

COMPLICATIONS OF AMPUTATION

The following are the common complications seen after amputation:
- Hematoma
- Infection
- Wound necrosis
- Pain
- Joint contractures
- Phantom limb sensation
- Stump neuroma formation
- Non-healing ulcers of stump.

COMMON LEVELS OF AMPUTATION/DISARTICULATION

Figure 48.10 shows common levels of amputation.

OPTIMUM LEVEL OF THE VARIOUS AMPUTATION STUMP

The optimal level of various stumps should be achieved to enable prosthesis fitting. The various level of amputation are shown in **Table 48.2**.

SPECIAL AMPUTATION STUMPS

- **Lisfranc's amputation** is a foot amputation *through the tarsometatarsal joint* while retaining the midfoot (navicular, cunieforms and cuboid) and hindfoot (calcaneus, talus and heel pad).
- **Chopart's amputation:** Foot amputation *through the midtarsal joint* while retaining the hindfoot (calcaneus, talus and heel pad).
- **Syme's amputation** is an ankle disarticulation, removal of malleoli, *BUT* heel pad is retained. The retained heel pad gives an excellent weight-bearing surface, and the patient can walk without a prosthesis. It is an example of end-bearing stump.

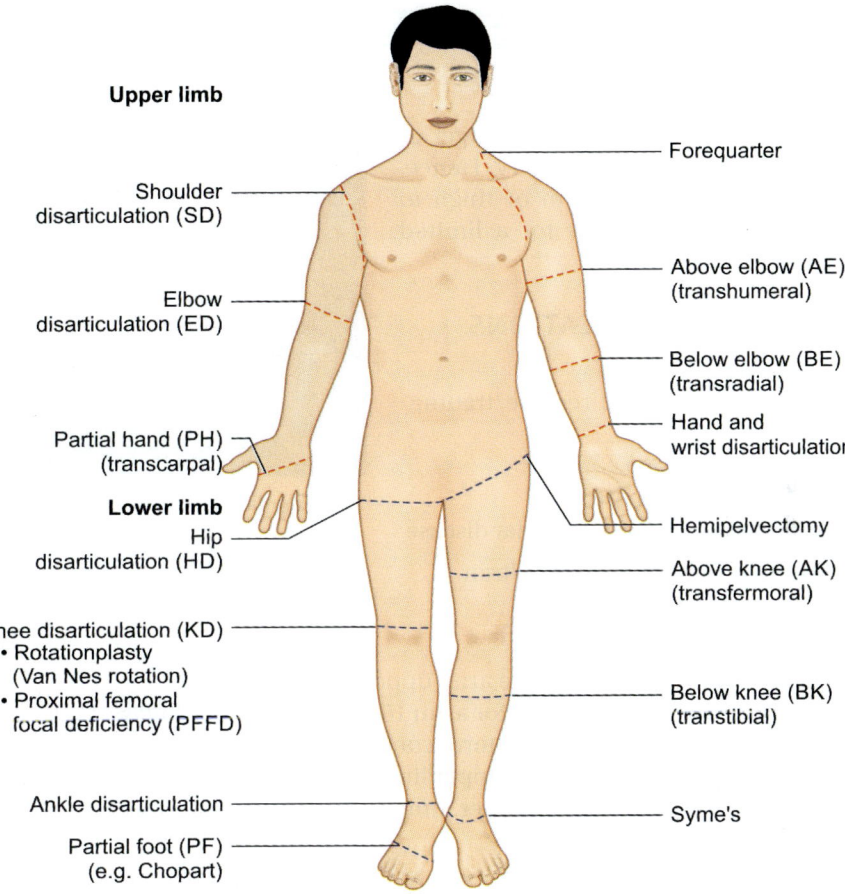

Fig. 48.10: Common levels of amputation.

Table 48.2: Optimum levels of the various amputation stump.			
Site of amputation	Optimum level	Shortest level	Longest level
Below elbow	Junction of proximal two-third and distal one-third of forearm	3 cm below the insertion of biceps brachii	5 cm above the wrist joint
Above elbow	Middle third of arm	4 cm below the anterior axillary fold	10 cm above olecranon
Above knee	Middle third of thigh	8 cm below pubic ramus	15 cm above medial joint line
Below knee	8 cm for every 1 m of height	7.5 cm below medial joint line	The level at which a myoplasty can be performed.

- **Pirogoff amputation:** It is a Syme's variant wherein ankle is disarticulated and malleoli is removed. However, the heel pad and posterior part of the calcaneum is retained.
- **Hindquarter amputation or external hemipelvectomy:** Entire lower limb with ipsilateral innominate bone is removed.
- **Forequarter amputation:** Entire upper limb with ipsilateral scapula and clavicle are removed.

TOURNIQUETS

INDICATIONS

The majority of upper/lower limb surgeries require a bloodless field during surgery. Hence, a tourniquet is applied to the arm or thigh to temporarily stop the blood flow for a limited time **(Fig. 48.11)**.

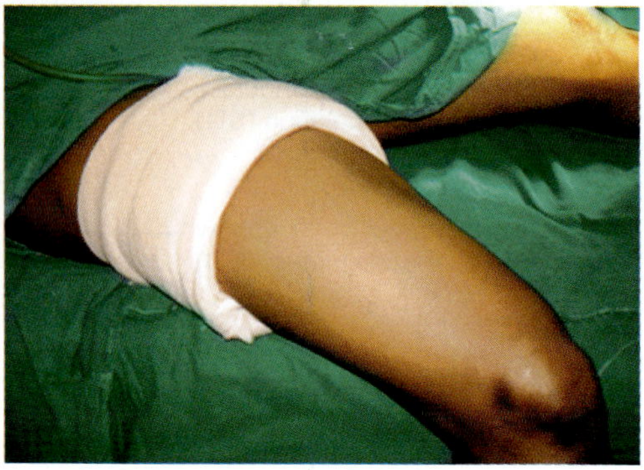

RELATIVE CONTRAINDICATIONS

- Limbs with severe infection
- Patients with poor cardiac reserve/traumatized limbs
- Peripheral neuropathy
- Deep vein thrombosis in the limb
- Raynaud's disease/peripheral vascular disease.

Fig. 48.11: Tourniquet on right thigh.

Extra precautions: Sickle cell disease/trait.

BASIC RULES OF TOURNIQUET

- **Site** of application: Upper part of the arm, upper thigh
- **Width** of the tourniquet pad: 10 cm for arm; 15 cm or larger for thighs
- Adequate **padding**: Two layers of cotton beneath the tourniquet
- **Optimal pressure**: 200–250 mm Hg upper limb; 300–350 lower limb
- **Timing:** In general NOT >2 hours upper limb; NOT >3 hours lower limb.

TYPES OF TOURNIQUET

- **Pneumatic tourniquet** is a type of pressure-regulated controlled unit tourniquet where the pressure over the arm/thigh can be controlled pressure through a machine. Hence, excess pressure can be avoided, which may result in muscle necrosis and neurovascular injury.
- **Non-pneumatic (Esmarch):** It is wrapped around the limb with *'manual control of adequate tightness'* to control the blood flow. So, the pressure under the tourniquet cannot be controlled. Hence, complications could be more.

COMPLICATIONS OF TOURNIQUET

- **Nerve injury** is one of the most common complications. It may result in nerve injury from mild transient loss of function to irreversible damage and paralysis.
- **Tourniquet pain:** If tourniquet has been there for long over the arm, the patient may complain of pain over the area of tourniquet possibly due to mild muscle necrosis and ischemia.
- **Compartment syndrome, rhabdomyolysis**: It occurs only if the tourniquet has been there for duration longer than permitted.
- **Post-tourniquet syndrome** is a syndrome of postoperative oedema and stiffness of the limb (not paralysis) due to reperfusion injury. It resolves over a few days-weeks.
- **Digital necrosis:** It can occur due to vascular occlusion.
- **Deep venous thrombosis**.

SYNOVIAL FLUID ANALYSIS

Often joint aspiration is performed to diagnose the clinical condition and differentiate between normal/degenerative arthritis/inflammatory/septic condition. Normal synovial fluid is highly viscous, clear, colorless, and nearly acellular. It forms a good mucin clot with low levels of LDH and lactic acid (<25 mg%).

The fluid is aspirated from the affected joint in a standard aseptic technique. The aspirated fluid is sent for examination for physical, microbiological and biochemical features.

- **Physical characteristics:** Clarity, color, and viscosity
- **Microbiological evaluation:** Cell count, type of cell, Gram stain, AFB stain, cultures
- **Biochemical analysis:** Protein, sugars, crystals. Table 48.3 summarizes the characteristics of various fluids.

The color of the aspirate can give a vital clues for underlying diagnosis:
- *Hemorrhagic:* Traumatic/bleeding disorders
- *Brownish:* Pigmented villonodular synovitis
- *Turbid:* Septic arthritis.

One of the major concerns about synovial fluid analysis is to differentiate between normal/inflammatory/septic fluid. Several criteria help differentiating between these conditions, such as assessment of 'glucose level' and cell count in fluid. **The glucose levels in septic fluid is always less than 1/2 to 1/3rd of current serum glucose levels, PMN > 75% and cell count > 75,000/mm³.**

Table 48.3: Characteristics of synovial fluid in normal and pathological conditions.

		Normal	Osteoarthrosis	Inflammatory	Septic	Hemorrhagic
Physical	Clarity	Transparent	Transparent	Translucent	Opaque	Bloody
	Color	Clear	Clear	Yellow	Turbid yellow/yellow-green	Bloody. Fat globules indicate #
	Viscosity	High	High	Low	Low	
Micro-biological	WBCs/mm³	<200	200–2000	2000–50,000	> 75–80,000	RBCs >>WBCs
	PMN%	<25%	<25%	50–60%	>75%	
	Gram stain				Positive	
	Cultures				Positive	
Bio-chemical	Sugars	>90% of the serum glucose level	>90% of the serum glucose level	50–90%	<50% of the serum glucose levels	
	Protein	<1/3rd of serum	<1/3rd of serum	Increased	Increased	
	Crystals	None	Sometimes CPPD	+ in crystal arthropathy	None	None

The LDH level is elevated in septic arthritis (>250 U/L), and lactic acid levels could be as high as 1000 mg%.

CHAPTER 49

Overview of Physiotherapy

The role of physiotherapy and occupational therapy in orthopaedics is paramount in rehabilitating patients and restoring their function. The major objective of rehabilitation and functional restoration is achieved by:
- Pain relief
- Joint mobilization
- Muscle strengthening
- Deformity prevention and correction (by stretching)
- Proprioceptive and gait training, return to sports.

PAIN RELIEF

There are a variety of modalities, such as cold therapy, heat therapy and tractions, which help relieving pain due to various musculoskeletal affections.
- **Local ice pack/cold therapy:**
    - Used in acute trauma, inflammation, and infective condition.
    - The application of ice helps reduce pain by reducing the blood flow to the affected area (vasoconstriction), thereby reducing inflammation and hematoma formation.
- **Heat therapies:** They are primarily used in relieving chronic pain. Various modalities are:
    - Moist heat **(Fig. 49.1)**
    - Wax bath
    - Shortwave diathermy: For diffuse pain **(Fig. 49.2)**
    - Local ultrasound massage: For local point tenderness, e.g., in tennis elbow **(Fig. 49.3)**.
    - Interferential therapy: For radicular pain, e.g., intervertebral disc prolapse with radicular pain **(Fig. 49.4)**

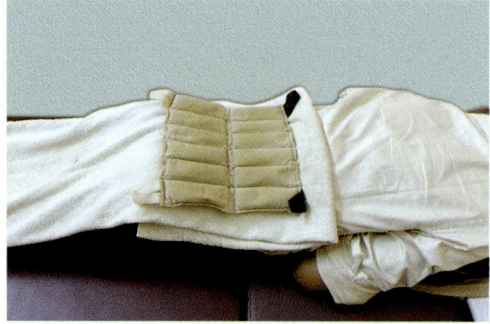

Fig. 49.1: Moist heat application over the lumbar area.

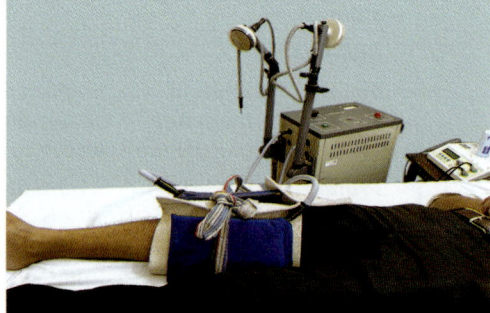

Fig. 49.2: Shortwave diathermy application over the right knee.

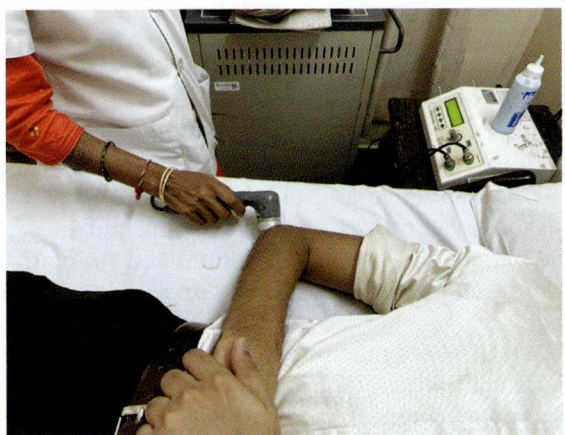

Fig. 49.3: Local ultrasound therapy over right elbow.

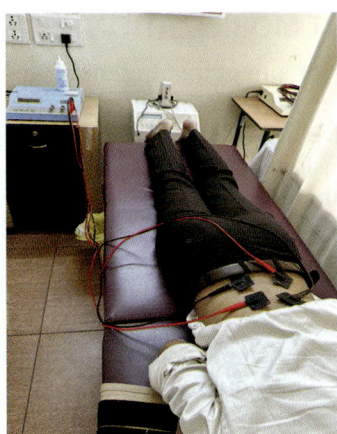

Fig. 49.4: Interferential therapy application over the lumbar area.

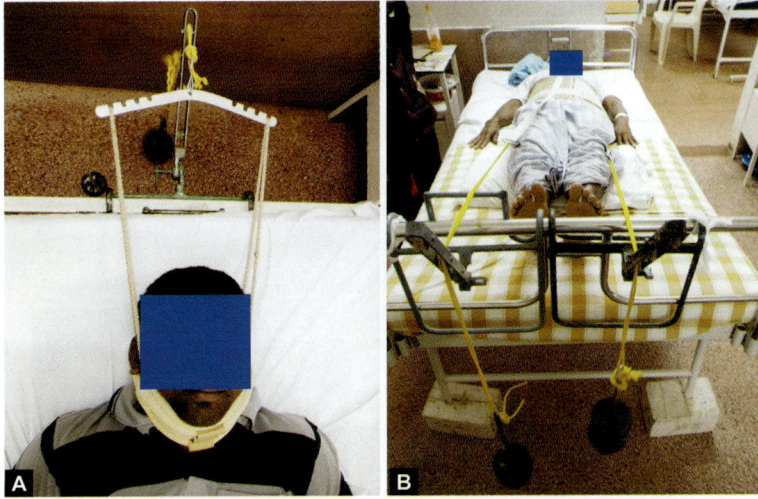

Figs. 49.5A and B: (A) Glisson's traction for neck pain; (B) Lumbar traction for back pain.

- Transcutaneous electrical nerve stimulation (TENS): TENS uses low voltage current to treat pain arising out of various conditions, such as osteoarthritis, tendinitis, fibromyalgia, bursitis, etc. TENS acts by several mechanisms, such as blocking pain pathways, raising local endorphin levels.

Note that heat therapies should be avoided in acute trauma, acute inflammation, infections, and tumors as that can increase blood flow to the affected region exacerbating pain. Furthermore, theoretically there is an increased risk of metastasis in a malignant bone tumor due to heat therapy induced increased blood supply.

- **Tractions:** Sometimes, intermittent traction is used to relieve pain and spasm, especially in cervical and lumbar spine disorders (IVDP, spondylitis) or in lower limb joint hip and knee pain (Perthes' disease, TB hip). Similar tractions can be applied in ward/home using static systems **(Figs. 49.5A and B)**. Tractions are also used to prevent and correct joint deformities.

JOINT MOBILIZATION

One major aim of treating musculoskeletal pathologies is the ***prevention and treatment of a stiff joint***. Joint mobilization can be achieved in various ways, such as:

- **Active joint mobilization:** The patient is encouraged to move their joints actively. Occasionally, patient cannot move their joint easily. In such a case, they can be assisted by the therapist in facilitating movement, known as active-assisted movement.
- **Passive joint mobilization:** The therapist passively moves the affected joint, and the patient does not use their effort. Later, once the patient gains some movement and strength, they are allowed active movements. *However, vigorous passive mobilization should be avoided for the risk of myositis ossificans.*
- **Continuous passive mobilization (CPM):** CPM is a machine that can passively move the joint without needing a therapist. CPM is used when joint motion is required, but active movement is not possible (due to pain) or not permitted to avoid muscle action. The limb is secured over the CPM machine and is calibrated to the predetermined degrees of intended motion. The machine is switched on, which then can bend and straighten the limb by moving the joint **(Fig. 49.6)**.
- **Hydrotherapy** is another way to reduce the stiffness in the joint, wherein the patient is encouraged to mobilize the joint in the pool of water. It helps relieve pain and spasms and encourages joint mobility and strength development.

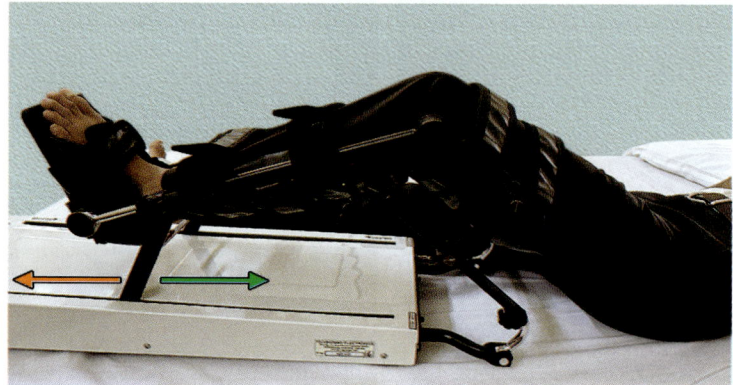

Fig. 49.6: CPM machine passively mobilizing the left knee.

MUSCLE STRENGTHENING

The strength of muscle is achieved by a combination of exercises as follows:

- **Isotonic exercises:** It is the most common form of muscle-strengthening exercise, wherein *the muscle tension remains constant (isotonic), but the length of the muscle and joint angle constantly changes.*
  Isotonic exercise is of two types: Concentric and eccentric. In concentric exercise, the external force is less than one generated in muscle, so muscle keeps shortening while contracting. In eccentric, the external force is larger than the force generated in muscle, so muscle tends to lengthen while lifting the load.
- **Isometric exercises:** In this, the joint angle and length of muscle remain constant (isometric), but tension changes, e.g., quadriceps strengthening isometric exercises while the knee is kept straight.

DEFORMITY PREVENTION AND CORRECTION

The therapist uses pain relief measures, passive and active mobilization techniques, splints and tractions to help prevent and correct the deformity.

PROPRIOCEPTIVE TRAINING

Once the fracture, ligament or injury is healed and enough ROM is achieved, the patient is trained to achieve balance and proprioception using balance boards.

Notes

CHAPTER 50

Basics of Imaging in Orthopaedics

INTRODUCTION

Besides the clinical examination, there is often a need to ask imaging departments for further investigation to understand the clinical problem or characterize the disorders. This chapter gives an overview of the different imaging techniques used on the musculoskeletal system, its strengths and limitations.

X-RAY OR PLAIN RADIOGRAPH

Mechanism of X-ray production: X-rays are produced in a so-called X-ray tube when a stream of electrons ejected from the cathode hits the anode.

While passing through the body, X-rays are absorbed by bony structures and calcifications. However, soft parts such as muscles, fat or gas absorb fewer X-rays. All the unabsorbed X-rays cause a blackening of the photographic film.

How body parts appear on the X-ray: As a function of different X-ray absorptions on the developed film:
- Gas and fat appear black
- Soft parts show shades of gray and
- Bones and calcifications appear white.

Imaging protocol: "Rule of two"
1. *Imaging in two planes,* preferably perpendicular to each other. For example, anteroposterior (AP), and lateral view **(Fig. 50.1)**
2. *One joint above and one joint below.*

How to read the image?
- *Name the region,* e.g., this is a plain X-ray of 'ankle'
- *Skin and soft tissues*: Intact/irregular; abnormal density? Gas?
- Displacement or effacement of *fascial planes?*
- *Form and contour of the bones.*
- *Description of articulation*: Normal, subluxated/dislocated.
- Any *irregularity of the cortex?*
- If the bone is fractured and displaced, *describe the displacement* of fragment in various planes. In long bones, the displacement mentioned is always of the 'distal' fragment, as the proximal fragment is supposed to be connected with the proximal stable torso. However,

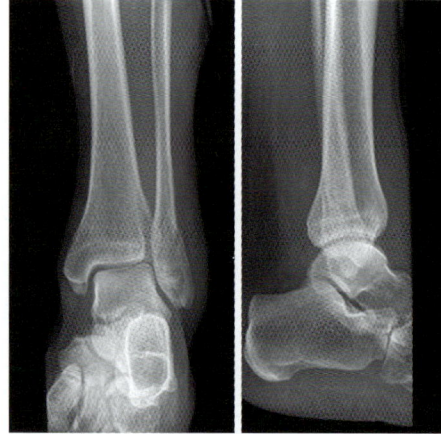

Fig. 50.1: Anteroposterior (AP), lateral X-ray of ankle.

in the spine, the displacement of a dislocated vertebra is always of the proximal vertebra (C5 dislocation over C6), as the distal fragment is fixed with a stable torso.
- *Abnormal density in the bone*, e.g., sclerotic or lytic area, thickening, abnormal line of radiolucency, etc.
- Fat-fluid level in the joint (lipohemarthrosis)? Indirect signs of a fracture? Any calcification or foreign material in the joint?

COMPUTED TOMOGRAPHY (CT)

One limitation of conventional plain radiography is that the understanding fracture pattern and displacements are difficult in certain situations, such as:
- **Intra-articular and periarticular fractures**
- **Areas with complex geometry:** Pelvis #, spine #
- **Superimposition of structures:** Chest overlapping scapula fracture makes it difficult to assess the exact fracture pattern. In such a situation, CT scan is very useful, which assesses a fracture in all three planes—axial, coronal, and sagittal **(Figs. 50.2 and 50.3)**. Moreover, a three-dimensional reconstruction of bones and joint help understand fracture pattern.

Mechanism of CT scan: CT scan also works on the principle of X-rays.

Advantages: CT scan is an advanced imaging technique which can illustrate all the complex areas of the bone and joints in all the planes. Another advantage of a CT scan is the 3D reconstruction of complex images. This makes operative planning easy.

Disadvantages: The imaging of soft tissue is not accurate. Also, the radiation dose is much higher than a regular X-ray.

MAGNETIC RESONANCE IMAGING (MRI)

A limitation of the CT scan is the lack of sufficient demonstration of soft tissue. MRI is the answer for *imaging soft tissues in the musculoskeletal system*.

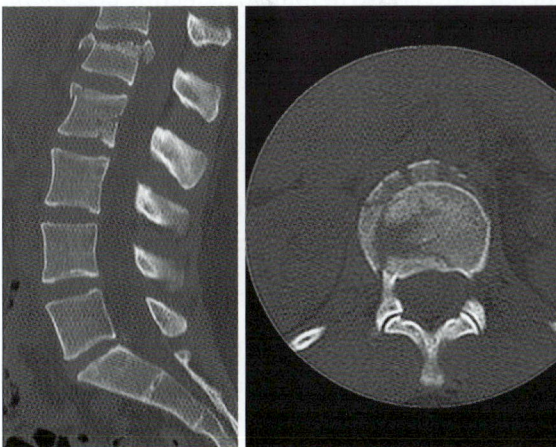

Fig. 50.2: Computed tomography (CT) scan of the lumbar spine (sagittal and axial image) showing fracture of L1 vertebra.

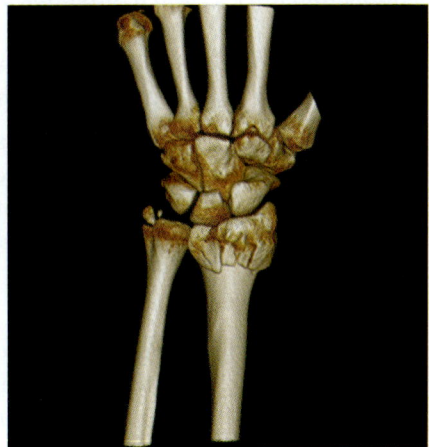

Fig. 50.3: 3D CT image of fracture distal radius showing comminution.

Technique: MRI is based on the behavior of our body's hydrogen nuclei (protons) when placed in a strong magnetic field. These protons, which are present in large numbers in water molecules and lipids, are forced by the strong magnetic field to align with it (vector in the axis of the magnetic field). Then the protons are stimulated by a radiowave frequency (RF) to resonate. They spin out of equilibrium and release energy by realigning with the magnetic field. The time of relaxation and the amount of energy released depend on the chemical nature of the molecule. The receiver coils placed around the body part to be examined detect the emitted signals. These signals are processed into the images.

The time protons take to fully relax after an RF pulse is measured as T1 and T2 relaxation. **(Figs. 50.4A and B)**.

T1 recovery is the time 63% of the atoms take to return to their original state after switching off the RF signals.

The T2 decay time is when only 37% of the atoms are under the influence of an RF pulse.

The shorter the relaxation times, the brighter the image (hyperintense vs hypointense signal). Fat appears white in T1 and T2, and fluids (water) appear white on T2 and dark in T1.

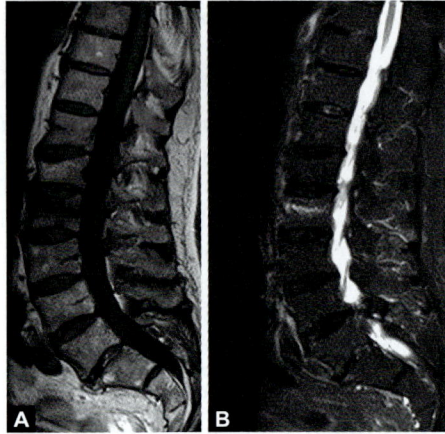

Figs. 50.4A and B: MRI of lumbosacral spine, sagittal images. (A) T1; (B) Fat suppressed T2 image.

Because of the fatty bone, the marrow bones appear white. Edema or metastasis changes the bright signal to a darker, hypointense signal. Gadolinium, an agent with paramagnetic properties, is often used for contrast detection or characterization of lesions.

Advantages of MRI: It is a great tool to image *soft tissue pathologies, such as injuries of ligament, tendon, and muscle, and assess bone marrow edema*. MRI is also helpful in detecting *occult and stress fractures and bone contusions*. It is also an excellent tool for detecting *spinal cord and nerve root compressions* due to any pathology in the spine. It is also an important tool to assess *soft tissue extension of bone tumors and bone marrow skip metastasis*.

Disadvantages: It is costly and creates a feeling of claustrophobia. Because of the strong magnetic field, an MRI cannot be done if there are pacemakers and stents in the body. However, pacemaker programming of MR can be done to circumvent the challenge. Regarding the presence of orthopaedic implants, there are MR-compatible titanium metallic implants.

ULTRASOUND

Ultrasound is widely used in medicine because it is readily available and cheap. The ultrasound can easily visualize soft tissues like tendons, muscles, nerves, bursae, or any other swelling or structure under the skin. Hence, it can diagnose joint effusion, tendinitis, paratendinitis, soft tissue swelling, bursitis, and changes in the rotator cuff.

Disadvantages: Since it is operator dependent, there is always a question about its accuracy. Further, it cannot detect the pathologies accurately within the joint, such as labral tears/meniscal injuries as USG rays cannot penetrate the joint.

RADIONUCLIDE IMAGING/BONE SCAN

For radionuclide imaging, radionucleotide substance is injected intravenously. Most radionuclides used in bone scans emit gamma radiation which a gamma camera can detect.

The most commonly used radionuclide is **Technetium-99m,** and others are **Gallium and Indium.** Technetium-99m-MDP (methylene diphosphonate) absorbs onto the hydroxyapatite crystals of bone.

The uptake depends upon the amount of abnormal blood flow and bone turnover and is seen as a "hot spot" in images. Such hot spots would be seen in trauma, tumor, infection and inflammatory conditions. So this makes the bone scan a sensitive modality but not specific **(Fig. 50.5)**.

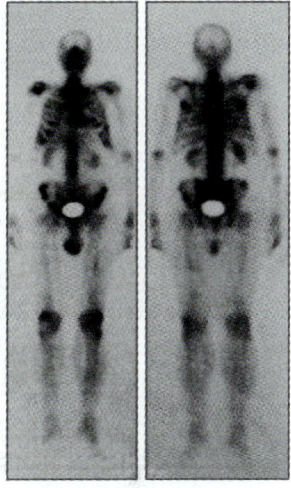

Fig. 50.5: Tc99 bone scan showing hot spot in ribs, spine, and pelvis.

Method: After intravenous injection, three different images can be produced:

I Phase = Flow phase: 2–5 second images are obtained for 60 seconds after injection to show arterial perfusion.

II Phase = Blood pool phase: An image is obtained 5 minutes after injection to show the venous pooling.

III Phase = Delayed phase: The image is obtained 2–4 hours later to evaluate skeletal metabolism.

Indications of bone scan: It has a wide range of indications, such as:
- Metastasis in a bone tumor
- Evaluating acute osteomyelitis when X-rays are normal
- Assessing complex regional pain syndrome
- Stress fracture.

SINGLE PHOTON EMISSION COMPUTED TOMOGRAPHY (SPECT)

It is *essentially a radionucleotide scan, but here the gamma camera is not fixed but moves around the patient's body and creates sectional images similar to CT and MRI.* It can also create a 3D image. With this, three-dimensional information on the pathological location is possible. The capillaries of the organ pick up the radionucleotide substance.

The basic indications of SPECT are the same as for the bone scan: Infection, inflammation or tumors.

It can provide accurate information about the organs too. So, it can be used for cardiac or brain function too.

POSITRON EMISSION TOMOGRAPHY (PET)

It is another type of radionucleotide scan, which is used to measure blood flow, oxygen flow and glucose metabolism. This makes it useful for tumor imaging **(Fig. 50.6)**.

The most commonly used pharmaceutical for PET is F-18 fluorodeoxyglucose (FDG), with fluorine-18 as a positron-emitting isotope. It is taken into cells and demonstrates increased glucose metabolism, e.g., in tumor cells. The PET scan is costlier than a single photon emission computed tomography (SPECT).

The PET can be combined with CT or MRI to assess the organ functioning.

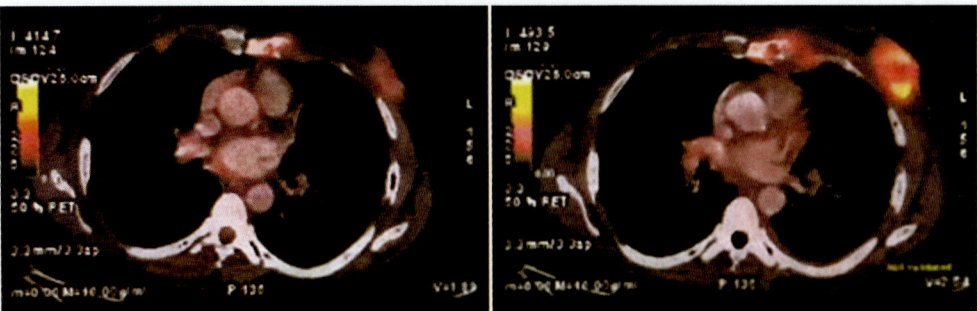

Fig. 50.6: Positron emission tomography (PET) scan.

It is useful in:
- Assessing bone tumor metastasis
- To differentiate between infections and aseptic loosening of the prosthesis
- To assess the response to the treatment of bone infection.

Index

Page numbers followed by *b* refer to box, *f* refer to figure, *fc* refer to flowchart, and *t* refer to table.

A

Abdomen 349, 404
    computed tomography scan of 231
    strapping 198
Abduction 313, 315, 537*f*, 548
Abductor
    digiti minimi 504
    hallucis 528
    pollicis
        brevis 503
        longus 140*f*, 575
Above elbow 655
    cast 615*f*, 618
Above knee 655
    cast 195, 618, 618*f*
        application 526*f*
    cylindrical cast 618*f*
    skin traction 199*f*, 317*f*, 630, 630*f*
Abscess
    cold 310, 313, 315, 319
    intramedullary 284*f*
    intraosseous 281*f*
    paravertebral 324, 324*f*
Acetabular
    fracture 173, 175, 175*f*
        classification of 174
        fixation 176
    index 534, 535*f*
    limbus 532
    socket 47
    trabeculae 180
Acetabulum 173, 174, 532, 536
    associated fracture of 51
    dysplastic 534
    fracture 173, 174*f*
    roof of 312
Acetaminophen 101
Achilles tendon 610
Achondroplasia 557, 557*f*, 558*f*, 601
Acid phosphatase 418
Acid-fast bacillus 328
    staining 316, 325
Acidosis
    lactic 18
    metabolic 228
Acromial spurs 567, 572
Acromioclavicular joint
    capsule 41, 42
    dislocation 41
        dog button stabilization of 43*f*
        treatment of 43, 43*f*
    surgical anatomy of 41
    X-ray of 41*f*
Acromion 35
Actinomycin-D 474
Acute anterior cruciate ligament
    bony avulsion 260
    tear 259
        clinical features of 258
Acute anterior dislocation
    shoulder, complications of 36
    treatment of 36
Acute flaccid asymmetric motor
    palsy 432
Acute hematogenous pyogenic
    osteomyelitis, pathogenesis
    of 280
Acute injury 20
    natural history of 23
Acute joint
    dislocations 222
    pain 102
Acute lung injury, transfusion-related 18
Acute monoarticular
    exacerbation 349
Acute neurovascular injury 55, 222
Acute osteomyelitis 286*fc*, 287, 299
    clinical features of 282
Acute posterior cruciate ligament
    tear 263
    clinical features of 262
Acute pyogenic osteomyelitis 280
    complications of 287
Acute respiratory distress syndrome 221
Acute traumatic anterior shoulder
    dislocation, clinical features
    of 34
Adalimumab 351
Adam's test 588, 589*f*
Adamantinoma 448
Adamkiewicz delivers vascular supply 155
Addisonian crisis 14
Adduction 39, 314, 315, 526
Adductor
    pollicis 504
    tenotomy 537
Adenovirus 296
Adequate pain control measures 237
Adriamycin 472
Adson's tests 593
Advanced trauma life support 3, 7, 16, 16*t*, 147, 173
    protocol 198
Air
    ambulance 7
    embolism 637
Airway 642
    adequacy of 642*f*
Albers-Schönberg disease 416
Alcohol 483
Alcoholism, chronic 483, 579
Alkaline
    phosphatase 63, 451
    phosphate 412
Alkalosis, metabolic 18
Allman classification 88
Allodynia 235, 236
Allograft 651
Allopurinol 365
Alopecia 403
Alpha-fetoprotein 557
American College of Rheumatism 346*b*
American College of Surgeons 7, 16
    Committee in Trauma 5
American Rheumatism Association 346*b*
American Spinal Injury Association
    Scoring 165
Amikacin 312
Amitriptyline 101
Amniotic band syndrome 522
Amplitude 492
Amputation 222, 455, 468, 472, 653
    common levels of 654, 655*f*
    complications of 654
    forequarter 655
    hindquarter 655
    indication for 653
    principles of 653
    site of 655
    stump 654
    types of 654
Amyloidosis 292
Anakinra 351
Analgesia 11
Analgesics 23, 251, 317, 341, 356, 362, 393
    adequate 237

Index

Andersson sign 356
Anemia 227, 238, 349, 476
Anesthesia
   general 125, 133, 567
   saddle 387
Anesthetic drugs 642
Aneurysm, traumatic 230
Aneurysmal sign 324
Angiogram 75
Angiography 54, 54*f*, 250
Angulation, degree of 122
Anhydrosis 515
Ankle 30, 164, 218, 441, 649, 653
   arthritis 220
   bimalleolar fracture of 217*f*
   binder 271*f*
   dislocation 619
   edema, persistent 271
   elevation of 23*f*
   foot 539
      compartment syndrome 209
      orthosis 510*f*
   fracture 217
      classification of 218
      Lauge-Hansen classification of 218*t*
   joint 521*f*, 524*f*
      osteology of 217
      space 22*f*
      surgical anatomy of 217
   lateral X-ray of 207*f*, 211*f*, 662*f*
   ligament injury 255, 269, 270, 271*fc*
      lateral 269*f*
      surgical anatomy of 269
   magnetic resonance imaging of 270
   medial side of 217
   mortise 217
   plain X-ray of 204*f*, 205, 207, 211, 270, 525
   plantar flexion 511
      loss of 510
   soft tissue injuries of 619
   sprain 21*f*, 269, 619
      grade of 270
      lateral 270
   swelling over lateral aspect of 270*f*
   X-ray of 553
Ankylosing spondylitis 334, 352, 353, 354*f*, 355*f*, 356*b*, 585, 650
Ankylosis 244, 648
   apophyseal 355
   painful fibrous 319
Annular ligament 123, 123*f*
Annulus fibrosus 377, 381
   structure of 377*f*
Anorexia 476
Anterior cord syndrome 156*f*
Anterior cruciate ligament 259-261, 264

blood supply of 258
bony avulsion 259*f*
bundles 257
function of 258
nerve supply of 258
reconstruction 260
repair 260
surgical anatomy of 257
tear 257, 258
   management of 261*fc*
Anterior dislocation 33, 45, 51
   types of 51
Anterior longitudinal ligament 377, 378, 378*f*, 381
Antibiotic 240, 292*f*, 361
   beads 253
   duration of 285
   impregnated bone cement beads 291
   laden bone cement beads 251*f*
   primary 251
   systemic 251
Antibody
   antinuclear 361
   monoclonal 413, 468
Anticoagulants disorders 7
Anticonvulsants 237
Antidepressants 101
Anti-inflammatory medication 23
Antipyretics 317, 433
Antirheumatoid drugs, disease-modifying 99, 350
Antiseptic solutions 635
Antitubercular drugs 312, 312*t*
Ape thumb deformity 503*f*
Apley's grinding test 265
Apophysis 62
   practical implication of 62
Appetite 310
   loss 449
Apprehension test 37
Arches
   bony component of 551
   soft tissue support of 552
Arm 539
   hyperabduction of 515*f*
   plain X-ray of 290*f*
Arnold-Chiari malformation 367, 556
Arrhythmias 228, 361, 637
Arterial blood gas analysis 227, 232
Arterial Doppler 109, 250
   scan 229
Arterial oxygenation 227
Arterial puncture 636
Artery
   axillary 94, 96
   brachial 104, 106, 109
   epiphyseal 66
   femoral 197, 637
   metaphyseal 66
   periosteal 66
   subclavian 592*f*

Arthritic joint 333*f*
   clinical manifestation of 333
Arthritis 149, 331, 333, 340, 346, 352, 370
   advanced 372
   alkaptonuric 372
   classification of 333
   crystal-induced 99
   degenerative 648
   enteropathic 361
   gouty 358
   hemophilic 370
   infective 352
   inflammatory 352, 648
   juvenile
      idiopathic 335, 373
      rheumatoid 334, 373
   later stages of 319
   mutilans 348, 357
   neoplastic 352
   neuropathic 552
   overview of 333
   paraneoplastic 352
   peripheral 362
   psoriatic 352, 357
   secondary degenerative 299
   seronegative 352, 352*b*
   severe 245
   stage of 296, 297, 297*fc*, 313, 314, 318, 343, 345*fc*, 389
   symmetric 346
Arthrocentesis 298
Arthrodesis 317, 317*f*, 320*f*, 342, 351, 370, 467, 488, 517, 596, 647-650
   position of 649
   triple 529, 529*f*
Arthrogryposis multiplex congenita 522, 562
Arthropathy 302, 648
   neuropathic 367
   seronegative 302, 334*fc*
Arthroplasty 455, 467, 647
   hemireplacement 183
   replacement 647
   resection 351
   types of 647
Arthroscopic debridement 341
Arthroscopic repair 38, 266
Arthroscopy 265*b*, 605*f*, 652
   diagnostic 259, 265, 652
   setup of 652*f*
Articular cartilage 295
   damage of 319
   destruction of 313
Articular pathology 343
Ascorbic acid, serum 427
Aseptic nonunion, treatment principles of 240
Aspirate pus 311
Aspiration 443, 461
Athetoid 440, 441
Athetosis 441

Index

Athletic pubalgia 275
Atresia, anal 589
Atrophy, disuse 432
Autograft, fresh 651
Autoimmune 343
    diseases 483
Autologous cartilage implantation 604*f*
Autonomic signs 516
Autosomal dominant 416, 559
    disorder 458
Autosomal recessive 416, 559
    disorder 403
Avascular necrosis 51, 53, 118, 139, 183, 184, 221, 301, 302, 594, 595*f*
    stage of 546
Aviator's astragalus 211
Aviator's fracture 211, 215
Avulsion injury 214
Axial compression 163
Axilla, front of 35
Axillary freckles 588
Axillary nerve 494, 497
    clinical assessment of 498
    motor supply of 497
    palsy 36, 498*f*
Axis deviation 594
Axis vertebra, traumatic spondylolisthesis of 170
Axon, structure of 482*f*
Axonotmesis 483, 484, 486, 487

B

Babcock's triangle 312
Back pain 412, 422, 659*f*
    generalized 411
Backfire fracture 137
Baclofen 442
Bado classification 127
Baker's cyst 340, 597, 597*f*, 598
Balloon
    inflation 415*f*
    sign 450
Bamboo spine 354, 355*f*
Band friction syndrome 275
Bankart lesion 34, 36, 37
    reverse 39
Bankart repair, open 38
Bar diagram 416*f*
Barbotage 569
Barlow's test 532, 533, 533*f*, 534
Barr's transfer 489
Barrington's nucleus 160
Barton fracture 136
Bartonella henselae 301
Baseball finger 140
Baseball pitcher's elbow 274
Batson's venous plexus, paravertebral 320
Baumann's angle 109
    measurement 109*f*

Bechterew's disease 353
Bedsore 221, 621
Behavioral disorders 440
Behavioral therapy 238
Beighton score 37*b*
Below elbow 655
    cast 618, 618*f*
Below knee 655
    cast 271*f*, 619*f*
    skin traction 628*f*
    slab 615*f*
Bence-Jones protein 475
Bennett's fracture 140, 140*f*
Biaxial traction 320*f*
Biconcave vertebra 408
Bigelow method, reverse 52
Bilateral genu valgum 599*f*, 600
    severity of 599
Bilateral genu varum 601, 601*f*
    deformity 339*f*
Bilateral tibial tuberosity, prominence of 606*f*
Bimalleolar fracture 217, 217*f*, 218
Biochemical analysis 657
Biofilm 240
    formation 240, 287
Biological agents 350, 351, 356
Biopsy 311, 316, 325, 451, 477
    closed 311
    excisional 452
    incisional 452
    open 311, 452
    principles of 452
    synovial 350
Bird nest appearance 324, 324*f*
Birth
    anoxia 439
    asphyxia 439
    injury 514*f*, 515*f*
    trauma 439
    theory 584
Bisphosphonates 413, 414, 421, 595
    long-term therapy of 200
Blackberry thumb 575
Bladder 388, 556
    atonic 169
    bowel normal 432
    care of 168
    dysfunction 387
    flaccid 162
    involvement of 165
Bleeding
    disorders 7, 101, 222, 334
    external 229
    gastrointestinal 101
    tendency, subcutaneous 560
    wound, presence of 249
Block elbow flexion 128
Blood
    components 230
    culture 284, 298

    flow 230
    investigations 418
    loss 251
    pressure 16, 154
        control 154
    supply 177, 258
    tests 10, 405, 424, 582
    transfusion 17, 251
        massive 17
    vessels 229
Blount's disease 601, 601*b*, 602
Body, joints of 68*f*
Bohler's angle 207, 208*f*
Bohler's Braun splint 623, 623*f*
Bone 221, 251, 254, 301, 316, 423, 424, 475, 552, 663
    aseptic necrosis of 545
    bag of 116
    biopsy 319, 420
    blood supply of 65*f*
    canal system 65*f*
    cancellous 63
    care of 168
    cells 64
    cement 292*f*, 467*f*
        injection 415*f*
        preparation of 292*f*
    compact 63
    computed tomography scan of 239
    cyst, aneurysmal 450, 454, 460, 461*f*, 468
    defective 418
        osteoclastic resorption of 416
    deposition 418
    destruction 471
    disease, metastatic 82
    disorder of 301, 418
    forearm 124*f*
    formation 63, 411
    forming cell 448
    function of 62, 63
    giant cell tumor of 465, 467
    graft 467, 467*f*, 650
        harvest 651*f*
        mechanism of action of 651
        open cancellous 291
        types of 650
    immature 416
    incidence of 309
    infarct 471
    infection 254, 279, 291
    loss 245, 248
    macroanatomy of 62
    marrow
        aspirate concentrate 477, 595
        injection 242
        transplant 418
    matrix 63
        defective mineralization of 408
        inadequate mineralization of 400
    metabolic diseases of 397, 399

microscopic structure of 64
mineral density 411
mineralization 421
morphogenetic protein 78, 242, 651
number of 450
ossification 66
Paget's disease of 418
pain 310, 419, 424
resorption 411 418
resorptive cells 64
scan 75, 75*f*, 234, 311, 324, 369, 420, 451, 464, 472, 477, 548, 665
   indication for 665
   indirect 369
spirochetal infections of 304
structural composition of 63, 63*fc*
subchondral 295, 333*f*, 336, 594*f*
tensile strength of 63
tuberculosis 309, 320, 327
tumor 445
   basics of 447
   benign 449*t*, 456
   classification of 447
   clinical features of 447
   diagnosis of 447
   investigations of 447
   malignant 449*t*, 453*t*, 470
   preexisting 471
   stage of 452
   types of 447, 447*fc*
   World Health Organization classification of 448*t*
types of 450
unit of 65*f*
von-Recklinghausen disease of 423
X-ray of 424
Bony
   ankylosis 245, 296, 297, 299, 321, 355*f*, 356
   Chance fracture 171
   correction 525
   crepitus 72
   deformity 289
   erosion 360
   factors, correction of 57
   lesion 318
   malunion 245
   surgery 528
   tenderness 129, 197, 282, 323
   trabeculae 177, 178*f*, 299*f*
      clinical importance of 178
Borderline leprosy 328
Borrelia burgdorferi sensu lato 305
Boston brace, modified 590, 591*f*
Botulinum toxin 442
Bouchard and Heberdon nodes 339*f*, 340
Boutonniere's deformity 347, 347*f*
Bow legs 601

Bowel 165
   care of 168
   control disturbance 556
   dysfunction 388
Bowler's thumb 273, 273*f*
Bowstringing test 385
Boxer's fracture 141, 141*f*
Braces 100, 166
Brachial artery 104, 106, 109
   kinking of 112*f*
Brachial plexus 92, 96, 97, 512, 592*f*
   formation 512*f*
   injury 97, 479, 512
      mechanism of 512
      types of 513
Brachial vessels, arterial Doppler of 109
Brachioradialis 499, 501
Bradycardia 161
Brain
   immature 439
   magnetic resonance imaging of 227, 441, 584
Breech delivery 532
Brim sign 420*f*
Bristow's procedure 39
Brittle bone disease 559
Brodie's abscess 279, 293, 293*f*
Broken skin 328
Broomstick cast 549*f*
Brown tumor 424, 425*f*
Brown-Séquard syndrome 158, 158*f*
Brucella 296
   abortus 280
   spondylitis 326
Bucket handle tear 265, 266
Budapest criteria 237
Bulbocavernosus reflex 387
Bumper fracture 193
Bunnell opponensplasty 489, 503
Burning sensation 236
Burns eschar around limb 222
Bursitis 99, 610
Bywaters syndrome 228

C

Café-au-lait spots 462, 588
Caisson's disease 593
Calcaneal apophysis 545
Calcaneal articular surface, restoration of 209*f*
Calcaneal K-wire 633*f*
Calcaneal traction 623*f*, 633
Calcaneocavus deformity 554
Calcaneocuboid joint 528*f*
Calcaneofibular ligament 269
Calcaneonavicular ligament 269
Calcaneotalar ligament 269
Calcaneum 206, 208*f*, 528, 628*f*
   axial view of 208*f*

fracture 75*f*, 206, 207*f*, 209*f*, 209*fc*, 242
traction 633
   risk of 633
Calcar femorale 179
Calcidiol-25 400
Calcification, white line of 407, 407*f*
Calcitonin 414, 421
Calcitriol 400
   high dose of 418
Calcium 399, 400, 403, 409, 412
   abnormalities 399
   absorption 399
   channel blockers 237
   deficiency rickets 403
   function of 399
   homeostasis cycle 401*f*
   intestinal resorption of 423
   oxalate deposition 365
   phosphate 66
   pyrophosphate crystal deposition 365
      arthritis, pathogenesis of 366*f*
   regulation 400
   role of 399
   serum 412
   stimulate
      calcitonin release, high levels of 400
      parathormone release, low levels of 400
   sulphate 253
   supplemental 406
Calf
   cramps 394
   pseudohypertrophy 434
Callus formation, stage of 77
Calve disease 545
Campanacci grading system 466
Campylobacter jejuni 359
Canal, urgent surgical decompression of 387
Cancellous bone 63
   grafting 242
Cannulation, indication for 634
Capitellum 107, 545
Caplan's syndrome 349
Capsular contracture 245, 345
Carbamazepine 237
Cardiac arrest 225
Cardiac conduction abnormality 354
Cardiac malformations 589
Cardiomyopathy 434
Cardiovascular system 14, 169
Caries
   exudata 327
   mobile 327
   sicca 327
   spine 309, 320
Carotid artery 637
Carpal tunnel

Index

contents of 577
entrapment 577*f*
floor of 577
roof of 577
syndrome 134, 301, 348, 493, 576, 577
Carpometacarpal joint arthritis 340
Cartilage
   damage 594*f*
      pathogenesis of 297*fc*
   forming cell 448
   growth 404
   layers of 336*f*
   loss of 340, 345*f*
   matrix synthesis 338
   reduced formation of 338
   surgery 653
Cartilaginous endplate 378
Cast 613, 616
   application, complications of 617
   orthopaedics use of 617
Catecholamines 14
Catheter
   insertion of 639
   malposition of 637
Catheterization 638
   contraindications of 638
   procedure 638
Catterall classification 547
Catterall group 549
Catterall sign 548
Cauda equina 152
   syndrome 159, 159*t*, 222, 385, 387
Cavity
   bone cement filling of 467
   curettage of 291, 467
Cavus 526
Cellular level dysfunction 15*fc*
Cellular proliferation 77
Central cord syndrome 157, 157*f*, 170
Central nervous system 16, 169, 432
Central nidus 464
Central prolapse 380, 381, 381*f*
Cerebral cortex, periventricular motor fibers of 439
Cerebral palsy 437, 439, 587, 599
   ataxic 441
   athetoid 441
   atonic 441
   classification of 440
   complications of 443
   pathogenesis of 439*fc*
Cerebro-pulmonary system 225
Cerebrospinal fluid 305, 433
Certolizumab 351
Cervical
   brace 166*f*, 585*f*
   canal stenosis, complications of 395
   cord myelopathy 395
   disc disease 386

discectomy, anterior 387
   myelopathy 384
   rib 457, 592, 592*f*, 593*f*
   spine 30, 165*f*, 348, 383, 387
      disc herniation, chronic 385
      fixation 167*f*
      hyperextension injury of 170
      injury 166
      magnetic resonance imaging of 165*f*, 369*f*
      X-ray of 165*f*, 584, 593
   spondylosis 388, 390
   traction 630
Cervico-thoraco-lumbo-sacral orthosis 590
Champagne glass pelvis 558
Chance fracture 171, 172*f*
   types of 171
Charcot's arthropathy 334, 367, 369, 369*f*, 370, 648
   hallmark of 368
   pathophysiology of 368
Charcot's elbow, X-ray of 369*f*
Charcot's foot 552
Charcot's joint 305, 369
Charcot-Marie-tooth disease 483
Charlston brace 590, 591*f*
Chauffeur fracture 137, 137*f*
Chemical 470, 483
   injury 483
Chemotherapy
   adjuvant 472, 473, 474
   multidrug 477
   neoadjuvant 472
Chest 206*f*, 404
   computed tomography scan of 466, 474
   X-ray 227, 227*f*, 232, 325, 466
Chiari malformation 590
Chickenwire pattern 453
Chills 298
Chinese letter
   appearance 462
   pattern 453
Chlamydia trachomatis 359
Cholecalciferol 400
Chondroblast 448
Chondroblastoma 448, 453, 469, 469*f*
Chondrocalcinosis 366
Chondrocytes 66
   secrete extracellular matrix 66
Chondroitin sulphate 341
Chondrolysis 544
Chondroma 468
Chondromalacia 607*f*
   patella 606
Chondromyxoid fibroma 448
Chondrosarcoma 448, 458, 458*f*, 477, 478*f*
   high-grade 478
   low-grade 478

primary 477
   secondary 477
Chopart's amputation 654
Chordoma 448
Chorea 441
Christmas disease 370
Chronic anterior cruciate ligament tear 260
   clinical features of 259
Chronic exertional compartment syndrome 275
Chronic osteomyelitis 221, 254, 287, 290*f*, 290*fc*, 471
   complications of 291
   pathogenesis of 288*fc*
   saucerized cavity of 291*f*
Chronic posterior cruciate ligament tear 263
   clinical features of 262
Cierny Mader classification 279
Circinate balanitis 360*f*
Cisplatin 472
Clarke's test 607
Claudication, neurogenic 394
Clavicle 35
   brace 89*f*
   fracture 79*f*, 91*f*
      common location of 88
      lateral third 90, 90*f*
      medial third 91
      mid-shaft 89*fc*
   peculiarities of 87
   surgical anatomy of 87
   X-ray of 87*f*
Clavicular brace 89
Claw
   hand 506*b*, 506*f*
   toe 610
Clergyman's knee 610
Clindamycin 299
Cloacae 288
Clonazepam 442
Closed reduction 76, 110, 125, 133, 645
   advantages of 645
   and internal fixation 133, 182, 186, 199, 203
   disadvantages of 645
Clotting time 371
Clubfoot
   idiopathic 523
   syndromic 523
Clutton's joint 304
Coagulation system 17
Coagulopathy 18
Coaptation splint 104
Cobb's angle 585, 589, 589*f*
Coccidioidomycosis 296
Cock up splint 489
Codfish vertebra 408, 412, 412*f*, 560
Codman's triangle 472, 472*f*
Codman's tumor 469

Colchicine 364
Cold
　abscess 310, 313, 315, 319
　　formation 322
　　　large paravertebral 322f
　extremity 229
　therapy 27, 351, 658
Coleman block test 554
Collagen cross-linking, abnormal 559
Collateral ligament
　injury 268
　lateral 44, 257, 266, 267, 267f
　tears, chronic 268
Colles' fracture 131, 131f, 133, 133fc, 135, 242, 618
　complications of 134
　malunited 650
Colloids, role of 17
Colonoscopy 362
Comminuted supracondylar fracture 193f
Common nerve injuries 494
　specific management of 489t
Common peroneal nerve 194, 329, 489, 508
　clinical assessment of 509
　injury, treatment of 509
　motor supply of 509f
　palsy 621
Compartment syndrome 31, 54, 55, 108, 109, 111, 112, 124, 125, 127, 196, 202, 221, 222, 224, 228, 617, 636, 656
　chance of 115, 615
　common sites of 222
　high incidence of 194
　pathogenesis of 223fc
Complete blood picture 284, 298, 315, 349
Complete ligament injury, chronic 255
Complex regional pain syndrome 23, 134, 212, 219, 221, 235, 236f
　Budapest criteria for 237
　pathophysiology of 235
Compression 23, 23f, 261
　acute 483
　distraction osteogenesis 246
　osteogenesis 246
　over spinal cord 165f
　principle 247
　stocking 231
　trabeculae
　　primary 178
　　secondary 178
Computed tomography 663
　angiogram 229
　guided radiofrequency ablation 464
　scan 54, 74, 94, 165, 234, 250, 256, 289, 290f, 293, 389, 392, 394, 413, 451, 464, 586
　　mechanism of 663

Condyle, lateral 117
Confusion 226, 476
Congenital talipes equinus varus 521, 522, 530
　boot 527f
　　characteristics 530
　foot 529f
　　management of 526
　treatment of 525
Conjunctivitis 360
Connective tissue hypothesis 522
Conservative treatment 356, 566, 580
Constipation 168, 424
Contractures 221, 440, 441, 490
Conus medullaris syndrome 159, 159t, 388
Convulsions, febrile 298
Coracoclavicular ligament 41, 42
Coracoid process 28f, 35
Core
　biopsy 451
　decompression 595, 595f
Coronoid fossa 106, 107
Corpus callosum 556
Cortical micturition centers 160, 161
Cortical window, opening of 286
Corticospinal tract 156
　anterior 152, 153
　lateral 152, 153, 157, 158
Corticosteroid, local 27, 608
Corticotomy 246f
Cortisol sensitizes cells 14
Costotransversectomy 326
Costovertebral ankylosis 355
Cotton bandages 4f
Coxa
　breva 548
　magna 548
　plana 548
　vara 540, 540f, 560, 560f
Coxsackie 296
Cozen's phenomenon 599
Cozen's test 573
　reverse 574
Cramer wire splint 623, 623f
C-reactive protein 302, 349, 473
Creases 523
Crepitus 333
　absence of 239
Critical compartment pressure 224
Crohn's disease 361
Crush injury 222, 228, 483
Crush syndrome 221, 222, 225, 228, 254
Crutchfield skull traction 633f
Cryoablation 464
Cryotherapy 102, 455
Crystalline arthritis 352, 362, 365
Crystalloids 17
Cubital fossa 617f
Cubital tunnel syndrome 504

Cubitus valgus 111, 118, 118f
　deformity 114
Cubitus varus 113, 114f, 242f, 650
　clinical features of 113
　deformity 111
Curopsy 461
Cyclooxygenase 100
　inhibitors 341
Cyclophosphamide 474
Cycloserine 312
Cysts
　aspiration 459
　hemophilic 371
　interosseous 580
　metaphyseal 548
　subchondral 338, 340
Cytomegalovirus 439

D

Dactylitis 357
　syphilitic 305
Dagger spine 355
Dancer's tendinitis 275
Dashboard injury 48f, 262f
De Quervain's disease 575, 575f
De Quervain's tenosynovitis 24, 575
Dead space, treatment of 289, 291
Decompression 326f
　anterolateral 326
Deep vein thrombosis 186, 230, 598, 656
　prevention of 168, 231
　risk 230b
　treatment of 231
Defibrillator 643
Deformity 72, 192, 239, 254, 292, 310, 314, 339, 340, 346, 419, 432, 441, 523
　correction 557, 649
　moderate 113
　prevention 658, 661
　severe 113, 407, 523
　site of 600, 602
　stage of 296, 297, 314, 345
　treatment of 561
Delirium tremens 221
Deltoid 498
　ligament 269
Denham pin 632, 632f
Dennis Brown splint 527f, 530
Density
　abnormal 663
　popcorn type of 478
Dental enamel formation 421
Depalma method 40
Depression 476
Dermatitis, exfoliative 362
Desmopressin 371
Dextropropoxyphene 101
Diabetes mellitus 238, 367, 483, 493, 565, 579

Index

Diacetylmorphine 101
Diaphyseal aclasis 458, 458f
Diaphysis 62, 405
Diarrhea, bloody 364
Diastematomyelia 590
Diazepam 442
Diclofenac 350
Digital necrosis 656
Dihydroxycholecalciferol 405
Dilwyn-Evans
    osteotomy 529
    procedure 528, 528f
Dimeglio score 524
Dinner fork deformity 132, 132f
    reverse 136
Diplegia 441
Disc
    degeneration 380, 385
        stage of 380f, 388
    dehydration 385
    extrusion 380
    herniation
        stage of 380
        types of 380
    prolapse 380
        level of 382
    protrusion 385
    replacement 387
    sequestration 380
Discectomy 387
Discoid meniscus 605, 605f
Disease-modifying agents 356
Dislocated acromioclavicular joint, X-ray of 41f
Dislocation 28, 45, 61, 440
    around
        knee 53
        shoulder 33
    atraumatic 29, 30
    classification of 29
    closed reduction of 50
    complex 28
    inferior 34
    management of 166
    open reduction of 50
    pathoanatomy of 30
    recurrent 28, 37, 50
    reduction of 36, 50
    site of 30
    stage of 314
    triple 318
    types of 30
    urgent reduction of 55
Distal femoral
    metaphyseal-diaphyseal junction 191
    nail 193
Distal femur
    exostosis of 457f
    fracture 191
    giant cell tumor of 468f
    megaprosthesis 468f
    osteosarcoma of 472f
    osteotomy 342
Distal forearm, X-ray of 129f
Distal humerus
    fracture site 78f
    intra-articular fracture of 115
Distal interphalangeal
    arthritis 358, 358f
    joint 273, 580
Distal phalanx 273, 273f
    avulsion of base of 274f
    enchondroma of 469
Distal radioulnar joint 129f, 132
    arthritis 130
    dislocation of 46, 128
    persistent dislocation of 130
    subluxation of 134
Distal radius 132
    fracture, closed reduction of 76f, 645f
Distal tibial articular surface 204
Distraction principle 247
Doppler scan 75
Dorsal
    carpal artery 138
    dislocation 530
    displacement 131
    interosseous 504
    kyphosis 411f
    rami, autonomic fibers of 482
    root 481
    spine 320, 411
        exaggerated kyphosis of 585f
        magnetic resonance imaging of 324f
        plain X-ray of 586
        tuberculosis 325f
    tendons 530
    tilt 131
Dorsolumbar spine 30, 326f
    scoliotic deformity of 589f
    X-ray of 355f
Dorsum, rest of 509
Dowager's hump 411, 411f
Drawer test, posterior 262
Drop arm test 570
Drowsy 226
Drugs 363
    sensitivity 311
Dual-energy X-ray absorptiometry scan 410, 412
Duchenne muscular dystrophy 434
Dunlop traction 111
Dupuytren's contracture 578, 579f
Durkan's test 578
Dwarfism, diastrophic 522
Dwyer's calcaneal osteotomy 528, 528f, 529
Dynamic cock-up splint 501, 501f
Dynamic compression plate 104, 105, 125, 128, 130

Dynamic hip screw 183, 184, 199
    fixation 186f
Dysmorphic face 560
Dysplasia, fibrous 450, 453, 461, 462, 463f, 471
Dyspnea 226
Dystonia 441
Dystrophin gene mutation 434

E

Ear 560
Echocardiography, transthoracic 232
Eclampsia 439
Edema control 237
Eichoff test 576
Elbow 30, 121f, 441, 539, 649, 653
    dislocation 44
        acute 46
        chronic 46
        terrible triad of 46
        types of 44, 45f
    extension 499
    joint 44f, 115f
        posterior dislocation of 44f, 45f, 114f
        secondary osteoarthritis of 121
        surgical anatomy of 44
    lateral view of 45f
    splint, lateral 624, 624f
    stiffness 111, 121
    supracondylar fracture of 106
    X-ray of 109f, 120f, 122f
Electrical injury 483
Electrical stimulation 487, 488
Electroconvulsive therapy 39
Electrolyte imbalance 228
Electromyography 32, 434, 491, 513
    pattern of 491
Elizabethtown classification, modified 546
Encephalitis 439
Enchondroma 448, 453, 469, 469f
Endocarditis 349
Endochondral ossification 66, 67fc
Endocrinal disorder 541, 543
Endotracheal intubation 640
Endotracheal tube 641f
Endplates 377
Enneking's staging 453t
Enophthalmos 515
Enteropathic arthritis 361
    pathogenesis of 361f
Enterovirus infection 431
Enthesitis 358, 360, 362
Enzyme-linked immunosorbent assay test 305
Enzymes, proteolytic 343
Epicondyles 106, 110f
    lateral 107, 267
Epicondylitis, lateral 24, 572
Epidural injections 386, 393, 395

Epilepsy 39, 440, 443
Epiphyseal lytic lesion 466
Epiphysis 85, 62, 281, 405, 548
Episcleritis 349
Equinus 526
Erb's palsy 514, 515*f*, 516, 516*t*
Erb's point 514, 514*f*
Erb-Duchenne palsy 514
Ergocalciferol 400
Erlenmeyer flask deformity 417, 417*f*
Erythema nodosum 362, 362*f*
Erythrocyte sedimentation rate 302, 315, 349, 356, 473
Escherichia coli 295
Etanercept 351
Ethambutol 311, 312, 317
Ethanol intoxication 39
Ethionamide 312
Ethyl alcohol 442
Etoposide 474
European League Against Rheumatism Criteria 346*b*
Evans' classification 185
Ewing's sarcoma 283, 448, 450, 451, 453, 473, 474*f*
Excision arthroplasty 317, 647
Exercises
    aerobic 100
    isometric 660
    isotonic 660
    strengthening 100
Exostosis
    multiple 458
    pedunculated 457*f*
    symptomatic 457
Extensor carpi
    radialis
        brevis 384
        longus 384
    ulnaris 499
Extensor digitorum 499
    longus 385, 508, 530
    tendon
        avulsion injury of 273
        bony avulsion of 273*f*
Extensor hallucis longus 385, 508, 530
Extensor lag 191
Extensor pollicis
    brevis tendons 575
    longus 499
        tendon rupture 135
External fixation 646
    advantages of 251
External fixator
    application over pelvis 147
    disadvantages of 646
    in situ 205*f*
External rotation 313-315
    deformity 197
Extra-articular manifestations 349, 354

Extracellular polymeric substance, matrix of 240
Extracorporeal shockwave therapy 27, 573, 608
Extraperiosteal excision 457
Eye 349, 354, 559
    features 362
    symptoms 358

F

Fabry's disease 483
Face 560
Facet
    injections 393, 395
    synovitis 388
Fairbank triangle 540
Fallen leaf sign 450, 459
Fanconi syndrome 404
Faradic current 491
Fascia 251, 552
    contracture, deep 245
Fasciculus
    cuneatus 153, 155-158
    gracilis 153, 155-158
Fasciocutaneous flaps 291
Fasciotomy 224, 225, 225*f*
Fat embolism 221, 227*t*
    cerebro-pulmonary features of 226
    syndrome 225
        Gurd's criteria of 227
        pathogenesis of 226*fc*
Fat macroglobulinemia 227
Febuxostat 365
Fejerine-Klumpke's palsy 515
Felty's syndrome 349
Femoral anteversion 540
    excess 57
Femoral artery 197, 637
Femoral condyle, lateral 257, 261
Femoral epiphysis 543*f*
Femoral head 47, 49, 177, 538*f*, 594*f*
    avascular necrosis of 50, 546, 593, 594*f*
    containment 550
    lateral extrusion of 548
    vascularity of 48, 178*f*
Femoral neck shaft angle 540
Femoral nerve 52, 197, 494, 505, 507
    clinical assessment of 507
    motor supply of 507*f*
Femoral varus derotation osteotomy 550, 550*f*
Femoral vessels, lateral circumflex 177
Femoroacetabular impingement 596
    types of 596*f*
Femur 318
    bony trabeculae of 299*f*
    bowing of 420, 420*f*
    diaphysis, Ewing's sarcoma of 474*f*
    dislocated head of 535*f*

Erlenmeyer flask deformity of 417*f*
    fracture neck of 177, 179*b*, 180, 182*fc*, 183*f*
    head and neck 532
    intertrochanteric 177, 181*b*
    neck of 312
    nonunion fracture neck of 184*fc*
    osteopetrosis of 417*f*
    subtrochanteric 197, 200*f*
    supracondylar level of 197
    thickening of 420
    X-ray of 178*f*
Fentanyl 101
Fever 226, 227, 283, 298, 310, 432, 449
    high-grade 282
    low-grade 230, 314
    relapsing 304
F-fluorodeoxyglucose 474
Fibrillin metabolism, abnormal 587
Fibrocartilage 337
Fibro-fatty tissue 434
Fibroma 448
    nonossifying 448
Fibromyalgia 409
Fibrosarcoma 448
Fibrosis, apical pulmonary 354
Fibrous ankylosis 313, 314, 321, 345
    stage of 313
Fibrous hamartoma formation 561
Fibrovascular inflammatory tissue 296
Fibula 651
    fracture 61*f*
        isolated 204
    length, restoration of 205
    neck 204
    open reduction of 77*f*
Fibular head 267
Fibulectomy 225
Ficat and Arlet classification 595
Fifth metatarsal base 545
    fractures 214*f*
Figure of eight bandage 89, 627
    application 627*f*
Finger
    extension 502
    metacarpophalangeal joints 127
    stiffness 134
Finkel-Biskis-Jinkins murine virus 470
Finkelstein test 576
First carpometacarpal joint, osteoarthritis of 576
First metatarsophalangeal joint 363
    Podagra of 363*f*
Fish mouth appearance 412
Fissures, anal 362
Fixation, internal 110, 133, 195*f*, 202, 645, 646
Flat foot 551
    types of 552
Flexed finger deformity 141
Flexible foot 553

Index

Flexion 163, 313-315, 537*f*, 596
    deformity 318, 348, 579
    distraction injury 171
    type supracondylar fracture 111
Flexor carpi
    radialis 384, 502, 503, 574
    ulnaris 384, 504
Flexor digiti minimi 504
Flexor digitorum
    brevis 528
    longus 528
    profundus 384
        avulsion of 142
    superficialis 384, 502
Flexor hallucis longus 528
Flexor retinaculum 577, 581*f*
Flexor tendon
    sheaths 580
    stenosing tenosynovitis of 581, 582*f*
    synovitis 581
Fluffy periosteitis 358
Fluids, intravenous 433, 635
Fluorodeoxyglucose 665
Fluorosis 421
    dental 421, 422*f*
    skeletal 422
Foley catheter 638, 639
Folic acid, peri-conceptional lack of 554
Foot 206*f*, 441, 556
    arches 551*f*
        surgical anatomy of 551
    arthritis of 552
    care of 557
    compartment syndrome 207
    computed tomography scan of 554
    deformities 348
    drop splint 168, 489, 490*f*, 510*f*
    magnetic resonance imaging of 554, 608
    muscles 508
    plain X-ray of 525
    sensory innervation of 510*f*
    small bones of 201
    soft tissue injuries of 619
    X-ray of 213*f*, 525*f*, 553
Footdrop 509
Footwear modification 341, 553
Foraminal disc prolapse 381*f*
Force, types of 19
Forearm
    bone
        fracture of 124
        X-ray of 124*f*
    compartment syndrome of 224*f*
    fracture 126*b*
        management 126
    interosseous membrane calcification 422*f*
    lateral cutaneous nerve of 498
    plain X-ray of 129

Forefoot 530
    adduction 521*f*, 529
    varus 529
Foucher's sign 597
Foveal vessels 178
Fracture 28, 59, 61, 69, 103, 144, 186*fc*, 221, 235, 248, 427, 648
    acetabulum 173
    blisters 194, 204, 205, 207, 209, 211, 218, 218*f*, 221
    calcaneum 75*f*
    characteristics of 74
    classification of 69, 69*b*
    clavicle 87, 88
    clinical features of 72
    clinical type of 69
    closed 69, 487
    common site of 88, 138
    complete 70, 180
    complications of 80, 221
    crosses physis 84
    delayed of 248
    dislocation 28*f*, 61*f*, 211
    displaced 90, 94, 98, 190, 211, 215
    displacement of 71, 107
    distal
        femur 191
        radius 663*f*
    extracapsular 185
    fibula 203
    fixation 228
    forearm 126*b*
    glenoid 98*f*
    Gustilo-Anderson type of 252
    incomplete 70, 180
    intercondylar 115, 116*f*
    internal fixation of 195*f*
    intertrochanteric 184, 185*f*, 242
    intertrochantric femur 184
    intra-articular 72*f*, 81, 81*f*, 115, 173, 189, 193, 205, 244, 663
    jumping 69
    lateral condyle 117*f*
    lateral one-third 88
    local complications of 221*t*
    malleolar 218, 218*f*
    malunion of 149
    management of 76, 166, 252
    metabolic 140, 141
    metatarsal 214, 237*f*
    middle one-third shaft 88
    nonunion of 90, 149, 238, 241*f*, 248
    oblique 104, 142*f*
    open reduction of 645*f*
    patella 187, 191*fc*
    periprosthetic 648
    prevention 561
    primary treatment of 146
    radiological classification of 70*f*
    retention 615
    scapula 97

    signs of 73
    site, dynamization of 242
    subtrochanteric femur 200
    supracondylar humerus 106, 242
    symptoms of 73
    systemic complications of 221*t*
    traumatic 69
    treatment 561
    undisplaced 90, 98, 190, 211, 215
    union 303
    vertebral 169, 412*f*, 415
    X-ray of 87*f*, 124*f*
Fracture around
    elbow 103
    hand 131
    knee 187
    shoulder 92
    wrist 131
Fracture femur 74*f*
    isolated 197
    neck 177
    treatment of 198
Fracture healing 79, 202, 650
    direct 78*f*
    stage of 77, 78*t*
    types of 77
Fracture line 107*f*, 108*f*
    direction of 107
Fracture midshaft
    clavicle 242
    humerus 104*f*, 105*f*
Fracture neck femur
    anatomical classification of 179*f*
    classification of 179
    complications of 183
    nonunion of 183
Fracture olecranon 119, 120*f*
    tension band wiring of 121*f*
    treatment of 120*fc*
Fracture pelvis 143
    eponyms for 149
    Tile's classification of 144*t*
    Young and Burgess classification of 145*f*
Fracture proximal humerus 92
    treatment of 95*fc*
Fracture shaft
    femur 197, 199*fc*
    humerus 103, 104*fc*, 239
    tibia 254*f*
        fibula 201*f*
Fragility fractures 411
Fragmentation 546
Fragments, number of 122
Frank compartment syndrome 224
Frankel's grading 165
Frankel's white line 427
Frax tool 412
Free fatty acid 226
Freezing stage 565, 566
Freiberg disease 545

French lateral closed wedge osteotomy, modified 114
French osteotomy 650
Fresh frozen plasma 18, 147
Friedreich's ataxia 483
Frontoparietal cortex 160
Frozen shoulder
   idiopathic 565
   secondary 96, 565
Frozen stage 565, 566
Fundoscopy 227

G

Gabapentin 237, 390
Gait 314, 540, 543, 547
   abnormality 434
   ataxic 441
   disturbances 440
   training 658
Galeazzi fracture 124, 129, 129f, 129, 130fc
   dislocation 128
Galeazzi sign 534, 534f
Galeazzi test 534
Gallow's traction 198f
Galvanic current 491
Gamekeeper's thumb 271, 272, 272f, 625
Gamer's thumb 575
Ganglion 579, 580
   block, sympathetic 237
   historical treatment of 580
   over dorsum 580f
Gangrene 229, 230
Garden's classification 180, 180f
Gardner-Wells
   skull traction 633f
   tongs 633
Garre's sclerosing osteomyelitis 279, 293
Gartland's classification 107, 108f, 109
Gas gangrene 221, 254
Gastrocsoleus 510
Gastrointestinal tract 310, 431
Gaucher's disease 593
Gaze sign 548
Genetic hypothesis 522
Genetic predisposition 361, 470
GeneXpert 311, 316
   test 325
Genitourinary tract 314
Gentamicin 292f
Genu valgum 340, 348, 348f, 598, 599, 600fc
   deformity 348f, 599
Genu varum 340, 340f, 348, 348f, 598, 601, 601f
   deformity 602
Gestations, multiple 439
Giant cell tumor 448-450, 453, 454, 461, 465, 466f, 467, 467fc

Gilmore groin 275
Girdlestone arthroplasty 317, 317f, 648
Gissane angle 207, 208f
Glasgow coma
   scale 5, 8
   score 9t
Glass holding position 139, 139f
Glenoid cavity 33f, 35
Glenoid dysplasia 33
Glenoid margin, anterior 37
Glisson's traction 631f, 659f
Glucosamine 341
Gluteal vessels, superior 50
Glycocalyx 287
Golfer's elbow 24, 574
Golimumab 351
Gout 362, 363f, 365
   acute 363, 364
   chronic 363, 365
   primary 362
   risk factors of 363
   secondary 362
Gower's sign 434, 435f
Graft, types of 651b
Great toe
   flexor hallucis longus 511
   gout of 363f
Greater trochanter 312
   group 178
Greater tuberosity 92f
   avulsion 36, 572
   fracture 96
   open reduction and internal fixation of 97f
   surgical anatomy of 96
Greenstick fracture 70, 71f, 83
Griffith's classification 323
Groans, abdominal 424
Ground glass
   appearance 462, 463f
   osteopenia 427
Growth 449
   hormone 541
   impairment 443
   skeletal 587
Growth disturbance 221, 440
   asymmetric 84
Growth plate 62, 245, 281, 299, 404, 405
   cartilage abnormality 400
   damage 287
   horizontal 548
Guanine nucleotide binding protein, mutation of 462
Guillain-Barré syndrome 432, 483
Gunstock deformity 113, 114f
Gurd's criteria 227
Gustilo-Anderson classification 203fc, 249, 250t, 252t

H

Haemophilus 280
Haglund's bump 609f
Haglund's deformity 609
Hair, tuft of 556, 599
Hallux rigidus 610
Hallux valgus 610
   deformity 650
Hammer toe 610
Hamstring strain 275
Hand 119, 558
   arthritis of 346, 357
   compartment syndrome 141
   metacarpophalangeal joints of 649
   syndrome 348b
   tendons, tenosynovitis of 347
   X-ray of 142f, 346, 358, 361
Handshake position 133
Hanging cast 104
Hangman's fracture 170, 170f
Hansen's disease 327, 367, 483, 486
   causes of 328
Hatchet lesion 355
Hawkins sign 212
Head 92f, 206b, 312
   splitting fracture 94
   temporary ischemia of 546
Headache 161
Head-on collision 171
Healing, signs of 548
Hearing disturbance 440, 441
Hearing impairment 420, 443
Hearing loss 419, 560
Heart 349, 354, 560
   rate 154
Heat therapy 351, 658
Heel
   lateral X-ray of 208f
   magnetic resonance imaging of 608
   pain 360
   varus 529
Hemagiosarcoma 448
Hemangioma 448, 556
Hemarthrosis 426
Hematologic disease 593
Hematoma 637, 654
   postsurgical 387
   stage of 77
Hemiepiphysiodesis 407, 407f, 601, 601f
Hemipelvectomy, external 655
Hemiplegia 440, 441
   double 441
Hemireplacement 647
   arthroplasty 183
Hemochromatosis 365
Hemoglobin 227
   low 349, 476
Hemophilia 334, 371f
   A 370

Index

B 370
  severity of 370
Hemorrhage 371
  control 371
  petechial 227f
Hemorrhagic shock 148, 221, 229
  clinical features of 16
  pathophysiology of 14fc
Hemothorax 637
Hepatitis 312
  A 296
  B 296, 439
  C 296
Hepatobiliary system 169
Herbert screw 139, 139f
Herniations, paracentral 380
Heroin 101
Herpes simplex 439, 483
Herring classification 547f
Herring lateral pillar classification 547
Heterotrophic ossificans 50
High median nerve injury 503
High tibial osteotomy 342, 342f, 650
High ulnar nerve
  injury 504
  weakness 119
High-flow oxygen 16
High-molecular-weight
  polysaccharide 102
High-velocity injury 48, 49, 51, 52, 54, 115, 162, 192, 194, 197, 200, 201, 204, 206, 210, 214, 248, 512
Hilgenreiner epiphyseal angle 541, 540
Hill-Sachs lesion 34, 36, 37
Hindfoot 531
Hinge knee brace 268f
Hip 30, 316, 404, 441, 539, 544, 556, 560, 649, 653
  abduction of 533f
  arthritis of 649
  avascular necrosis of 544
  bilateral developmental dysplasia of 538
  central fracture dislocation of 52
  developmental dysplasia of 337, 531, 532f, 536f
  dislocated 316
  dysplasia of 535f
  magnetic resonance imaging of 316
  motion 549
  movements of 173, 540
  osteoarthritis 183, 544
  pain 314, 541f
  plain X-ray of 412, 534, 540, 543, 594
  septic arthritis of 300
  unilateral developmental dysplasia of 538
  X-ray of 315, 355, 535f, 540f, 560f

Hip dislocation 47, 48, 49f
  teratologic 531
  types of 48
Hip joint 47, 49f, 355f
  anterior dislocation of 51
  articular surface of 173
  capsule of 532
  fibrous ankylosis of 313
  fusion of 596
  line tenderness 315
  posterior dislocation of 48
  secondary osteoarthritis of 53
  surgical anatomy of 47
  tuberculosis of 312
  unstable 533
Hip spica 537f, 619
  cast 619f
Hip tuberculosis
  clinicopathological staging of 314t
  pathologico-clinical stages of 313
  pathology of 313
  sequalae of 313
Hippocratic method 36, 37f
Histamine test 513
Histiocytoma
  benign fibrous 448
  malignant fibrous 448
Histoplasma 296
Hoffa syndrome 275
Hoffman sign 486
Holles' fracture 133f
Holstein-Lewis fracture 103, 104, 106, 106f
  humerus, X-ray of 106f
Homer Wright rosette 453
  formation 474
Homogentisic acid 372
Honeycomb appearance 461
Hong-Kong procedure 326
Horn cell, anterior 153, 154, 431, 432
Horner's syndrome 513, 515
Horse tail configuration 152
Hot pack 27
Housemaid's knee 610
Human immunodeficiency virus 301, 303, 483, 579
  infections 301
Humeral capitellar angle 109
Humeral head 35
  dislocation of 35
  proximal migration of 571f
Humerus 107, 123
  chronic osteomyelitis of 290f
  fracture
    greater tuberosity of 96, 97f
    of head of 31
  gross swelling of mid-shaft 473f
  head of 92f
    avascular necrosis of 95
  intercondylar fracture of 115
  lower lateral shaft of 106f

shaft of 92f
  courses posterior aspect of 103
  supracondylar fracture of 108f
  surgical neck of 71f
  upper-end of 469f
Hungry bone syndrome 425, 425b
Hutchinson's fracture 137
Hutchinson's triad 304
Hyaline cartilage 297f, 335
Hyaluronic acid 335
  injection 102
Hydration 364
Hydrocephalus 556
Hydrostatic pressure 104
Hydrotherapy 660
Hydroxyapatite crystals 63
Hydroxychloroquine 350
Hydroxycholecalciferol 400
Hydroxylysine 412
Hydroxyproline 412
Hyperabduction injury 515
Hyperalgesia 235, 236
Hypercalcemia 476
Hypercalciuria 425
Hypercoagulable states 230, 593
Hyperextension, metatarsophalangeal 610
Hyperkalemia 228
Hyperparathyroidism 81, 365, 423
  classification of 423
  pathophysiology of 424f
  primary 424, 425
  secondary 424, 425
Hyperphosphatemia 228
Hyperreflexia, autonomic 161
Hypertension 161
Hypertrophy 343
Hyperuricemia 18, 312, 364, 420
Hypocalcemia 228
Hypocapnia 232
Hypogonadism 541
Hypokalemia 18
Hypophosphatemia, renal loss-related 403
Hypophosphatemic rickets 403, 404, 406
  clinical features of 406
  investigations of 406
Hypothermia 18
Hypothesis
  developmental arrest 522
  mechanical 522
  positional 522
Hypothyroidism 238, 541
Hypotonia 440, 441
Hypovolemic shock 13, 16, 147, 222
  pathophysiology of 14
  treatment of 198
Hypoxanthine-guanine
  phosphoribosyl transferase disease 362
Hypoxia 232

Index

I

Ice pack 27
  over injured ankle 23*f*
Ifosfamide 472, 474
Iliac crest 173, 651
Iliac spine 173
  anterior
    inferior 144
    superior 144, 313, 315, 315*f*
Ilizarov fixator 246*f*
Ilizarov frame application 246*f*
Ilizarov method 240, 529
Ilizarov technique 246
Immobilization 36
Immune system, activation of 360
Implants, internal 646
Index finger abduction 489
Index thigh 197
Indwelling urinary catheterization 639*f*
Infanthood varus, progression of 598*f*
Infection 225, 238, 244, 248, 418, 483, 602, 637, 640, 648, 654
  duration of 279
  etiological type of 279
  gastrointestinal 304
  maternal 439
  musculoskeletal 277
  preexisting 471
Inferior vena cava filter 231
Inflammatory bowel disease 361
Infliximab 351
Infraclavicular lesions 514
Infraspinatus 497
  function of 496
Injections
  intra-articular 102, 361
  therapy 442
Injury
  acute 20
  direct 70, 163
    penetrating 296*f*
  eversion 270
  grade of 256
  grading severity of 20
  hyperextension 170, 610
  indirect 70
  inversion 270
  ischemic 483
  level of 489
  life-threatening 197
  low-velocity 115, 162, 192, 214
  mechanism of 70, 70*t*, 163*t*, 258, 261, 264, 267, 270, 489, 514*f*, 515*f*
  meniscal 257, 263
  mode of 162, 516
  multiple 198
  neurological 170
  postganglionic 513*f*
  preganglionic 513*f*

reperfusion 222
scene of 11
site of 162
types of 5, 144
undisplaced 86
urethral 221
vascular 97, 112, 221, 230*fc*
velocity of 97, 249, 250
vertebral 162
Insecticides 483
Intensive care unit 227
Intercondylar extension 115*f*, 193*f*
Interferential therapy 386, 658
  application 659*f*
Interleukins 78
Intermalleolar distance 599, 600
Internal fixation 110, 133, 195*f*, 202, 645, 646
  advantages of 646
  disadvantages of 646
  surgery 183
Interosseous membrane, calcification of 422
Interscalene triangle, contents of 592
Intersection syndrome 576
Intervertebral disc 377, 378, 378*f*
  biomechanics of 378
  calcification of 372, 372*f*
  central prolapse of 381*f*
  cross section of 377*f*
  prolapse 377, 378, 386, 592
    pathogenesis of 379*fc*
  space involvement 353
  surgical anatomy of 377
Intra-articular
  adhesion 245
  comminuted fracture 208*f*
  extension 192*f*-195*f*
  steroid injection 102, 341, 566
Intra-articular fracture 72*f*, 81, 81*f*, 115, 173, 189, 193, 205, 244, 663
  accurate reduction of 195
  principles of 173
Intra-articular hyaluronic acid 102
  injection 341
Intracapsular metaphysis 282
Intralesional excision 454
Intramedullary abscess 284*f*
  fate of 281
Intramedullary interlocking nail 199*f*, 202
Intramedullary nail 105
Intraosseous metaphyseal vessels 178
Intraosseous pus, aspiration of 284
Intrauterine crowding, theory of 583
Intravenous cannula 634, 634*f*, 635, 642
  parts of 634
  procedure of 635*f*
  size of 634
Intravesical pressure 162

Involucrum 288, 290*f*
Iritis 354, 360, 362
Irradiation 593
Ischemia 229
Ischemic contracture 230
Iselin's disease 545
Isoniazid 311, 312, 317
Ixodes ricinus 305

J

J needle biopsy 472, 474, 478
Jack test 553
Jackknife fracture 171
Jaundice 227
Javelin Thrower's elbow 274
Jaw-thrust 4
Jefferson's fracture 169, 170, 170*f*
Jersey finger 142, 273, 274*f*
Joint 251, 371
  arthritis of 571*f*
  capsule, pathological laxity of 33
  care of 168
  cartilage 333
  computed tomography scan of 366
  contracted capsule of 523
  contractures 654
  debridement of 317
  dislocation of 28, 44, 90, 539
  disorders 301, 302
  distribution 346
  effusion 426
  extensive destruction of 368
  hip 47, 49*f*, 355*f*
  hyaline cartilage 297
  hypothesis 522
  instability of 255
  line tenderness 265, 333, 339
  midtarsal 654
  mobilization 351, 658, 660
  neuropathic 305
  painless destructive arthropathy of 367
  pathological fusion of 648
  peripheral 321
  permanent surgical fusion of 648
  replacement 351, 648
  secondary osteoarthritis of 81
  space 340, 368
  spirochetal infections of 304
  stabilization 433, 443
  stiffness 168, 169, 221, 244, 254, 289, 292, 300
  surgical debridement of 299
  swelling of 298
  tuberculosis of 309, 327
  types of 67, 67*fc*
  X-ray of 298
Joint aspiration 298, 360, 364, 369
  diagnostic 366
Joint destruction 318
  severe 369*f*

Index

Joint disease 418
    degenerative 418, 421
Joint pain 422
    pathogenesis of 99
    relief of 99
Joint reconstruction 647t
    methods of 647
Joint surface
    congruity, accurate restoration of 81
    incongruent 81, 173
Jones fracture 214f, 215, 216f
Jones tendon transfer, modified 105, 489, 502
Jordan's sign 371
Joshi's external stabilization system 526, 529
Judet and Letournal classification 174
Jumper's knee 275

K

Kahler's disease 475
Kanamycin 312
Kaposi sarcoma 301, 302
Kashin Beck disease 373
Keratoderma blennorrhagicum 360, 360f
Kernicterus 439
Kidney 475
Kienbock's disease 545
Kirschner wire 631, 632, 632f
    fixation 110, 110f, 133f
Kite's method 527, 527t
Klebsiella pneumoniae synovitis 354
Klein line 543, 543f
Klippel-Feil syndrome 589
Klumpke's palsy 515, 515f, 516, 516t
Knee 30, 404, 441, 539, 556, 649, 653
    arthroscopy of 605f
    bilateral congenital dislocation of 562f
    bony ankylosis of 299f
    collateral ligaments of 266
    computed tomography scan of 194
    coronal illustration of 257f
    deformities 348
    dislocated 53f
    extension 187, 267, 507
    flexion 267, 508
    fracture dislocation of 28f
    lateral X-ray of 259f, 606
    ligament injury of 255, 257
    medial collateral ligament of 21f
    medial side of 610
    meniscal injury of 257
    meniscus of 257
    plain X-ray of 189, 192, 259, 263, 265, 268, 340, 340f, 600
    posterior dislocation of 53f
    posterolateral corner of 262
    primary degenerative osteoarthrosis of 338
    replacement, unicompartmental 342
    stabilizing structures of 54
    stiffness 191, 193
    tuberculosis, pathological stages of 318
    tunnel view of 603
    X-ray of 53f, 192f-195f, 259f, 319, 366, 427, 466f, 597
Knee dislocation 53
    congenital 562
Knee joint 191, 457f
    aspiration 298f
    congruity 264
    flexion deformity of 318
    posterior subluxation of 318
    swelling of 366f
    tuberculosis of 318
Knee ligament 257f
    injury 50, 194
Knock knee 599
Knuckle bender splint 489, 490f, 506f
Kocher's method 36
Kocher-Langenbeck approach 176
Kohler's disease 545
Kyphoplasty 415, 415f
Kyphoscoliosis 556
Kyphosis 150, 324, 412, 419, 585
Kyphotic deformity 322
Kyphotic vertebra, correction of 415f

L

Laceration 483
Lamina 150
    dura, loss of 425
Laminectomy 326
Laminotomy 387
    exploratory 148
Larsen's syndrome 562
Laryngoscope 641, 641f
Lasegue test 385
Latarjet procedure 38, 38f
Latency 492
Lateral condyle 117
    fracture 117, 118fc
Lateral cord syndrome 158
Latissimus dorsi, function of 496
Lauge-Hansen classification 218, 218t
Lead 483
Leflunomide 351
Leg 206
    angiography of 54f
    anteroposterior X-ray of 201f
    external rotation of 318
    length discrepancy 287
    splint, posterior 622
    X-ray of 71f, 73f
Legg-Calve-Perthes disease 545
Lelli's test 258
Leontiasis ossea 462
Leprosy 367
    indeterminate 328
    infection 328
    lepromatous 328
Leptospirosis 304
Lesch-Nyhan syndrome 362
Lesion
    excision of 467
    margins of 450
    symptomatic 463
Lesser toe flexor digitorum longus 511
Leukemia 451, 475, 593
Leukocyte count 473
Leukocytosis 298
Leukomalacia, periventricular 439, 441
Leverage technique 36
Ligament 47, 245, 255, 552
    anterior syndesmotic 217
    around ankle joint 217
    complex, lateral 217
    function of 255
    lateral side 269
    medial side 269
    sacrospinous 143
    stretching 345
    syndesmotic 269
Ligament injury 59, 255, 257
    general clinical features of 255
    general description of 255
    grade of 256, 256t
    treatment of 256
Ligament laxity 532, 553
    assess features of 56
Ligamentous chance fracture 171
Ligamentum teres 532
Light bulb sign 40f
Limb
    attitude of 51
    compartment 223
    defects 589
    deformity 287
        management of 407
    elevation 231
    external rotation of 185
    gangrene of 221
    injuries 12
    ischemia reperfusion injury of 228
    length 543
        discrepancy 51, 289, 291, 586
    lower 229, 404, 539, 650
    motor examination of 73
    neurovascular assessment of 72
    plain radiograph of 224
    prolonged compression of 223
    reconstruction 246
    salvage 454, 472
        surgery, indication for 454
    sensory examination of 73
    shortening 72, 245, 432
    vascular injury of 230fc

Limp 540, 543, 594
    painless 547
Lipid cell 448
Lipoma 448, 556
Liposarcoma 448
Lisfranc's amputation 654
Lisfranc's injury 212, 213, 213*f*
Liston's long splint 622, 622*f*
Little leaguer's
    elbow 274, 545
    shoulder 274
Liver disease 101
Lobstein Vrolik disease 559
Local contiguous infection 296*f*
Local corticosteroid 27, 608
    injection 573, 575
Local ice pack therapy 658
Local ultrasound
    massage 658
    therapy 242, 659*f*
Local visceral injury 221
Loder classification 542
Long arm posterior splint 624
Long bone 293, 558, 560
    blood supply of 64
    metaphysis of 460
    parts of 62, 62*f*
Long leg view 600
Long thoracic nerve 494, 495
    motor supply of 495*f*
    palsy, clinical features of 495
Loose body 340
    removal 652
Loosen tight bandage 229
Lordosis 150
    lumbar 534
Lover's fracture 206
Low back pain 357, 360, 362, 377, 384, 387, 394
    mechanical 391
Low median nerve palsy 503
Low ulnar nerve palsy 504
Lower limb 229, 404, 539, 650
    disorders 583
    shortening of 49, 197
    sites 632
    splint 620
    vessels, arteriogram of 75*f*
Lower motor neuron 153, 154
Lower tibia, open fracture of 253*f*, 646*f*
Low-molecular-weight heparin 231
Lumbar canal stenosis 385, 387, 393, 394*f*
    diagnosis of 393
Lumbar nerve root compression 384
Lumbar spine 355*f*, 382*f*, 384, 387, 392*f*
    axial section of 394*f*
    computed tomography scan of 663*f*
    coronal section of 381*f*
    extension 391

injury 166
involvement, tests for 353
lateral X-ray of 386*f*
plain X-ray of 392
X-ray of 355*f*, 409*f*
Lumbar spondylosis 388, 389, 389*f*
    lumbosacral corset for 390
Lumbar traction 630, 631*f*, 659*f*
Lumbar vertebra fixation 167*f*
Lumbodorsal spine, X-ray of 354
Lumbosacral spine
    magnetic resonance imaging of 664*f*
    plain X-ray of 387
    X-ray of 394
Lunate dislocation 46, 47*f*
Lung 310, 349, 354
    snow-storm appearance of 227*f*
Luxatio erecta 34, 34*f*
Lyme's borreliosis 305
Lyme's disease 304, 305, 483
Lymph nodes, cervical 314
Lymphadenopathy 345
Lymphoma 451, 475, 593

M

Macintosh curved blade 641*f*
Maffucci syndrome 469
Magnesium 399, 400
    role of 399
Magnetic resonance imaging 31, 55, 74, 165, 256, 265, 268, 284, 299, 289, 293, 311, 369, 387, 389, 392, 394, 457, 458, 461, 466, 472, 474, 516, 543, 566, 568, 570, 574, 578, 586, 595, 663
    advantages of 664
    disadvantages of 664
Maisonneuve fracture 203
Malabsorption syndromes 426
Malaise 310, 432
Malar rashes 370
Malformations, genitourinary 589
Malignant peripheral nerve sheath tumor 448
Malignant transformation 468
    chance of 458
    higher chance of 458
Mallampati test, modified 642, 642*f*
Malleolar fracture 218, 218*f*
    management of 219*fc*
    undisplaced 619
Malleoli
    double 404
    nonunion of 219
Malleolus leads
    malunion of 220
    nonunion of 220
Mallet finger 140, 141*f*, 273, 273*f*
    splint 273*f*
Mallet toe 610, 649

Malnutrition 238
Malunion 90, 106, 111, 134, 186, 193, 221, 242, 254, 418
    common sites of 242
Malunited fracture supracondylar humerus 242*f*, 650
Mannerfelt syndrome 348
Mantoux test 310, 311, 315
Marble bone disease 416
March fracture 69
Marfan's sign 404
Marginal excision 454
Marie-Strümpell disease 353
Marrow 475
    cells 448
Martel sign 364*f*
Massive blood transfusion 17
    complications of 18
Massive multilevel cervical disc herniation 384
Matrix metalloproteinases 338
Mazabraud syndrome 463
McCune-Albright syndrome 462
McLaughlin procedure, modified 40
McMurray's test 265
Meary's angle 553, 553*f*
Mechanical pain, recurrent 265
Mechanoreception 64
Medial calcaneal tuberosity 608*f*
Medial circumflex femoral vessels 177
Medial collateral ligament 21*f*, 257, 266, 267, 267*f*
Medial displacement 74*f*
Medial epicondyle 107, 267
Medial epicondylitis 24, 574
Medial femoral condyle 257, 260, 261, 266, 603*f*
    lateral surface of 602
Medial joint space 22*f*
Medial longitudinal arch 551
Medial malleolus 218
Medial meniscus 264*f*, 266
Medial patellofemoral ligament 56, 187, 257
Medial talonavicular subluxation 523
Medial tibial plateau 260, 261, 266
Median nerve 329, 489, 494, 502
    clinical assessment of 503
    compression 137
        higher risk of 136
    injury 490*f*, 503
    treatment of 503
Medications, antiepileptic 579
Megaprosthesis in situ 468*f*
Melatonin 587
Meningitis 439
Meningocele 555, 556, 556*f*
Meningomyelitis, tubercular 323
Meniscal allograft replacement 266
Meniscal calcification 367*f*
Meniscal tears, morphological type of 265*f*

Index

Meniscal vascular zones, practical application of 264
Meniscectomy
  arthroscopic partial 266
  complications of 266
Meniscus
  function of 264
  lateral 264*f*
  repair of 266*f*
  vascular zones of 264*f*
Mental functions, higher 556
Mental retardation 440, 441
Meralgia paresthetica 507
Mermaid splint 407*f*
Mesenchymal cells 66
  transform 66
Metabolic factors, correction of 609
Metacarpal fracture, X-ray of 141*f*
Metacarpophalangeal joint 272, 579
  subluxation 347
Metaphyseal capillary, hairpin loop structure of 280
Metaphyseal fragment 85*f*
Metaphyseal lesion 471
Metaphysis 62, 85, 246*f*, 280, 405, 456, 459*f*
Metastasis 449, 474
  pulmonary 468
Metatarsals
  fracture of 214
  specific fractures of 214
  stress fracture of 214
  undisplaced fracture of 215
Methotrexate 350, 351, 356, 472
Methylprednisolone, intracystic injection of 459
Meticulous neurovascular examination 54
Meyerding's scale 391
Microbes 295
  anaerobic 296
Milch classification 117*f*
Milch method 36
Milwaukee brace 590, 591*f*
Mineral homeostasis 64
Miosis 515
Mirel's score criteria 82, 450, 451*t*
Mirror therapy 237
Mitral valve 560
Mobility, abnormal 72
Mobilize joints 237
Modular endoprosthesis 455
Moist heat 341, 658
  application 658*f*
Mommy thumb 575
Monoarthritis 335
Mononeuropathy 482, 493
Monoplegia 440
Monteggia fracture 124
  dislocation 126, 127, 128*fc*
Morel-Lavallée lesion 149, 149*f*, 173, 173*f*, 174, 176

Morning stiffness 346
Morrant-Baker's cyst 597
Morton's neuroma 609, 609*f*
Mosaicplasty 604*f*
Mother's wrist 575
Motion
  radiological types of 265
  severe restriction of 569
Motor anatomical cerebral palsy, types of 440*f*
Motor assessment 164, 498, 503, 504, 507-509, 511
Motor control, loss of 440
Motor examination 485
Motor features 105
Motor function test 494-497
Motor impairment 236
Motor innervation 496, 497, 498, 499, 503, 504, 507, 508, 510
Motor march 486
Motor palsy 329
Motor power 164
Motor system 152
Motor tracts 156
Motor weakness 323, 327
Movement 173, 323
  loss of 566
  noxious types of 99
  painful restriction of 339
  range of 548, 566
Mseleni joint disease 373
Mucocutaneous lesions 360, 360*f*, 362
Mulder's click 609
Multilevel lumbar disc prolapse 387
Multiple congenital contracture 539, 539*f*
Multiple exostosis 458
  hereditary 458
Multiple myeloma 409, 448, 450, 453, 475
Muscle 221, 251, 371, 432
  around hip 532
  atrophy 490
    inspection for 26
  biopsy 434
  cover around joint 29
  denervated 491, 492*f*
  disease of 433
  function of 499
  motor assessment of 501
  palsy 329
  paralysis 649, 652
  spasm 310, 345, 586
  strain 20
  wasting 314, 485, 570
  weakness 345
Muscle strengthening 658, 660
  exercises 351
Muscle tendon
  complex 245
  injury 221

Muscular attachments 210
Muscular dystrophies 493
Musculocutaneous nerve 494, 498, 499*f*
  clinical assessment of 498
Musculoskeletal birth defect, congenital 521
Musculoskeletal disorders, degenerative 101
Musculoskeletal effects 440
Musculoskeletal manifestations 348
Musculoskeletal pathologies 442
Musculoskeletal signs 404
Musculoskeletal system 169, 440, 663
Myalgia 426
Mycobacterium
  demonstration of 311
  leprae 328
  tubercle bacilli 321
  tuberculosis 240, 310
Mycoplasma genalium 359
Mycotoxin contamination 373
Myelocele 555, 556
Myelodysplasia 522
Myelomeningocele 555, 556
Myelopathy 385
Myeloschisis 555
Myocarditis 349
Myocutaneous flaps 291
Myofibroblast, preponderance of 579
Myoglobin, release of 228
Myopathy 301, 302, 433, 493
Myositis
  mass 245
  non-infectious 302
Myositis ossificans 46, 51, 111, 114, 221, 232, 233
  pathophysiology of 233*fc*
  prevention of 234

N

Nail
  changes 357
  involvement 358
  pitting 358
Nalgonda technique 422
Napoleon hat sign 392, 392*f*
Naproxen 350
Narath vascular sign 49, 534
Nausea 432, 476
Neck
  femur, fracture of 650
  magnetic resonance imaging of 584, 593
  movement 642
  pain 383, 592
  shaft angle measurement 177*f*
  stiffness 432
  sudden violent hyperextension of 170*f*
Necrosis 221

Necrotic muscles, debridement of 225
Needle biopsy 461, 462
    aspirate 473
Neer's classification 92, 93, 93*f*
Neoplasm 301, 302
Nerve 54, 221, 251, 371
    anterior interosseous 502
    axillary 494, 497
    basic unit of 482
    cell 448
    compression 617
    failed regeneration of 490
    microanatomy of 482*f*
    palpation of 485
    palsy, chronic 329
    recovery, signs of 486
    types of 489
Nerve conduction
    study 119, 492
    velocity 32, 55, 486, 513, 593
    test 578
Nerve injury 30, 30*t*, 174, 221, 225, 235, 489, 516, 656
    axonotmesis type of 105
    classification of 483
    clinical assessment of 485
    complications of 490
    specific 494
    treatment of 486
    types of 484*t*, 488
Nerve repair 517
    primary 488
    secondary 488
Nerve root 377, 378, 381, 385
    compression of 382*f*
    involvement 382
Nervous system, parasympathetic 154
Neural tube defect 554
Neurectomy 442
Neuritis
    optic 312
    stage of active 329
    traumatic 432
Neurofibroma 448
Neurofibromatosis 462, 588
Neurogenic disorders 522
Neurolysis 488
Neuromuscular disorders 429, 431, 587
Neuromuscular junction 153
Neuropathy
    compressive 483
    peripheral 312, 395
Neuropraxia 105, 483, 484, 486, 487, 492
Neurorrhaphy 105, 488
Neurotization 488, 517
Neurotmesis 484, 486-488
Neurovascular assessment 31
Neurovascular bundle 637
Neurovascular deficit 108, 197

Neurovascular examination 51, 113, 125
Neurovascular injury 94, 194, 196, 254
    chance of 115
Neurovascular structures 104, 149
Neutrophilia 298
Nevus, pigmented 556
Night cries 310
Night splints 608
Nitisinone 372
Nonadhesive skin traction 629, 629*f*
Non-end bearing amputation 654
Non-Hodgkin's lymphoma 301, 303
Nonosseous signs 405
Nonsteroidal anti-inflammatory drugs 100, 256, 341, 350
    classification of 100
Nontraumatic nerve injury 487
Nonunion 118, 186, 206, 221, 254
    causes of 206*b*
    common sites of 238
    site, atrophic 247*f*
    treatment of 239, 240
Noradrenaline absorption 101
Normal osteoclastic bone resorption, failure of 416
Nortriptyline 101, 237
N-terminal propeptide 412
Nucleic acid amplification
    method 311
    tests 311
Nucleus pulposus 377, 381
Nursemaid elbow 122
Nutrient artery 66, 320
Nutrition 411
Nutritional rickets 406
    treatment of 406

O

Ober's circumtibial transfer 489
Obesity 541
Occupational therapy 351, 442
Ochronosis 372
Ochsner's clasping index 503
Olecranon 107, 120, 120*f*, 610
    fossa 107
    fracture, complications of 121
Oligoarthritis 335
    asymmetric non-erosive 360
Oligohydramnios 532
Ollier's disease 469
Onion peel appearance 450, 474
Onychodystrophy 358
Onycholysis 358
Open femur fracture 249*f*
Open fracture 69, 201, 222, 248, 248*f*, 250, 253*f*, 646*f*
    complications of 254
    side of 249
Open reduction 76, 244, 645
    advantages of 646

and internal fixation 89, 95, 95*f*, 104, 105, 110, 125, 128, 130, 133, 148, 176, 182, 186, 190, 199, 206, 209, 212, 219
    indication for 126*b*
    disadvantages of 646
Opera glass deformity 357
Opioids 101
Opisthotonus 441
Opponens digiti minimi 504
Opponens pollicis 503
Oral phosphates 408
Oral steroids 365, 434
Oral vitamin C supplementation 427
Oropharyngeal structures 641*f*
Orotracheal intubation 643*f*
Orthopaedics 301, 620, 662
    basics of 61
    common terminologies in 61
    emergencies 222, 250
    procedures 645
    surgery 301, 303, 442
    treatment 418
Orthopantomogram 294
Orthosis 390, 393, 395, 442, 573, 575, 576
    support 386
Orthotics 27, 100, 341, 608
Ortolani's tests 532, 533, 533*f*, 534
Osgood-Schlatter disease 545, 606, 606*f*
Ossification
    center, primary 66
    centers around elbow 107*f*
    intramembranous 66, 67
Osteitis
    deformans 418
    fibrosa cystica 423, 424
Osteoarthritis 99, 186, 221, 334, 335, 576, 597, 601
    classification of 337*t*
    hip 183, 544
    post-traumatic 193
    primary 338
    radiocarpal 135
    secondary 50, 53, 81, 121, 422
Osteoarthrosis 335, 338*fc*657
    classification of 337
    knee 333
    patellofemoral 191
    primary 337
    secondary 266
Osteoarticular plugs 604*f*
Osteoblast 64, 66, 448
    activity stimulators 413
    secrete rank ligand 64
    stimulator 413
Osteoblastoma 448, 465
Osteochondritis dessicans 545, 602-604
Osteochondroma 448, 456, 456*f*
Osteochondrosis 544

Index

Osteoclasis 243
Osteoclast 64
    inhibitors 413
Osteoconduction 651
Osteocyte 64
Osteogenesis
    distraction 246, 246*f*
    imperfecta 559, 560*f*
        types of 559
Osteoid osteoma 448, 463, 464, 464*f*
Osteoinduction 651
Osteolytic lesions 319*f*, 324
Osteoma 448, 465
    frontal bone 465*f*
Osteomalacia 81, 408, 410, 416
Osteomyelitis 240, 248, 279, 287, 296*f*, 298, 301, 475, 633
    acute 286*fc*, 287, 299
        bacterial 280
    chronic 221, 254, 287, 290*f*, 290*fc*, 471
        hematogenous 288
    metaphyseal 282
    non-tubercular 301
    pathogenesis of 283*fc*
    primary subacute 293
    pyogenic 280
    tubercular 309, 327
Osteonecrosis 302
Osteopenia
    diffuse 408
    disuse 221
    periarticular 350*f*
Osteopetrosis 416, 417*t*
    congenita 416
Osteophyte 389*f*
    formation 338, 340
    medial 340*f*
Osteoporosis 81, 168, 301, 409, 410, 414*b*, 416, 416*f*, 443, 585
    clinical features of 412*b*
    risk factors for 410, 410*b*
    severe 560*f*
Osteoporotic fracture treatment 414
Osteoporotic spine, X-ray of 412*f*
Osteoporotic vertebral collapse 415
Osteosarcoma 448, 451, 453, 470, 471, 472*fc*
    intramedullary 470, 473
    periosteal 473
    primary 470
    secondary 421, 470, 471
    telangiectatic 461, 468, 473
    types of 473
Osteosclerosis 416, 416*f*
    disorders 416
Osteosclerotic myeloma 475
Osteotomy 351, 649
    common examples of 650
    corrective 243, 407, 650
    derotation 650
Otosclerosis 560

P

Packed red blood cells 17
    transfusion of 147
Paget's disease 362, 418, 420*f*, 421, 471
Pain 236, 283, 322, 339, 449, 473, 543, 566, 570, 636, 654
    atraumatic 280
    character 449
    control therapies 237
    effective control of 237
    hip 314, 541*f*
    management of 99
    neuropathic 490
    region of 384, 385
    relief 568, 569, 573, 575, 576, 608, 658
        surgery for 517
    relieve 27, 371
    severe 282, 298
Painful arc syndrome 571, 572*f*
Painful articular syndrome 302
Pallidum, subspecies 304
Palmar aponeurosis, contractures of 579
Palmar ganglion, compound 581, 581*f*
Palmaris brevis 504
Palpation 289
Palsy
    clinical features of 498
    early 329
Panner's disease 545
Pannus chokes articular cartilage 343
Pannus over femoral cartilage, arthroscopic image of 297*f*
    condyle 344*f*
Papineau technique 291
Para-aminosalicyclic acid 312
Paracentral prolapse 380
Paracetamol 101, 341
Paralytic dislocation 29
Paralyzed muscle, electrical stimulation of 488
Paraplegia
    early-onset 323
    late-onset 323
    time of onset of 323
Paraspinal muscle spasm 323
Paratenonitis 24
Parathormone 414
    function of 423
Parathyroid hormone 64, 399, 411, 418
Parenthesis 516
Parosteal osteosarcoma 234, 473
Parrot's beak 265
Parrot's nodes 305
Pars interarticularis 392*f*
Passive joint mobilization 660
Passive movements 485
Patchy osteoporosis 237*f*
Patella 30

accurate reduction of 189
alta 57
articular surfaces of 187*f*
cartilage 607*f*
function of 187
lower pole of 545
non-articular surfaces of 187*f*
surfaces of 187
surgical anatomy of 187
Patella dislocation 55
    acute 56
    primary 57
    recurrent 56, 57
Patella fracture 188, 191
    complications of 191
    treatment of 190
Patellar apprehension sign 56
Patellar clonus 164
Patellar retinacula 188
Patellar tendinitis 24, 275*f*
Patellar tendon bearing 203
    cast 202, 618*f*, 619
Pathological dislocation 29, 300
Pathological fracture 69, 81, 82, 82*f*, 291, 287, 412, 419-421, 455, 468, 478*f*
    increased incidence of 422
    intramedullary nail fixation of 82*f*
Pauwel's osteotomy 650
Pauwels' angle 179, 184
    practical implication of 179
Pauwels' classification 179, 180*f*
Pavlik harness 198, 537*f*
Peak bone mass 411*b*
Pediatric capable trauma centers 7
Pediatric disorders 519, 521
Pedicle screw system 167*f*
Peg-leg gait 531
Pelkin spur 427
Pellegrini-Stieda disease 268*f*
Pelvic
    binder 147
        application 148*f*
    floor 143
    girdle 143
    osteotomies 538*f*, 550
    sheet 147
        application 147*f*
    tilt 586
Pelvis 197, 206, 404, 409, 420, 558, 665*f*
    bone, fracture of 146
    computed tomography scan of 231
    external fixator 148*f*
    fracture 147*f*-149*f*, 173, 197
        classification of 144
    Judet iliac view of 175*f*
    Judet obturator view of 175*f*
    osteopetrosis of 417*f*
    plain X-ray of 145*f*
    surgical anatomy of 143

X-ray of 48*f*, 52*f*, 145*f*, 146*f*, 174*f*,
185*f*, 186*f*, 316*f*, 354*f*, 409*f*, 548,
558*f*, 590
Pencil in-cup deformity 358
Pencil thin cortex 427
Pentazocine 101
Penumbra sign 293
Peptic ulcer disease 101
Pericardial effusion 349
Pericarditis 349
Perilunate dislocation 46
Perineal care, difficult 621
Perineural abscess, stage
of 329
Perineural fibrosis 273*f*, 345
Periosteal collar 66
Periosteal reaction 284*f*, 427, 450
Periosteal vessels 281
Peripheral nerve 328, 479, 483
injuries 481, 492
involvement 329
supply of 481*f*
surgical anatomy of 481
Perkins line 535*f*
Peroneal nerve
component 494
deep 508, 510
Peroneus brevis 385
Peroneus longus 385, 509
Perthes' disease 544, 545, 548*f*, 549*fc*,
550, 650, 659
acute 549
prognostic factors of 551
Pes anserinus 610
Pes cavus 554, 554*f*
Pes planus 551
foot 551*f*
Petechiae 226
Pethidine 101
Phalangeal fracture 140, 142
Phalen's test 578
reverse 578
Phantom limb sensation 654
Pharmacologic therapy
100, 442
Phemister triad 311, 315
Philadelphia collar 625, 625*f*
Pholcodine 101
Phosphate 405
abnormalities 399
deficiency 403
function of 399
Phosphopenic rickets 403
treatment of 408
Phosphorus 399, 412
role of 399
Physeal injury 83, 85*f*, 221
classification 84
complications of 86
Physical force, adverse effect of 3
Physiological flat foot 553

Physiotherapy 27, 237, 341, 351, 356,
386, 390, 393, 395, 433, 568,
573, 575, 608
overview of 658
Physis 62, 84*f*, 85, 281, 405
accurate reduction of 86
function of 84
sparing procedure 455
surgical anatomy of 84
Piece of pie sign 46, 47*f*
Piedmont's fracture 128
Pilon fracture 205*f*
treatment of 206*fc*
Pirani score 524
Pirogoff amputation 655
Plain X-ray 234, 239, 243, 250, 256,
289, 324, 405, 408, 417, 420,
457, 459, 461, 462, 464, 466,
471, 474, 476, 478, 531, 560, 569
Plantar fasciitis 24, 362, 607
tenderness spot 608*f*
Plantar flexion 270, 511, 521*f*
Plantar plate 610
Plasma cell 477
tumor 475
Plasmacytoma, solitary 475
Plaster of Paris
bandage 613*f*
cast 613
material
advantages of 613*t*
disadvantages of 613*t*
Plaster, application of 615
Plastic deformity 71
Plastic surgical procedures 244
Plate fixation 244
Platelet 147
calmodulin defects 587
count 227
Platelet-rich plasma 575
injections 608
intra-articular injection of 341
local injection of 27
Pneumonia 221
Pneumothorax 637
Pointing index sign 503
Policeman's tip position 515*f*
Poliomyelitis 431, 433*b*, 587
acute 431, 432
pathogenesis of 432*fc*
Poliovirus antibodies 433
Polyarthritis 327, 335, 373
symmetric 346
Polycythemia vera 593
Polydioxanone 603
Polydipsia 476
Polymerase chain reaction
316
Polymethylmethacrylate 292*f*
bone cement 253
Polyneuropathy 482, 483, 493

Polyostotic fibrous dysplasia, triad
of 462
Polytrauma 1
Polyurethane polymer 613
Polyuria 476
Ponseti's method 526, 527, 527*t*
Pontine center 160, 161
Popliteal artery 54*f*, 75*f*
Popliteal fossa 339*f*
Popliteal vessels 194
Porter's tip position 515*f*
Positive end-expiratory pressure 227
Positron emission tomography scan
665, 666
Post-correction bracing 527
Postdiphtheria palsy 432
Posterior column 151, 153, 173
tracts 157
Posterior cord syndrome 157, 157*f*
Posterior cruciate ligament 257, 260,
261, 264
avulsion, acute displaced 263
function of 261
surgical anatomy of 261
tear 261
Posterior dislocation 33, 34, 44*f*, 45,
45*f*, 114*f*
shoulder, complications of 40
Posterior glenoid margin erosion 39
Posterior interosseous nerve palsy
127, 128, 501
clinical features of 501
Posterior longitudinal ligament 377,
378, 378*f*, 381, 394
Posterior sacroiliac ligament complex
144
Posterior syndesmotic ligaments 217
Posterior talofibular ligament 269
Posterior tibial nerve 329
Posteromedial bundle 261
Post-fasciotomy 225
Postganglionic lesion 513, 514
Post-head injury 233
Post-menopausal osteoporosis 413
Postpolio residual palsy 431
Post-tourniquet syndrome 656
Post-traumatic stress disorder 221
Postvascular repair 222
Potassium, release of 228
Pott's fracture 217, 218, 219*f*
Pott's paraplegia 323
classification of 323
Pott's spine 309, 320
Prednisolone 365
Pregabalin 237, 390
Preganglionic lesion 513
Preiser's disease 545
Pressure over cortex 281
Pressure sores 621
Pressure ulcer 617*f*
Primary osteoarthrosis 337
pathophysiology of 338

Index

Procalcitonin 284, 298
Pro-inflammatory cytokines 235
Pronation abduction 218
Pronator teres 503, 574
Prophylactic fixation 82
Propionibacterium acnes 296
Prostate
   metastasis 451
   specific agent 451
Prosthesis 179
Prosthetic joint 296
   dislocation of 648
Proteoglycan synthesis stimulator 341
Protrusio acetabuli 316, 409
Protrusion 380
Provisional amputation 654
Provocative test 593
Proximal carpal row 577
Proximal femoral nail 185
Proximal femur 178*f*
   chondrosarcoma of 478*f*
   epiphysis 545
   fibrous dysplasia of 463*f*
   nail fixation 186*f*
Proximal fragment, abduction of 200*f*
Proximal humerus
   comminuted fracture of 94, 94*f*
   gross swelling of 478*f*
   minimally displaced fracture of 94
   surgical anatomy of 92
   X-ray of 459*f*
Proximal humerus fracture 92, 93, 93*f*
   classification of 93
   open reduction and internal fixation of 95*f*
Proximal interphalangeal
   flexion 610
   joints 579
Proximal muscle weakness 434
Proximal phalanx, oblique fracture of 142*f*
Proximal radius 127*f*
Proximal tibia 187, 425*f*
   chondrosarcoma of 458*f*
   fracture of 193, 194*f*
   intra-articular fracture of 81*f*
   metaphysis 284*f*, 293
   physis 407*f*
   varus deformity of 243*f*
Pseudarthrosis 116, 562*f*
Pseudoarthrosis coxae 316
Pseudobulbar palsy 441
Pseudogout 365, 366, 366*f*, 367*f*
   acute 367
   chronic 367
   clinical features of 366
Pseudo-Jones avulsion fracture 215*f*
Pseudomonas aeruginosa 280, 295
Pseudoparalysis 283, 298
Pseudotumor 371
Psoriasis 358*f*, 362

   nail features of 357*f*
   over elbow 357*f*
Psoriatic lesions 357*f*
Psoriatic skin lesions 357
Psychic moans 424
Psychotherapy 238
Ptosis 515
Puberty, precocious 462
Pubic diastasis 145*f*, 146*f*, 149*f*
Pubic ramus, superior 143*f*
Pubic type 51
Pubis 173
Pulmonary function test 356, 590
Pulse rate 16
Punched out lesion 450
Purine-rich food, dietary excess of 363
Pus 311
   aspiration 316, 319
Putti-Platt procedure 39
Pyoderma gangrenosum 362
Pyogenic spondylitis 326
Pyomyositis, infectious 302
Pyrazinamide 311, 312, 317
Pyrophosphate arthropathy, chronic 366

Q

Q angle 56, 600
Quadriceps 507
   active tests 262
   muscle 191
   strengthening exercises 341
   wasting 265
Quadriplegia 441
Quantitative D-dimer assay 231

R

Radial cutaneous nerve 329
Radial deviation 347, 347*f*, 499
Radial displacement 135*f*
Radial fossa 106, 107
Radial head 107, 123
   fracture 121, 122*f*
   subluxation of 123*f*
Radial interosseous nerve palsy,
   clinical features of 501
Radial nerve 103, 104, 489, 494, 498, 501
   close relation of 106*f*
   palsy 490*f*, 501*f*
   clinical features of 105
   repair of 105
Radial styloid 575
   intra-articular oblique fracture of 137
Radial tear 265
Radial tunnel syndrome 574
Radiation 483
Radical excision 454
Radiculopathy 493

Radiological parameters 549
Radiology 371
Radionuclide imaging 665
Radiotherapy 468, 470
Radiowave frequency 664
Radius 107, 481
   fracture of distal end of 131
   metaphysis, aneurysmal bone cyst of 461*f*
   normal angulations of lower-end 132*f*
   torus fracture of 71*f*
   ulna shaft, fracture of 124
Raloxifene 413
Rapid growth 280
Rash, petechial 227
Rat fever 304
Reactive arthritis 352, 359
   classic triad of 359
Rear-end collision 170
Red rubber catheter 638
Reflex 164
   deep 164
   persistent neonatal 441
   superficial 164
   sympathetic dystrophy 134, 212, 219, 235
Regeneration 546
   process of 485
Regurgitation 354
   aortic 361, 560
Rehabilitation 32, 36, 77, 111, 169, 259, 263, 434, 487
Reinnervation polyphasic motor unit potentials 491
Reiter's disease 334
Reiter's syndrome 352, 359, 359*f*, 360*f*
Relocation-release test 37
Renal calculi 221
Renal cell carcinoma 82*f*
Renal disease 101
   chronic 409
Renal failure 225, 228, 476
Renal osteodystrophy, chronic 541
Renal parenchyma 423
Renal phosphate wasting 403
Renal stones 424
Renal tubular acidosis 404
Renal tubules 423
Replacement arthroplasty 647
   complications of 648
   contraindications of 648
   indication for 648
Residual sensorimotor deficit 388
Residual urine, large amount of 162
Respiratory care 168
Respiratory muscle palsy 432
Respiratory rate 16
Respiratory system 14
Respiratory tract 328
   infection 169, 186

Restlessness 226
Retention 76
Retinoblastoma gene 470
Retrocalcaneal bursitis 609
Retrocalcaneal spur 610*f*
Rhabdomyolysis 656
　　traumatic 228
Rheumatoid arthritis 102, 334, 335, 343, 346*b*, 349, 365, 483, 581, 597, 599
　　pathogenesis of 344*f*, 344*fc*, 345*fc*
Rheumatoid factor 349, 361
　　serum 346
Rheumatoid knee 344*f*
　　X-ray of 350*f*
Rheumatoid nodules 346, 349, 349*f*
Rhizomelic dwarfism 557, 557*f*
Rib 651, 665*f*
　　hump 587
RICE
　　protocol 22
　　therapy 102
Rich blood supply 185
Rickets 400, 404, 406*t*, 410, 416, 416*f*
　　calcipenic 400, 403, 405
　　causes of 403*t*
　　healing phase of 407*f*
　　hypocalcemic 400
　　hypophosphatemic 403, 404, 406
　　types of 403*t*
Rifampicin 311, 312, 317
Rigid foot 553
Rind sign 462
Ring diameter 621
Risser's sign 590
Road traffic accident 124, 141, 197, 201, 218, 258, 261
Rocker bottom
　　chair 530*f*
　　foot 530*f*
Romanus sign 356
Ronaldo's fracture 140, 140*f*
Root 481
　　orientation 382, 382*t*
　　value 495, 497, 498, 502, 504, 509
Rotationplasty 455, 455*f*
Rotator cuff
　　arthropathy 570
　　strength of 566
　　tear 94, 569, 572
　　　massive 648
　　tendinitis 567
　　tendinopathy 24, 567, 572
Rotatory deformity 587
Round back
　　deformity 354
　　kyphosis 411*f*
　　kyphotic deformity 354*f*
Rubella 439
Rugger jersey spine 417, 417*f*, 425
Rule of 1-2-3 642, 642*f*

Rule out foot compartment syndrome 211
Runners' fracture 69
Rush rod application 562*f*
Rutherford-Morrison aphorism 280

S

Sacral dimples 588
Sacral spinal micturition center 160
Sacroiliac joint
　　inflammation of 352
　　space 354*f*
Sacroiliitis 357, 360
Sacrum 143
Sag sign 262
Salmonella 280
　　osteomyelitis 280
　　typhi 295
Salt and Pepper appearance 425
Salter-Harris
　　classification 84
　　injury 117
　　physeal injury 85*f*
　　　classification 86
Sarcoidosis 483
Sarcoma, pleomorphic 448
Saucerization 290
Sausage digits 357
Scaphoid 138, 545
　　blood supply of 138*f*
　　occult fractures of 139
　　tubercle 577
　　waist, fracture of 139*f*
Scaphoid fracture 138, 139*f*, 625
　　internal fixation of 139*f*
　　site of 138*f*
Scapula
　　body of 98*f*
　　medial winging of 495
Scapular manipulation 36
Scheuermann's disease 545, 585, 585*b*
Schwann cells 488
Schwannoma 448
Sciatic list 384
Sciatic nerve 50, 197, 494, 507, 508
　　clinical assessment of 508
　　injury 50, 490*f*
　　motor supply of 508*f*
Scleritis 349, 360
Scleromalacia 349
Sclerosis 354*f*, 369*f*
　　subchondral 338, 340
Scoliosis 434, 464, 501*f*, 561, 586, 589*f*, 591*f*
　　classification of 586, 587*fc*
　　postural 384, 586, 587, 587*t*
　　structural 586, 587, 587*t*
　　surgical correction of 591
　　types of 586
Scorbutic knee, X-ray of 427*f*
Scorbutic rosary 426

Scurvy 283, 426
Seat belt injury 171
Seddon's classification 483
Segond fracture 259
Segond sign 259*f*
Seizures 228
Selective estrogen receptor modulator 413
Selective nerve root block 386
Selenium deficiency 373
Semmes Weinstein testing 578
Sensation over dorsum, loss of 501
Sensitization, local 235
Sensorimotor deficit 329, 383, 387
Sensory abnormalities 236
Sensory assessment 164, 498, 501, 503, 504, 507-509, 511
Sensory deficit 384, 385
Sensory examination 73, 485
Sensory features 105
Sensory fibers 481
Sensory innervation 497, 498, 499, 503, 504, 507, 508, 510, 510*f*
Sensory loss 327, 329, 432, 516
Sensory nerve action potential 492
Sensory system 153
Septic arthritis 222, 254, 282, 283, 287, 295, 296*f*, 300-302, 365
　　debridement 653
Septicemia 221, 254, 287, 292, 299
Sequestration, stage of 282, 282*f*
Sequestrectomy 290
Sequestrum 288, 290*f*, 291*f*
　　types of 289
Serological tests 409
Serology 472, 474
Serratiopeptidase 256
Serratus anterior 495
　　function of 495
Sesamoid bone, largest 187
Sever's disease 545
Sexual dysfunction 149, 388
Shaft fractures 204
Shaft tibia 201
　　fibula, fracture of 201
Shanmugasundaram classification 316*b*
Shenton line 49*f*, 534, 535*f*
Shepherd crook deformity 450, 462, 463*f*
Shin splint 274
Shock 13, 15*fc*, 228
　　absorber 264
　　anaphylactic 14
　　cardiogenic 14
　　classification of 13
　　compensated 15
　　decompensated 15
　　distributive 14
　　electric 39
　　endocrine 14

Index

hemorrhagic 148, 221, 229
hypovolemic 13, 16, 147, 222
neurogenic 14
obstructive 14
septic 14
severity of 15, 16, 16*t*
spinal 156
types of 13*t*
Shortwave diathermy 341, 386, 393, 658
   application 658*f*
Shoulder 30, 441, 610, 649, 653
   anterior dislocation of 28*f*, 31*f*, 35*f*
   dislocation of 41*t*, 92
   dystocia 513
   frozen 301, 565
   function of 96
   hemireplacement of 95*f*
   pain, acute 569
   recurrent anterior dislocation of 37
   replacement, reverse 570, 571*f*
   stiffness of 90, 96
   tuberculosis of 327
   X-ray of 33*f*, 71*f*, 355, 568
Shoulder dislocation
   acute 35
   anterior 33*f*
   atraumatic 33
   traumatic 33
   types of 33
Shoulder joint
   acute anterior dislocation of 34
   arthritis of 372*f*
   posterior dislocation of 39
Sickle cell anemia 280, 593
Simple bone cyst 449, 450, 459, 459*f*, 461
Sinding-Larsen-Johansson disease 545
Singh's index 412
Single anterior spinal artery 155
Single photon emission computed tomography 665
Sinogram 289
Sinus
   formation 282, 282*f*
   multiple 288
   single 288
Sinus tract
   excision 290
   formation 288
   malignancy 292
Skeletal dysplasia 557, 599, 601
Skeletal traction 1, 623*f*, 628, 628*f*, 631, 632, 633*f*
   advantages of 631
   care of 633
   complications of 633
   site of 632

Skeletal tuberculosis 309, 310
   clinical features of 310
   etiopathology of 310
   treatment of 311
Skier's thumb 271
Skin 221, 251, 357, 560, 636
   changes 237
   contractures 245
   disorders 362
   epidermal layer integrity 19
   injury 221
   involvement 328
   lesion 328
   loss 253*f*
   ulceration 617
Skin traction 628-630
   adhesive 629
   complications of 630
   contraindications of 631
   problems of 630
Skull 404, 420, 560, 632
   cotton wool appearance of 420*f*
   traction 633
Slipped capital femoral epiphysis 337, 541
   pathogenesis of 542*fc*
Sluggish reflex 384, 385
Small blue round cells 453
Small joints, arthritis of 357
Smith's fracture 111, 135, 136, 618
Snake bite 223
Soap bubble appearance 450, 466
Soft cervical collar 390
Soft tissue 290
   injury 19, 24, 235
      types of 19
   interposition of 238
   local 248, 254
   loss 248, 254
   necrosis 636
   reconstruction 57
   release, posteromedial 526, 528*t*
   stabilizers 29
   surgery 528
Sole, convex contour of 530
Solitary asymptomatic lesions 457
Solitary exostosis 456
   chondrosarcoma of 458
Southwick angle 542-544
   measurement 544*f*
Spastic diplegia 441
Spastic paraparesis 422
Spasticity 440, 441
Speech
   disturbance 440
   therapy 442
Spilled teapot sign 46
Spina bifida 522, 554, 555, 556*f*, 587, 588
   aperta 555
   classification of 555

cystica 556, 557
occulta 555, 557
types of 555*f*
Spina ventosa 327
Spinal accessory nerve 494
   motor supply of 495*f*
   palsy, clinical features of 494
Spinal artery
   anterior 153, 155-157
   posterior 153, 155-157
   thrombosis 323
Spinal brace 415, 415*f*
Spinal canal 382, 394*f*
   branch, anterior 320
   stenosis 422
   stenosis, features of 419
Spinal column
   clinical importance of 151
   function of 152
Spinal cord 150, 150*f*, 153, 155, 169, 323, 381, 431, 485, 590
   arterial supply of 155*f*
   blood supply of 155, 155*t*
   compression 384
   cross-section of 153*f*
   injury 150, 155, 169, 172
      acute 155, 161, 165
      level of 154
      syndromes 156, 156
   major sensory-motor tracts of 153*t*
   malformation 589
   surgical anatomy of 152
Spinal fusion 591
Spinal hyperextension, anterior 167
Spinal instrumentation 326*f*
Spinal muscular atrophy 587
Spinal osteotomy 356, 650
Spinal segment 152*f*
Spinal tuberculosis
   complications of 326
   principles of 326
   surgical treatment of 326
Spine 206*f*, 404, 408, 441, 558, 560, 583, 625, 665*f*
   anatomy of 150
   axial section of 381*f*
   board 625
   columns of 151*f*
   computed tomography scan of 590
   degenerative conditions of 375
   dorsolumbar scoliotic deformity of 586*f*
   infections 296
   injuries of 150, 163*f*
   kyphosis of 419
   ligament of 422
   magnetic resonance imaging of 360, 362, 385, 433, 531, 557, 590, 284*f*
   normal curvature of 150
   plain X-ray of 385, 412

posterior aspect of 556
specific fractures of 169
surgical anatomy of 150
traumatic 164
tuberculosis of 320, 321
X-ray of 360, 362, 389, 557, 589
Spine injury 162, 168*t*
classification of 162
clinical features of 164
complications of 169
management of 166
principles of 166*b*
pattern of 172
Spinothalamic tract 156
anterior 153
lateral 153, 156-158
Spinous process 150, 378
Spiral groove 103
Spirochetes 304
Splenomegaly 345
Splint 489, 623*f*
function of 620
length of 621
material 620
Splintage 509, 510, 503, 504
Split skin graft 203
Split thickness skin graft 254*f*
Spondylitis 388
Spondyloarthropathy 335
seronegative 352, 352*b*
Spondyloepiphyseal dysplasia 599
Spondylolisthesis 170*f*, 390, 391*f*, 392
classification of 390
grade of 391
Spondylolysis 390, 392
Spondylosis 388
lumbar 388, 389, 389*f*
Sports
hernia 275
injuries 255, 258, 271
Sprain 62, 23*fc*
grade of 20*f*, 20*t*
wrist 138
Spring ligament 269
Spurling sign 383
Stabilize long bone fracture 17
Stable cardiovascular status 232
Stable spine 164
Staphylococcus
aureus 280, 293, 295, 301, 302
epidermidis 296
Static restraints 33, 44
Static stabilizers 255
Steinmann pin 631, 632*f*
Stem cell 341
transplantation 477
Stener lesion 272
Stenosis, aortic 354
Sternal occipital mandibular immobilizer 166

Sternocleidomastoid 494
function of 494
Z-plasty lengthening of 585
Sternomastoid tumor 584
Steroids 350, 361, 477
anabolic 414
intra-articular injections of 361
Stiff joint, adhesiolysis for 652
Stiffness 46, 130, 141, 422
early 245
late 245
types of 244
Stimson's method 36, 37*f*
Stomatitis, aphthous 361
Stone 424
Stool analysis 360
Stoss therapy 406
Straight leg raising test 385
Strains 23*fc*, 62
grade of 21*f*, 20*t*
Streeter's dysplasia 522
Strength duration curve 491, 492*f*
Streptococcus pyogenes 280, 295
Streptomycin 312
Stress 69, 363
fracture 69, 214 274, 419
radiograph 22
X-ray 256
Strontium ranelate 414
Structural scoliosis 586, 587, 587*t*
types of 588*t*
Student's elbow 610
Stump neuroma formation 654
Stump, non-healing ulcers of 654
Subacromial bursitis 572
Subchondral bone 295, 333*f*, 336, 594*f*
changes 338
Subclavian vessels 97
Subluxated hip 534
Subluxation 28, 61, 134
Subperiosteal abscess formation, stage of 281, 281*f*
Subperiosteal elevation 427
Subscapularis, attachment of 92
Subtalar joint, arthritis of 212
Sudeck's dystrophy 141, 212, 219, 235
form of 134
Sudeck's osteodystrophy 134
Sulfasalazine 351, 356
Sunburst appearance 471
Sunderland classification 484
Sunlight exposure, adequate 406
Superficial palmar artery 138
Superficial peroneal nerve 508, 510
Superior facet 378
Superior radioulnar joint 126
Supraclavicular lesions 514
Supracondylar fracture 106, 107*f*-109*f*, 110*fc*, 111, 114*t*, 115*f*, 193*f*
complication of 112
extension type 111

humerus, complications of 111*b*
malunion of 113
Supracondylar humerus 103, 107*f*
fractures 650
Kirschner wire fixation of 110*f*
Supraolecranon hollowing 45*f*
Suprascapular nerve 494, 496
motor supply of 496*f*
Supraspinatus 497
function of 496
repair of 571*f*
tear, arthroscopic image of 571*f*
tendinitis 24
Surgery 235, 341, 358, 387, 390, 472, 474, 516, 573, 576, 586
role of 433*b*
Surgical excision 465, 580
Surgical local sympathetic ganglion sympathectomy 237
Swan neck deformity 347, 347*f*
Sweating 161
Swelling 72, 192, 280, 282, 283, 310, 319*f*, 339, 456, 471*f*, 473, 593
appearance 449
hourglass shape 581
painful bony 426
surface 449
Syme's amputation 654
Sympathetic nervous system 154
Sympathetic skin response 485
Syndesmophyte 354, 355*f*
Synovectomy 317, 344*f*, 351, 652
Synovial chondromatosis 604, 605*f*
Synovial fluid
analysis 350, 657
characteristics of 657*t*
content 295
function of 335
Synovial hypertrophy 319, 344*f*, 605*f*
Synovial inflammation 343
Synovial joint
osteoarthrosis of 338*fc*
surgical anatomy of 335, 335*f*
Synovitis
chronic 372
stage of 296, 297*fc*, 313, 314, 318, 343, 344*fc*, 546
Synovium 313, 316, 318, 335
Synthetic cast 613
advantages of 614, 614*t*
disadvantages of 614, 614*t*
Synthetic graft 651
Synthetic plaster 613*f*
Syphilis 304, 367, 439
adult 305
congenital 304, 305
early 305
congenital 304
infectious 304
late 304, 305
congenital 304

Index

latent 304
primary 304
secondary 304
treatment of 305
Syringomyelia 323, 367, 590
Systemic lupus erythematosus 334, 365, 483, 593
Systemic steroid 361
therapy 593

T

Tabes dorsalis 367
Tabetic arthropathy 305
Tachycardia 14, 226, 227, 298
Tachypnea 14, 226, 298
Talipes equinus varus, congenital 521, 522, 530
neurogenic 525
Talocalcaneal tarsal coalition 553f
Talofibular ligament, anterior 269
Talus 210, 528, 531
blood supply of 210
body, avascular necrosis of 212
fracture 210, 212fc
neck of 211
neck fracture, nonunion of 212
vascularity of 210f
vertical orientation of 530
Tardy ulnar nerve palsy 118, 221
pathophysiology of 119fc
Tarsal bone 206
Tarsal coalition 552, 553
Tarsal tunnel syndrome 348, 511
Tarsometatarsal dislocation 212
Tarsometatarsal joint 654
dislocation of 369f
Tear
complete 272
complex 265
horizontal 265
longitudinal 265
morphological type of 265b
partial 272
Technetium bone scan 237, 284
Teeth 559
Telescopy test 315, 534
Tenderness 51, 136, 173, 310, 575
Tendinitis 24, 274
Tendinopathy 24-26, 99
chronic 27
pathogenesis of 25fc
severe 27
Tendinosis 24
Tendo-Achilles 511, 528, 553
contracture 530
tendinitis 24, 362
tendon 610f
Tendon 251, 552
anatomy, facts of 24
healing 27
hypovascularity of 567

injury 24
lengthening 528
repair 351
rupture 345, 348
transfer 329, 351, 442, 488, 503, 505, 509, 517, 652
principles of 488b
procedure 651
Tennis elbow 24, 572
splint 573f
tenderness 573f
Tennis leg 275
Tenosynovitis 348
Tenotomy 528
Tensile stresses 378
Tensile trabeculae
primary 178
secondary 178
Tension band wiring 120, 121f, 190
Teratologic disorders 522
Teres minor 498
function of 497
Tetanus 221, 254
prophylaxis 251
Tetany 424
Tethered cord syndrome 556, 590
Thawing stage 565, 566
Therapeutic intra-articular procedures 296f
Thermal injury 483, 617
Thessaly test 265
Thiazide 410
Thigh, X-ray of 197f
Thioacetazone 312
Thiocolchicoside 390
Thixotropic properties 335
Thomas knee splint 197f, 199f, 620, 621, 622f
Thomas splint, parts of 621, 622f
Thoracic kyphosis 585
Thoracic spine tuberculosis 324f
Thoracodorsal nerve 494, 495
injury, clinical features of 496
motor supply of 496f
Thoracolumbar braces 167f
Thoracolumbar region 322f
Thoraco-lumbo-sacral orthosis 590
Thrombocytopenia 227
Thromboembolism, pulmonary 221, 231
Thrombophlebitis 636
Thrombosed vessel 229
Thumb
abduction splint 490f, 503f
adduction 489
drop 135
enchondroma of 469f
extension 502
spica splint 624, 625f
splint 576f
Stener lesion of 272

ulnar digital nerve of 273f
Z deformity of 347
Thurston-Holland sign 84, 85f
Thyroid dysfunction 565
Tibia 318
anterolateral bowing of 561
bowing of 420, 561
computed tomography scan of 464f
congenital pseudoarthrosis of 561, 561f
fibula fracture 72f
fracture of 61f, 249f
open fracture of 69f
osteoid osteoma of 464f
progressive bowing of 419
pseudoarthrosis of 562f
Sabre shin appearance of 560f
shaft transverse undisplaced fracture 71f
thickening of 420
vara 601
varus malunion of 243f, 650f
Tibial hemimelia 522
Tibial nerve 509, 510
motor supply of 511f
Tibial osteotomy 650f
Tibial plafond
articular surface, accurate restoration of 205
fracture of 204, 205
Tibial plateau
fracture 193, 195fc
classification of 194
lateral third 261
Tibial spines, prominence of 340, 340f
Tibial tuberosity 545
apophysis, fragmentation of 606
Tibialis anterior 385, 508, 509
Tibialis posterior 385, 510, 511, 528, 552
dysfunction 552
tendinitis of 274
Tight tendo-achilles 530
Tile's classification 144, 144t
Tinel's sign 486
Tinnitus 419
Tissue
devitalization of 249, 250
hyperlaxity of 552
perfusion 13
Tizanidine 390
Toe
deformity 610
types of 610
plantar flexion of 510
Tom Smith arthritis 300
Tone, abnormal 440
Tophaceous chalky deposits 363
Torn anterior cruciate ligament 75f

Torticollis 583, 583*f*
　congenital 583
　secondary 583
　types of 583
Torus fracture 71, 71*f*, 83
Total elbow arthroplasty 116
Total hip
　arthroplasty 176
　replacement 183, 184, 317, 317*f*, 596, 596*f*
Total joint
　arthroplasty 370
　replacement 647, 342, 342*f*, 647*f*
Total parenteral nutrition 636
Total white blood cell count 349
Tourniquet
　basic rules of 656
　complications of 656
　pain 656
　types of 656
Toxins 483
Toxoplasmosis 439
Tracheoesophageal fistula 589
Traction 166, 317, 483, 628, 659
　countertraction technique 36
　horizontal component of 320*f*
　methods of 628
　objective of 628
　principles of 628
　types of 628
Traction injury 163
　severe 512
Tramadol 101
Transcutaneous electrical nerve stimulation 102, 386, 566, 659
Transformation, malignant 468
Transiliac biopsy 413
Trans-scaphoid perilunate dislocation 46
Transverse arch 551
Trapdoor sign 459
Trapezius 494
　function of 494
　weakness 494
Trapezoid 41, 87
Trauma 379
　direct 39, 103, 188
　indirect 39, 103, 188
　mode of 124, 144
Traumatic dislocation 29, 30
　acute 32
　clinical features of 30
　complications of 32
Traumatic nerve injury 486, 493
　management of 487
Traversing root 382
Trefoil pelvis 409, 409*f*
Tremor 441
Trendelenburg gait 434
Trendelenburg sign 543
Trendelenburg test 315, 547
　positive 534

Treponema pallidum 304
Treponematoses, endemic 304
Trethowan sign 543
Triage, principles of 3
Triangular fibrocartilage complex injury 135
Triceps 499, 501
Tricyclic antidepressants 101, 237
Trident hand 558
Trigger finger 581
Triple axon reflex 513
Triple deformity, stage of 318
Triple lumen catheter 637*f*
Trochanteric bursa 312
Trochanters 184
Trochlea 107
Trochlear dysplasia, high-grade 57
Trochlear torticollis 583
Trolley track sign 354, 355*f*
Trophic skin changes 235
True cut needle biopsy 466
True neoplastic stromal cells 465
True shortening, stage of 314, 315
Trunk sternum 87
Tubercle granuloma, presence of 311
Tubercular arthritis 309
Tubercular hip, radiological types of 316*b*
Tubercular infection 301
　types of 309
Tubercular lesions 318
Tubercular paraplegia 323
Tubercular spine, pathogenesis of 321*fc*
Tubercular spondylitis 309
Tuberculoid leprosy 328
Tuberculosis 321*f*, 581
　around hip, site of 313*f*
　arthritis 327
　bone 309, 320
　cervical 322
　dactylitis 327
　incidence of 309
　knee 318
　lumbar 322
　musculoskeletal 327
　osteomyelitis 327
　skeletal 309, 310
　thoracic 322
Tuberosity
　ischemic 144, 610
　lesser 92*f*
Tuli's middle path regime 325
Tumor 387, 453, 602
　benign 453*t*
　bone 445
　chemotherapy of 362
　fungation of 455
　like lesion 456, 459, 460, 461
　location of 456
　matrix 450

metastatic 81
necrosis factor 78
prosthesis 648
Turf toe 275
Tyrosine 372

U

Ulcer, trophic 368*f*
Ulna 107, 123
　dorsal subluxation of 347
　greenstick fracture of 71*f*
　shaft 70
　triangular fibrocartilage complex of 132
Ulnar collateral ligament 122, 271, 272
　avulsion injury of 272*f*
　injury 272*f*
　lateral 44
Ulnar digital nerve, neuroma of 273
Ulnar nerve 329, 489, 494, 504, 505*f*
　anterior transposition of 119, 119*f*
　clinical assessment of 504
　injury 490*f*
　treatment of 504
Ulnar paradox 506*b*
Ulnar styloid process 136
Ultrasonography 22, 535, 543, 566, 568, 570, 574, 576, 578, 582
Ultrasound 299, 664
Unicameral bone cyst 459
Unicondylar replacement 342*f*
Upper cervical spine 345
Upper end humerus, X-ray of 84*f*
Upper limb 87, 119, 229, 539, 650
　characteristic position of 516
　disorders 565
　sites 632
　splint 624
Upper motor neuron disease 154, 439
Upper tibial traction 632, 632*f*
　risk of 633
Urea, serum 405
Uremia 476
Urethra 148, 640
Urethral sphincter
　external 160
　internal 160
Urethritis 360
Urge incontinence 161
Uric acid 358, 363, 364
　filtration of 362
　high production of 362
Uricase 365
Uricosurics 365
Urinary bladder 148, 159, 161
　dysfunction 161
　function 161
　innervation 159
　outline of 160*t*
　neurological control 160, 160*f*
Urinary calcium 405

Index

Urinary catheters 17, 147, 638, 640
    types of 638
Urinary retention 387
Urinary system 14
Urinary tract infection 186, 640
Urine 227, 372, 476
    analysis 360, 425
    examinations 311
    uric acid excretion 364
Uveitis 354, 362

V

VACTERL syndrome 589
Vague pain 594
Valgum 339
Valgus osteotomy, rationale of 184
Valgus stress 272f
Valgus test 267
Van ness 455, 455f
Vancomycin 299
Varum 339
Varus 526
    deformity 242f, 243f
    derotation osteotomy 537f
    test 267
Vascular cells 448
Vascular claudication 395
Vascular Doppler scan 73
Vascular endothelial growth factor 78
Vascular hypothesis 522
Vascular injury 97, 112, 221, 230fc
    common sites of 229
Vasculitis 345, 349
Vasoconstriction, peripheral 14
Vasodilatation, peripheral 14
Vaughan-Jackson syndrome 348
Velpeau bandage 626, 626f
    application 626f
Vena cava filter, inferior 231
Venous congestion 593
Venous thrombosis 221
Ventilation-perfusion scan 232
Ventral rami, autonomic fibers of 482
Ventral root 481
Vertebra 460
    squaring of 354
Vertebral artery 155
Vertebral biopsy 325
Vertebral body 377, 378
    blood supply of 378f
Vertebral central epiphysis 545
Vertebral column 150, 150f
    denis three columns concept of 151
    function of 152
    injury 164
    stability of 151
Vertebral motion segment 388

Vertebral pathological fractures 82
Vertebral ring epiphysis 545
Vertebroplasty 415
Vertical talus 531f
    congenital 525t, 530
Vessel 52
    axillary 92
    computed tomography guided selective embolization of 148
    injury 230
Vincristine 474
Virchow's triad 230
Visceral organs 144, 146
Viscosupplementation 102
Visual impairment 443
Vitamin
    B_{12} deficiency 483
    B_6 317
    C 237, 426
        deficiency 426
    D 400, 403
        deficiency 302, 403
        levels 412
        low dose 406
        role of 399
        supplement 409
        synthesis 400
    D dependent rickets 403, 407
        type 1 403, 406
        type 2 403, 406
    D regulation 400
        cycle 420f
    D_2 400
    D_3 400
        supplementation 406
    deficiency 483
Volkmann ischemia 112, 221, 222, 483
    contracture 111, 112, 221, 225, 230
Volkmann sign 112
Vomiting 432, 476
von Rosen splint 537f
von Willebrand disease 370
von-Recklinghausen disease 423

W

Waist 138
Waiter's tip position 515f
Wallenberg syndrome 170
Wallerian degeneration 483, 484
    direct 485
    regeneration, neuronal 484
Wartenberg's syndrome 576
Washerwoman's sprain 575
Watkins transfer 489
Weaver's bottom 610
Wedge tarsectomy 528, 529
Weight bearing joint 337
Weight loss 100, 310

Weight reduction 608
Well's clinical probability tool 231
Whiplash injury 170, 171, 171f
White blood cells 298
Wick catheter method 224
Wide excision 454, 472, 478
Wilson's disease 365
Wimberger's sign 304, 427
Wind swept deformity 348, 348f
Wormian bones 560
Wound
    area 251
    closure of 252
    coverage 252
    debridement 225
    management of 251
    necrosis 654
    over proximal leg 248f
    size of 249
Wright and Moll's diagnostic criteria 358
Wright tests 593
Wrist 30, 119, 404, 441, 539, 649, 653
    arthritis of 346
    dorsum of 580
    drop 104
    extension 499
    lateral view of 132
    lateral X-ray of 136f
    movements 575
    osteoarthritis 139
    pain 130
    plain X-ray of 578
    posteroanterior view of 132
    radial deviation of 347, 347f
    stiffness 134
    X-ray of 131f, 135f, 346, 527, 576

X

Xanthine oxidase inhibitors 365
X-linked recessive disorder 370, 434
X-ray 229, 237, 293, 300, 311, 350, 362, 364, 422, 469, 557, 566, 570, 608
    production, mechanism of 662
Xylocaine jelly 639f

Y

Young and Burgess classification 144, 145f

Z

Z deformity 347
Zanca view 42
Zancolli's capsulodesis 489
ZN stain 311